T0139302

Sleep and Psychiatric Disorders in Children and Adolescents

SLEEP DISORDERS

Advisory Board

Antonio Culebras, M.D.
Professor of Neurology
Upstate Medical University
Consultant, The Sleep Center
Community General Hospital
Syracuse, New York, U.S.A.

Anna Ivanenko, M.D., Ph.D.
Department of Psychiatry and Behavioral Sciences
Feinberg School of Medicine, Northwestern University, Chicago
Division of Child and Adolescent Psychiatry, Children's Memorial Hospital
Chicago
Alexian Brothers Medical Center, Elk Grove Village
and Central DuPage Hospital, Winfield, Illinois, U.S.A.

Clete A. Kushida, M.D., Ph.D., RPSGT
Director, Stanford Center for Human Sleep Research
Associate Professor, Stanford University Medical Center
Stanford University Center of Excellence for Sleep Disorders
Stanford, California, U.S.A.

Nathaniel F. Watson, M.D.
University of Washington Sleep Disorders Center
Harborview Medical Center
Seattle, Washington, U.S.A.

Sleep and Psychiatric Disorders in Children and Adolescents

Edited by

Anna Ivanenko

Feinberg School of Medicine, Northwestern University
Children's Memorial Hospital
Chicago, Illinois, USA

Alexian Brothers Medical Center
Elk Grove Village, Illinois, USA

Central DuPage Hospital
Winfield, Illinois, USA

informa
healthcare

New York London

Informa Healthcare USA, Inc.
52 Vanderbilt Avenue
New York, NY 10017

© 2008 by Informa Healthcare USA, Inc.
Informa Healthcare is an Informa business

No claim to original U.S. Government works
Printed in the United States of America on acid-free paper
10 9 8 7 6 5 4 3 2 1

International Standard Book Number-10: 1-4200-4807-4 (Hardcover)
International Standard Book Number-13: 978-1-4200-4807-0 (Hardcover)

This book contains information obtained from authentic and highly regarded sources. Reprinted material is quoted with permission, and sources are indicated. A wide variety of references are listed. Reasonable efforts have been made to publish reliable data and information, but the author and the publisher cannot assume responsibility for the validity of all materials or for the consequence of their use.

No part of this book may be reprinted, reproduced, transmitted, or utilized in any form by any electronic, mechanical, or other means, now known or hereafter invented, including photocopying, microfilming, and recording, or in any information storage or retrieval system, without written permission from the publishers.

For permission to photocopy or use material electronically from this work, please access www. copyright.com (http://www.copyright.com/) or contact the Copyright Clearance Center, Inc. (CCC) 222 Rosewood Drive, Danvers, MA 01923, 978-750-8400. CCC is a not-for-profit organization that provides licenses and registration for a variety of users. For organizations that have been granted a photocopy license by the CCC, a separate system of payment has been arranged.

Trademark Notice: Product or corporate names may be trademarks or registered trademarks, and are used only for identification and explanation without intent to infringe.

Library of Congress Cataloging-in-Publication Data

Sleep and psychiatric disorders in children and adolescents / edited by Anna Ivanenko.
    p. ; cm. – (Sleep disorders ; 5)
  Includes bibliographical references and index.
  ISBN-13: 978-1-4200-4807-0 (hardcover : alk. paper)
  ISBN-10: 1-4200-4807-4 (hardcover : alk. paper) 1. Sleep disorders in children. 2. Sleep disorders in adolescence. 3. Child psychiatry. 4. Adolescent psychiatry. I. Ivanenko, Anna. II. Series: Sleep disorders (New York, N.Y.) ; 5.
  [DNLM: 1. Sleep Disorders–complications. 2. Sleep Disorders–psychology. 3. Adolescent. 4. Child. 5. Mental Disorders. WM 188 S63126 2008]
  RJ506.S55S572 2008
  618.92'8498–dc22

                                        2007049955

For Corporate Sales and Reprint Permissions call 212-520-2700 or write to:
Sales Department, 52 Vanderbilt Avenue, 16th floor, New York, NY 10017.

Visit the Informa Web site at
www.informa.com

and the Informa Healthcare Web site at
www.informahealthcare.com

Preface

This volume provides the first rigorous attempt to integrate our current knowledge on sleep, emotional, and behavioral development in children and adolescents. Pediatric sleep medicine has made significant progress from the first description of sleep states in newborns in the mid-1960s, to an almost distinct clinical discipline that offers a comprehensive assessment and treatment of children with a wide array of sleep and circadian disorders in the context of their neurobehavioral, emotional, and cognitive development.

In the past two decades, there have been a growing number of research studies exploring sleep characteristics in children with various psychiatric disorders as well as investigating the impact of primary sleep disorders on the neurocognitive, behavioral, and affective development in children. This book explores and defines the complex relationship between the field of sleep medicine and child psychiatry in a cogent synthesis of prevalence, etiology, assessment, and treatment.

The book is written for a large audience of clinical professionals involved in caring for children and adolescents, especially mental health professionals, general pediatricians, child neurologists, and sleep specialists with an interest in pediatric aspects of sleep medicine.

I would like to acknowledge an outstanding panel of authors that made this book project possible. They conducted state-of-the-art research on every aspect of pediatric sleep development, providing readers with detailed overview of biological, psychological, socio-cultural and pharmacological aspects of pediatric sleep and its interface with psychiatric pathology in children and adolescents.

Although there are many areas of pediatric sleep medicine and child psychiatry that still remain controversial and not very well defined, evaluation and treatment of pediatric sleep problems present a pressing need for thousands of clinicians and millions of parents. This book serves to provide guidance and to disseminate information regarding accurate assessment, pathophysiology, and effective treatments to practitioners faced with the challenges to help children and their families achieve a better night's sleep.

Anna Ivanenko

Contents

Contributors

Candice A. Alfano Department of Psychiatry, Children's National Medical Center, The George Washington University School of Medicine, Washington, D.C., U.S.A.

Rupali Bansal Division of Pediatric Pulmonology, Phoenix Children's Hospital, Phoenix, Arizona, U.S.A.

Dean W. Beebe Division of Behavioral Medicine and Clinical Psychology, Cincinnati Children's Hospital Medical Center and Department of Pediatrics, University of Cincinnati College of Medicine, Cincinnati, Ohio, U.S.A.

Kathy L. Bradley-Klug University of South Florida, Tampa, Florida, U.S.A.

Joseph A. Buckhalt Department of Counselor Education, Counseling Psychology, and School Psychology, Auburn University, Auburn, Alabama, U.S.A.

Melissa M. Burnham Department of Human Development and Family Studies, University of Nevada, Reno, Nevada, U.S.A.

Daniel P. Cardinali Department of Physiology, Faculty of Medicine, University of Buenos Aires, Buenos Aires, Argentina

Samuele Cortese Child and Adolescent Psychopathology Unit, Robert Debré Hospital, Paris VII University, Paris, France and Child Neuropsychiatry Unit, G.B. Rossi Hospital, Department of Mother-Child and Biology-Genetics, Verona University, Verona, Italy

Flavia Cortesi Center of Pediatric Sleep Disorders, Department of Developmental Neurology and Psychiatry, University "La Sapienza," Rome, Italy

Lynn A. D'Andrea Department of Pediatrics, Medical College of Wisconsin and Children's Hospital of Wisconsin, Milwaukee, Wisconsin, U.S.A.

Mona El-Sheikh Department of Human Development and Family Studies, Auburn University, Auburn, Alabama, U.S.A.

Margaret T. Floress Munroe-Meyer Institute, Department of Pediatric Psychology, University of Nebraska Medical Center, Omaha, Nebraska, U.S.A.

Jane F. Gaultney Department of Psychology, University of North Carolina, Charlotte, North Carolina, U.S.A.

Erika E. Gaylor Center for Education and Human Services, Policy Division, SRI International, Menlo Park, California, U.S.A.

Flavia Giannotti Center of Pediatric Sleep Disorders, Department of Developmental Neurology and Psychiatry, University "La Sapienza," Rome, Italy

Jeannine L. Gingras Department of Psychology, University of North Carolina and United Sleep Medicine Centers, Charlotte, North Carolina, U.S.A.

Dmitriy Gromov   Center for Addiction Medicine, Massachusetts General Hospital, Boston, Massachusetts, U.S.A.

Irina Gromov   Matrix Alliance, Inc., Dallas, Texas, U.S.A.

Reut Gruber   Department of Psychiatry, McGill University, Douglas Research Center, Montreal, Quebec, Canada

Mary Lou Gutierrez   Department of Psychiatry, Loyola Medical Center, Maywood, Illinois, U.S.A.

Anna Ivanenko   Department of Psychiatry and Behavioral Sciences, Feinberg School of Medicine, Northwestern University, Chicago, Division of Child and Adolescent Psychiatry, Children's Memorial Hospital, Chicago, Alexian Brothers Medical Center, Elk Grove Village, and Central DuPage Hospital, Winfield, Illinois, U.S.A.

Kyle P. Johnson   Department of Psychiatry, Oregon Health & Science University, Portland, Oregon, U.S.A.

Peggy S. Keller   Department of Human Development and Family Studies, Auburn University, Auburn, Alabama, U.S.A.

Lukasz M. Konopka   Clinical Psychology Department, Chicago School of Professional Psychology and Department of Psychiatry and Behavioral Neuroscience, Loyola University Medical Center, Chicago, Illinois, U.S.A.

Suresh Kotagal   Center for Sleep Medicine and Departments of Neurology and Pediatrics, Mayo Clinic, Rochester, Minnesota, U.S.A.

Brett R. Kuhn   Munroe-Meyer Institute, Department of Pediatric Psychology, University of Nebraska Medical Center, Omaha, Nebraska, U.S.A.

Jennifer Kurth   Department of Child and Adolescent Psychiatry, Children's Memorial Hospital and Department of Psychiatry and Behavioral Sciences at Feinberg School of Medicine, Northwestern University, Chicago, Illinois, U.S.A.

Michel Lecendreux   Pediatric Sleep Disorders Center and Child and Adolescent Psychopathology Unit, Robert Debré Hospital, Paris VII University, Paris, France

Daniel S. Lewin   Pediatric Behavioral Sleep Medicine and Department of Pediatrics and Psychiatry, Children's National Medical Center, The George Washington University School of Medicine, Washington, D.C., U.S.A.

Marsha Luginbuehl   Child Uplift, Inc., Fairview, Wyoming, U.S.A.

Susan G. McGrew   Department of Pediatrics and Kennedy Center, Vanderbilt University and Monroe Carell Jr. Children's Hospital, Nashville, Tennesssee, U.S.A.

Valerie McLaughlin Crabtree   Division of Behavioral Medicine, St. Jude Children's Research Hospital, Memphis, Tennessee, U.S.A.

Beth A. Malow   Department of Neurology and Kennedy Center, Vanderbilt University, Nashville, Tennessee, U.S.A.

Lisa J. Meltzer   Children's Hospital of Philadelphia and University of Pennsylvania School of Medicine, Philadelphia, Pennsylvania, U.S.A.

Jodi A. Mindell   Department of Psychology, Saint Joseph's University and Children's Hospital of Philadelphia, Philadelphia, Pennsylvania, U.S.A.

Hawley E. Montgomery-Downs   Department of Psychology, West Virginia University, Morgantown, West Virginia, U.S.A.

Louise M. O'Brien   Sleep Disorders Center, Departments of Neurology and Oral and Maxillofacial Surgery, University of Michigan, Ann Arbor, Michigan, U.S.A.

Edward B. O'Malley   Sleep Disorders Center, Norwalk Hospital, Norwalk, Connecticut, U.S.A. and NYU School of Medicine, New York, New York, U.S.A.

Mary B. O'Malley   Sleep Disorders Center, Norwalk Hospital, Norwalk, Connecticut, U.S.A. and NYU Department of Psychiatry, New York, New York, U.S.A.

Judith A. Owens   Division of Pediatric Ambulatory Medicine, Rhode Island Hospital, Providence, Rhode Island, U.S.A.

Seithikurippu R. Pandi-Perumal   Division of Clinical Pharmacology and Experimental Therapeutics, Department of Medicine, College of Physicians and Surgeons of Columbia University, New York, New York, U.S.A.

Cindy Phillips   Drexel University and Children's Hospital of Philadelphia, Philadelphia, Pennsylvania, U.S.A.

Giora Pillar   Pediatric Sleep Clinic, Meyer Children's Hospital, Rambam Medical Center and Technion Faculty of Medicine, Haifa, Israel

Sigita Plioplys   Department of Child and Adolescent Psychiatry, Children's Memorial Hospital and Department of Psychiatry and Behavioral Sciences at Feinberg School of Medicine, Northwestern University, Chicago, Illinois, U.S.A.

Teresa J. Poprawski   Clinical Psychology Department, Chicago School of Professional Psychology and Department of Psychiatry and Behavioral Neuroscience, Loyola University Medical Center, Chicago, Illinois, U.S.A.

Sarit Ravid   Pediatric Neurology, Meyer Children's Hospital, Rambam Medical Center and Technion Faculty of Medicine, Haifa, Israel

Teresa Sebastiani   Center of Pediatric Sleep Disorders, Department of Developmental Neurology and Psychiatry, University "La Sapienza," Rome, Italy

Stephen H. Sheldon   Northwestern University, Feinberg School of Medicine and Division of Pulmonary Medicine, Children's Memorial Hospital, Chicago, Illinois, U.S.A.

Dana Sheshko   Attention, Behavior, and Sleep Research Laboratory, Douglas Research Center, Montreal, Quebec, Canada

Darryn M. Sikora   Oregon Health & Science University, Portland, Oregon, U.S.A.

Marcel G. Smits   Centre for Sleep-Wake Disorders and Chronobiology, Hospital Gelderse Vallei, Ede, The Netherlands

D. Warren Spence   Sleep and Alertness Clinic, University Health Network, Toronto, Ontario, Canada

Venkataramanujan Srinivasan   Department of Physiology, School of Medical Sciences, University Sains Malaysia, Kelantan, Malaysia

Riva Tauman   Sleep Disorders Center, Dana Children's Hospital, Tel Aviv Medical Center, Tel Aviv University, Tel Aviv, Israel

Cristina Vagnoni   Center of Pediatric Sleep Disorders, Department of Developmental Neurology and Psychiatry, University "La Sapienza," Rome, Italy

Kristiaan B. van der Heijden   Leiden University, Centre for the Study of Developmental Disorders, Leiden, The Netherlands

Lisa A. Witcher   Division of Pediatric Sleep Medicine and Kosair Children's Hospital Research Institute, Department of Pediatrics, University of Louisville, Louisville, Kentucky, U.S.A.

1 Sleep and Behavior in Children and Adolescents: A Multi-System, Developmental Heuristic Model

Dean W. Beebe

Division of Behavioral Medicine and Clinical Psychology, Cincinnati Children's Hospital Medical Center and Department of Pediatrics, University of Cincinnati College of Medicine, Cincinnati, Ohio, U.S.A.

INTRODUCTION

Recorded observations on human sleep date back to antiquity (1), but it was not until the nineteenth century that Western medicine began to explore the potential for sleep problems in children. Perhaps the first published account of a specific childhood sleep problem affecting daytime behavior in the Western medical literature was from Dr. William Hill, who in 1889 wrote that nocturnal breathing problems could cause "backwardness and stupidity" in schoolchildren (2). By the early twentieth century, advice on appropriate childhood sleep practices proliferated in popular books and magazines (3). Much of this was grounded in presumed causal relationships between sleep and daytime behavior, with the Journal of the National Education Association in 1928 declaring that chronic fatigue was "one of the major causes of school failure and breakdown" (3, p. 351). While this basic premise—that children's sleep and daytime behavior are linked—remains widely held in the lay and scientific communities, rigorous scientific methods to test and explicate the nature of this link have been applied only within the past half-century.

The chapters in this book attest to the fact that the links between sleep and daytime behavior in children are more complex than was reflected in early writings. In the face of such complexity, the goals of this chapter are broad. First, it will provide a context for the rest of the book by presenting a heuristic model for understanding the relationships between sleep, behavior, and other factors intrinsic within and external to a child. It will then emphasize the importance of viewing these factors in a developmental context. Finally, it will highlight several implications of considering sleep and behavior in a dynamic, multifaceted, systemic, and developmental manner.

A MULTI-SYSTEM HEURISTIC MODEL

Figure 1 summarizes a heuristic model of the relationships between sleep and daytime functioning in children. Immediately apparent in the model are its proposed bidirectional and mediational relationships. For example, sleep and family functioning are assumed to have bidirectional links: A child's sleep-related behaviors can impact upon parental functioning, and family functioning can influence a child's sleep (see chap. 5). As an example of mediation, the daytime behavioral problems that have been associated with pediatric sleep-disordered breathing (SDB) are believed to be mediated by neurologic dysfunction (4,5). Though not

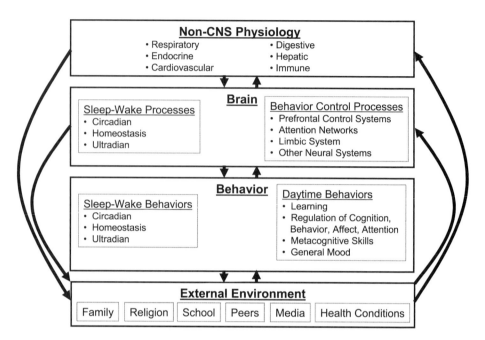

FIGURE 1 A multi-system heuristic model that relates sleep and daytime behaviors with other factors intrinsic within and external to a child.

indicated with arrows in the figure, the model assumes that elements within each level are systemically interrelated. For example, neural systems that regulate sleep and arousal overlap with, or are closely linked to, those that regulate attention (6). What follows is a brief explanation of each component of the model, accompanied by illustrative examples.

Non-Brain Physiology

This component of the model recognizes that pediatric sleep and behavior problems can stem from primary medical conditions outside of the brain. These include conditions that affect physiological systems as diverse as pulmonary (e.g., asthma, SDB), rheumatologic (e.g., fibromyalgia, arthritis), endocrine (e.g., diabetes), cardiovascular (e.g., cardiomyopathy), digestive (e.g., gastroesophogeal reflux), immunological (e.g., lupus), and others. Aberrations in these non-brain physiological systems are believed to have two paths by which they can impact sleep and daytime behaviors. First, as in the above example of obstructive SDB, a largely non-brain respiratory condition can impact the brain via sleep disruption and intermittent hypoxia, leading to daytime behavioral dysfunction (see chap. 11). For other medical conditions, associated treatments (e.g., use of steroids to treat severe asthma) may affect neural functioning, leading to changes in sleep and daytime behaviors (e.g., 7). Medical disorders and their treatments may also impact environmental conditions, which in turn can result in behavior changes. For example, recurrent hospitalizations can significantly disrupt routines associated with sleep, academic, family, and social functioning (e.g., 8). Even in non-hospitalized children, the presence of a medical condition can alter a child's relationships with parents and teachers, potentially altering both sleep and waking behaviors.

Conversely, non-brain physiology can be modified by both brain and environmental factors. Several neural networks involved in behavior regulation also affect distal physiologic systems. For example, the limbic system plays a key role not only in memory and emotion, but also in modulating the endocrine, respiratory and cardiovascular systems. Kleine-Levin Syndrome, described more fully by Pillar (chap. 13) is an example of a neuroendocrine disorder that affects both sleep and daytime behaviors. In addition, a number of environmental health conditions (e.g., toxicants) have been identified that place children at risk for disorders of both brain and non-brain systems (e.g., 9,10). Further, among children with medical disorders, environmental factors such as parent management of treatments can shape disease presence and severity (11). This, in turn, can affect sleep quality and/or behavioral functioning.

The Brain

In mainstream Western medicine, it is well-recognized that the brain controls all but the most rudimentary behaviors. Readers who are interested in learning more about waking brain–behavior relationships in children are referred to excellent neuropsychology texts written or edited by Anderson and colleagues (12), Yeates and colleagues (13), Baron (14), and Hunter and Donders (15). Similar tomes on the relationships between the brain and sleep have been authored or edited, for example, by Steriade and McCarley (16), and Luppi (17), and the topic is also addressed in several broad-scoped sleep texts (e.g., 18–20) Although the rapid pace of progress in this area suggests the need for an update, an excellent text was edited in 2003 by Maquet and colleagues (21) that is particularly relevant to those who are interested in the relationship between sleep and behavior in children, as it focuses on the importance of sleep in neural development and plasticity. These books highlight the fact that, although they are the primary domains of inquiry for neurologists and neuroscientists, brain structure and function are relevant for all professionals who are interested in human behavior, including sleep.

In the model, a conceptual distinction is made between neural systems related to sleep and daytime behavior. Historically, systems thought to modulate sleep have focused on the brain stem through the diencephalon, whereas systems associated with daytime behavior regulation have been described almost exclusively in the neocortex. However, as highlighted in several chapters in this book, the neural systems that regulate sleep and waking behaviors in fact overlap or are closely linked. For example, abnormalities in the dopaminergic system may result in symptoms of both restless leg syndrome and attention-deficit/hyperactivity disorder (22).

Three neural systems have received particular attention in research on the impact of sleep deprivation on human behavior. First, a substantial literature suggests that the prefrontal cortex is unusually sensitive to sleep deprivation and dyssomnias (e.g., 5,23–26). Second, because prominent attention deficits have been identified in sleepy adults, there is also interest in attention-related neural networks. These include the prefrontal cortex, but also extend extrafrontally, most notably to portions of the parietal lobes (27). Finally, recent research on learning and memory suggests that there should be greater consideration of the effect of sleep deprivation and dyssomnias on the limbic system, especially the hippocampus (e.g., 28–31). Unfortunately, nearly all of the relevant research on sleep and brain functioning has been on adults. Because of the unique neurodevelopmental status of children, there is a pressing need to better understand the neural mechanisms that underlie sleep, waking behavior, and their interrelationships in pediatric populations.

Behavior

This level of the model encompasses the overt behaviors of the child, as well as covert thought processes (e.g., memory) and emotions that may have behavioral manifestations (e.g., acquisition and exhibition of skills in the classroom, outward signs of anxiety). With some exceptions, this is the primary domain for pediatric sleep medicine and child mental health. In both disciplines, due consideration is given to physiological processes (including brain processes), but patients' present-ing concerns and clinical histories often focus upon observable behaviors. Because this is the level at which most research on sleep–behavior relationships has occurred, the reader will find rich coverage in the subsequent chapters.

It is worth noting that, although it is assumed that the brain underlies nearly all human behavior, there are points at which feedback from behavior can modify the brain. First, as Hebb predicted 60 years ago (32), behavioral repetition results in a change in neural connectivity. Second, in an extension of Hebb's model, connec-tivity is affected by life experiences, which are in part determined by behaviors. Third, internally directed cognitions can have an influence. Consider the romantic infatuations of adolescence. Not only can these result in observable behavior changes, but the intense ruminative and affective components of infatuation can temporarily dysregulate sleep and arousal (33,34). Fourth, contextual factors often determine whether a given behavior or outcome will be expressed. Leaders in neuropsychology (35,36) and sleep medicine (26,37) have noted that individuals who are prone to functional deficits may show them only when faced with certain environmental demands (e.g., sleepiness tends to affect driving most on long, monotonous trips). Finally, behavioral sleep treatments such as chronotherapy are predicated upon the ability of externally directed behavior changes to, over time, modify sleep-related brain processes.

External Environment

This level of the model acknowledges that the child functions within a dynamic set of interconnected contextual structures, some of which are inherently social (e.g., family, school, peer networks) while others are less directly so (e.g., built environ-ment and public health conditions). Collectively, these reflect the cultural milieu in which a child functions. This is the primary operational domain of anthropologists, sociologists, environmental engineers, and toxicologists. It has also become a key domain of interest for sleep specialists. On a basic level, there is increasing appreci-ation of the role of culture in defining sleep and behavioral health and pathology (see chaps. 3 and 4). Beyond this, the influence of school start times on both sleep and behavior, while fodder for public speculation as early as the 1920s (3), has undergone more scientific scrutiny in the past 25 years (see chap. 7). Although parent functioning has long been known to have reciprocal relationships with child sleep and daytime behaviors, advances in our scientific knowledge of these relationships recently warranted dedicated attention to the topic in an entire issue of the *Journal of Family Psychology* (21(1); see also chap. 5). Finally, the rapidly evolving peer and technological landscape which envelops today's children has also received recent scientific attention (e.g., 38,39).

In addition to the long-term influence of normative environmental conditions, extreme conditions can quickly cause marked changes in behaviors, the central nervous system (CNS), and non-CNS physiology. In other cases, environmental health conditions (e.g., neurotoxicants) can have a significant impact across multiple physiological systems.

DEVELOPMENTAL CONSIDERATIONS

In presenting reciprocal relationships, the above multi-system model is not completely static; it implies at least a limited form of temporal progression. However, it fails to do justice to the influence of developmental factors that, although also present in adults, are particularly dramatic during childhood. Figure 2 makes that development more explicit. In this figure, functioning at any given time point is seen both as (a) an aggregate product of the relevant events which occurred developmentally prior to that time, and (b) the context in which development will play out to determine future functioning.

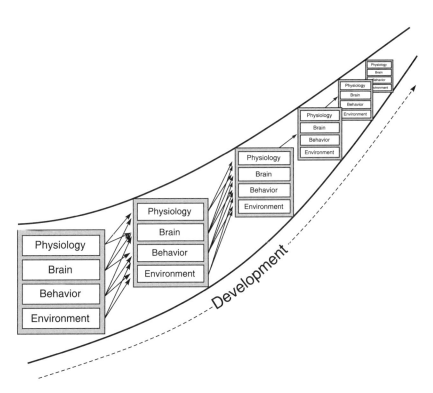

FIGURE 2   The heuristic model viewed in the context of human development.

As a starting point, it is useful to examine the "typical" developmental changes observed in each system. A detailed account of these changes extends beyond the scope of the current chapter, but Montgomery-Downs' chapter (chap. 2) summarizes the typical development of children's sleep on the neural and behavioral levels. Readers seeking even more details are referred to Marcus et al (40). Those seeking an overview of neural, behavioral, and environmental elements of neurobehavioral development are directed to Anderson and colleagues' text (12), as well as papers focusing on specific developmental periods, such as adolescence (33,41,42).

Though such understanding of "typical" development is important, by necessity it blurs important individual differences in developmental course and trajectory. Although at least some of these individual differences may be accounted for by genetic variation, there appear to be very few instances of complete genetic determinism. Even seemingly innate or preprogrammed developmental phenomena can often be modified by altering key elements in the environment (43). For example, although the development of the feline visual system is remarkably consistent under typical conditions—on first inspection following a genetically determined innate pattern—relatively simple manipulations in the nature and timing of visual stimulation, *as well as the presence, nature, and timing of sleep,* have been shown to alter the connectivity of this system (c.f., 44). Similarly, in a rodent model of SDB, the experimental induction of intermittent hypoxia during sleep in an immature animal has been demonstrated to result in lasting neural and behavioral changes (45,46).

There are serious ethical constraints to performing similar studies in humans, but findings such as these are reminders that development does not reflect the inexorable genetic unfolding of a preprogrammed sequence of events, but rather the result of a complex interplay of genetics and the relevant context of the developing cell, tissue, organ, system or organism. Two identical cells, tissues, organs, systems, or organisms, if faced with different circumstances, can respond differently (43). While in many cases this response is adaptive in the long run, in others the response may be in the direction of long-term maladaptation. In both situations, the response forms part of the immediate context for the next stage in development. Over time, despite the shared starting point, this process can result in very different outcomes (47). When a stressor is extreme (e.g., toxicity resulting in widespread organ damage), prolonged (e.g., persisting over many iterations of development), or unfortunately timed (e.g., during a critical or sensitive period of development), the developmental process can go particularly awry.

Although this developmental interaction between genetics and the environment can be generalized to a range of systems (e.g., baroreceptor development (48)), many of these are functionally mature by birth or soon afterwards. In contrast, neurodevelopment occurs throughout childhood, resulting in a protracted period of heightened plasticity during which adverse events could result in aberrant neural organization (43,47,49). For example, if indeed the prefrontal cortex is particularly sensitive to inadequate sleep, this could be profoundly important for children and adolescents, as the prefrontal cortex has a prolonged period of maturation that extends through the second decade of life (33,50–52). Given that this brain region appears critical to higher-level cognitive and social abilities, one might speculate that—even without obvious neural damage—inadequate or otherwise compromised sleep over time could result in unusual and/or suboptimal development of the microarchitecture of the brain and, consequently, in compromised long-term daily functioning.

IMPLICATIONS AND CONCLUSIONS

Having sketched out the basic skeleton of a heuristic model, I will close with several of its implications for research and clinical care.

1. Perturbations on one level (e.g., a respiratory abnormality) may result in significant changes in others (e.g., altered neurological functioning resulting in behavior changes that impact the family). Conversely, effectively treating problems on one level (e.g., SDB treated with adenotonsillectomy) might result in changes on another (e.g., improved family functioning). That stated, when developing an intervention on one level, it is important to consider whether interventions are also needed on others to maximize the impact. For example, continuous positive airway pressure for SDB may fail due to poor adherence unless the child's parents are supportive and proficient in the necessary behavior management skills.

2. For any given outcome, there may be multiple sources of interacting risk and resilience. A child from a socioeconomically disadvantaged family who experiences significant environmental stress, is of suboptimal health (e.g., significantly overweight), and does not have access to compensatory resources (e.g., effective tutoring) is probably at greater risk for a negative outcome from inadequate or disordered sleep than a child with similar sleep problems who is of more optimal health and environmental circumstances.

3. The nature of the relationship between two factors may vary developmentally. For example, the neurobehavioral effects of SDB may vary developmentally, with young children being more prone than adults to show behavioral dysregulation (5,53). Similarly, the nature of peer/social pressures in determining sleep patterns likely varies across childhood.

4. The timing of a developmental insult affects the kinds of problems that can result. Maureen Dennis has published an influential framework for conceptualizing the impact of brain insults on developing skills (54). She suggests that this impact will differ depending on whether, at the time of the insult, a skill is just emerging (resulting in abnormal skill onset or order of emergence), is in the process of developing (resulting in abnormalities in rate, strategy, or mastery of the skill), or has been established (resulting in problems with skill control and upkeep).

5. Developmental psychopathology often reflects not only a child's immediate circumstances, but also the influence of past events which may no longer be evident (47). As detailed in the chapters by Johnson (chap. 24), and Malow (chap. 25), sleep and behavioral concerns often co-occur in children with neurodevelopmental disorders. This co-occurrence may represent short-term causal or maintaining relationships, symptoms of a shared neurological abnormality, or the "downstream" results of a past neurodevelopmental insult or abnormality.

6. There is an ongoing need to identify events or circumstances that can push a child's development in a maladaptive direction. The goal would be to avoid these triggers or, via early identification and treatment, to minimize their impact in a targeted manner. Conversely, events or contexts that tend to result

in corrective or more adaptive developmental paths should be identified and maximized.

7. Treatment is not futile. There is the potential to change developmental trajectory after an adverse event or events. Indeed, in some cases, the development of an adversely affected child will, with treatment, converge upon what is considered "normal." However, for most conditions, the degree of residual post-treatment risk remains largely unknown.

8. For these and other reasons, developmental and contextual issues must be considered in research, ideally using prospective longitudinal methods.

The reader will no doubt be able to generate additional examples and implications of the model, especially after reviewing the other chapters in this book. The intent here was not to be comprehensive, but rather to lay the foundation for those chapters and for future work in the area. As a field, we now have a much better understanding of the relationship between children's sleep and their daytime behaviors than we did even a few decades ago. The challenge, moving forward, is to build upon these scientific advancements and to apply this emerging understanding for the betterment of public health and the clinical care of children with sleep and behavioral disorders.

REFERENCES

1. Thorpy MJ. History of sleep and man. In: Thorpy MJ, Yager J, eds. The Encylopedia of Sleep and Sleep Disorders. New York, NY: Facts on File, Inc., 1991.
2. Hill W. On some causes of backwardness and stupidity in children: And the relief of these symptoms in some instances by nasopharyngeal scarifications. British Medical Journal 1889; 2:711–12.
3. Stearns PN, Rowlands P, Giarnella L. Children's sleep: Sketching historical change. Journal of Social History 1996; 30:345–66.
4. Beebe DW. Neurobehavioral Effects of Childhood Sleep–Disordered Breathing (SDB): A comprehensive review. Sleep 2006:1115–34.
5. Beebe DW, Gozal D. Obstructive sleep apnea and the prefrontal cortex: Towards a comprehensive model linking nocturnal upper airway obstruction to daytime cognitive and behavioral deficits. Journal of Sleep Research 2002; 11:1–16.
6. Oken BS, Salinsky MC, Elsas SM. Vigilance, alertness, or sustained attention: Physiological basis and measurement. Clinical Neurophysiology 2006; 117:1885–901.
7. Bandla H, Splaingard M. Sleep problems in children with common medical disorders. Pediatric Clinics of North America 2004; 51:203–27.
8. Hinds PS, Hockenberry M, Rai SN, et al. Nocturnal awakenings, sleep environment interruptions, and fatigue in hospitalized children with cancer. Oncology Nursing Forum 2007; 34:393–402.
9. Guidotti TL, Gitterman BA. Global pediatric environmental health. Pediatric Clinics of North America 2007; 54:335–50.
10. Suk WA, Murray K, Avakian MD. Environmental hazards to children's health in the modern world. Mutation Research 2003; 544:235–42.
11. DiMatteo MR, Giordani PJ, Lepper HS, Croghan TW. Patient adherence and medical treatment outcomes: A meta-analysis. Medical Care 2002; 40:794–811.
12. Anderson V, Northam E, Hendy J, Wrennall J. Developmental Neuropsychology: A clinical approach. Philadelphia, PA: Psychology Press, 2001.
13. Yeates KO, Ris MD, Taylor HG. Pediatric Neuropsychology: Research, Theory, and Practice. New York: Guilford, 2000.

14. Baron IS. Neuropsychological Evaluation of the Child. New York: Oxford University Press, 2004.
15. Hunter SJ, Donders J. Pediatric Neuropsychological Intervention. Cambridge: Cambridge University Press, 2007.
16. Steriade MM, McCarley R. Brain Control of Wakefulness and Sleep. New York: Springer, 2005.
17. Luppi P-H. Sleep: Circuits and Functions. Boca Raton, FL: CRC Press, 2004.
18. Lee-Chiong TL. Sleep: A Comprehensive Handbook. Hoboken, NJ: Wiley-Liss, 2005.
19. Sheldon HS, Kryger M. In: Principles and Practice of Pediatric Sleep Medicine. Philadelphia: Saunders, 2005.
20. Kryger M, Roth T, Dement WC. In: Principles and Practice of Sleep Medicine. Philadelphia: Saunders, 2005.
21. Maquet P, Smith C, Stickgold R. Sleep and Brain Plasticity. New York: Oxford, 2003.
22. Picchietti DL, Underwood DJ, Farris WA, et al. Further studies on periodic limb movement disorder and restless legs syndrome in children with attention-deficit hyperactivity disorder. Movement Disorders 1999; 14:1000–7.
23. Horne JA. Why We Sleep. Oxford: Oxford University Press, 1988.
24. Horne JA. Human sleep, sleep loss, and behaviour. British Journal of Psychiatry 1993; 162:413–19.
25. Harrison Y, Horne JA. The impact of sleep deprivation on decision making: A review. Journal of Experimental Psychology: Applied 2000; 6:236–49.
26. Durmer JS, Dinges DF. Neurocognitive consequences of sleep deprivation. Seminars in Neurology 2005; 25:117–29.
27. Posner MI, Petersen SE. The attention system of the human brain. Annual Review of Neuroscience 1990; 12:25–42.
28. Ellenbogen JM, Payne JD, Stickgold R. The role of sleep in declarative memory consolidation: passive, permissive, active or none? Current Opinion in Neurobiology 2006; 16:716–22.
29. Born J, Rasch B, Gais S. Sleep to remember. Neuroscientist 2006; 12:410–24.
30. Stickgold R. Sleep-dependent memory consolidation. Nature 2005; 437:1272–8.
31. Stickgold R, Walker MP. Sleep-dependent memory consolidation and reconsolidation. Sleep Medicine 2007; 8:331–43.
32. Hebb DO. The Organization of Behavior. New York: Wiley, 1949.
33. Dahl RE. The regulation of sleep-arousal, affect, and attention in adolescence: Some questions and speculations. In: Carskadon MA, ed. Adolescent Sleep Patterns: Biological, social, and psychological influences. Cambridge, UK: Cambridge University Press, 2002: pp. 269–84.
34. Brand S, Luethi M, von Planta A, Hatzinger M, Holsboer-Trachsler E. Romantic love, hypomania, and sleep pattern in adolescents. Journal of Adolescent Health 2007; 41:69–76.
35. Satz P. Brain reserve capacity on symptom onset after brain injury: A formulation and review of evidence for threshold theory. Neuropsychology 1993; 7:273–95.
36. Dennis M. Childhood medical disorders and cognitive impairment: Biological risk, time, development, and reserve. In: Yeates KO, Ris MD, Taylor HG, eds. Pediatric Neuropsychology: Research, Theory, and Practice. New York: Guilford, 2000:3–22.
37. Dorrian J, Rogers NL, Dinges DF. Psychomotor vigilance performance: neurocognitive assay sensitive to sleep loss. In: Kushida C, ed. Sleep Deprivation: Clinical Issues, Pharmacology, and Sleep Loss Effects. New York: Marcel Dekker, 2005: pp. 39–70.
38. Carskadon MA. Factors influencing sleep patterns of adolescents. In: Carskadon MA, ed. Adolescent Sleep Patterns: Biological, Social, and Psychological Influences. Cambridge, UK: Cambridge University Press, 2002: pp. 4–26.
39. Olds T, Ridley K, Dollman J. Screenieboppers and extreme screenies: The place of screen time in the time budgets of 10–13 year–old Australian children. Australian and New Zealand Journal of Public Health 2006; 30:137–42.
40. Marcus CL, Loughlin GM, Carroll JL, Donnelly D. Breathing During Sleep in Children, 2nd Edn.: Informa Healthcare, 2008.

41. Sadeh A, Gruber R. Stress and sleep in adolescence: A clinical-developmental perspective. In: Carskadon MA, ed. Adolescent Sleep Patterns: Biological, Social, and Psychological Influences. Cambridge, UK: Cambridge University Press, 2002: pp. 236–53.

42. Blakemore SJ, Choudhury S. Development of the adolescent brain: Implications for executive function and social cognition. Journal of Child Psychology and Psychiatry 2006; 47:296–312.

43. Michel GF. A developmental-psychobiological approach to developmental neuropsychology. Developmental Neuropsychology 2001; 19: pp. 11–32.

44. Frank MG, Stryker MP. The role of sleep in the development of central visual pathways. In: Maquet P, Smith C, Stickgold R, eds. Sleep and Brain Plasticity. New York: Oxford University Press, 2003:190–206.

45. Row BW, Kheirandish L, Neville JJ, Gozal D. Impaired spatial learning and hyperactivity in developing rats exposed to intermittent hypoxia. Pediatric Research 2002; 52:449–53.

46. Gozal E, Row BW, Schurr A, Gozal D. Developmental differences in cortical and hippocampal vulnerability to intermittent hypoxia in the rat. Neuroscience Letters 2001; 305:197–201.

47. Courchesne E, Townsend J, Christopher C. Neurodevelopmental principles guide research on developmental psychopathologies. In: Cicchetti D, Cohen DJ, eds. Developmental Psychopathology, Vol 1: Theory and Methods. Oxford, England: John Wiley and Sons, 1995: pp. 195–226.

48. Bavis RW. Developmental plasticity of the hypoxic ventilatory response after perinatal hyperoxia and hypoxia. Respiratory Physiology & Neurobiology 2005; 149:287–99.

49. Gottesman, II, Hanson DR. Human development: Biological and genetic processes. Annual Review of Psychology 2005; 56:263–86.

50. Dahl RE. The impact of inadequate sleep on children's daytime and cognitive function. Seminars in Pediatric Neurology 1996; 3:44–50.

51. Dahl RE. The regulation of sleep and arousal: Development and psychopathology. Development and Psychopathology 1996; 8:3–27.

52. Dahl RE, Lewin DS. Pathways to adolescent health sleep regulation and behavior. J Adolesc Health 2002; 31:175–84.

53. Beebe DW. Neurobehavioral effects of obstructive sleep apnea: An overview and heuristic model. Current Opinion in Pulmonary Medicine 2005; 11:494–500.

54. Dennis M. Language and the young damaged brain. In: Boll T, Bryant BK, eds. Clinical Neuropsychology and Brain Function: Research, Measurement and Practice. Washington, DC: American Psychological Association, 1989: pp. 85–124.

2 Normal Sleep Development in Infants and Toddlers

Hawley E. Montgomery-Downs

Department of Psychology, West Virginia University, Morgantown, West Virginia, U.S.A.

INTRODUCTION

Evidence for the deleterious consequences of pediatric sleep disruption and disorders is growing. Several chapters of this volume review the cumulative findings suggesting that long-term developmental consequences may result from untreated sleep disorders during early childhood. While pediatric sleep medicine and research are rapidly expanding and tremendous advances have been made, this increasing appreciation of the importance of sleep and the effects of sleep disorders emphasizes the need for a broader understanding of normative aspects of sleep.

This chapter is formatted to cover several unique aspects of normative sleep during the first two years of life. First, because sleep during infancy is distinct from any other life span period, the unique nature of sleep during the first year of life is reviewed. Next, although the 1996 mandate by the American Thoracic Society (1) to develop normative polysomnographic reference values in children has been largely accomplished for preschool and older children (2,3), such data on infants and toddlers are lacking. One reason for this is that polysomnographic measurement itself causes dramatic interference with normal sleep in young children. Because of this, the reference values described herein rely upon parental report and a brief discussion of the current methodology and its shortcomings is included. Following the description of the current normative values, the effects that "sleeping like a baby" can have on new parents are discussed. Finally, environmental considerations, including a review of the current recommendations, for safe sleeping are reviewed.

BEHAVIORAL AND SLEEP STATES

A "state" is an arbitrary but precisely defined set of behavioral and physiologic characteristics. States in the young infant include crying, active alert, quiet alert, active sleep, and quiet sleep. Active sleep is characterized by phasic eye movements, irregular respiratory rates and patterns, and frequent large and small skeletal muscle group movement. Conversely, quiet sleep is characterized by a lack of eye movement and gross motor movement with the exception of occasional startle responses and by the presence of slow, regular respiratory rates and patterns. Young infants lack the neural mechanisms that induce atonia, or paralysis, during sleep. Thus, their states are easily identified by direct observation, the "gold standard" at this age. Although relatively minimal training allows identification of state, sleep behaviors including open-eyed rapid eye movements, gross body movements, and vocalizations are easily misunderstood by parents as waking behaviors requiring intervention.

Young infants enter active sleep first at the beginning of a sleep period. Beginning around six months there is a shift to beginning the sleep cycle with quiet sleep. The ratio of active to quiet sleep is initially about 50:50, a ratio that decreases dramatically during the first year of life with an increase in the proportion of quiet sleep. Likewise, the infant sleep cycle duration is roughly from 50 to 60 minutes, unlike the approximate 90 minute sleep cycle of older children and adults. Thus, infants' sleep is both qualitatively and quantitatively distinct from any other age group. Perhaps the most remarkable aspect of early infant sleep is its polyphasic nature. As originally quantified by Kleitman in 1963, relatively brief sleep periods are spread roughly equally through the diurnal and nocturnal periods during the first several weeks after birth (4).

MEASUREMENT OF SLEEP STATE

There are many methods used to measure infant and toddler sleep (5). The costs and benefits of each method should be considered in terms of the effects they have on the sleep state under assessment. As described above, direct observation is the gold standard for identification of sleep state during early infancy. Other standard methods include motility monitoring, actigraphy, videosomnography, and polysomnography.

Motility monitoring uses a thin capacitance-type sensor pad placed under the infant's bedding to transmit a single digitized channel representing the infant's respiration pattern and body movements. This signal is used to score wake, sleep, and transitional states while the infant is in the bed (6). Motility monitoring has shown measurement reliability and validity with electroencephalogram (EEG) and other recording procedures (7–10). The lack of instrumentation of the infant with this system and its ability to provide naturalistic information recorded in the home make this technology very attractive for use with young infants. Its disadvantage is that data are available only when the infant is in the crib.

Actigraphs are small, watch-type devices worn around the young child's ankle. They digitally record gross motor activity using highly sensitive accelerometry to provide a nonintrusive, home-based method for monitoring sleep/wake state, sleep quality and maintenance, insomnia, and locomotor activity levels in children (11). Several manufacturers produce competing brands of actigraphy that use different algorithms to identify sleep periods. Not all of these have been specifically validated for use with infants and/or toddlers. This is a rapidly changing technology and those interested in investing in actigraphy should consult manufacturing representatives and current users to determine which system has been validated for the population of intended use. At this point, actigraphy only provides sleep/wake state, not individual sleep states.

Time-lapse videosomnography, based on the principles of direct observation, is another nonintrusive method for identifying infant state using video technology which is later coded. Videosomnography is vulnerable to the same limitation as motility monitoring in that it only records periods when the infant is in the crib. Unlike motility monitoring, it does not provide respiratory rate and pattern data. However, in addition to state, videosomnography also provides information about the sleep environment so evaluation can also be made about the use of sleep aids and parent interactions with the child such as during night awakenings (12,13).

Polysomnography, Latin for "many sleep writings," is a method whereby multiple sensors are attached to the infant's head, face, neck, chest, and legs. These are used to collect physiologic information including electroencephalogram (EEG), electrooculogram (EOG), electromyogram (EMG), respiratory and cardiac output to identify brain, eye, muscle, and cardiorespiratory activity consistent with definitions of active sleep, quiet sleep, or indeterminate sleep in young infants (14,15) until approximately one year of age. For toddlers, the differentiated sleep stages 1, 2, 3, 4, and rapid eye movement (REM) sleep can be identified (16). Polysomnography has become the gold standard for clinical evaluation of sleep disorders. However, it is quite expensive, and home-based validation has not yet been performed for infants and toddlers. Further, laboratory-based polysomnography interferes with normal sleep in a phenomenon called "first-night effects." Actigraphy values in the home preceding and during a single night of laboratory polysomnography in 14-month-olds showed that although sleep onset times were preserved, sleep in the laboratory was disrupted on every other measure compared to their sleep at home. When testing was performed the morning after the sleep study, these differences did not affect standardized scores on a behavioral assessment, but the magnitude of difference between home nights and laboratory nights was associated with impaired emotional regulation (17). Whether these effects of sleep in the laboratory affect clinical diagnosis, and whether an adjustment night in the laboratory would reduce the differences in this age group are currently unknown.

NORMAL NIGHTTIME AND TOTAL SLEEP DURATIONS

Despite the technologies available, parental report questionnaires have provided the large-scale normative values about sleep times and durations for infants and toddlers described in this section.

Several recent studies report normative data for infant and toddler sleep. Results from the Zurich Longitudinal Study on 460 children from 1 month through adolescence born between 1974 and 1978 were reported in 2003. Twenty-four-hour sleep duration in this group decreased from an average of 14.2 hours at 6 months to 13.2 hours at 2 years. Consolidation of nocturnal sleep and a decrease in daytime napping occurred during the first year, resulting in a small increase in nighttime sleep duration by one year (18).

We recently reported on a cross-sectional sample of 944 infants and toddlers from two weeks through two years. Average 24-hour sleep duration across these two years was 12.5 hours (Fig. 1). Of note, the total 24-hour sleep durations did not change from birth through two years, yet daytime naps accounted for a greater proportion of 24-hour sleep among younger infants (Fig. 2) (19). These values were about an hour longer at the same ages than those found by Iglowstein and colleagues. This was despite a possible cohort effect for the Zurich Longitudinal Study which compared groups begun almost 20 years apart showing that total sleep duration decreased from 1974 to 1993 due to later bedtimes (but unchanged wake times) (18).

Consistent values were also reported by the National Sleep Foundation's (NSF) 2004 Sleep in America Poll (20). This report was based on phone interviews with the parents of 210 infants and 239 toddlers. Total daily sleep times were reported to decrease from 13.2 hours at 0–2 months to 11.4 at 2 years. The summary of nocturnal and 24-hour daily sleep times from two weeks through two years from these three recent studies are represented in Table 1.

The normative 24-hour sleep durations for infants and young toddlers reported in these recent studies are notably shorter than the historically recommended values. Methodological differences between these current studies and those

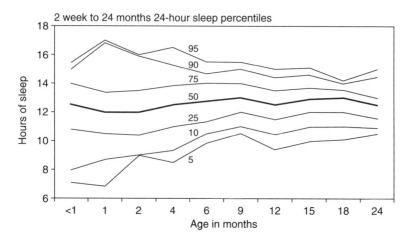

FIGURE 1   Fifth through ninety-fifth percentiles for parental-reported (N=944) hours of daily sleep (inclusive of nocturnal sleep and diurnal naps) for infants and toddlers 2 weeks through 2 years of age.

used for reference values in parenting books may explain some of their discrepancies. The studies by Iglowstein et al. (18) and Montgomery-Downs and Gozal (19) elicited values separately for nocturnal sleep and daytime naps; nocturnal sleep duration was further verified by asking parents to report current nocturnal bed and rise times. Queries regarding daytime naps were broken down into both the usual number of naps and their typical duration. Napping has previously been shown to have a reliable pattern (21) and the mean values from current data are consistent

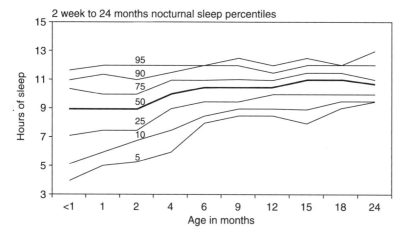

FIGURE 2   Fifth through ninety-fifth percentiles for parental-reported (N=944) hours of nocturnal sleep for infants and toddlers 2 weeks through 2 years of age.

TABLE 1 Reference Values for Nocturnal and 24-Hour Daily Sleep Times from Two Weeks Through Two Years

Age in months	0.5		1		2		4		6		9		12		15		18		24	
	Noc	TST	Noc	TST	Noc	TST	Noc	TST	Noc	TST	Noc	TST	Noc	TST	Noc	TST	Noc	TST	Noc	TST
Iglowstein et al.									11.0	14.2	11.2	13.9	11.7	13.9			11.6	13.6	11.5	13.2
NSF			7.8*	13.2*			9.3[a]	13.1[a]	9.7[b]	12.8[b]	9.3[c]	12.1[c]			10.1[d]	12.5[d]	9.7[e]	11.6[e]		
Montgomery-Downs et al.	8.7	12.2	8.4	12.1	8.7	12.0	9.6	12.4	10.3	12.6	10.5	13.0	10.3	12.4	10.6	12.7	10.8	12.7	10.7	12.5

Noc = Nocturnal sleep time.
TST = 24-hour total sleep time.
*0–2 months.
[a]3–5 months.
[b]6–8 months.
[c]9–11 months.
[d]12–17 months.
[e]18–23 months.

with this previous report in terms of both the number of naps and the nap duration, although most studies find large individual differences among subjects. In other words, the values in these studies were calculated from reported bed and rise times, and from typical numbers and durations of naps. This method may give very different results than simply asking parents how many hours out of 24 they think their child typically sleeps. Likewise, the current methods may avoid a social desirability effect. The lack of change in total 24-hour sleep times from two weeks through two years was consistent across these studies. However, some reported differences in 24-hour sleep times may also be culturally related; Italian infants from birth to five months have been reported to have the same total sleep time as described in these data, although that group was reported to have a significant decline in total sleep time across the first years, which the studies described above did not find (22).

Since there is no conclusive evidence to indicate that sleep duration below a certain threshold in this age range is nonoptimal or imposes particular morbidities, it is difficult to justify the recommendation often made to parents that their infant should sleep 16 hours each day. Indeed, such *a priori* excessive expectations may lead parents to manage their child's sleep routines inappropriately, and consequently induce sleep problems, or potentially lead to the erroneous belief that their child suffers from a sleep disorder.

NIGHTTIME AWAKENINGS

Brief awakenings between sleep cycles during the night are a normal part of sleep at all ages. Infants are reported by their parents to have an average of 1.3 (range 0–6, SD ± 1.1) awakenings at night and toddlers are reported to have an average of .73 (range 0–5, SD ± 1.0). These awakenings are generally so short that they are not remembered the following morning. If, however, something in the environment is amiss, the waking period will persist. The effect this can have on infant awakenings at night is well-explained by Ferber (23) using the "comfy pillow" analogy. Briefly, an adult who discovers during a normal waking following a sleep cycle that his or her pillow is gone will not simply return to sleep. Rather, he or she will search for the pillow and ultimately become agitated thinking someone has tricked him or her. This analogy is consistent with our interpretation of infant responses when they fall asleep in their parent's arms or during a feeding only to awaken later in their crib. The crib may be a reasonable sleeping location, but if it's not where they fell asleep originally then it may not be where they expect to awaken.

Using this principle infants are often categorized as "self-soothers" or "signalers." Self-soothers are infants who are able to return to sleep without parental intervention, whereas signalers are those who require parental intervention to return to sleep. One common recommendation is that parents encourage their infants to self-soothe by putting them down in their crib while they are still awake but drowsy and allowing them to fall asleep in the location where they will awaken later so that they will then be able to use the same resource during normal nighttime awakenings between sleep cycles. There are certainly data to support this. Anders and colleagues use longitudinal time-lapse videosomnography in the home to report that at three weeks of age most infants are put into their cribs already asleep both at the beginning of the night and following nighttime awakenings. By three months infants who were put into their cribs awake at the beginning of the night were more likely to self-soothe following nighttime awakenings than infants of the same age who were put into their cribs asleep at the beginning of the night (24). This research group recently identified that spending more sleeping time in the crib during the first year and having a parent who took longer to respond to nocturnal signaling when the infant was three months of age were predictors of self-soothing at 12 months (25). The cumulative findings from this research program support viewing the development of "sleeping through the night" from a transactional model, or systems approach, in order to understand the nocturnal relationship between the parent and the child's status as a self-soother or signaler.

These findings are particularly important because approximately 19% of 2-year-olds are reported by their parents to have a "sleep problem" (26), consistent with the 15% to 35% of children reported to have some form of sleep disturbance in their first five years (27,28). This high prevalence rate may indeed reflect problematic sleep among infants and toddlers, but there is also an emerging paradigm suggesting that perhaps parental and societal expectations of young children and how much they should sleep are unreasonable. It is often reported by behavioral sleep medicine specialists that simply having the parent fill out a sleep diary and discussing with them the results in the context of reasonable expectations is an effective intervention. Behavioral sleep medicine is graining strength as a highly effective therapy for solving many pediatric sleep problems (29).

EFFECTS ON MATERNAL SLEEP

Although fascinating from an empirical, developmental perspective, infants' polyphasic sleep and young children's frequent need for parental intervention is in sharp contrast to the sleep needs of the parents themselves. Interrupted parent sleep is a biological necessity in that young infants require nutrition, and perhaps physical contact with their parent, during the night. Yet sleep disruption is considered one of the key factors contributing to difficulties with maternal postpartum adjustment. It is important to briefly review the effects of normal infant sleep on new parents.

Postpartum mood disturbance is common, with 85% of women in the first week following childbirth experiencing the "baby blues" (30), a known risk factor for the onset of postpartum depression (31), which is diagnosed in 10% to 15% of women within four weeks after delivery (32,33). The children of women with untreated postpartum depression are more likely to fail to thrive, have reduced cognitive abilities and greater behavior, emotional, and social problems (34). An association between the infant's polyphasic sleep, maternal sleep disturbance, and maternal depression has been consistently reported. The fatigue reported by most women during the initial postpartum period is considered a major factor contributing to the onset of affect and mood disturbance (35–37). Postpartum fatigue plays such a major modifying role in distress that it has been suggested that negative postpartum affect is a spectrum disorder with fatigue as major factor (38).

It has been difficult to disentangle the cause–effect relations between sleep disruption and negative affect (39). However, recent studies suggest a causal effect of sleep deprivation leading to affect changes. Lee and colleagues found that at one month after delivery, a negative affect group had an average of 1.7 fewer hours of sleep per day than during their third trimester and 1.3 hours less than the positive affect group whose sleep remained unchanged from their third trimester (30). Researchers have also shown that improving the infant's sleep leads to improvements in maternal depression scores (39,40–42). A new study suggests strong benefits for using a preventative behavioral-educational intervention with first-time mothers to promote maternal and infant sleep (43). So, within "normal" it may be possible to improve the sleep of infants and to improve the mother's sleep and affect as a result.

ENVIRONMENTAL CONSIDERATIONS
Safe Sleeping

A full discussion of the current information pertaining to sudden infant death syndrome (SIDS) is beyond the scope of this chapter. However, in the context of normal infant sleep, it is important to briefly note that several independent risk factors for SIDS have been well-established. These include: sleeping in the prone position, sleeping on a soft surface, maternal smoking during pregnancy, infant overheating, late or no prenatal care, young maternal age, preterm birth and/or low birth weight for gestational age, and male gender (44).

In light of these risks, the American Academy of Pediatrics (AAP) (44), the National Institute of Child Health and Human Development (45), and the United States Consumer Product Safety Commission (46,47) have made consistent recommendations for safe sleeping environments and practices for healthy infants. These recommendations include: always placing sleeping infants in a completely supine position on a firm crib mattress covered by a tight-fitting sheet. Soft materials (including pillows, comforters, stuffed toys, "pillow-like" bumper pads, etc.) should not be placed in the crib with the infant. When a blanket is used the infant should be positioned "feet to foot" with the infant's feet at the foot of the crib and a thin blanket tucked around the crib mattress reaching only as far as the infant's chest to avoid having the head become covered. Infants should sleep in a separate bed in the same room as the mother. Women should not smoke during pregnancy, and infants should never be exposed to environmental tobacco smoke. The use of a pacifier should be considered at the beginning of sleep periods (though not by force, and should not be coated in sweet solutions), should be cleaned and replaced regularly, and may be delayed until one month of age for breastfed infants. To avoid overheating, the infant should be lightly clothed and the sleeping room should be a comfortable temperature for a lightly clothed adult. Commercial devices marketed to reduce SIDS and home monitors should not be used and measures should be taken to avoid development of positional plagiocephaly. The rationales for these recommendations have been thoroughly described and the reader is encouraged to review the latest AAP policy statement (44).

Co-Sleeping

The AAP recommendation regarding co-sleeping described above is particularly controversial. The practice of co-sleeping, or bed-sharing, refers to having the infant sleep in the same bed as the parent. Despite the recommendation that this practice be avoided, co-sleeping is commonly reported. One out of every 10 children between the ages of two weeks and two years are reported to sleep exclusively in the parents' bed, and an additional 5% to 16% are reported to sleep in their parents' bed at least part of the night (19,20).

It remains unclear from these studies what proportion of co-sleeping in this age range is occurring by choice or by perceived necessity. A comprehensive discussion of co-sleeping issues is clearly beyond the scope of this chapter. However, the relatively high proportion of children reported to co-sleep with their parents further emphasizes the need for community education regarding safe co-sleeping practices and greater sensitivity to the cultural and family dynamics surrounding this parenting decision (see reference 48 for review).

ABNORMAL INFANT AND TODDLER SLEEP

In closing, there are certain sleep behaviors that are not normal but that are not usually identified as such by parents and thus are not reported to healthcare professionals. Specifically, parental knowledge about symptoms of pediatric sleep-disordered breathing is lacking. Sleep-disordered breathing and its physiological and behavioral consequences is reviewed extensively in other chapters (also see reference 49 for review). In an exit survey of parents of older children, only 8% of parents of children with a significant history of snoring, the cardinal symptom of sleep-disordered breathing, mentioned this symptom during a routine checkup (50). However, it should be noted in particular that snoring is not considered a normal part of sleep at any age. The AAP has recommended that children one year and older be screened for snoring at well-child visits (51).

REFERENCES

1. American Thoracic Society. Standards and indications for cardiopulmonary sleep studies in children. Am J Respir Crit Care Med 1996; 153:866–78.
2. Traeger N, Schultz B, Pollock AN, Mason T, Marcus CL, Arens R. Polysomnographic values in children 2–9 years old: Additional data and review of the literature. Pediatric Pulmonology 2005; 40(1):22–30.
3. Montgomery-Downs HE, O'Brien LM, Gulliver TM, Gozal D. Polysomnographic characteristics in normal preschool and early school-age children. Pediatrics 2006; 117(3):741–53.
4. Kleitman N. Sleep and Wakefulness. Chicago, IL: University of Chicago Press, 1963.
5. Thoman ET, Acebo C. Monitoring of sleep in neonates and young children. In: Ferber R, Kryger M, eds Principles and Practice of Sleep Medicine in the Child. Philadelphia: W.B. Saunders Company, 1995: pp. 55–68.
6. Thoman EB, Glazier RC. Computer scoring of motility patterns for states of sleep and wakefulness: Human infants. Sleep 1987; 10:122–29.
7. Booth CL, Morin VN, Waite SP, Thoman EB. Periodic and nonperiodic sleep apnea in premature and fullterm infants. Developmental Medicine and Child Neurology 1983; 25: 283–96.
8. Thoman EB, Miano VN, Freese MP. The role of respiratory instability in SIDS. Developmental Medicine and Child Neurology 1978; 19:748–56.
9. Thoman EB, Zeidner LP, Denenberg VH. Cross-species invariance in state related motility patterns. American Journal of Physiology 1981; 241:R312–R315.
10. Waite SP, Thoman EB. Periodic apnea in the full-term infant: Individual consistency, sex differences, and state specificity. Pediatrics 1982; 70:79–86.
11. Sadeh A, Hauri PJ, Kripke DF, Lavie P. The role of actigraphy in the evaluation of sleep disorders. Sleep 1995; 18:288–302.
12. Anders T, Sostek A. The use of time-lapse video recording of sleep-wake behavior in human infants. Psychophysiology 1976; 13:155–8.

13. Anders T, Keener M. Developmental courses of nighttime sleep-wake patterns in full-term and pre-term infants during the first year of life. Sleep 1985; 48:173–92.
14. Anders T, Emde R, Parmelee A. (eds). A Manual of Standardized Terminology, Techniques and Criteria for the scoring of States of Sleep and Wakefulness in Newborn Infants, Los Angeles: UCLA Brain Information Services, 1971.
15. Sheldon SH. Polysomnography in infants and children. In: Sheldon SH, Ferber R, Kryger MH. (eds.) Principles and Practice of Pediatric Sleep Medicine. Elsevier, 2005.
16. Rechtschaffen A, Kales A. (eds.) A Manual of Standardized Terminology, Techniques and Scoring System for Sleep Stages of Human Subjects. Los Angeles, California: Brain Information Services/Brain Research Institute; University of California, 1968.
17. Montgomery-Downs HE, Gozal D. Toddler behavior following polysomnography: Effects of unintended sleep disturbance. Sleep 2006; 29(10):1282–7.
18. Iglowstein I, Jenni OG, Molinari L, Largo RH. Sleep duration from infancy to adolescence: Reference values and generational trends. Pediatrics 2003; 111(2):302–7.
19. Montgomery-Downs HE, Gozal D. Sleep habits and risk factors for sleep-disordered breathing in infants and young toddlers in Louisville, Kentucky. Sleep Medicine 2006; 7(3):211–19.
20. National Sleep Foundation. Sleep in America Poll available at: www.sleepfoundation.org
21. Weissbluth M. Naps in children: 6 months–7 years. Sleep 1995; 18(2):82–7.
22. Ottaviano S, Giannotti F, Cortesi F, Bruni O, Ottaviano C. Sleep characteristics in healthy children from birth to 6 years of age in the urban area of Rome. Sleep 1996; 19(1):1–3.
23. Ferber R. Solve Your Child's Sleep Problems. New York, NY: Simon & Schuster, Inc, 1985.
24. Anders TF, Halpern LF, Hua J. Sleeping through the night: A developmental perspective. Pediatrics 1992; 90(4):554–60.
25. Burnham MM, Goodlin-Jones BL, Gaylor EE, Anders TF. Nighttime sleep-wake patterns and self-soothing from birth to one year of age: A longitudinal intervention study. Journal of Child Psychology and Psychiatry 2002; 43(6):713–25.
26. Gaylor EE, Burnham MM, Goodlin-Jones BL, Anders TF. A longitudinal follow-up study of young children's sleep patterns using a developmental classification system. Behavioral Sleep Medicine 2005; 3(1):44–61.
27. Lozoff B, Wolf AW, Davis NS. Sleep problems seen in pediatric practice. Pediatrics 1985; 75(3):477–83.
28. Richman N. A community survey of characteristics of one- to two- year-olds with sleep disruptions. J Am Acad Child Psychiatry 1981; 20(2):281–91.
29. Mindell JA, Kuhn B, Lewin DS, Meltzer LJ, Sadeh A, American Academy of Sleep Medicine. Behavioral treatment of bedtime problems and night wakings in infants and young children. Sleep 2006; 29(10):1263–76.
30. Kendell RE, McGuire RJ, Connor Y, Cox JL. Mood changes in the first three weeks after childbirth. J Affect Disord 1981; 3:317–26.
31. Cox JL et al. Prospective study of the psychiatric disorders of childbirth. Br J Psychiatry 1982; 140:111–17.
32. Boyce P, Stubbs JM. The importance of postnatal depression. Med J Aust 1994; 161(8):471–2.
33. O'Hara M, Swain A. Rates and risk of postpartum depression—a meta-analysis. Int Rev Psychiatry 1996; 8:37–54.
34. Bell AJ, Land NM, Milne S, Hassanyeh F. Long-term outcome of post-partum psychiatric illness requiring admission. J Affect Disord 1994; 31:67–70.
35. Swain AM, O'Hara MW, Starr KR,Gorman LL. A prospective study of sleep, mood, and cognitive function in postpartum and nonpostpartum women. Obstet Gynecol 1997; 90:381–6.
36. Gardner DL. Fatigue in postpartum women. Appl Nurs Res 1991; 4:57–62.
37. Hiscock H, Wake M. Infant sleep problems and postnatal depression: A community-based study. Pediatrics 2001; 107(6):1317–22.
38. Fisher JRW, Feekery CJ, Rowe-Murray HJ. Nature, severity and correlates of psychological distress in women admitted to a private mother-baby unit. J Paediatr Child Health 2002; 38:140–5.

39. Armstrong KL, O'Donnell H, McCallum R, Dadds M. Childhood sleep problems: Association with prenatal factors and maternal distress/depression. J Paediatr Child Health 1998; 34(3):263–6.
40. Lee K, Zaffke ME, McEnany G. Parity and sleep patterns during and after pregnancy. Obstet & Gynecol 2000; 95:14–18.
41. Armstrong KL, Van Haeringen AR, Dadds MR, Cash R. Sleep deprivation or postnatal depression in later infancy: Separating the chicken from the egg. J Paediatr Child Health 1998; 34:260–2.
42. Dennis CL, Ross L. Relationships among infant sleep patterns, maternal fatigue, and development of depressive symptomatology. Birth 2005; 32(3):187–93.
43. Stremler R, Hodnett E, Lee K, MacMillan S, Mill C, Ongcangco L, Willan A. A behavioral–educational intervention to promote maternal and infant sleep: A pilot randomized, controlled trial. Sleep 2006; 29(12):1609–15.
44. American Academy of Pediatrics Task Force on Sudden Infant Death Syndrome. The changing concept of sudden infant death syndrome: Diagnostic coding shifts, controversies regarding the sleeping environment, and new variables to consider in reducing risk Pediatrics 2005; 116(5):1245–55.
45. National Institute of Child Health and Human Development statement on SIDS prevention information available at: http://www.nichd.nih.gov/publications/pubs/BTS_QA_Healthproviders.cfm
46. Scheers NJ, Dayton CM, Kemp JS. Sudden infant death with external airways covered Case-Comparison Study of 206 Deaths in the United States Arch Pediatr Adolesc Med 1998; 152:540–7.
47. Scheers NJ, Rutherford GW, Kemp JS. Where should infants sleep? A comparison of risk for suffocation of infants sleeping in cribs, adult beds, and other sleeping locations. Pediatrics 2003; 112(4):883–9.
48. McKenna JJ, McDade T. Why babies should never sleep alone: A review of the co-sleeping controversy in relation to SIDS, bedsharing and breast feeding. Paediatr Respir Rev 2005; 6(2):134–52.
49. Beebe DW. Neurobehavioral morbidity associated with disordered breathing during sleep in children: A comprehensive review. Sleep 2006; 29(9):1115–34.
50. Blunden S, Lushington K, Lorenzen B, Wong J, Balendran R, Kennedy D. Symptoms of sleep breathing disorders in children are underreported by parents at general practice visits. Sleep and Breathing 2003; 7(4):167–76.
51. Section on Pediatric Pulmonology, Subcommittee on Obstructive Sleep Apnea Syndrome. American Academy of Pediatrics. Clinical practice guideline: Diagnosis and management of childhood obstructive sleep apnea syndrome. Pediatrics 2002; 109(4):704–12.

3 Behavioral Sleep Disorders in Infants and Toddlers

Melissa M. Burnham[a] and Erika E. Gaylor[b]

[a] Department of Human Development and Family Studies, University of Nevada, Reno, Nevada, U.S.A.
[b] Center for Education and Human Services, Policy Division, SRI International, Menlo Park, California, U.S.A.

INTRODUCTION

Infant and toddler sleep "problems" are among the most commonly reported complaints of parents to their pediatricians (1). In fact, a recently published community survey of mothers in Melbourne, Australia revealed that a full 34% reported a sleep problem in their three- to six-month-old infants; with 31% of these indicating that the problem was "severe" (2). These findings are consistent with classic research into the prevalence of sleep problems in the infant and toddler population, as these studies typically have reported that around 25% of parents indicate that their young children experience some type of sleep disturbance (3–5). Contrary to these data, a large poll conducted in 2004 by the National Sleep Foundation in the United States (6) found that only 6% of parents of infants and 11% of parents of toddlers reported that their child had a sleep problem. In this poll, parents were more likely to report a sleep problem if their child slept significantly less than his/her peers, took 30 minutes or longer to fall asleep, or woke up two or more times per night. Differences in prevalence rates found between studies may be due to the sampling methods used. The Sleep in America poll randomly sampled households with a child under the age of 10, while most other investigations that report prevalence rates recruited families for a study specifically related to sleep. It is possible that families who sign up for such studies may already have a problem with their child's sleep, thus possibly inflating the prevalence rates obtained. Clearly, more representative data need to be collected in order to determine accurate prevalence rates.

Notwithstanding the differences in prevalence rates found between studies, sleep disruptions in infants and toddlers are clearly problematic for some parents, and may be problematic for the infants themselves (e.g., 7). Yet, a closer look into the issues surrounding such disturbances reveals a plethora of external, mediating, and moderating factors that make defining a "sleep problem" in this population problematic in itself. Factors such as normative developmental changes, intra-individual variation, inter- and intra-cultural variation, as well as who reports the problem, are just some of the issues that complicate the definition of a sleep disorder in infants and toddlers. An additional concern relates to the impact of the sleep disturbance on the child's behavior, and on the child's family. This chapter will engage the reader in a presentation of these issues, will describe the varying methods that have been used to classify sleep disorders in this age group, and will end with a discussion of the major categories of behavioral sleep disorders, specifically focusing on research into their causes and correlates.

FACTORS COMPLICATING THE DEFINITION OF A SLEEP DISORDER IN INFANTS AND TODDLERS

Any review of behavioral sleep disorders in infants and toddlers would be remiss in not including a detailed discussion of the issues that obscure clear understanding of what does and does not constitute a disorder. Three sets of specific issues will be presented in an attempt to reveal the complexity of defining sleep disorders in this population.

Normative Developmental Changes and Individual Variation

First, as discussed by Montgomery-Downs in Chapter 2, during the age span of 0 to 3 years, children experience substantial developmental changes in sleep habits and patterns. Infants gradually develop a clear diurnal sleep–wake rhythm, the proportion of time spent in and distribution of stages within sleep change over time, and the longest period of uninterrupted sleep gradually increases (8–11). It is clear that the majority of infants and toddlers continue to wake up at night throughout this developmental period; what changes is that a proportion of very young children develop the ability to soothe themselves back to sleep following these awakenings (12). It should be noted as well that the traditional definition of "sleeping through the night" involves sustaining sleep between the hours of midnight and 5 a.m. (13). Without awareness of these definitions and research findings, many parents may hold unrealistic expectations for their young infants' sleep.

In addition to the developmental changes that the "average" baby experiences, research has revealed substantial amounts of individual variation in sleep–wake patterns (e.g., 11). A recent cross-sectional study of children aged one to five years demonstrated significant inter-individual variability, especially in comparison to previous studies (14). Indeed, not only do infants sleep differently from each other, but infant sleep differs quite dramatically from night to night within individuals as well (15–16), especially among young children in families of low socioeconomic status (14). Thus, focusing on measures of central tendency and ignoring measures of dispersion gives only a partial picture of the reality of infant/toddler sleep. It is essential for clinicians to hold these individual differences in mind when disseminating normative data to parents. The developmental changes and variability in sleep patterns across time make it difficult to describe objectively "normal" versus "problematic" sleep. This complexity needs to be acknowledged in any assessment or diagnosis of a sleep disorder.

Culture

In addition to ontogenetic differences in sleep, it is equally important, when making a judgement about whether or not sleep is problematic, to examine the culture within which sleep develops. In their comparative analysis of human sleep, Worthman and Melby (17) concluded that "the peculiarities of Western sleep ecologies may contribute to the patterns and prevalence of sleep disorders observed in those settings" (p. 109). For every practice and expectation that one finds typical in one culture or subculture, the opposite is likely to be found in another. Although differences are typically greater between different types of societies around the world, they exist within Western culture as well. For instance, Italian, Japanese, and American families each have very different views of where, when, how, and with whom infants and toddlers should sleep (18). Jenni and O'Connor (18) note that "many 'problems' with sleep during childhood, such as difficulties falling asleep alone or waking at night and seeking parental attention, are based on culturally constructed definitions and expectations that are not necessarily rooted in sleep biology" (p. 205). Without a shared sleep norm across—or, indeed, within—cultures, it is difficult to decide what is a problem. There are clear socioeconomic, ethnic, and other subgroup differences within any given culture that make clinical decisions and definitions challenging.

Family

In the American Psychiatric Association's (19) *Diagnostic and Statistical Manual of Mental Disorders* (revised 4th edition; DSM-IV-TR), one criterion for the diagnosis of primary insomnia in adults is that the sleep problem must cause clinically significant distress or impairment in the patient. One of the major problems in defining a sleep disorder in the infant and toddler population is that the person voicing the complaint is not the patient him/herself, but rather a family member. The consequences of perceived infant sleep problems on the family are real and cannot be dismissed, but the issue of whose problem it is makes classification of a sleep disorder more complicated for the infant/toddler clinician, compared to the assessment of adults. Because infants and toddlers are unable to voice a complaint about their own sleep disturbances, clinicians must rely on parent report. Thus, "problems" are defined by family members—presumably due to the negative impact of the child's sleep behavior on the family. In addition, each family has a different threshold for what is considered a problem. One family may not find their six-month-old's habitual night waking pattern disruptive or abnormal while another family might consider even one awakening problematic in this age group. In one study comparing different definitions of a sleep problem in young children, only one family reported that their child currently had a sleep problem, although 11 children met the suggested criteria for one (20). In a follow-up to this investigation, approximately 25% of children were reported to be co-sleeping with a parent, yet only a third of these parents reported it as problematic (21). In an epidemiological investigation, 25% of one- to two-year-olds were found to be habitually waking up at night at least five times per week, but only half of the parents considered this pattern to be a problem (22). When accompanied by each of the other potential complicating factors discussed above, then, threshold differences make a single definition of problematic sleep virtually impossible to deduce.

Each of the three sets of factors described above contributes to the difficulty that clinicians face in defining and diagnosing sleep problems in very young children, and should be considered when interacting with families who have a complaint about their young child's sleep. The complexities in defining and diagnosing sleep problems in infants and toddlers discussed above illustrate the difficulty in defining and diagnosing *any* disorder during the infant/toddler period. Clinicians should keep in mind these complexities, as well as the fact that symptoms in the very young child occur within the context of the parent–infant relationship. Indeed, adding to an already complicated set of influential factors is the fact that sleep disturbances can be seen as the product of a disturbed infant–parent relationship, and can themselves negatively impact the parent–infant relationship (23,24). The correlates of infant/toddler sleep disturbances will be discussed in more detail following the presentation of different methods used to classify sleep problems in this population.

CLASSIFICATION OF SLEEP DISORDERS

Complicating the matter further still is the fact that several clinical and research classification schemes, or nosologies, exist, and each defines sleep disorders somewhat differently (24–27). The most commonly used classification scheme in pediatric sleep medicine is the second edition of the *International Classification of Sleep Disorders* (ICSD-2), published by the American Academy of Sleep Medicine (28). Under this most recent revision, a pediatric sleep problem is classified as "Behavioral Insomnia of Childhood," which includes three sub-classifications: Sleep-onset association type, limit-setting type, or combined type (27). These will be discussed in more detail below. Other classification schemes used clinically include the *Diagnostic and Statistical Manual of Mental Disorders* (DSM-IV-TR) (19) and the *Diagnostic Classification of Mental Health and Developmental Disorders of Infancy and Early Childhood*—revised (DC: 0-3R) (29). The DSM-IV-TR does not parse out childhood sleep disorders as distinct from the adult criteria for diagnosis and is thus considered less helpful in describing disrupted sleep in infants and toddlers. The DC 0-3R, although specifically designed for use with the infant/toddler population, is rarely used by sleep clinicians, and does not include quantitative metrics to classify sleep problems (30).

It is significant to note that research investigations generally have not used these clinical classification schemes to identify sleep problems in their study populations. An entirely different set of schemes has been used for research purposes. The most common of these include simple parent report of a sleep problem (yes/no), and the more specific criteria identified by Richman (5) and Anders et al. (30). Screening tools have also been used by pediatricians and researchers to detect severe problem sleep in a normative population (e.g., bedtime issues, excessive daytime sleepiness, night awakenings, regularity and duration of sleep, and snoring) (31–34), although for the very young child under three years, the Brief Infant Sleep Questionnaire (34) is the most appropriate. Using an investigator-derived algorithm (total sleep time, sleep onset latency, and night awakenings), Sadeh and colleagues (35) found that 19% of children in the first three years of life were classified as having poor sleep using this measure.

Of each of the research classification schemes used, perhaps the closest match to the most commonly used clinical criteria (ICSD-2) is the Anders classification scheme (30). The Anders scheme classifies sleep onset and night waking as two separate problems, similar to the ICSD-2 sub-classifications (Table 1). These problems are labeled "protodyssomnias" to differentiate them as developmentally distinct from the adult dyssomnia categorization used in the DSM-IV. The ICSD-2 classification of "limit-setting type" refers to issues surrounding bedtime delay or refusal, similar to Anders' "sleep onset protodyssomnia." The ICSD-2 classification of "sleep-onset association type" is manifested by night waking issues, and is generally caused by the constellation of parent-provided factors present while the infant initially falls asleep. If these factors are not present during the middle of the night when the infant wakes up, the infant signals the parent and requires the same set of factors to fall back to sleep. Not surprisingly, this sub-classification most closely aligns with Anders' "night waking protodyssomnia." According to Mindell and

TABLE 1   Classification Scheme for Sleep Protodyssomnias in Toddlers and Preschoolers

Sleep onset protodyssomnia	
(Child must meet any 2 of the 3 criteria listed)	
12–24 months	(1) > 30 minutes to fall asleep; (2) parent remains in room for sleep onset; (3) more than three reunions[a]
> 24 months	(1) > 20 minutes to fall asleep; (2) parent remains in room for sleep onset; (3) more than two reunions
Night waking protodyssomnia	
12–24 months	1 or more awakenings[b]/night, totaling $\geq$ 30 minutes[c]
> 24 months	1 or more awakenings/night, totaling $\geq$ 20 minutes
> 36 months	1 or more awakenings/night, totaling $\geq$ 10 minutes

Note. A protodyssomnia is not diagnosed before 1 year of age. The criteria pertain to solitary sleeping infants. Duration criteria are subdivided. Perturbations (one episode/week for at least 1 month) are considered variations within normal development. Disturbances (two to four episodes/week for at least 1 month) are considered as possible risk conditions that may be self-limiting. Disorders (five to seven episodes/week for at least 1 month) most likely are continuous and require intervention.
[a] Reunions reflect resistances in going to bed (e.g., repeated bids, protests, struggles).
[b] Awakenings must require parental intervention and occur after the child has been asleep for >10 minutes.
[c] A criterion of $\geq$ 30 minutes is applied to the whole night regardless of the number of awakenings.
Source: Ref. (30).

colleagues (27), both ICSD-2 sub-classifications require specific symptoms, a defined level of severity, a time length, and must result in impairment of either the child or parent in order to be diagnosed. The Anders classification scheme also has severity criteria, specific criteria for different age groupings, and frequency and duration criteria. Notably, the Anders classification scheme does not consider co-sleeping, in and of itself, a problem, does not recommend classifying infants under 12 months of age, and does not require parent complaint of a problem in order for a child to be classified (30). These exceptions distinguish the Anders scheme from the ICSD-2 clinical classification. Although problematic sleep certainly exists in some children before the age of one, relationship, family, and developmental contexts within which the sleep problem is manifested may require more attention during this age span.

TYPES OF SLEEP DISORDERS IN INFANTS/TODDLERS AND THEIR ETIOLOGY
This section will attempt to describe the two main types of behavioral sleep disorders found in infants and toddlers and their etiology. Each of the two main categorizations of sleep disorders will be discussed separately, with specific reference to its respective ICSD-2 and Anders' classification.

Limit-Setting Sleep Disorder (Anders' Sleep Onset Protodyssomnia)
As mentioned briefly above, limit-setting sleep disorder (Anders' sleep onset disorder) involves problems with the delay and/or resistance of bedtime, and is typically seen in 5% to 10% of children aged two and above (36). It is manifested in prolonged bedtime routines and strong resistance to going to bed. This type of sleep disorder generally increases during childhood, as children gain more independence

and experience more fears (37–39) and thus is not found in the infant population and is just beginning to appear in some toddlers. It is thought to be exacerbated by parents' inadequately enforcing bedtimes and/or responding to (and thus reinforcing) children's "curtain calls" (requests, after bedtime, for one more story, one more drink of water, one more hug, five more minutes, and the like). The most robust research in this area comes from older children but demonstrates a significant correlation between bedtime resistance and daytime resistance to parental behaviors (40). Both problems are considered the result of parents' inability to set clear limits during the day and at bedtime. These problems may also reflect a mismatch between the parents' expectations and the child's predisposition (27).

Sleep Onset Association Disorder (Anders' Night Waking Protodyssomnia)

The second type of behavioral sleep disorder, which is the most common for infants and toddlers, is "sleep onset association disorder" or Anders' "night waking protodyssomnia." This type of disorder affects as many as 15% to 20% of children under the age of three (36). It should be noted, however, that not all parents consider an infant or toddler needing their assistance to be problematic. The factors discussed above (culture, expectations, etc.) mediate between the symptoms displayed by the child and the interpretation of these symptoms as problematic. Sleep onset association disorder is characterized by the pairing of a certain set of circumstances or objects introduced by a parent (e.g., a pacifier, rocking, nursing, etc.) with bedtime. When the child wakes up at night and these circumstances or objects are not present, the child needs them to be reintroduced in order to fall back to sleep. This type of disorder is typically manifested in difficulty falling asleep without these objects or circumstances and frequent night waking (27,36). Infants and toddlers with a sleep onset association disorder have been referred to as "non-self-soothers" (41) because they cannot reinitiate sleep following a nighttime awakening without assistance.

Sleep onset association disorder is thought to be exacerbated by parents' providing a bedtime environment that cannot be reproduced by the infant when he/she wakes up in the middle of the night. One group of researchers found that these types of "nonadaptive sleep associations" were associated with significantly higher odds of night waking in six-month-old to four-year-old children referred from a sleep clinic, compared to a matched control group who did not have night waking problems (42). While sleep associations are certainly part of the cause of this particular type of sleep disorder, there are apparently other reasons that night waking develops. Interestingly, active physical comforting at bedtime only explained 3% of the variance in infant sleep problems at one year when examined with other variables such as maternal cognitions, temperament, and maternal anxiety/depression, but it did explain more variance in the continuity of problematic sleep from the first to the second year of life (43).

IMPACT OF SLEEP DISORDERS

The two main behavioral sleep disorders that are commonly seen in the infant/toddler period have different causes and appear within a rich context of other factors that need to be considered before diagnosis and treatment. The impact of these sleep disorders on families and on the children themselves is significant and also needs to be considered. It is to these specific correlates of infant/toddler sleep disturbances that this review now turns. Because research in this area is relatively new, includes small investigations, and has rarely been longitudinal in nature, the term "correlates" will be used instead of "outcomes" to discuss the purported impacts of infant/toddler sleep disorders on families and the children themselves.

Family Correlates

Some of the correlates of infant/toddler sleep problems in families include: maternal depression, parental fatigue, general disruptions to family life, poor maternal mental and physical health, and less parental well-being (2,44–49). In one investigation, resolving the sleep problems of 6–12-month-old infants resulted in significant improvement in parents' sleep quality, cognitions about infant sleep, depression, and marital harmony (48). One must consider the direction of effect in any of these investigations; it is entirely possible that some of these correlates preceded the child's sleep disruption or the two are related to a completely different, unstudied factor. In a prospective study, persistent sleep disruptions, defined by the parent across the first 2 to 24 months of life, were uncommon (6%) but were associated with maternal depression and parenting stress at 24 months (49). In contrast, at least one investigation has reported that once maternal sleep quality was controlled, the relationship between infant sleep problems and maternal mental health was eliminated (2). It is important to keep in mind that in most investigations, both child sleep and parental well-being were measured by parent report, which potentially confounds any reported relationships.

Child Correlates

Clearly, infant/toddler sleep disruptions are correlated with, and indeed may cause, several negative family outcomes. Less clear is whether or not there is a negative impact on the child him/herself. While studies on older children, adolescents, and adults have found relationships between sleep problems and daytime behavior (e.g., 50–53), data are virtually nonexistent for the infant/toddler population. Studying children under three years of age is particularly challenging because it is normative for children in this age group to nap at least once, if not several times per day. Thus, any daytime behavioral effects of a nighttime sleep problem may be diminished by the child's use of daytime sleep to "make up for" a restless or short night. Literature on the effects of sleep loss in humans and other animals suggests that transient sleep loss is made up either by sleeping longer or more intensely; this is most likely true for young children as well.

Notwithstanding the lack of research with infants and toddlers, research with older children and adults has found that sleep loss over a significant period of time can have serious consequences. What those consequences are, for whom, and under what conditions, are still the subject of intense research. For example, recent research provides some evidence that rapid eye movement sleep helps consolidate memory and promotes advanced cognitive functioning (54). Sleep quantity and architecture also may play a critical role in promoting brain plasticity (55). These lines of research in animals and adults suggest that understanding the inter- and intra-individual variation in a young child's sleep is important because optimal sleep may provide the foundation for neurocognitive development and growth (56,57).

Any problem that results in significant sleep loss for infants and toddlers may impact their cognitive functioning, but developmental human research in this age period is sorely lacking. An understanding of how sleep contributes to brain development, as well as the normative range and limits to individual variability in sleep, is essential in order to explore possible maladaptive cognitive outcomes in this age range.

A growing body of work has found associations between sleep and older children's cognitive and emotional functioning and physical well-being. For instance, amount of sleep is associated with maladjustment in preschoolers (40) and experimental studies have found that even a small amount of sleep loss (one hour) is associated with impaired daytime cognitive and behavioral functioning in school-age children (58). In addition, shorter daytime sleep between three and five years of age (59), as well as shorter nighttime sleep at three years (60) have been linked to obesity during middle childhood.

In older children, there also appears to be an interaction between the temperamental characteristic of resistance and sleep loss that predicts a child's ability to effectively manage sleep loss. In one series of investigations, preschoolers' sleep problems were more strongly associated with behavior problems in children high in resistance to control than in children low in resistance (61,62). Preliminary evidence suggests that temperamental resistance is predictive of persistent sleep problems in toddlers as well (63). Although the literature on sleep and temperament is inconsistent, some studies have shown that infants with night waking problems are described as more temperamentally difficult (64,65), less adaptive (66,67), and more irritable (66). Infants who take longer to fall asleep are described as more withdrawn (67). The direction of these effects is hard to discern for several reasons, including the parallel development of physiological, cognitive, and emotional regulatory systems, problems with parent report, and the inherent bidirectionality of such behaviors (i.e., sleep affects emotional processing but emotional processing affects sleep).

Although waking up at night is considered a behavioral sleep disorder, the consequences of sleep fragmentation in infants and toddlers are much less well-known than the effects of such fragmentation in older children and adults. When behavioral sleep problems result in sleep loss and/or deprivation, the possibility exists that neurodevelopmental processes are at risk (68). Studies in older children (described above) suggest that sleep disruption compromises executive functioning and self-regulatory abilities, skills necessary to perform complex cognitive tasks. Other studies have shown that severe and chronic infant night waking predicts later disorders including attention-deficit/hyperactivity disorder diagnosis (ADHD) at five years (69). Finally, there is some evidence to suggest that limit-setting and sleep onset association sleep disorders are distinct and impact—or are manifestations of—dysregulation in distinct domains of functioning. In particular, Bruni and colleagues (70) found that frequent nighttime awakenings (sleep onset association disorder) were associated with higher externalizing scale scores, and greater bedtime resistance (limit-setting sleep disorder) was related to higher internalizing scale scores in preschool-age children.

Several studies have reported modest relationships between disturbed sleep and later behavior problems in very young children (e.g., 71, 72). It should be acknowledged that other stable factors could contribute to the appearance of later behavior problems as well, but these are rarely considered. A recent study elucidated this possibility in its finding that night waking in infancy predicted only 3% of the variance in behavioral scores at 42 months (73). Persistent night waking and enduring settling problems were better predictors of later negative behavior than was night waking during the infancy period. A study by Wake and colleagues (49) provides further evidence that it is persistent, rather than transient, problems during the infant/toddler period that relate to subsequent child behavior problems. A final set of evidence pointing to a relationship between infant/toddler sleep disruption and daytime behavior comes from intervention studies with clinical populations. These investigations have found a relationship between treatment of the sleep problem and an improvement in daytime behavior, as measured by parent report (e.g., 7). It seems safe to conclude that severe, persistent sleep problems during the infant/toddler period appear to impact daytime behavior; what is less clear is the potential impact of less severe problems.

TREATMENT

Later chapters of this volume focus on specific treatment approaches; a brief overview is provided here. Research on the development of clinical guidelines for problematic sleep has focused on nonpharmacological treatments (27,74–76). As a general rule, pharmacological interventions have been found to be ineffective in children under two years of age (27,77). Many clinical interventions are based on the assumption that decreasing parent involvement at sleep onset/bedtime will facilitate self-soothing behaviors in the infant/toddler and will lead to better sleep (78,79). Recent prospective intervention studies using objective measures of sleep focused on educating parents about normal sleep variation, providing behavioral techniques to promote self-soothing, and supporting parents in implementing the techniques find decreases in infant night awakenings, nighttime crying, and longer uninterrupted sleep periods (80,81). Instituting a consistent bedtime routine improves multiple aspects of infant sleep, especially the amount of time it takes to fall asleep and the longest continuous sleep period for 7–18-month-olds (82).

Treatment approaches that consider individual differences in parenting cognitions may help to resolve the issues related to the definition of a sleep problem that currently exist. Parental cognitions (i.e., beliefs, expectations, attributions, and interpretation) influence parents' behavior towards infants' sleep. Parents who present to a sleep clinic with complaints about their infants' night waking are more likely to endorse difficulties in accepting "limit-setting" as an explanation for night waking (35). These parents experience a conflict about what they think they should be doing and what they actually do in response to their child's sleep.

CONCLUSION

The sleep concerns of parents of very young children often reflect a discrepancy between parental expectations and developmentally appropriate sleep behaviors or parental misinterpretation of normal behaviors. In addition, several mediating and external factors influence parents' perceptions. Coupled with great individual variability and the backdrop of typical ontogenetic change, the definition of what constitutes a sleep problem becomes exigent. It is thus challenging to reach a conclusion with regard to the potential effects of a sleep problem on the child when research relies upon different definitional criteria. Only with accepted definitions of and criteria for sleep disorders and the delineation of what is considered normal sleep in this population will knowledge in this area progress.

Theoretically, however, there is reason to speculate that severe, persistent sleep problems that result in accumulated sleep deficits can have severe consequences for children in this age group. The transition from infancy to early childhood is marked by the development of self-regulatory competencies that are hypothesized to reflect the continuing maturation of the brain. These competences include the ability to sustain attention despite distractions and to inhibit prepotent responses and are supported by the capacity for effortful control. Because similar areas of the brain control both effortful regulation of behavior and arousal regulation, we might expect that young children with a more developed capacity for effortful control may exhibit more mature or optimal patterns of sleep. Theory suggests that sleep should allow an individual to perform better and with greater ease because of the integration and consolidation of information that occurs during sleep. Further research in the area of behavioral sleep disorders in infants and toddlers and their potential effects is critical to furthering our understanding of this important period in the lifespan.

REFERENCES

1. Thiedke CC. Sleep disorders and sleep problems in childhood. American Family Physician 2001; 63(2):277–84.
2. Bayer JK, Hiscock H, Hampton A, et al. Sleep problems in young infants and maternal mental and physical health. Journal of Paediatrics & Child Health 2007; 43: 66–73.
3. Bixler EO, Kales JD, Scharf MB, et al. Incidence of sleep disorders in medical practice: A physician survey. Sleep Research 1976; 5, 62.
4. Lozoff B, Wolf AW, Davis NS. Sleep problems seen in pediatric practice. Pediatrics 1985; 75:477–83.
5. Richman N. A community survey of characteristics of one to two year olds with sleep disruptions. J Am Acad Child Psychiatry 1981; 20:281–91.
6. National Sleep Foundation. 2004 Sleep in America Poll. Retrieved from http://www.kintera.org/atf/cf/%7BF6BF2668–A1B4–4FE8–8D1A–A5D39340D9CB%7D/2004 SleepPollFinalReport.pdf.
7. Minde K, Faucon A, Falkner S. Sleep problems in toddlers: Effects of treatment on their daytime behavior. J Am Acad Child Adolesc Psychiatry 1994; 33(8):1114–21.
8. Anders TF, Keener M. Developmental course of nighttime sleep-wake patterns in full-term and premature infants during the first year of life: I. Sleep 1985; 8(3):173–92.
9. Coons S, Guilleminault C. Development of consolidated sleep and wakeful periods in relation to the day/night cycle in infancy. Dev Med Child Neurol 1984; 26:169–76.
10. Jacklin CN, Snow ME, Gahart M, et al. Sleep pattern development from 6 through 33 months. J Ped Psychol 1980; 5(3):295–303.
11. Burnham MM, Goodlin-Jones BL, Gaylor EE, et al. Nighttime sleep-wake patterns and self-soothing from birth to one year of age: A longitudinal intervention study. J Child Psychology and Psychiatry 2002; 43:713–25.
12. Anders TF. Night-waking in infants during the first year of life. Pediatrics 1979; 63:860–4.
13. Moore T, Ucko LE. Night waking in early infancy: Part I. Archives of Disease in Childhood 1957; 32:333–42.
14. Acebo C, Sadeh A, Seifer R, et al. Sleep/wake patterns derived from activity monitoring and maternal report for healthy 1- to 5-year-old children. Sleep 2005; 28(12):1568–77.
15. Burnham M, Anders TF, Gaylor EE, et al. Night-to-night consistency of sleep variables over the first year: A preliminary analysis. Poster presented at the International Conference for Infant Studies, April 1998.

16. Sadeh A, Acebo C, Seifer R, et al. Activity-based assessment of sleep-wake patterns during the 1st year of life. Infant Beh & Dev 1995; 18:329–37.
17. Worthman CM, Melby MK. Toward a comparative developmental ecology of human sleep. In: Carskadon MA, ed. Adolescent Sleep Patterns: Biological, Social, & Psychological influences. New York: Cambridge University Press, 2002: pp. 69–117.
18. Jenni OG, O'Connor BB. Children's sleep: An interplay between culture and biology. Pediatrics 2005; 115:204–216.
19. American Psychiatric Association. Diagnostic and Statistical Manual of Mental Disorders, 4th edn, text revision (DSM-IV-TR). Arlington, VA: APA, 2000.
20. Gaylor EE, Goodlin-Jones GL, Anders TF. Classification of young children's sleep problems: A pilot study. J Am Acad Child Adolesc Psychiatry 2001; 40(1):61–7.
21. Gaylor EE, Burnham MM, Goodlin-Jones BL, et al. A longitudinal follow-up study of young children's sleep patterns using a developmental classification system. Behavioral Sleep Medicine 2005; 3(1):44–61.
22. Scott G, Richards MPM. Night waking in one-year-old infants in England. Child: Care, Health & Development 1990; 16:283–302.
23. Goodlin-Jones BL, Burnham MM, Anders TF. Sleep and sleep disturbances: Regulatory processes in infancy. In: Sameroff AJ, Lewis M, Miller SM, eds. Handbook of Developmental Psychopathology, 2nd edn New York: Kluwer Academic/Plenum Publishers, 2000: pp. 309–25.
24. Minde K. Sleep disorders in infants and young children. In: Maldonado-Duran JM, ed. Infant and Toddler Mental Health: Models of Clinical Intervention with Infants and Their Families. Washington, DC: American Psychiatric Publishing, 2002: pp. 269–307.
25. Glaze DG, Rosen CL, Owens JA. Toward a practical definition of pediatric insomnia. Curr Ther Res Clin Exp 2002; 63(Suppl B):B4–B17.
26. Middlemiss W. Infant sleep: A review of normative and problematic sleep and interventions. Early Child Development & Care 2004; 174(1):99–122.
27. Mindell JA, Kuhn B, Lewin DS, et al. Behavioral treatment of bedtime problems and night wakings in infants and young children. Sleep 2006; 29(10):1263–76.
28. American Academy of Sleep Medicine. International Classification of Sleep Disorders, 2nd ed. Westchester, IL: American Academy of Sleep Medicine, 2005.
29. Zero to Three. Diagnostic Classification of Mental Health and Developmental Disorders of Infancy and Early Childhood, Revised. Washington, DC: Zero to Three: National Center for Infants, Toddlers, and Families, 2005.
30. Burnham MM, Gaylor EE, Anders TF. Sleep disorders. In: Luby JL, ed. Handbook of Preschool Mental Health: Development, Disorders, and Treatment. New York: Guilford, 2006: pp. 186–208.
31. Owens J, Spirito A, McGuinn M. The Children's Sleep Habits Questionnaire (CSHQ): Psychometric properties of a survey instrument for school-age children. Sleep 2000; 23(8):1043–51.
32. Bruni O, Ottaviano S, Guidetti V, et al. The Sleep Distrance Scale for Children (SDSC): Construction and validation of an instrument to evaluate sleep disturbances in childhood and adolescence. J Sleep Res 1996; 5:251–61.
33. Chervin R, Hedger K, Dillon J, et al. Pediatric Sleep Questionnaire (PSQ): Validity and reliability of scales for sleep-disordered breathing, snoring, sleepiness, and behavioral problems. Sleep Medicine 2000; 1(1):21–32.
34. Sadeh A. A brief screening questionnaire for infant sleep problems: Validation and findings for an internet sample. Pediatrics 2004; 113:e570–e577.
35. Sadeh A, Flint-Ofir E, Tirosh T, et al. Infant sleep and parental sleep-related cognitions. Journal of Family Psychology 2007; 21(1):74–87.
36. Mindell JA. Sleep disorders in children. Health Psychology 1993; 12(2):151–62.
37. Crowell J, Keener M, Ginsburg N, et al. Sleep habits in toddlers 18 to 36 months old. J Amer Acad Child Adolesc Psychiatry 1987; 26:510–15.

38. Jenkins S, Owens C, Bax M, et al. Continuities of common behavior problems in pre-school children. J Child Psychol Psychiatry 1984; 25(1):75–89.
39. Salzarulo P, Chevalier A. Sleep problems in children and their relationship with early disturbances of the waking sleep-wake rhythms. Sleep 1983; 6(1):47–51.
40. Bates JE, Viken RJ, Alexnader DB, et al. Sleep and adjustment in preschool children: Sleep diary reports by mothers relate to behavior reports by teachers. Child Development 2002; 73:62–75.
41. Goodlin-Jones BL, Burnham MM, Gaylor EE, et al. Night waking, sleep-wake organization and self-soothing in the first year of life. J Dev Behav Pediatr 2001; 22(4):226–33.
42. Fehlings D, Weiss S, Stephens D. Frequent night awakenings in infants and preschool children referred to a sleep disorders clinic: The role of nonadaptive sleep associations. Children's Health Care 2001; 30(1):43–55.
43. Morrell J, Steele H. The role of attachment security, temperament, maternal perception, and care-giving behavior in persistent infant sleeping problems. Infant Mental Health Journal 2003; 24(5):447–68.
44. Lam P, Hiscock H, Wake M. Outcomes of infant sleep problems: A longitudinal study of sleep, behavior, and maternal well-being. Pediatrics 2003; 111:e203–e207.
45. Eckerberg B. Treatment of sleep problems in families with young children: Effects of treatment on family well-being. Acta Paediatr 2004; 93:126–34.
46. Meijer AM, van den Witenboer GLH. Contribution of infants' sleep and crying to marital relationship of first-time parent couples in the 1st year after childbirth. Journal of Family Psychology 2007; 21:49–57.
47. Meltzer LJ, Mindell JA. Relationship between child sleep disturbances and maternal sleep, mood, and parenting stress: A pilot study. Journal of Family Psychology 2007; 21:67–73.
48. Hall WA, Clauson M, Carty EM, et al. Effects on parents of an intervention to resolve infant behavioral sleep problems. Pediatric Nursing 2006; 32(3):243–50.
49. Wake M, Morton-Allen E, Poulakis Z, et al. Prevalence, stability, and outcomes of cry-fuss and sleep problems in the first 2 years of life: Prospective community-based study. Pediatrics 2006; 117:836–42.
50. Smedje H, Broman JE, Hetta J. Associations between disturbed sleep and behavioural difficulties in 635 children aged six to eight years: A study based on parents' perceptions. European Journal of Child & Adolescent Psychiatry 2001; 10:1–9.
51. Wolfson AR, Carskadon MA. Sleep schedules and daytime functioning in adolescents. Child Development 1998; 69(4):875–87.
52. Owens-Stively J, Frank N, Smith A, et al. Child temperament, parenting discipline style, and daytime behavior in childhood sleep disorders. Developmental & Behavioral Pediatrics 1997; 18(5):314–21.
53. Buckhalt JA, El-Sheikh M, Keller P. Children's sleep and cognitive functioning: Race and socioeconomic status as moderators of effects. Child Development 2007; 78(1):213–31.
54. Stickgold R. Sleep-dependent memory consolidation. Nature 2005; 437(7063):1272–8.
55. Frank MG, Issa NP, Stryker MP. Sleep enhances plasticity in the developing visual cortex. Neuron 2001; 30:275–87.
56. Stickgold R, James L, Hobson JA. Visual discrimination learning requires sleep after training. Nature Neuroscience 2000; 3(12):1237–8.
57. Cheour M, Martynova O, Naatanen R, et al. Speech sounds learned by sleeping new-borns. Nature 2002; 415:599–600.
58. Sadeh A, Gruber R, Raviv A. The effects of sleep restriction and extension on school-age children: What a difference an hour makes. Child Development 2003; 74:444–55.
59. Agras WS, Hammer LD, McNicholas F, et al. Risk factors for childhood overweight: A prospective study from birth to 9.5 years. Journal of Pediatrics 2004; 145:20–5.
60. Reilly JJ, Armstrong J, Dorosty AR, et al. Early life risk factors for obesity in childhood: A cohort study. British Medical Journal 2005; 330:1357–62.

61. Bates JE, Viken RJ, Williams N. Temperament as a moderator of the linkage between sleep and preschool adjustment. Paper presented at the meeting of the Society for Research in Child Development. Tampa, FL, April 2003.
62. Goodnight JA, Bates JE, Staples AD, et al. Temperamental resistance to control increases the association between sleep problems and externalizing behavior development. Journal of Family Psychology 2007; 21(1):39–48.
63. Staples AD, Bates JE, Kuwabara M. Linking temperament and increased sleep disruption during toddlerhood. Paper presented at the meeting of the Society for Research in Child Development. Boston, MA, March 2007.
64. Weissbluth M. Sleep duration and infant temperament. J Pediatr 1981; 99(5):817–19.
65. Weissbluth M. Liu K. Sleep patterns, attention span, and infant temperament. J Dev Behav Pediatr 1983; 4(1):34–6.
66. Van Tassel EB. The relative influence of child and environmental characteristics on sleep disturbances in the first and second years of life. J Dev Behav Pediatr 1985; 6(2):81–6.
67. Scher A, Epstein R, Sadeh A, et al. Toddlers' sleep and temperament: Reporting bias or a valid link? A research note. J Child Psychol Psychiatry 1992; 33(7):1249–54.
68. Dahl R. Sleep and arousal: Development and psychopathology. Dev Psychopathol 1996; 8:3–27.
69. Thunstrom M. Severe sleep problems in infancy associated with subsequent development of attention deficit/hyperactivity disorder at 5.5 years of age. Acta Paediatr 2002; 91(5):584–92.
70. Bruni O, Lo Reto F, Miano S, et al. Daytime behavioral correlates of awakenings and bedtime resistance in preschool children. Suppl Clin Neurophysiol 2000; 53:358–61.
71. Dearing E, McCartney K, Marshall NL, et al. Parental reports of children's sleep and wakefulness: Longitudinal associations with cognitive and language outcomes. Infant Beh and Dev 2001; 24:151–70.
72. Gregory AM, Eley TC, O'Connor TG, et al. Etiologies of associations between childhood sleep and behavior problems in a large twin sample. J Am Acad Child Adolesc Psychiatry 2004; 43(6):744–51.
73. Scher A, Zukerman S, Epstein R. Persistent night waking and settling difficulties across the first year: Early precursors of later behavioural problems? J Reprod and Infant Psychology 2005; 23(1):77–88.
74. Kuhn BR, Elliott AJ. Treatment efficacy in behavioral pediatric sleep medicine. Journal of Psychosom Res 2003; 54:587–97.
75. Mindell JA, Owens JA. Clinical Guide to Pediatric Sleep: Diagnosis and management of sleep problems. Philadelphia: Lippincott Williams & Wilkins, 2003.
76. Ramchandani P, Wiggs L, Webb V, et al. A systematic review of treatments for settling problems and night waking in young children. British Medical Journal 2000; 320:209–13.
77. Merenstein D, Diener-West M, Halbower AC, et al. The trial of infant response to diphenhydramine: The TIRED study—A randomized, controlled, patient-oriented trial. Arch Pediatr Adolesc Med 2006; 160:707–12.
78. Ferber R. Solve Your Child's Sleep Problems. New York: Simon & Schuster, 1985.
79. Owens JL, France KG, Wiggs L. Behavioural and cognitive-behavioural interventions for sleep disorders in infants and children: A review. Sleep Medicine Reviews 1999; 3(4):281–302.
80. Hall WA, Saunders RA, Clauson M, et al. Effects of an intervention aimed at reducing night waking and signaling in 6- and 12-month-old infants. Behav Sleep Med 2006; 4(4):242–61.
81. Stremler R, Hodnett E, Lee K, et al. A behavioral-educational intervention to promote maternal and infant sleep: A pilot randomized, controlled trial. Sleep 2006; 26(12):1609–15.
82. Mindell J, Luedtke K, Wiegand B, et al. Effects of a consistent bedtime routine on infant sleep. Sleep 2007; 30(Abstract Supplement):A91.

4 Sleep Practices and Habits in Children across Different Cultures

Flavia Giannotti, Flavia Cortesi, Teresa Sebastiani, and Cristina Vagnoni

Center of Pediatric Sleep Disorders, Department of Developmental Neurology and Psychiatry, University "La Sapienza," Rome, Italy

INTRODUCTION

Sleep characteristics in children vary not only with age but also with ethnic and sociocultural influences. In fact, lifestyle issues, as well as cultural beliefs and family values, might influence sleep too. Cultural differences are not random events, they occur because cultures with different geographies, climates, economies, religions, and histories exert unique influences. Individualism–collectivism is the major dimension of cultural variability used to explain differences and similarities in communication across cultures (1). They represent conflicting views of beliefs, attitudes, norms, rules, and values, reflecting the nature of humans, society, and the relationship between them. In individualistic cultures, people are viewed as independent and possessing a unique pattern of traits that distinguish them from other people; on the contrary, individuals in collectivistic cultures view themselves as inherently interdependent within the group to which they belong. Children both actively shape and are shaped by the social worlds in which they live. Primarily, the immediate family environment represents the microsystems into which the parents bring their own background development. The family is in turn embedded within the wider community and cultural networks of a macrosystem, representing overriding norms, cultural beliefs, and values in any particular society. Although these may vary both between and within different societies and cultures, consistencies in the beliefs, attitudes, and actions of particular social groupings can be identified and can help us to understand how children's sleep habits develop.

Most work looking at influences on children's sleep development has tended to focus on individual factors in children and their parents, family interactions, and the impact of sociodemographic factors. Nevertheless, cultural factors are vitally important in creating the context within which different, more proximal factors interact to affect a child's health, development, and well-being. Thus, child sleep development is the result of complex interrelationships of biological, psychological, environmental, and social influences, the relative contributions of which are often difficult to separate. The biology of sleep, including sleep homeostatic mechanisms and chronobiological factors, is a determinant in children's sleep. Individual characteristics such as temperament, large individual differences in the ability to regulate sleep, cultural beliefs about the function and meaning of sleep, and cultural norms for sleep practices and social interactions impact sleep patterns as well. The ways in which culture and biology interact play a major role in the establishment of sleep patterns, developmental norms and expectations regarding normal and problematic children's sleep development. The evolution of sleep behaviors across childhood is particularly sensitive to this interplay. So many variables that affect sleep patterns are highly culturally based: How we sleep, with whom we sleep, where we sleep, sleeping and waking times—all are influenced by diverse cultures.

Variability among cultures concerning sleep-patterning expectations and interpretations is enormous and for almost any preference or norm, its opposite can be found in other cultural settings. According to Triandis (1) individualistic societies, such as the U.S.A. and Western Europe, emphasize autonomy and emotional independence; on the other hand collectivist societies, such as Africa and Latin America, stress collective identity, emotional dependence, and strong interpersonal bonds. In Asian societies, cultural values that emphasize the group are translated into specific rearing practices such as prolonged body contact between mother and child, while encouragement of child autonomy and independence is the typical trait of child rearing in individualistic cultures. Moreover, cultures that display considerable interpersonal closeness or immediacy are labeled "high-contact cultures " because people in these countries stand closer, touch more, and prefer more sensory stimulation than do people in "lower-contact cultures" (2). High-contact cultures, such as South America, Southern and Eastern European, and Arab countries, create immediacy by increasing sensory input, whereas low-contact cultures, such as Asian and Northern European countries, prefer less sensory involvement (3). More recent research has shown that North America is probably a high-contact culture, whereas, as already stated, Asia is a low-contact culture (4).

There is a growing interest in the study of children's sleep behavior in different cultures, both within and between countries. However, few works have focused on the influences of cultural factors on children (5,6).

Furthermore, in recent years, we have witnessed dramatic demographic changes in many countries; consequently health professionals and pediatricians have been confronted with families of widely differing cultural origins. A growing literature is documenting differences between ethnic groups in child-rearing values, beliefs, and goals (7). Thus, it becomes more important in evaluating etiologic factors and planning interventions for the individual child and the family to incorporate pediatric sleep disorders in their specific cultural context.

This chapter will try to provide an overview of some specific sleep issues that are highly influenced by cultural context based on the review of previous epidemiological surveys carried out in different sociocultural contexts.

BEDTIME ROUTINES

Child and parent sleep-related behavior in Anglo–European countries consists of distinct bedtime rituals that in these cultures are meant to enhance a child's sleep. It consists of a set of activities, which usually take place in the child's bedroom, including wearing nightclothes, using a transitional object to take to bed with the child, telling stories or singing songs, leading to a gradual diminution of external stimuli in the environment, and providing reassurances to the child from parents before the child is left alone in his/her bedroom.

These bedtime routines, however, are not always similar to all Western industrialized societies. In a comparison study on infant care practices in U.S. families from the Boston area and Italian families from a small town, New and Richman (8) found that while American bedtime rituals were well established and children were required to go to bed regardless of their resistance, Italian children were allowed to fall asleep in the carriage or someone's lap instead of their own bed.

In this study, Italian parents were less concerned about their child's sleep habits than Americans were.

In another study on the sleeping habits of about 3000 Italian children, aged from birth to six years, in the urban area of Rome, Ottaviano (9) noted a high incidence of active parental involvement at bedtime in respect of about 50% of children across all age groups. Even though a similar incidence has been reported in Australian toddlers (10) and in Portugal, where more than 40% of parents stay with their children until they fall asleep (11), this bedtime settling practice is less common in Swedish (12) and U.S. children (13).

In a recent study on sleep in German infants, Valentin reported that, even though the majority of parents believe that some assistance is necessary to help a child to fall asleep only one in five parents stays with the child until he or she has fallen asleep (14). In the Italian sample, parental involvement at the time to fall asleep was significantly associated with longer sleep latency, a higher incidence of nightwakings and, probably as a consequence, a reduction of nighttime sleep (9). This childrearing practice seems to reflect, mainly in the first years of life, the attitude of Italian parents, who are often afraid to leave little children awake alone in their own bed. A recent study on children's sleep habits in India (15) reported that less than half of children had a specific bedtime routine, such as a bedtime story, bottle of milk, and cuddly toys, similar to those reported for children belonging to Western societies; but two-thirds of them refused to sleep without the presence of their parents. Similar habits at bedtime are reported by almost 80% of Southern French parents of 12–24-month-olds and about 50% of them use to remain with children until they fell asleep (16).

In sharp contrast, another study, carried out regularly in an urban area of France, reported that even the traditional practice of singing lullabies is slowly giving way to the use of recorded music as a sleep aid, reflection of a more distant approach even in infancy to bedtime routines (17). This variance may be due to different sociocultural contexts even within the same country.

Regarding school-aged children, recent studies pointed out that sleeping habits and disturbances were negatively impacted by a number of lifestyles habits that might be culturally mediated (18, 19).

In a recent study, Spilsbury (20) demonstrated in a sample of 8–11-year old U.S. children that a parenting style that encourages development of self-care routines and the enforcement of family rules is linked to a healthier sleep pattern and longer sleep duration. On the other hand, an epidemiological survey (21) in Italy, pointed out a relatively high incidence of parental presence at bedtime that decreased with age, but surprisingly still includes 7% of Italian children aged 10–12 years. An increasing number of Italian children used to fall asleep before going to their bed, mainly in the sitting room watching TV. The parental television viewing habit that consists usually in watching TV during dinner might encourage the habit of children falling asleep in front of television. As already stated, for U.S. school-aged children (22), bedtime television viewing adversely affects their sleep, encouraging bedtime refusal, and the delayed onset of sleep.

Consistent with these results Thompson and Christakis (23) reported that in about 30% of children 4–35 months old, irregular naptime and bedtime schedules significantly correlated with the number of hours of TV viewing. A recent survey (19) found that poor sleep hygiene practices are common in Italian school-aged children. More than 30% of Italian children having a TV set in their bedroom used television as a sleep aid. These children went to bed and woke up significantly later on weekdays and on weekends, and slept significantly less on weekdays than those without a TV set in their bedroom. In terms of specific bedtime-related television behaviors, Owens et al. (18) reported that about 26% of U.S. children had a television set in their bedroom, and even though only 3% of them needed television as an aid to falling asleep, about 76% of them reported TV viewing as a part of the child's usual bedtime routine. Importantly, the majority of parents though that TV had little or no effect on their child's sleep. Paavonen et al. (22) reported a significant correlation between frequent TV viewing at bedtime and sleep onset problems in Finland too. Gaina pointed out that an increase in the duration of watching TV was associated with prolonged sleep latency, as was playing videogames in Japanese 12-year-old children (24). More recently, BaHamman et al. (25) reported shorter sleep duration in Saudi school children who watched TV at bedtime and played computer games after 8 p.m. In India, TV viewing interfered with the child's sleep routine leading to delayed sleep in 39% of children (15). Moreover, it has been reported that more than 40% of Brazilian children aged seven to 10 used to drink milk before bedtime, and about 28% of them watched TV as an aid to sleep (26). Even in China, almost 20% of school-aged Chinese children had their own television set and computer in their bedrooms (27).

In contrast to Western societies, in other cultures there is no specific preparation of children for sleep. In a study on the use of bed mosquito nets in malaria control in a rural area of Gambia, Aikins et al. (28) pointed out the difficulty of establishing children's sleeping habits. Young children usually sleep with their mother and are thus protected by her bed net, while older children usually sleep with a parent, another adult relative, other siblings, or (rarely) on their own. Similarly, in Uganda children less than five years use mosquito nets primarily because they share a bed with their parents (29). Moreover, adolescent boys may sleep outdoors (30) and are thus much less likely to have access to a net.

In Nigeria, many children are flooding the streets of major towns, struggling to cope with social and economic problems at home. In a study on the life habits of these street children, Dareng (31) pointed out that, no matter where they wandered during the day, they returned to the same place to sleep and seemed to fall asleep in a regular routine. Many at times go to their sleeping places around 10 to 11 p.m. The majority sleep outside the stores and are usually awoken by a watchman between 5 and 6 a.m.

In a comparative study on the sleeping habits of U.S. children and Mayan Indian communities in Guatemala, Morelli et al. (32) described children falling asleep when they were sleepy, usually in someone's arms, or when they were taken to bed along with a parent. No bedtime routines were reported, no stories or songs. Differences in attitude toward sleep in general were equally clear between the two cultures. American parents used lullabies, stories and toys to ritualize the sleep experience, whereas Mayan parents simply let their babies fall asleep when they wanted to, without any rules. We would like to underline that Mayan mothers interviewed in this study reported no bedtime resistance or sleep problems. In the more complex Balinese society, infants are held continuously by a variety of adults, so they fall asleep easily in noisy situations (33).

SLEEPING ARRANGEMENTS

In many parts of the world where the unit of economic production is the family, such as in Asia, Africa, and among the indigenous populations of the Americas, children are encouraged to sleep with their mothers, grandparents, or older siblings even when ample space is available. Co-sleeping in childhood promotes closeness and togetherness in cultures where interdependency and solidarity is the goal for the family or where children are thought to be fragile, particularly in the context of high infant mortality rates. On the other hand, in European and American contexts, where autonomy is greatly valued, infants are encouraged to sleep alone from an early age, which promotes individualism. Co-sleeping is almost universal in India for 93% of children aged 3–10 years and 91% at six years (15). It is interesting to note that sleeping on the floor is a typical practice in some Asian countries, such as Korea and Japan, while the use of beds is universal in urban and most rural areas of China (34).

Even though Western cultural practices of nonparental care are becoming increasingly common in Japan, the traditional arrangement of sleeping, parents and children next to each other on mattresses or futons on the floor or on adult beds, is still common. The Japanese crib is defined as a dedicated "child bed," similar to the Western-style crib; the parents typically sleep immediately next to the child bed, on another bed or futon. Alternatively, the child shares the adult bed. The child bed is primarily used in infancy and is thought to be protective in the vulnerable neonatal period, because parents are concerned about hurting the neonates if they share the bed, while the use of a mattress/futon is more common among toddlers and preschoolers. Fukumizu et al. (34) reported that in Japan 80% of infants co-sleep with their parents and 20% of them used a dedicated bed. Asian mothers believe that children are too young to sleep alone. Thus, bed-sharing is considered part of the fabric of the close-knit relationships of family members. Child-rearing practices emphasize the development of interdependence and family closeness, thus child–parent bed-sharing up to school age is accepted in many families.

In a study on Korean 1–7-year-olds, Yang and Hahn reported a bed-sharing rate of 45% (35). Even with the radical sociocultural changes in contemporary Chinese society, there is still a strong emphasis on the parent–child bond in the child-rearing practice (36). Parents tend to be overprotective and almost 18% of Chinese children regularly co-sleep (37). Co-sleeping is also very common in Brazil, either in the isolated community of African-Brazilians living in Mato Grosso-Brazil, where more than 80% of children are sharing a bed until 10 years old (38), or among the Brazilian indigenous population of Terena and Bororo (39), or even in the urban area of Sao Paulo City, where there are more than 90% of 7–10-year-olds sharing (26). Moreover, Mayan babies too used to sleep with their mothers in all cases for the first and sometimes the second year. In more than half of the cases, the father was there as well, or he was sleeping with older children in another bed. Mayan mothers saw that their own sleeping arrangements provided closeness at night between mothers and babies (32). In the Balinese society, sleeping alone is considered undesirable for persons of any age (33).

Thus, in almost all cultures around the world, babies sleep with an adult, while older children sleep with parents or other siblings. It is only in industrialized Western societies, such as those in North America and in some parts of Europe, that sleep has become a private affair. In these countries, people generally believe that a child should sleep separately from its parents as soon as possible, to foster the development of autonomy and independence. The conviction that an individual has to become independent early to succeed later in life greatly influences parent–child interaction and child-rearing practice. In the U.S.A. the incidence of co-sleeping largely varies depending on the ethnicity and geographical areas; while up to 70% of black families used to co-sleep, 21% of Hispanic-American and less than 10% of white middle-American urban children shared parents' beds (40–43).

In Northern Europe the trend toward adopting a more distant behavioral style in sleep practices is very common. Such countries are considered "low-contact cultures," which prefer less sensory involvement (4). In Finland less than 10% of children sleep in their parents' bed (44). In Lyon, a large town in southern France, less than 1% of infants regularly co-sleep (16). Surprisingly, recent research reported that in Sweden, also considered as a "low-contact" country, more than 60% of children used to co-sleep. In fact, the practice of co-sleeping in Sweden is perceived as a normal family activity, important for children's well-being and development, proposed as good practice for providing the child with the environment of closeness and security that he/she requires (45). Approaching Southern Europe, sleep practices seem to become globally more proximal. In Portugal, co-sleeping is very common (11). In Italy this sleep practice, almost absent during the first year of life, increases significantly from the second year for about 10% to 14% of toddlers and 17% of preschoolers (9). Consistent with other studies (40,46), this sleep practice decreases with age, but it is still high for Italian pre-adolescents for almost 4% of them (47).

SLEEP PATTERNS

Several studies suggested that social pressure, television, internet, and late night movies compete with sleep, resulting in a rather drastic change in sleep habits and sleep time in children, with a tendency for getting insufficient sleep (48–50). A cross-cultural study of Dutch and American families with infants and young children carried out in the early 1990s (51) showed that Dutch babies were getting more sleep in a regular schedule that included earlier bedtimes than American babies of the same age. In this study Dutch parents stressed the importance of maintaining a regular and restful routine for infants and young children, a code of child-rearing expressed as the three Rs ("rust"—rest, "regelmaat"—regularity, and "reinheid"—cleanliness), which includes plenty of sleep, considered essential for children's healthy development.

American parents, on the other hand, stressed the roles of development and inborn individual differences among children in influencing their children's sleep patterns. Consequently, they considered maintaining a regular sleep schedule as less important and talked more about strategies for getting baby to sleep. With time at home so limited for American working parents, getting the child to bed on time often takes second or third place after spending time playing with the child (52). In another study on cultural influences on bedtime behavior in two- to seven-year-old children, McLaughlin Crabtree found that African-Americans had later bedtimes than Caucasians with similar risetimes, resulting in significantly short sleep duration and more excessive daytime sleepiness, independent of socioeconomic status (SES) and age (53). Kohyama et al. found that about 50% of three-year-old children in Japan fell asleep at 10 p.m. or later (54). Italian infants and preschoolers were reported to have a late bedtime too (9). Comparison with other parental report surveys showed that Italian children have a later bedtime than Australian, Swedish, Swiss, and U.S. children of the same age (12,55–58). This may reflect sociocultural and climate influences as well as certain social habits of Italian families, such as allowing their children to participate in the family's evening life, including the late dinner. As already stated for American families, as well as in Anglo-European societies, bedtime has become an integral part of the "quality time" that many working middle-class parents devote to children.

Another study comparing sleep habits of two large European towns in Belgium and in Italy confirmed a later bedtime in Italian children, who shared late dinner with parents, compared to those reported for Belgian children (59). Comparison with other studies showed that Italian preschoolers sleep less than children of the same age living in other countries (56,57,60). Similarly, the results of an epidemiological survey on Italian school-aged children pointed out that also in this age group there was a shorter sleep duration and a later bedtime than those reported for children of the same age in different countries (27,56,57,61–64). Only Japanese children, who also showed a similar late bedtime, reported shorter sleep time probably due also to an early wake-up time (65). Chinese and Japanese schoolchildren reported a late bedtime and early risetimes as a result of academic pressures that lead social and familial emphasis on study time. In China bedtimes range from 9 p.m. at five to six years to 9:45 p.m. for 11-year-olds during weekdays (28). In a recent study on the sleep habits of Saudi elementary school children, BaHamman et al. (25) reported that the average bedtime was around 9:30 p.m. and risetime around 6 a.m. Sleep duration in this study was even lower than that reported in other studies in Western countries. An even later bedtime, around 10 p.m., was reported for Indian children, significantly associated with longer daytime naps and shorter nighttime sleep duration (15). Similarly, Brazilian school-aged children used to fall asleep around 10 p.m. (26).

Interestingly, a comparison study of parental attitudes and expectations in Norway showed that Sami, a minority people living in the circumpolar region, were more lenient about bedtime rules than Norwegian mothers were. Particularly, they were more permissive in letting their child stay up late if they wanted to and bedtime was later on average at 9 p.m. compared to 8 p.m. for Norwegian children. Similarly, more Norwegian mothers regulated bedtime according to the seasons, letting the child stay up much longer during the summer (66). Notably, in developing countries, all children and adolescents are enrolled in daily subsistence tasks, but girls generally work longer hours than boys. They participate more frequently in heavy duties at home, have shorter rests and sleep times than do girls from industrialized countries (67).

DAYTIME SLEEP

Ethnic and sociocultural factors too may influence daytime sleep procedures in early childhood. Most studies pointed out that the percentage of children napping regularly decreases gradually with age. The age-related reduction in daytime sleep is closely related to maturation of chronobiological and homeostatic mechanisms, which regulate sleep/wake cycling and sleep structure, with an adult-like sleep architecture emerging by approximately the age of five years. Several studies showed that the percentage of children napping regularly drops gradually from close to 100% at the age of two years to less than 10% at six years of age (56,68,69). However, cultural preference may play an important role in the regulation of napping habits. Several factors influencing when children stop napping, such as regulatory systems, home routines, school schedules, etc., have not been systematically investigated. In Italy, the frequency of naps dropped off sharply, with less than 10% of children still regularly napping at 4–5 years (9), whereas in the U.S.A. (68) more than 50% of children were still napping at the same age and in Iceland children stop napping at three years (70).

As well as cultural differences, ethnic and racial factors may influence napping too. In a study of 2–5-year-old U.S. children, Lavigne pointed out that a minority (Hispanic, African-American, and others) were found to report longer daytime naps than non-Hispanic white children (71). A more recent study showed remarkable racial differences in napping in African-American and Caucasian two- to eight-year-old U.S. children. In this study, African-American children were found to be more likely to continue napping at older ages than Caucasian children, resulting in less nightttime sleep but with similar amounts of sleep across a 24-hour period (72). A recent study on the sleep habits of Saudi school-aged children reported that 25% to 45% of 6–13-year-olds used to nap during weekdays. Interestingly nap duration in this study is quite long, lasting around 95 minutes.

However, in the last 20 years we have witnessed dramatic changes in sleep patterns; and even in those countries where a biphasic sleep pattern was dominant, such as populations living around the Mediterranean Sea, in South America, Africa and Asia, daytime napping behavior appears to be slowly disappearing, probably as result of globalization.

CONCLUSION AND FUTURE IMPLICATIONS

This review indicated that there are as many ways to sleep as there are cultural variations. As stated by Triandis (73) "We are not aware of our culture unless we come in contact with another one." In this increasingly globalized world, it is becoming more and more necessary that people be aware of other traditions and beliefs and be more accepting of each other's differences. Sleep practices among infants and children is a topic that often stimulates discussion and controversy among child specialists, all obviously sharing the same goal: the child's psychological and physical well-being. After many decades of research, there is still no consensus regarding the "best" sleeping arrangements for children and the "optimal" way to prepare a child for a restful night's sleep. Thus, none of the different sleep practices is "better" but each is contingent on what is the required competency for that society. We would like to reiterate the importance of a cross-cultural approach in broadening and deepening our understanding of child sleep behavior. In contrast to working intensively within a single culture, a comparative approach allows researchers and practitioners to obtain a richer understanding of the phenomena under inquiry and to understand broader patterns of relationships between behavioral and cultural variables. Cultural comparisons are of intrinsic value because they allow us not only to better understand children and adolescents' sleep in different contexts but also to evaluate the eventual benefits and consequences of different cultural sleep practices. This kind of understanding about how parents from different backgrounds organize their children's "developmental niches" can help in developing a culturally more informed and therefore more sensitive approach in pediatric sleep care. Finally, not all children respond similarly to the same culturally structured environments. Thus, cross-cultural studies of how individual variances are differentially accommodated in various cultural systems can offer new ideas for how to improve the "developmental niche." Given that cultures are not static but dynamic, responsive, and changing, the end point of the debate is less likely to be how cultures differ, than how we study culture and how we work with diversity. In clinical practice the cultural background should be taken into consideration, and treatment plans should also be adjusted in a way that best accommodates the child's and his or her family's value systems and the cultural environments in which they are embedded.

REFERENCES

1. Triandis HC. Individualism and Collectivism. Nisbett RE, ed. Boulder, CO: Westview Press, 1995.
2. Hall ET, ed. The Hidden Dimension. Garden City, NY: Doubleday, 1966.
3. Sussman NM, Rosenfeld HM. Influence of culture, language, and sex on conversational distance. J Pers Soc Psychol 1982; 42(1):66–74.
4. Andersen PA, Hecht ML, Hoobler GD, et al. Non verbal communication across cultures. In: Gudykunts WB, ed. Cross-cultural and Intercultural Communication, 2nd edn California State university, Fullerton, CA: Sage publications, 2003: pp. 73–90.
5. Jenni OG, O'Connor B. Children's sleep: Interplay between culture and biology. Pediatrics 2005; 115(1 Suppl):204–16.
6. Owens JA. Sleep in children: Cross-cultural perspectives. Sleep Biol Rhythms 2004; 2(3):165–73.
7. Harkness S, Super CM, eds. Parents' Cultural Belief Systems: Their Origins, Expressions and Consequences. New York: Guilford Press; 1996.
8. New RS, Richman AL. Maternal beliefsand infant care practices in Italy and United States. In: Harkness S, Super CM, eds. Parents' Cultural Belief Systems: Their Origins, Expressions and Consequences. New York: Guilford Press, 1996: pp. 385–404.
9. Ottaviano S, Giannotti F, Cortesi F, et al. Sleep characteristics in healthy children from birth to 6 years of age in the urban area of Rome. Sleep 1996; 19(1):1–3.
10. Armstrong KL, Quinn RA, Dadds MR. The sleep patterns of normal children. Med J Aust 1994; 161(3):202–6.
11. Pereira Ramos MN. Maternage en Milieu Portugais Autochtone et Immigré. De la tradition de la Modernité: Une Étude Ethnopsychologique. Paris France: Institut de Psychologie, University de René Descartes, 1993. Unpublished thesis.
12. Smedje H, Broman JE, Hetta J. Sleep disturbances in Swedish preschool children and their parents. Nord J Psychiatry 1998; 52(1):61–9.
13. Crowell J, Keener M, Ginsburg N, et al. Sleep habits in toddlers 18 to 36 months old. J Amer Acad Child Adol Psychiatry 1987; 26(4):510–15.
14. Valentin SR. Commentary: Sleep in German infants—the "cult" of independence. Pediatrics 2005; 115(1 Suppl):269–71.
15. Bharti B, Malhi P, Kashyap S. Patterns and problems of sleep in school going children. Indian Pediatr 2006; 43(1):35–8.
16. Louis J, Govindama Y. Sleep problems and bedtime routines in infants in a cross cultural perspective. Arch Pediatr 2004; 11(2):93–8.
17. Brisset C. Le Coucher du Jeune Enfant. Etude Psycho-Antropologique Iconograppique et Clinique des Représentations Parentales et Culturelles. Paris France: Institut de Psychologie Unversity de Rene Descartes 1997. Unpublished thesis.
18. Owens J, Maxim R, McGuinn M, et al. Television-viewing habits and sleep disturbance in school children. Pediatrics 1999; 104(3):e27.
19. Giannotti F, Cortesi F, LeBourgeois MK, et al. Abstract of Papers, 18th Annual Meeting of Associated Professional Sleep Societies, Philadelphia, PA, June 5-10, 2004. Sleep Abstract Supplement 2004, 27, A94.

20. Spilsbury JC, Storfer-Isser A, Drotar D, et al. Effects of the home environment on school-aged children's sleep. Sleep 2005; 28(11):1419–27.
21. Giannotti F, Cortesi F, Ottaviano S. Abstract of Papers, 11th Annual Meeting of Associated Professional Sleep Societies, San Francisco, CA, June 10–15, 1997. Sleep 1997, 20, Abstract Supplement.
22. Paavonen EJ, Pennonen M, Roine M, et al. TV exposure associated with sleep disturbances in 5- to 6-year-old children. J Sleep Res 2006; 15(2):154–61.
23. Thompson DA, Christakis DA. The association between television viewing and irregular sleep schedules among children less than 3 years of age. Pediatrics 2005; 116(4):851–6.
24. Gaina A, Sekine M, Xiaoli C, et al. Weekly variation in sleep patterns: Estimates of validity in Japanese schoolchildren. Sleep Biol Rhythms 2005; 3(2):80–5.
25. BaHammam A, Bin Saeed A, Al-Faris E, et al. Sleep duration and its correlates in a sample of Saudi elementary school children. Singapore Med J 2006; 47(10):875–81.
26. Silva TA, Carvalho LBC, Silva L, et al. Sleep habits and starting time to school in Brazilian children. Arq Neuropsiquiatr 2005; 63(2B):402–6.
27. Li S, Jin X, Wu S, et al. The impact of media use on sleep patterns and sleep disorders among school-aged children in China. Sleep 2007; 30(3):361–7.
28. Aikins MK, Pickering H., Alonso PL, et al. A malaria control trial using insecticide-treated bed nets and targeted chemoprophylaxis in a rural area of the Gambia, West Africa. Perception of the causes of malaria and of its treatment and prevention in the study area. Trans R Soc Trop Med Hyg 1993; 87(2):25–30.
29. Mugisha F, Arinaitwe J. Sleeping arrangements and mosquito net use among under-fives: Results from the Uganda Demographic and Health Survey. Malar J 2003; 2(1):40.
30. Aikins MK, Pickering H, Greenwood BM. Attitudes to malaria, traditional practices and bednets as vector control measures: A comparative study in five west African countries. J Trop Med Hyg 1994; 97(2):81–6.
31. http://ospiti.peacelink.it/npeople/apr99/pag7april.html (accessed April 2007).
32. Morelli G, Rogoff B, Oppenheim D, et al. Cultural variation in infants' sleeping arrangements: Questions of indipendence. Dev Psychol 1992; 28(4):604–13.
33. Mead M. Children and ritual in Bali. In: Belo J, ed. Traditional Balinese Culture. New York: Columbia University Press, 1970: 198–211.
34. Fukumizu M, Kaga M, Kohyama J, et al. Sleep-related nighttime crying in Japan: A community-based study. Pediatrics 2005; 115(1 Suppl):217–24.
35. Yang CK, Hahn HM. Cosleeping in Young Korean children. Developmental and Behavioral Pediatrics 2002; 23(3):151–7.
36. Chao RK. Beyond parental control and authoritarian parenting style: Understanding Chinese parenting through cultural notion of training. Child Dev 1994; 65(4):1111–19.
37. Liu X, Liu L, Wang R. Bed sharing, sleep habits and sleep problems among Chinese school-aged children. Sleep 2003; 26(7):839–44.
38. Reimao R, Rosa Pires DeSouza JC, Vilela Gaudioso CE. Sleep habits in native Brazilian Bororo children. Arq Neuropsiquiatr 1999; 57(1):14–17.
39. Reimao R, Rosa Pires DeSouza JC, Vilela Gaudioso CE, et al. Sleep characteristics in children in the isolated rural African-Brazilian descendant community of Furnas do Dionisio, state of Mato Grosso do sul, Brazil. Arq Neuropsiquiatr 1999; 57(3-A):556–60.
40. Lozoff B, Wolf AW, Davis NS. Cosleeping in urban families with young children in the United States. Pediatrics 1984; 74(2):171–82.
41. Lozoff B, Askew GL, Wolf AW. Cosleeping and early childhood sleep problems: Effects of ethnicity and socioeconomic status. J Dev Behav Pediatr 1996; 17(1):9–15.
42. Weimer SM, Dise TL, Evers PB, et al. Prevalence, predictors, and attitudes toward cosleeping in an urban pediatric center. Clin Pediatr 2002; 41(6):433–8.
43. Fuchs Schachter F, Fuchs ML, Bijur PE, et al. Cosleeping and sleep problems in Hispanic-American urban young children. Pediatrics 1989; 84(3):522–30.
44. Sourander A. Emotional and behavioral problems in a sample of Finnish three-year-olds. Eur Child Adolesc Psychiatry 2001; 10(2):98–104.

45. Welles-Nystrom B. Cosleeping as a window into Swedish culture: Considerations of gender and health care. Scand J Caring Sci 2005; 19(4):354–60.
46. Jenni OG, Zinggler Fuhrer H, Iglowstein I, et al. A longitudinal study of bedsharing and sleep problems among Swiss children in the first 10 years of life. Pediatrics 2005; 115(1 Suppl):233–40.
47. Cortesi F, Giannotti F, Sebastiani T, et al. Cosleeping and sleep behavior in Italian school-aged children. J Dev Behav Pediatr 2004; 25(1):28–33.
48. Wolfson AR, Carskadon MA. Sleep schedules and daytime functioning in adolescents. Child Dev 1998; 69(4):875–87.
49. Gau SF, Soong WT. Sleep problems of junior high school students in Taipei. Sleep 1995; 18(8):667–73.
50. Shin C, Kim J, Lee S, et al. Sleep habits, excessive daytime sleepiness and school performances in high school students. Psychiatry Clin Neurosci 2003; 57(4):451–53.
51. Super CM, Harkness S, van Tijen N, et al. The three R's of Dutch child rearing and the socialization of infant arousal. In: Harkness S, Super CM, eds. Parents' Cultural Belief System: Their Origin, Expressions and Consequences. New York: Guiford Press, 1996: pp. 447–66.
52. Harkness S, Super CM. The developmental niche: a model for understanding culture, child health and development. In: Silverman E, ed. Child Health in the Multicultural Environment. Report of the thirty-first Ross Rountable on Critical Approaches to common pediatric problems. Columbus, Oh: Columbus Ross Products Division, Abbott laboratories, 2000: pp. 50–9.
53. McLaughlin Crabtree V, Beal Korhonen J, Montgomery-Downs HE, et al. Cultural influences on the bedtime behaviors of young children. Med 2005; 6(4):319–24.
54. Kohyama J, Shiiki T, Ohinata-Sugimoto J, et al. Potentially harmful sleep habits of 3-years-old children in Japan. J Dev Behav Pediatr 2002; 23(2):67–70.
55. Armstrong KL, Quinn RA, Dadds MR. The sleep patterns of normal children. Med J Aust 1994; 161(3):202–6.
56. Iglowstein I, Jenni OG, Molinari L, et al. Sleep duration from infancy to adolescence: Reference values and generational trends. Pediatrics 2003; 111(2):302–7.
57. Owens JA, Spirito A, McGuinn M, et al. Sleep habits and sleep disturbance in elementary school-aged children. J Dev Behav Pediatr 2000; 21(1):27–36.
58. Fukuda K, Sakashita Y. Sleeping pattern of kindergartners and nursery school children: Function of daytime nap. Percept Mot Skills 2002; 94(1):219–28.
59. Bruni O, Proietti C, De Luca K, et al. Abstracts of Papers, 14th European Congress on Sleep Research of the European Sleep Research Society, Madrid, Spain, September 9–12, 1998. Abstract 32.
60. Richman N. A community survey of characteristics of one- to two-year-olds with sleep disruptions. J Am Acad Child Psychiatry 1981; 20(2):281–91.
61. Saarenpaa-Heikkila OA, Rintahaka PJ, Laippala PJ, et al. Sleep habits and disorders in Finnish schoolchildren. J Sleep Res 1995; 4(3):173–82.
62. Laberge L, Petit D, Simard C, et al. Development of sleep patterns in early adolescence. J Sleep Res 2001; 10(1):59–67.
63. Clarisse R, Testu F, Maintier C, et al. A comparative study of nocturnal sleep duration and timetable of children between five- and ten-years-old according to their age and socio-economic environment. Arch Pediatr 2004; 11(2):85–92.
64. Liu X, Liu L, Owens JA, et al. Sleep patterns and sleep problems among school-children in the United States and China. Pediatrics 2005; 115(1 Suppl):241–9.
65. Takemura T, Funaki K, Kanbayashi T, et al. Sleep habits of students attending elementary schools, and junior and senior high schools in Akita prefecture. Psychiatry Clin Neurosci 2002; 56(3):241–2.
66. Javo C, Ronning JA, Heyerdahl S. Child-rearing in an indigenous Sami population in Norway: A cross-cultural comparison of parental attitudes and expectations. Scand J Psychol 2004; 45(1):67–78.

67. Torun B, Davies P, Paolisso M, et al. Energy requirements and dietary energy recommen-
     dations for children and adolescents 1 to 18 years old. Eur J Clin Nutr 1996; 50(1 Suppl):
     S37–S81.
68. Weissbluth M. Naps in children: 6 months–7 years. Sleep 1995; 18(2):82–7.
69. Anders TF. Neurophysiological studies of sleep in infants and children. J Child Psychol
     Psychiatry 1982; 23(1):75–83.
70. Thorleifsdottir B, Bjornsson JK, Benediktsdottir B, et al. Sleep and sleep habits from
     childhood to young adulthood over a 10-year period. J Psychosom Res 2002;
     53(1):529–37.
71. Lavigne JV, Arend R, Rosenbaum D, et al. Sleep and behavior problems among
     preschoolers. J Dev Behav Pediatr 1999; 20(3):164–69.
72. Crosby B, Lebourgeois MK, Harsh J. Racial differences in reported napping and noctur-
     nal sleep in 2- to 8-Year-old children. Pediatrics 2005; 115(1 Suppl):225–32.
73. Triandis HC, ed. Culture and Social Behavior. New York: McGraw-Hill, 1994.

5   Links Between Family Functioning and Children's Sleep

Peggy S. Keller,[a] Joseph A. Buckhalt,[b] and Mona El-Sheikh[a]

[a]*Department of Human Development and Family Studies, Auburn University, Auburn, Alabama, U.S.A.*
[b]*Department of Counselor Education, Counseling Psychology, and School Psychology, Auburn University, Auburn, Alabama, U.S.A.*

INTRODUCTION

Sleep is a social phenomenon (1). This may especially be the case for children, for whom decisions regarding when and where to sleep are made by others. Few historical reviews have been done, but available evidence indicates that societal changes in the way families live has affected children's sleep (2,3). In considering generational changes in Western cultures, Anders and Taylor (2) trace changes in practices concerning children's sleeping spaces, and suggest that the development of the infant cradle may have been a first step in having children sleep apart from adults. And while separate beds and bedrooms for infants, toddlers, and children are the norm for most middle- to upper-class Western families, a large percentage of children sleep with parents and other family members on a regular or an occasional basis.

A recent special issue of the *Journal of Family Psychology* (4) highlighted the importance of studying sleep in the family context for several reasons: (a) The social dimension of sleep often means that family members' sleep amount and quality are interrelated; (b) Parents can influence children's sleep in much the same way that they influence children's waking behavior, by creating rules, setting limits, and providing an environment that is more or less conducive to obtaining high quality sleep; and (c) Because sleep and vigilance represent opponent processes (5), characteristics of the family that create concern, worry, anger, or insecurity for children (e.g., conflict, insensitive parenting) are likely to prevent children from obtaining adequate sleep (6).

The focus of this chapter is on how family stress might disrupt children's sleep. We begin with a discussion of why family stress is associated with the development of sleep problems in children. Next, we review the literature on associations of general family stress and more specific types of family problems (poor parenting, marital conflict) with children's sleep parameters (duration and quality of sleep). Finally, we present evidence that links between family stress and children's sleep are bidirectional.

SLEEP AND VIGILANCE AS OPPONENT PROCESSES

According to Dahl (5), it is useful to think of sleep as a state of rest and relaxation that is opposed to a state of arousal and vigilance. During sleep, the individual lacks a clear awareness of the environment and therefore has a reduced ability to monitor and respond to threat. During periods of wakeful arousal, on the other hand, the individual has activated attentional and other resources in order to attend to any potential threat and therefore has a reduced ability to relax and achieve sleep. Adults and children cycle between periods of wake and sleep over the course of the day, but emotional arousal and attentional demands can disrupt this cycle.

Family stress has important implications for children's ability to regulate emotion, which includes emotional arousal and attentional processes. For example, Emotional Security Theory (EST) (7,8) proposes that family stress undermines children's sense of security about the family. According to EST, multiple family relationships (see (9–11) for consideration of security in the parent–child relationship; see (12,13) for consideration of security in the interparental relationship) serve as sources of security for the child, meaning that the quality of these relationships either promotes or undermines children's sense of safety, family stability, and support. Children who are secure are confident in the supportiveness of their environment, have few concerns for the long-term stability of the family, and have close, warm relationships with other family members. Children view destructive conflict, neglect, and intrusiveness as threats to their security. When children are insecure, they lack confidence in the family's ability to meet child needs and provide a safe environment, have negative expectations for family functioning and stability over the long term, and distant, conflict-ridden, or enmeshed relationships with other family members. An important point is that emotional security directs and organizes children's affect and behavior. Insecure children are motivated to maintain vigilance for any potential threats that arise within relationships (e.g., conflict or separation), have intense negative emotional reactions to these events, and attempt to regulate their exposure to the threat (e.g., avoidance, acting out).

Although little research has directly explored links between emotional security and children's sleep, the implications for children's sleep are clear. Children who are secure should be able to easily transition from a period of wakefulness during the day to one of rest and relaxation at night. As a result, they are more likely to obtain adequate sleep. Children who are insecure may be too worried or concerned about the family to reduce their arousal at bedtime. As a result, these children may experience difficulty falling and staying asleep. In summary, there are clear theoretical reasons to expect that family stress can help or hinder children's ability to obtain adequate, high quality sleep.

GENERAL FAMILY CLIMATE AND CHILDREN'S SLEEP

In addition to strong theoretical justification for the role of family functioning in children's sleep, there is also empirical evidence demonstrating the link between general family stress and children's sleep problems (14,15). For example, adolescent perceptions of a good home atmosphere are related to good perceived sleep quality (16). Family disorganization has also been found to correlate with preschoolers' sleep problems based on mother report (17). Bates and colleagues (18) found that mothers' reports of stressful life events were associated with children's greater variability in sleep times and later bedtimes, based on maternal diary reports. When mothers' perceived daily parenting hassles (children not listening to parents, needing to change plans due to child needs) as stressful, asthmatic children were more likely to experience wakings during the night based on mother interview (19). This study was particularly startling in that the effect of family stress on night wakings in asthmatic children was as strong as the effects of allergen exposure in other studies. This finding is consistent with additional research showing that family stress, in comparison to academic and social/peer stress, is more consistently associated with increased insomnia in undergraduates over a three-week period, and that other forms of stress were only associated with insomnia when family stress was high (20). Thus, even when children have left home for college, the family continues to influence the quality of their sleep. The authors suggest that the family is especially important for the formation of personal identity, a key developmental goal for this period, and therefore family disruptions may be more distressing than more normative social and academic stress. This interpretation is supported by research assessing 8–11-year-old children's family environment: Greater encouragement of maturity was linked to longer sleep duration and earlier bedtime (21). The evidence therefore suggests that low stress, highly encouraging family climates are associated with better sleep than family climates characterized by stress and lack of encouragement.

However, effects may be particularly negative for those children who demonstrate emotion-focused coping in response to stress (22). That is, children who ruminate and worry about the family climate may be at greater risk for sleep disruptions than are children who adopt more adaptive coping strategies. This is consistent with the hypervigilance (5) and emotional security (8) frameworks for understanding the development of sleep problems. Family stress may lead to sleep disruptions to the extent that it is threatening to children's feelings of security and safety.

THE PARENT–CHILD RELATIONSHIP AND CHILDREN'S SLEEP

Additional research has documented relations between problems specific to the parent–child relationship and children's disrupted sleep. For example, studies have shown that different forms of parental abuse are associated with sleep problems for children. In one study, physically or sexually abused children were found to be twice as physically active during the night than controlled or depressed children (23). Based on actigraph-derived sleep parameters, abused children experienced a longer sleep latency (period of time between lying down in bed and actually falling asleep) and reduced sleep efficiency (percentage of sleep period spent asleep). Physically abused children suffered greater sleep disruptions than sexually abused children. The increased vulnerability of physically abused children in comparison to other forms of abuse has been observed in other studies as well (24).

More normative forms of parenting have also been linked to children's sleep. For example, a comparison of children with and without sleep disorders revealed that parenting problems such as lax discipline were more likely to predict poor sleep quality in the control group than in the clinical group (25). Thus, parent–child relations may be important to sleep for a very large number of children in the general population. A study of a treatment program for sleep disturbances in adolescents with a history of substance abuse reported significant indirect effects of parental involvement (number of activities with adolescents) on adolescent sleep quality (26). Parental involvement predicted less psychological distress in adolescents, which was associated with increased sleep efficiency. The study also found that lower parental involvement was directly related to later adolescent wake times after controlling for adolescent distress.

Further, there is evidence that the link between parenting and children's sleep changes as children develop. Even after controlling for several potential confounds [including gender, race, socioeconomic status (SES), family structure, school start and end times, daily activities such as television watching, sports, homework and work], parental warmth predicted 5–12-year-old children's greater sleep duration, but general parental monitoring predicted 12–19-year-old children's greater sleep duration (27).

However, additional research suggests that it may be best for parents to temper warmth with limit setting during the night for children of all ages. In a study of children with severe learning disabilities (aged 5–20 years), Quine (28) found that problems with falling asleep and waking at night were more common when mothers were more responsive toward children during the night, attending immediately to child cries with comfort and affection and failing to encourage self-soothing skills. Similarly, the ability of infants to self-soothe and regain sleep is associated with parents waiting longer before responding to infant cries at night and removing the infant from the crib for shorter periods of time (29). For this reason, behavioral sleep interventions typically encourage parents to refrain from quickly responding to children's wake episodes and instead give children the opportunity to successfully regain sleep on their own. Interestingly, parents of infants with clinical sleep problems are more likely to view hypothetical vignettes of infant night waking as excessively demanding behavior and endorse limit setting (e.g., letting the child cry rather than intervening) as the appropriate approach, while at the same time reporting greater problems setting limits for their own infants (30). According to the authors of this study, it is possible that infants of parents who have difficulties with setting limits may develop sleep problems because they become increasingly reliant on parental intervention during the night; alternatively, irritable and demanding babies may present difficulties for parents' ability to set limits for their infants. An additional finding of interest was that fathers were more likely to endorse imposing limits on wakeful babies than mothers. Mothers were more likely to focus on the distress experienced by their infants and at the same time expressed greater anger toward the infant. Other studies have also found that maternal cognitions regarding setting limits, anger towards infants, and concerns regarding parental efficacy are associated with infant sleep problems (31). The implication is that fathers may be especially beneficial for altering patterns of parental behavior that prevent children from learning to self-soothe and obtain sleep on their own. Unfortunately, most of the research on child sleep in the family context has focused on mothers only.

There has been a very limited number of studies addressing the link between children's security in the parent–child relationship (attachment security) and children's sleep. El-Sheikh and colleagues (32) found that children's perceived attachment security was not associated with child-reported or actigraph-measured sleep. However, the link between perceived insecure attachment and children's poor socio-emotional functioning was stronger for children experiencing sleep problems (33). Scher (34) reported an association between attachment security and infant night waking: Infants categorized as ambivalently attached to mothers were more likely to wake during the night than securely attached infants, based on maternal report of night waking. Morrell and Steele (35) found that after controlling for infant age, maternal depression, maternal cognitions regarding limit setting and anger toward infant demands, infant temperament, and maternal physical comforting during the night, ambivalent attachment was a significant predictor of infant sleep problems at one year and persistent sleep problems at age two. McNamara, Belsky and Fearon (36) compared 15-month-old toddlers classified as insecure-avoidant or insecure-ambivalent and found that ambivalently attached experienced greater night wakings than avoidantly attached children, and that ambivalently attached children were more likely to suffer from clinical sleep problems than avoidantly attached children. There is also some evidence that attachment security in adulthood (security to one's romantic partner rather than parent), which is closely tied to childhood attachment security, is associated with sleep. Anxious attachment appears to be more predictive of poor sleep quality based on a questionnaire measure of sleep, than does avoidant attachment (37), even after controlling for depressive affect and behavioral inhibition (38). Furthermore, Benoit and colleagues (39) found that 100% of mothers with children suffering from sleep disorders reported an insecure adult attachment, compared to 57% of mothers with children not suffering from sleep disorders.

Taken together, these studies seem to indicate that anxious or ambivalent, in comparison to avoidant, attachment classifications may be particularly disruptive for children's sleep. This is highly consistent with vigilance (5) and emotional security (7,8) frameworks for understanding sleep problems. That is, children who focus on family concerns, experiencing high levels of anxiety, should be more likely to have problems attaining and maintaining sleep than children who are dismissive and avoidant of family problems. McNamara, Belsky and Fearon (36) further speculate that sleep problems may contribute to ambivalent attachment because rapid eye movement (REM) sleep is important for the development of emotion regulation. Specifically, they propose that ambivalent children will evince higher percentages of REM sleep, which activates proximity seeking behavior and provokes a preoccupation with obtaining parental contact rather than self-soothing during night wakings. Thus, bidirectional relations between attachment insecurity and sleep disruptions may be possible.

MARITAL FUNCTIONING AND CHILDREN'S SLEEP

Although marital conflict is a normative experience in many families and the quality of the marital relationship is an important predictor of child functioning (40), there have been very few studies exploring how marital functioning or children's exposure to marital conflict is related to their sleep. In a study of over 150 third-grade children, it was found that children's exposure to marital conflict was linked to sleep problems assessed via both child reports of subjective sleepiness and sleep problems and actigraphic measures of percent sleep and activity during the night (41). Further, in another study, children's emotional insecurity about the marital relationship was found to be an intervening variable that fully accounted for the association between marital conflict and children's sleep disruptions (42). Thus, findings suggested that children's concerns about the stability of the marital relationship may prevent them from transitioning from wakeful to relaxed states and obtaining adequate sleep. Sleep disruptions that were associated with emotional insecurity predicted parent reports of greater emotional and behavioral problems, teacher reports of emotional problems, behavioral problems, and poor academic performance, as well as reduced performance on standardized tests (32,42,43). Further, it appears that these relations may be stronger for African-American children or children in lower SES families. It is possible that marital conflict and sleep disruptions are most likely to be associated with children's maladjustment and poor cognitive functioning when they are associated with additional risks.

According to the Health Disparity view (44) children from minority or low-income backgrounds experience an increased burden for physical and mental health problems, due to social factors such as discrimination and economic factors such as reduced access to health care and other resources. Thus, the combination of marital problems and health disparity may represent an exacerbation of risk that increases the likelihood of sleep problems over the likelihood associated with the presence of either risk factor alone.

EVIDENCE FOR BIDIRECTIONAL RELATIONS

Just as family problems including poor parenting and marital conflict have been associated with children's ability to obtain adequate sleep, there is also research demonstrating that children's sleep problems are associated with effects on parents, particularly their ability to obtain adequate sleep and their mood. For example, longer sleep latency and greater sleep disruptions in children (based on maternal report) are correlated with greater mother fatigue and sleepiness (45,46). An examination of families with children seeking treatment at a sleep disorders clinic also found that child sleepiness and sleep problems were correlated with mother sleepiness; similarly, child sleep duration was associated with mother sleep duration (47). There were similar findings regarding fathers' sleep. Additionally, even after controlling for mother sleep duration, father sleep duration, and child sleep duration, and child age, children's disrupted sleep was linked to maternal daytime sleepiness. Finally, this study found that parents of children with multiple sleep disorders reported more sleepiness than children with only behavioral sleep disorders, parasomnias, or sleep-disordered breathing. Studies of children suffering from epilepsy (48), atopic eczema (49), and clinical sleep problems (50,51) have each found that children's night wakings and poor sleep quality are associated with parental night wakings, anxiety, depression, and perceived stress. Poor adolescent sleep quality has even been found to predict parental divorce or separation over time, possibly because adolescent sleep quality and family relations are closely tied (52).

Especially cogent evidence that children's sleep problems may have negative effects on other family members comes from studies of sleep problem interventions. Specifically, when children's sleep problems are successfully treated, parental sleep quality, mood, perceptions of stress, and marital satisfaction have been found to improve (53–55). For example, Adams and Rickert (56) designed a treatment for bedtime tantrums that involved putting toddlers to bed when they naturally fell asleep and having parents and children engage in several enjoyable activities before bedtime. Bedtime was gradually made earlier until it reached the time parents desired. This treatment was effective in reducing toddlers' bedtime tantrums and improved parents' marital satisfaction. An extinction intervention in which parents were instructed to systematically avoid contact with their child after placing him or her to bed was shown to significantly reduce child night wakings and increase child amount of time awake at night and amount of sleep, all within two weeks (57). These improvements in child sleep were accompanied by parental decreases in subjective feelings of tiredness, parenting stress, and depression, as well as increases in feelings of hopefulness. Unfortunately, much of this research has been limited by a reliance on parent report of child and parent sleep, and thus it is possible that relations reflect shared method variance.

FUTURE DIRECTIONS

There is strong evidence linking family problems to children's sleep disruptions. Studies of general family stress, problems specific to the parent–child relationship, and marital conflict each demonstrates that families can provide an environment that can either promote or hinder children's sleep amount and quality. Given that sleep represents the antithesis of vigilance and arousal, it is possible that family problems prevent children from obtaining adequate sleep because they reduce children's security about the family and create feelings of worry or concern that are incompatible with rest and relaxation.

At the same time, there is a clear need for additional research. Few studies have explored the links between marital functioning and children's sleep. Similarly, many studies have excluded fathers and siblings. Furthermore, families are embedded within a social and cultural milieu that affects family relationships and functioning. Some studies have shown that family sleep behavior differs across cultural contexts (58) and ethnic groups (59). For example, the prevalence of co-sleeping varies along ethnic and socioeconomic lines, with lower income/education and American ethnic minority families showing more co-sleeping (60). Weimer and colleagues (61) reported that children under the age of five had an 88% rate of co-sleeping with a parent in an urban sample of predominantly African-American mothers. Further, co-sleeping was strongly related to single parenthood, lower education, and fewer bedrooms in the house.

Co-sleeping is just one family practice that varies not only among individual families, but also by culture. Setting and maintaining consistent bedtimes constitutes a major area in which families affect children's sleep. Here again, cultural practices appear to differ, with African-American families having been found to allow later, and less regular, bedtimes for children (62,63). However, additional questions regarding the impact of family stress on children's sleep and functioning for different cultural and ethnic backgrounds remain. In particular, it is not clear whether some forms of parenting problems or marital conflict may be more or less detrimental depending on the context.

One particularly fruitful avenue for future research is in exploring how sleep disruptions may help account for the development of children's psychopathology in the context of family risk. Family problems such as parental abusiveness, poor parenting practices, and marital conflict have each been linked with children's increased risk for emotional and behavioral problems. Recently, research indicates that this association between family dysfunction and child maladjustment is at least partially due to children's disrupted sleep (41,42). In addition, sleep may serve as an intervening variable for reduced functioning in domains that have been less frequently studied in the context of parenting and marital problems. For example, to the extent that family dysfunction disrupts children's sleep, children may experience cognitive problems (43), increased susceptibility to illness (64), and obesity (65). Thus, increased study of the role of sleep may improve understanding of the full spectrum of effects of family dysfunction on children's physical and mental health. Furthermore, and in addition to mediating the link between family problems and children's adjustment and development, sleep problems may function to exacerbate the connection between familial risk factors and child functioning. For example, whereas child–mother attachment was not directly related to sleep, the two variables interacted to exacerbate child adjustment and cognitive functioning (33). Thus, when children had an insecure attachment in conjunction with sleep disruptions, they were at risk for adjustment and cognitive difficulties. Finally, future research is needed to test theoretical models of the processes involved in the effects of family problems and child sleep, and characteristics that place children at greater or lesser risk for sleep disruptions must be identified.

Methodological limitations of current research should also be noted. Many studies suffer from very small sample sizes, and are cross-sectional in nature. Furthermore, many studies rely on potentially inaccurate parent-report of sleep problems rather than more objective actigraphic or polysomnographic measures. Continued research on the effects of family stress on children's quality and quantity of sleep therefore stands to make an important impact on the field, providing increased specification for the etiology of sleep disorders, a greater understanding of the impact of various forms of family risk in multiple contexts, and improved models of the link between family problems and the development of psychopathology in children.

ACKNOWLEGMENTS

This work was supported by National Science Foundation grants 0339115 and 0623936 awarded to Mona El-Sheikh and Joseph Buckhalt.

REFERENCES

1. Meadows, R. The "negotiated night": An embodied conceptual framework for the sociological study of sleep. The Sociological Review 2005; 53:240–54.
2. Anders, TF, Taylor, TR. Babies and their sleep environment. Children's Environments 1994; 11:66–84.
3. Stearns, PN. Children's sleep: Sketching historical change. Journal of Social History 1996; 30:345–66.
4. El-Sheikh, M, Dahl, RE. Special issue: Carpe noctem: Sleep and family processes. Journal of Family Psychology 2007; 21.
5. Dahl, RE. The regulation of sleep and arousal: Development and psychopathology. Development and Psychopathology 1996; 8:3–27.
6. Dahl, RE, El-Sheikh, M. Considering sleep in a family context: Introduction to the special issue. Journal of Family Psychology 2007; 21:1–3.
7. Cummings, EM, Davies, PT. Emotional security as a regulatory process in normal development and development of psychopathology. Development and Psychopathology 1996; 8:123–39.
8. Davies, PT, Cummings, EM. Marital conflict and child adjustment: An emotional security hypothesis. Psychological Bulletin 1994; 116:387–411.
9. Bowlby, J. Attachment and Loss: Vol 1. Attachment. New York: Basic Books, 1969.
10. Colin, VL. Human Attachment. New York: McGraw-Hill, 1996.
11. Waters, E, Cummings, EM. A secure base from which to explore close relationships. Child Development 2000; 71:164–72.
12. Davies, PT, Harold, GT, Goeke-Morey, MC, et al. Child emotional security and interparental conflict. Monographs of the Society for Research in Child Development 2002; 67(3).
13. Davies, PT, Forman, EM. Children's patterns of preserving emotional security in the interparental subsystem. Child Development 2002; 73:1880–903.
14. Liu, X, Uchiyama, M, Okawa, M, et al. Prevalence and correlates of self-reported sleep problems among Chinese adolescents. Sleep 2000; 23:27–34.

15. Sadeh, A, Raviv, A, Graber, R, et al. Sleep patterns and sleep disruptions in school-age children. Developmental Psychology 2000; 36:291–301.
16. Tynjälä, J, Kannas, L, Levälahti, E, et al. Perceived sleep quality and its precursors in adolescents. Health Promotion International 1999; 14:155–66.
17. Gregory, AM, Eley, TC, O'Connor, TG, et al. Family influences on the association between sleep problems and anxiety in a large sample of pre-school aged twins. Personality and Individual Differences 2005; 39:1337–48.
18. Bates, JE, Viken, RJ, Alexander, DB, et al. Sleep and adjustment in preschool children: Sleep diary reports by mothers relate to behavior reports by teachers. Child Development 2002; 73:62–74.
19. Fiese, BH, Winter, MA, Sliwinski, M, et al. Nighttime waking in children with asthma: An exploratory study of daily fluctuations in family climate. Journal of Family Psychology 2007; 21:95–103.
20. Bernert, RA, Merrill, KA, Braithwaite, SR, et al. Family life stress and insomnia symptoms in a prospective evaluation of young adults. Journal of Family Psychology 2007; 21:58–66.
21. Spilsbury, JC, Storfer-Isser, A, Drotar, D, et al. Effects of the home environment on school-aged children's sleep. Sleep 2005; 28:1419–27.
22. Sadeh, A, Keinan, G, Daon, K. Effects of stress on sleep: The moderating role of coping style. Health Psychology 2004; 23:542–5.
23. Glod, CA, Teicher, MH, Hartman, CR, et al. Increased nocturnal activity and impaired sleep maintenance in abused children. Journal of the American Academy of Child and Adolescent Psychiatry 1997; 36:1236–43.
24. Sadeh, A, McGuire, JP, Sachs, H, et al. Sleep and psychological characteristics of children on a psychiatric inpatient unit. Journal of the American Academy of Child and Adolescent Psychiatry 1995; 34:813–19.
25. Owens-Stively, J, Frank, N, Smith, A. et al. Child temperament, parenting discipline style, and daytime behavior in childhood sleep disorders. Developmental and Behavioral Pediatrics 1997; 18:314–21.
26. Cousins, JC, Bootzin, RR, Stevens, SJ, et al. Parental involvement, psychological distress, and sleep: A preliminary examination in sleep-disturbed adolescents with a history of substance abuse. Journal of Family Psychology 2007; 21:104–13.
27. Adam, EK, Snell, EK, Pendry, P. Sleep timing and quantity in ecological and family context: A nationally representative time-diary study. Journal of Family Psychology 2007; 21:4–19.
28. Quine, L. Severity of sleep problems in children with severe learning difficulties: Description and correlates. Journal of Community and Applied Social Psychology 1992; 2:247–68.
29. Burnham, MM, Goodlin-Jones, BL, Gaylor, EE, et al. Nighttime sleep-wake patterns and self-soothing from birth to one year of age: A longitudinal intervention study. Journal of Child Psychology and Psychiatry 2002; 43:713–25.
30. Sadeh, A, Flint-Ofir, E, Tirosh, T, et al. Infant sleep and parental sleep-related cognitions. Journal of Family Psychology 2007; 21:74–87.
31. Morrell, JMB. The role of maternal cognitions in infant sleep problems as assessed by a new instrument, the Maternal Cognitions about Infant Sleep Questionnaire. Journal of Child Psychology and Psychiatry 1999; 40:247–58.
32. El-Sheikh, M, Buckhalt, JA, Keller, PS, et al. Child emotional insecurity and academic achievement: The role of sleep disruptions. Journal of Family Psychology 2007; 21:29–38.
33. El-Sheikh, M, Keller, PS, Buckhalt, JA. Children's perceived attachments to parents and their socio-emotional and academic functioning: Sleep disruptions as moderators of effects. European Journal of Development, under review.
34. Scher, A. Attachment and sleep: A study of night waking in 12 month old infants. Developmental Psychobiology 2001; 38:274–84.

35. Morrell, J Steele, H. The role of attachment security, temperament, maternal perception, and care-giving behavior in persistent infant sleeping problems. Infant Mental Health Journal 2003; 24:447–68.
36. McNamara, P, Belsky, J, Fearon, P. Infant sleep disorders and attachment: Sleep problems in infants with insecure-resistant versus insecure-avoidant attachments to mother. Sleep and Hypnosis 2003; 5:7–16.
37. Scharfe, E, Eldredge, D. Association between attachment representations and health behaviors in late adolescence. Journal of Health Psychology 2001; 6:295–307.
38. Carmichael, CL, Reis, HT. Attachment, sleep quality, and depressed affect. Health Psychology 2005; 24:526–31.
39. Benoit, D, Zeanah, CH, Boucher, C, et al. Sleep disorders in early childhood: Association with insecure maternal attachment. Journal of the American Academy of Child and Adolescent Psychiatry 1992; 31:86–96.
40. Cummings, EM, Davies, PT. Effects of marital conflict on children: Recent advances and emerging themes in process-oriented research. Journal of Child Psychology and Psychiatry 2002; 43:31–63.
41. El-Sheikh, M, Buckhalt, JA, Mize, J, et al. Marital conflict and disruption of children's sleep. Child Development 2006; 77:31–43.
42. El-Sheikh, M, Buckhalt, JA, Cummings, EM, et al. Sleep disruptions and emotional insecurity are pathways of risk for children. Journal of Child Psychology and Psychiatry 2007; 48:88–96.
43. Buckhalt, JA, El-Sheikh, M, Keller, PS. Children's sleep and cognitive functioning: Race and socioeconomic status as moderators of effects. Child Development 2007; 78:213–31.
44. Carter-Pokras, O, & Baquet, C. What is a "health disparity?" Public Health Reports 2002; 117:426–34.
45. Meltzer, LJ, Mindell, JA. Impact of a child's chronic illness on maternal sleep and daytime functioning. Archives of Internal Medicine 2006; 166:1749–55.
46. Meltzer, LJ, Mindell, JA. Relationship between child sleep disturbances and maternal sleep mood and parenting stress: A pilot study. Journal of Family Psychology 2007; 21:67–73.
47. Boergers, J, Hart, C, Owens, JA, et al. Child sleep disorders: Associations with parental sleep duration and daytime sleepiness. Journal of Family Psychology 2007; 21:88–94.
48. Cottrell, L, Kahn, A. Impact of childhood epilepsy on maternal sleep and socioemotional functioning. Clinical Pediatrics 2005; 44:613–16.
49. Moore, K, Davies, TJ, Murray, CS, et al. Effect of childhood eczema and asthma on parental sleep and well-being: A prospective comparative study. British Journal of Dermatology 2006; 154:514–18.
50. Lam, P, Hiscock, H, Wake, M. Outcomes of infant sleep problems: A longitudinal study of sleep, behavior, and maternal well-being. Pediatrics 2003; 111:203–7.
51. Thome, M, Skuladottir, A. Changes in sleep problems, parents' distress and impact of sleep problems from infancy to preschool age for referred and unreferred children. Scandinavian Journal of Caring Sciences 2005; 19:86–94.
52. Vignau, J, Bailly, D, Duhamel, A, et al. Epidemiologic study of sleep quality and troubles in French secondary school adolescents. Journal of Adolescent Health 1997; 21:343–50.
53. Hiscock, H, Wake, M. Randomised controlled trial of behavioural infant sleep intervention to improve infant sleep and maternal mood. British Medical Journal 2002; 324:1062–5.
54. Mindell, JA, Durand, VM. Treatment of childhood sleep disorders: Generalization across disorders and effects on family members. Journal of Pediatric Psychology 1993; 18:731–50.
55. Thome, M, Skuladottir, A. Evaluating a family-centered intervention for infant sleep problems. Journal of Advanced Nursing 2005; 50:5–11.
56. Adams, LA, Rickert, VI. Reducing bedtime tantrums: Comparison between positive routines and graduated extinction. Pediatrics 1989; 84:756–61.

57. Eckerberg, B. Treatment of sleep problems in families with young children: Effects of treatment of family well-being. Acta Paediatrica 2004; 93:126–34.
58. Worthman, CM, Brown, RA. Companionable sleep: Social regulation of sleep and cosleeping in Egyptian families. Journal of Family Psychology 2007; 21:124–35.
59. Milan, S, Snow, S, Belay, S. The context of preschool children's sleep: Racial/ethnic differences in sleep locations, routines, and concerns. Journal of Family Psychology 2007; 21:20–8.
60. Lozoff, BA, Wolf, A, Davis, N. Co-sleeping in urban families with young children in the United States. Pediatrics 1984; 74:171–82.
61. Weimer, SM, Dise, TL, Evers, PB, et al. Prevalence, predictors, and attitudes toward cosleeping in an urban pediatric center. Clinical Pediatrics 2002; 41:433–8.
62. Crabtree, VM, Korhonen, JB, Montgomery-Downs, HE, et al. Cultural influences on the bedtime behaviors of young children. Sleep Medicine 2005; 6:319–24.
63. Lozoff, BA, Askew, GL, Wolf, AW. Cosleeping and early childhood sleep problems: Effects of ethnicity and socioeconomic status. Journal of Developmental and Behavioral Pediatrics 1996; 17:9–15.
64. Bryant, PA, Trinder, J, Curtis, N. Sick and tired: Does sleep have a vital role in the immune system? Nature Reviews: Immunology 2004; 4:457–67.
65. Snell, EK, Adam, EK, Duncan, GJ. Sleep and the body mass index and overweight status of children and adolescents. Child Development 2007; 78:309–23.

6 Circadian Sleep Disorders and Comorbid Psychiatric and Behavioral Disorders in Children and Adolescents

Reut Gruber[a] and Dana Sheshko[b]

[a]Department of Psychiatry, McGill University,
Douglas Research Center, Montreal, Quebec, Canada
[b]Attention, Behavior, and Sleep Research Laborarory,
Douglas Research Center, Montreal, Quebec, Canada

INTRODUCTION

As the earth spins on its axis once a day, and completes an orbit around the sun within a year, most regions experience changes in environmental lighting conditions, and major temporal structures are created. This includes the day–night cycle, the lunar cycle and the seasons. The regular alternation between light and dark, and the seasonal changes in their relative durations, impose major constraints on living organisms. This has led to the key evolutionary feature of predictive adaptation to the cycles. These adaptive mechanisms have evolved to promote survival and reproduction, utilize the solar cycle, and are termed "circadian rhythms" (*circa* about, *diem* a day). The most evident manifestation of human adaptation to day / night alternation is the diurnal temporal organization of behavior into periods of wakefulness during the day and sleep during the night. These rhythms are regulated by the circadian timing system, and depend on genetically controlled rhythmic molecular events that control a wide range of rhythms in cellular, systemic, and behavioral processes. The circadian timing system is a fundamental homeostatic process that powerfully influences human behavior and physiology throughout development. The present chapter reviews information regarding the basic neurobiology of the circadian timing system, its ontogenesis, circadian disorders commonly seen in children and adolescents along with their comorbidities, and treatment of these sleep disorders in youth.

THE CIRCADIAN TIMING SYSTEM

The circadian timing system provides temporal organization for most neurobehavioral, physiological, and biochemical variables, including the sleep–wake cycle (1). It consists of a biological clock, input pathways, and output pathways (1,2).

The Biological Clock

A circadian clock is a self-sustaining oscillator that exhibits endogenous rhythmicity, has a period of ~24 hours, and controls many physiological (e.g., endocrine regulation) and behavioral (e.g., attention, psychomotor performance and memory) systems. Circadian pacemakers, which are the paired suprachiasmatic nuclei (SCN) in the anterior hypothalamus (1), are clocks that regulate the temporal organization of function in other circadian or brain systems or tissues. When humans or animals are placed in temporal isolation (i.e., an environment without time cues), the pacemaker is responsible for the maintenance of free-running rhythms (3). Under free-running conditions, circadian rhythms remain extremely accurate, usually varying from 23 to 25 hours, depending on the species and context.

Because SCN oscillations do not occur over exactly 24 hours, it is necessary to realign the circadian pacemaker each day with the light–dark cycle (4). The absence of such alignment results in the drifting of clock oscillations (or free-running) out of phase with the light–dark cycle. The alignment process is called entrainment (5). Successful entrainment of sleep–wake rhythms to a 24-hour day requires the biological clock to be "reset" by an average of one hour each day. The endogenous clock is reset predominantly by light, which is the major environmental *zeitgeber* (time giver) (5). It is accomplished by coupling molecular feedback loops to the control of neuronal membrane potential (6), and results from rhythmic expression of transcriptional activating factors which form long feedback loops in SCN cells (2). Light exposure at times that reset (phase shift) the clock increases the metabolic activity in the SCN, which in turn activates positive and negative transcriptional feedback loops. This activation then leads to periodic activation of transcription by a set of clock genes, including *timeless* (*tim*), *clock* (*clk*), *cycle* (*cyc*), *doubletime* (*dbt*), *cryptochrome* (*cry*), *Bmal1* (*Mop3*), and *vrille* (*vri*) (7–11). Oscillating circadian gene products regulate their own expression through a complex system of transcription, translation, and posttranslational processes (12,13). This provides the fundamental basis for underlying circadian rhythms.

Entrainment by the light–dark cycle is complemented by a feedback loop involving the rhythmic release of melatonin (7). Melatonin is secreted into the cerebrospinal fluid and bloodstream by the pineal gland (14). Its release distributes photic information throughout the body by linking the perception and transduction of photic information to the dissemination of time-coding signals. High melatonin receptor expression is found in the SCN itself and in the hypophyseal pars tuberalis (PT), allowing the central nervous system (CNS) to mediate clock information to the periphery (15,16). High receptor expression is also found in other brain structures and peripheral tissues. The circadian rhythm of plasma melatonin levels closely follows the core body temperature cycle, with the minimum core body temperature occurring just after the peak level of plasma melatonin. The timing of these body temperature events corresponds to the increase in evening sleep propensity in humans (17).

Input Pathways

Input pathways relay photic information from the retina to the SCN to synchronize (or entrain) the oscillations of the clock to the 24-hour light–dark cycle. The entrainment pathway is initiated by specific photoreceptors: a set of ganglion cells that contain photopigments, particularly melanopsin (18). These ganglion cells project to the SCN core through the retinohypothalamic tract originating in the retina, and monosynaptically terminate in the SCN (19,20). Another pathway from the intergeniculate leaflet to the SCN modulates clock entrainment and appears to modulate the effect of retinal input on the SCN (21).

Output Pathways

Several discrete neural pathways projecting from the SCN control various functional systems (22,23). The circadian system exerts its influence over neural physiology and various systems through these pathways that project predominantly from the hypothalamus (22,23). Output pathways of the circadian system also regulate the rhythmic production of several hormones, including melatonin and cortisol (24). In addition, there is a hierarchy of pacemakers and oscillators that extend from the SCN pacemaker to other brain pacemakers and oscillators, and then to a large chain of peripheral clock genes in many tissues and organs (25).

THE ONTOGENESIS OF THE CIRCADIAN SYSTEM AND ITS REGULATION
Prenatal Development of the SCN
In primates, the SCN circadian clock is formed, and begins to oscillate, in utero. While it remains unknown when the SCN first appear in primates, at gestation week 18, the SCN are formed and already possess melatonin receptors (26), and may thus generate self-sustained and entrainable oscillations. Several circadian rhythms which are driven by the SCN in adults are present prenatally, including rest–activity, breathing movements, heart rate, and urine production (27). While there is some evidence that these rhythms are controlled by the fetal SCN, it is possible they are actually controlled by the maternal SCN. However, by the late embryonic stage the elements constituting the molecular clock are present and rhythmic gene expression is inducible as the systems involved are equipped to do so.

Prenatal Entrainment of the SCN
It appears that a biological clock begins to oscillate in the mammalian SCN from the late embryonic stage. However, such a clock would generate a rhythm slightly different from 24 hours, as shown in adult organisms. Therefore, a continual correction by environmental periodicities, or *zeitgebers*, is necessary. The main *zeitgeber* in mammals is the light–dark cycle. However, non-photic cues seem to be more effective in the early developmental stages, terminal embryonic span, and initial postnatal days. Studies using rats and golden hamsters show that the fetal clock is entrained by maternal time cues, such as the effect of environmental lighting on the maternal circadian system. When mothers are blinded, the fetal SCN metabolic activity synchronizes with the free-running rhythm of the mother (28). The maternal-to-fetal clock pathway may involve dopamine signaling and/or melatonin. However, the maternal SCN can merely entrain; they do not generate the fetal rhythms.

Sladek et al. (29) investigated prenatal development in the rat SCN molecular clockwork. The circadian profiles of five clock gene mRNAs, namely *Per1*, *Per2*, *Cry1*, *Bmal1*, and *Clock*, were examined on embryonic day 19 (E19). E19 was chosen because neurogenesis in the fetal SCN is completed by this time (30), and a circadian rhythm in metabolic activity is present by this stage (31). All of the above-mentioned five clock genes were found to be expressed in the SCN at E19. However, expression was not observed to be linked to a circadian rhythm, possibly because SCN rhythmicity has only just begun at E19 (31,32), and therefore the amplitude of the clock gene expression rhythms might be too small to be detected. In addition, clock gene expression rhythms might be present in individual SCN neurons, but the neurons might not be sufficiently synchronized because of the very low number of synapses present at E19 (30).

Postnatal Entrainment of the SCN

Recent evidence shows that the circadian system in primate infants is responsive to light at very premature stages, and that low-intensity lighting can regulate the developing clock. In rodents such as rats, mice, and hamsters, newborn neonates are totally dependent on their mothers. In the laboratory, the influence of maternal entrainment of newborn rhythmicity becomes less important after the first week of life, at which time photic entrainment begins to override maternal entrainment. As the clock rhythmicity strengthens, maternal cues may lose their entraining ability, and light, the stronger entraining agent, may take their place.

Additional factors other than the light–dark cycle may contribute to the entrainment of the circadian sleep–wake rhythms in newborns. Absence of the mother may strongly entrain the neonatal clock. When newborn pups are deprived of their mothers during the light phase (i.e., at the time when they usually suckle milk), the rhythmic SCN expression of *Per1* and *Per2* genes is completely phase-reversed within six days (33). In contrast, in adult rodents, non-photic time cues such as restricted feeding and methamphetamine injection significantly altered the phases of the behavioral rhythms, but had no effect on the circadian expression rhythms of the clock genes in the SCN (34,35). Studies using adult hamsters showed that only physical exercise suppressed *Per1* and *Per2* clock gene expression in the SCN (36). Those findings suggest that the sensitivity of the neonatal SCN to non-photic time cues differs from that of the adult SCN. Gradually, photic entrainment of the SCN clock prevails.

Over time, additional factors other than the light–dark cycle may contribute to the circadian sleep–wake rhythms in humans. These factors include knowledge of the time of day, social contacts, the timing of food availability, and scheduling of bed rest and activity.

Development of Diurnal Temporal Organization of Behavior

The organization of the sleep–wake system in a diurnal pattern that corresponds to the day–night cycle involves a shift from multiphasic sleep distributed across the day and night, to a monophasic event of consolidated sleep concentrated during the dark hours of the night. This developmental process of sleep consolidation is linked to the functioning of a circadian system, and to the gradual reduction of sleep needs accompanied by a significant increase in waking time as humans mature. In humans, the most rapid shift in sleep consolidation occurs during the first year of life (37). After birth, there is progressive maturation of the circadian system with day–night rhythms in activity and hormone secretion developing between one and three months of age. At six weeks of age, infants are awake more during the day-time than at night. At 12 weeks of age, daytime sleep duration decreases further, and far greater sleep occurs at night (38). Importantly, although consolidated periods of rest and activity are not apparent until one to two months after birth, day–night differences in activity can be detected as early as one week of age in some infants. At the age when day–night differences in infant activity become apparent, day–night rhythms in hormone production are observed. Day–night rhythms in melatonin production can be detected at 12 weeks of age. Circadian variations in cortisol levels appear between three and six months of age. With advancing age, the release of other hormones and circulating factors based on circadian rhythms is reported to occur. At one year of age, more of the waking time shifts to the daylight hours and more of the sleep time shifts to the night. Although morning and afternoon naps continue to occur, total sleep time decreases to about 14 to 15 hours per day, with the majority occurring during the night, and the remainder obtained during one to two daytime naps (39,40).

Following the rapid developmental period during the first year, later development of the sleep–wake system manifests as a slow monotonic process. The decline in daytime napping and consolidation of sleep into one period at night is a gradual process that occurs between early and middle childhood, and is associated with the disappearance of daytime naps (41), delayed evening bedtime, and a resulting reduction in sleep time (42).

Developmental changes in sleep–wake (light–dark) patterns occur again as children move into adolescence. Puberty is a critical maturational phase during which a major shift occurs (43,44). As individuals progress through pubertal development during adolescence, they tend to become characterized by an evening preference. This shift in bedtime and wake preference has been ascribed to psychosocial factors that promote a later bedtime, such as increased academic demands, social relationships and autonomy, extracurricular activities, and media (45–47). However, similar adolescent sleep patterns across cultures suggest that biological processes, rather than changes in the psychosocial milieu, regulate the sleep phase delay in teens (e.g., 46). This view is supported by studies that strictly controlled psychosocial influences (48–50).

CIRCADIAN RHYTHM SLEEP DISORDERS

Optimal sleep quality is achieved when the desired sleep time is aligned with the timing of the endogenous circadian sleep–wake schedule. When there is a misalignment between the endogenous circadian timing and the external 24-hour social and physical environment, circadian rhythm sleep disorders (CRSD) may arise. The present discussion focuses on CRSD in children and adolescents, with an emphasis on comorbid disorders that may precede the development of a CRSD, or may arise as a consequence.

The classification and diagnostic criteria for CRSD and its subtypes discussed throughout this chapter are based on published criteria from the *International Classification of Sleep Disorders* (ICSD-2) (51) and the *Diagnostic and Statistical Manual of Mental Disorders* (DSM IV-TR) (52). In general, CRSD are characterized by failure to adjust the sleep–wake pattern to a socially appropriate schedule. This in turn leads to complaints of insomnia and/or excessive daytime sleepiness and impairment in important areas of functioning and quality of life (53).

Diagnosis of CRSD requires that the sleep disruption cannot be more accurately explained by another current disorder or by the use of medication, and that the preferred pattern is sustained for at least seven days. Potential etiological factors in CRSD include behavioral, physiological, and genetic factors.

Specific Circadian Rhythm Sleep Disorders
Delayed Sleep Phase Disorder (DSPD)
DSPD is characterized by an inability to fall asleep and to wake at desired or socially acceptable times (51). The major sleep period is delayed in relation to desired sleep and wake times. Patients complain of chronic or recurrent inability to

fall asleep and wake up according to a socially acceptable schedule. However, once sleep is achieved, its quality and quantity are normal if the individual is not forced to wake earlier than desired (51). Diagnosis requires that the preferred pattern maintains a stable, albeit delayed, phase of entrainment to the 24-hour sleep–wake pattern, and is sustained for at least seven days. A delay in other circadian rhythms (e.g., core body temperature or melatonin) may also be used to determine the presence of the delayed phase.

The reported prevalence of DSPD in the general population varies. While an early proposal that DSPD is "common at all ages" (54) has been supported by more recent studies (53), others suggest its general prevalence is actually unknown (51). DSPD is estimated to occur in 2% to 10% of the children to adolescent age range (55), and in 7% to 16% of adolescents (51), demonstrating an increasing prevalence with age. In contrast to those figures, a large-scale epidemiological study of 10,000 participants in Scandinavia reported a prevalence of only 0.72% in the general population (56). However, these results may be an underestimation due to the constraints of the self-reported sleep logs that were utilized (53). DSPD appears to occur equally in both genders (53). In children and adolescents, DSPD has been associated with depression, attention-deficit/hyperactivity disorder (ADHD), and personality disorders.

Advanced Sleep Phase Disorder (ASPD)

Similarly to DSPD, ASPD patients are not able to follow a socially acceptable sleep–wake schedule, but the body's "clock" is set too early. The major sleep period is advanced in relation to desired sleep and wake times. Patients complain of a chronic or recurrent inability to fall asleep and wake up according to socially acceptable schedules. While patients feel the need to go to sleep and rise earlier than is conventional, sleep quality and duration are within normal ranges when uninterrupted (51).

The prevalence of ASPD in the general population has yet to be determined. ASPD is believed to be very rare in adolescence and young adulthood (57), affect approximately 1% of middle-aged and older adults, and increase in prevalence with age (51). The Scandinavian study of 10,000 people mentioned previously did not identify any ASPD cases (56).

Irregular Sleep–Wake Disorder

While both DSPD and ASPD are typified by sleep–wake schedules that are incongruent with environmental demands, such patients can maintain a distinct day-to-day schedule. In contrast, irregular sleep–wake disorder is characterized by a tremendously variable and idiosyncratic sleep–wake pattern. This may result in a different major sleep interval for each 24-hour period, potentially with sleep time broken into numerous shorter periods without an easily identifiable major sleep period. Sleep occurs at irregular intervals (at least three) in any given 24-hour period for at least seven days. While the sum total of these sleep periods over 24 hours may be within the normal range, sleep is in a disordered pattern (51). Irregular sleep–wake disorder is characterized by insomnia or excessive sleepiness, either alone or in combination.

Although precise prevalence rates for irregular sleep–wake disorder are unknown, it is speculated to be more common in adolescents and young adults. Irregular sleep–wake disorder has been associated with severe intellectual disabilities, blindness, and psychiatric disorders (53). Blindness limits awareness of the environment and thus interferes with the recognition of entrainment cues (58).

Free-Running Sleep Disorder

Irregular sleep–wake disorder patients are capable of entrainment to "reset" their circadian system (53). In contrast, free-running sleep disorder patients experience a variable sleep–wake schedule because their internal circadian "pacemaker" is either at odds with a 24-hour timetable, or follows a longer schedule (e.g., 25 hours) (51). The sleep–wake pattern typically becomes progressively later each day while following a period of longer than 24 hours. A diagnosis requires this drift in sleep–wake pattern to be documented for at least seven days (preferably longer to determine the daily drift) using actigraphy and sleep logs. Free-running sleep disorder patients complain of insomnia or excessive daytime sleepiness associated with an endogenous circadian sleep–wake rhythm incongruent with the exogenous 24-hour light–dark cycle.

Free-running sleep disorder appears to be quite rare in people without vision impairment, although specific prevalence rates are unknown (51). Free-running disorder, also known as non-24-hour sleep–wake disorder, is most common among the vision-impaired, as the circadian system cannot become entrained by environmental cues to follow the community's established 24-hour timetable (51).

Common Comorbidities of Circadian Rhythm Sleep Disorders in Children and Adolescents

Sleep disturbances often occur in tandem with behavioural and psychiatric disorders in children and adolescents. These relationships likely work bidirectionally in that sleep deprivation may cause changes in affect and behaviour. In turn, emotional and psychiatric problems may prompt sleep disturbances. Both relationships have been described as reciprocal, as the symptoms of each contribute to the severity and clinical presentation of the other (59–61). The exact nature of the interactions of these psychiatric comorbidities with CRSD—and whether there is a causal link—has yet to be determined empirically. A number of the most common comorbidities of CRSD will now be discussed.

Depression

Adolescents are increasingly presenting with overlapping phase delay and/or other sleep–wake disorders with depression (62). Depressed adolescents complain of difficulty falling asleep, unwillingness to wake up and/or go to school, extreme daytime sleepiness, and appear to demonstrate an increasingly delayed sleep–wake preference over time. Dahl and Lewin (62) suggest that a common conundrum for clinicians is to disentangle all the potential factors that may be contributing to the adolescent's behavior, including reduced motivation, school refusal or anxiety, difficulties in attention, delayed circadian phase, and depressive symptoms.

Bipolar Disorder

Once believed to be primarily an adult disorder, the occurrence of bipolar disorder and bipolar spectrum disorder in children and adolescents has become increasingly recognized, along with its deleterious effects within this age group (63). Literature reviews of circadian issues and bipolar disorder in adults state that while there are indications that the circadian pacemaker is involved in bipolar disorder, very little information exists regarding the influence of the circadian system upon sleep organization within bipolar disorder. Harvey et al. (64) highlighted the importance of pursuing such research, since there appears to be a high incidence of sleep difficulty in youth with bipolar disorder, and sleep is vital for emotion regulation and learning. Further understanding of the relationship between bipolar disorder and circadian dysfunction in children and adolescents is critical, as the impairment generated by bipolar disorder is of growing concern (63), and the potential amplification of impairment due to comorbid sleep problems could lead to more severe negative outcomes.

Attention-Deficit/Hyperactivity Disorder (ADHD)

DSPD is characterized by chronic inability to fall asleep at desired times, which leads to excessive daytime sleepiness.

Objective studies assessing fatigue/alertness using the Multiple Sleep Latency Test (MSLT) found that ADHD children exhibited more daytime sleepiness than controls. (65,66). The inability to fall asleep at a desired time has also been associated with ADHD, as reflected in bed-time refusal and long sleep latencies reported by parents of ADHD children. It is possible that a circadian phase delay may contribute to bedtime refusal (59) and to increased fatigue during the day in youth with ADHD. Bedtime could become aversive if a child is sent to bed before he or she feels the need to sleep due to a phase delay. Such discord may lead parents to attribute their child's conduct to disruptive behavior disorders such as ADHD, when the true culprit may be an underlying circadian disorder. Future research differentiating between symptoms specific to ADHD and circadian disorders, along with symptoms that may contribute to one another, would improve detection and treatment of such disorders.

Personality Disorders

In adults, CRSD are more common in people with personality disorders compared to those without personality disorders (67). It has been suggested that CRSD and personality disorders share diagnostic and etiological factors, in that both are characterized by a disparity between an individual's needs and behavior, and the expectations of their society (68). It was further posited that while a relationship between the two appears to exist, the causal direction of that relationship remains uncertain. It may be that having an abnormal sleep–wake pattern due to a circadian sleep disorder reinforces the disregard for societal expectations present in personality disorders. Conversely, the social and functional impairment associated with personality disorders may be aggravated by a deviant sleep–wake pattern (68). Dagan and colleagues (67) further hypothesized that the congenital misalignment of the circadian pacemaker, and the consequent divergence from societal expectations of an appropriate sleep–wake schedule, may result in emotional, social, and functional problems.

These difficulties may then intensify as a person gets older, leading to the development of a personality disorder later in life.

In adolescents, comorbidity has been demonstrated between CRSD and personality disorders in an inpatient sample (68), although that sample of 13–23 year olds included young adults. These results suggested that there was an increased prevalence of CRSD (delayed sleep phase syndrome specifically) in patients diagnosed with a personality disorder compared to patients diagnosed with any other psychiatric disorder. The applicability of those findings to the general population remains uncertain given the data were generated from a clinical sample. However, the data further suggested that the presence of delayed sleep phase disorder may play a significant role in the emergence of the functional difficulties associated with personality disorders. While no personality disorder in particular has been clearly associated with CRSD, it has been suggested that individuals with avoidant or schizoid personality disorders prefer nighttime for its seclusion (53). There appears to be a paucity of research examining the comorbidity of CRSD and personality disorders in adolescence.

Neurodevelopmental Disorders

Jan and Freeman (69) found that children with severe neurodevelopmental disorders (such as visual impairment, intellectual disabilities, and autism) have a higher prevalence of CRSD compared to children with other disabilities. In addition, while there is a positive relationship between the number of neurodevelopmental factors, and sleep disorder severity and incidence within this population of children (70), the underlying sleep disorders often appear to be unidentified or left untreated (71,72).

Jan and Freeman (69) contend that the increased CRSD prevalence in neurodevelopmental disorder patients reflects an inability to respond to environmental entrainment cues that instruct the body when to sleep. The ramifications of these maladaptive sleep–wake patterns are significant for both the child and the family since a persistent pattern of fragmented sleep may result in the development of a CRSD, with ensuing sleep deprivation. A child with a severe neurodevelopmental disability requires a great deal of family care and supervision. A concomitant circadian problem leading to sleep disruption will increase the stress on the family, resulting in a diminished ability to provide care (69).

Conclusions

The relationship between CRSD and concomitant psychiatric and behavioral disorders in children and adolescents remains inadequately understood. When circadian and psychiatric or behavioral disorders are comorbid, it is possible that one disorder may be overlooked and remain untreated due to the masking effect of the other (71,72). Considering the evident impact of both sleep disturbances and comorbid psychiatric or behavioral disorders on functioning in children and adolescents, it is necessary to determine the effect of each in order to properly identify all potential factors contributing to the individual's impairment and quality of life.

DIAGNOSIS AND TREATMENT

The aim of CRSD assessment is to characterize the abnormal sleep pattern and identify potential behavioral and psychological factors that might be contributing to its presence and exacerbation. The aim of subsequent therapy is to synchronize the circadian clock with the environmental light–dark cycle. This review will now discuss some of the most common methods of CRSD assessment and treatment.

Diagnostic Procedures
1. Obtaining Symptom Information
Patient and parent evaluations can be used to determine the presence of CRSD symptoms as defined by the *International Classification of Sleep Disorders* (revised) (51).

2. Assessment of One-Week Interval of Sleep–Wake Data
Assessments over at least seven days should be made using sleep diaries. Important data to record include clock times for "lights off" and "lights on" (to estimate the time in bed), sleep latency, number of awakenings, time spent awake after initial sleep onset, terminal time spent awake prior to arising from bed, and total sleep time. Concurrent objective verification can be obtained over this period using wrist actigraphy to gather data on patterns of estimated sleep and wakefulness (73).

3. Objective Assessment of Sleep and the Circadian Phase
Ideally, a CRSD diagnosis involves objective assessment of the circadian phase via hourly sampling of plasma or saliva to determine melatonin levels.

4. Examination of Sleep Hygiene
Detailed description of bedtime routine, caffeine or alcohol consumption, drug use, exercise habits, and the child's sleep environment should be used to determine the contribution of factors related to sleep hygiene to the presenting symptoms.

5. Assessing Comorbid Psychiatric Problems
Because of the comorbidity with psychiatric disorders, it is critical to be aware of the potential contribution of psychiatric illness. A detailed history of psychiatric symptoms and psychoactive substance use should be part of the routine evaluation (74).

6. Assessing Psychological and Emotional Factors that Might Contribute to the Presenting Symptoms
When assessing a child or adolescent for CRSD, it is necessary to distinguish a legitimate circadian problem from a school avoidance issue. Both CRSD and school avoidance can manifest as a reluctance to wake in time for school. A key to a differential diagnosis is that the child can fall asleep earlier in the night when required if experiencing school avoidance, but cannot if he or she has a CRSD (58).

Treatment
CRSD therapies aim to synchronize the circadian clock of the individual with the environmental light–dark cycle. Various therapies have been used that target either the schedule itself (chronotherapy) or the mechanisms which can reset the circadian

timing system (i.e., light, melatonin), and non-photic time cues. Changing the circadian rhythm implies major lifestyle changes, and requires the patient to sleep at times when he or she was previously alert. Therefore, treatment can be more effective if the therapist can identify motivating factors that will assist the patient in making such lifestyle changes. In addition, treatment must address other factors such as the severity of the disorder, comorbid psychopathology, ability and willingness of the patient to comply with treatment, school schedules, work obligations, and social pressures. Therefore, a multimodal treatment approach is recommended.

Chronotherapy

Chronotherapy is an intervention that targets the sleep–wake schedule. The process involves sleep and wake times being progressively delayed by approximately two to three hours every two days until an appropriate earlier bedtime and wake time has been reached, after which it is maintained (75). Since the endogenous circadian rhythm in humans is usually > 24 hours, it is generally easier to delay than to advance the sleep–wake cycle. A phase-delaying protocol should take into consideration any necessary social and work activities. Once the target bed period is achieved, it is important to ensure bright light exposure in the morning and dim light in the evening in order to maintain the desired sleep–wake schedule.

The practicality and acceptability of chronotherapy has been criticized due to its strict requirements that can be imposed on social and professional obligations, and the prolonged duration of the treatment (76). However, chronotherapy can be particularly useful in children and adolescents as it takes advantage of their natural tendency to delay sleep, thereby increasing the likelihood of success. Such success can serve as a motivating factor that encourages therapy compliance.

Phototherapy

Bright light has been successfully used to realign the circadian phase, and has been demonstrated to be effective in producing both forward (phase advance) and backward (phase delay) phase shifting. In general, DSPD patients should undergo light exposure in the morning to advance circadian rhythms, whereas ASPD patients should undergo light exposure in the evening to delay the rhythms to achieve a more appropriate sleep–wake timetable (77–81).

Ideally, core body temperature and/or plasma or salivary melatonin levels should be measured under controlled conditions to determine the initial circadian phase, and these measurements should be repeated after treatment to characterize the altered circadian phase (82). [But see Lack and Wright (83).]

Phototherapy can be associated with compliance problems as it is a demanding treatment for many children and parents. Therefore, a phototherapy treatment plan should include a behavioral component addressing the motivation and the collaborative efforts of the child.

Melatonin

Melatonin administration has been used as a means to exert phase-shifting, and as a hypnotic for relieving sleep onset insomnia in DPSD patients (84–86). Melatonin doses of 0.3 or 0.5 mg can be administered two hours prior to the estimated DLMO (dim light melatonin onset), or four hours prior to the average sleep onset time.

Despite its potential for treating some CRSD, the clinical effectiveness and guidelines for melatonin use (e.g., length of treatment, dosing parameters, and timing of administration) have not been established. Studies examining the use of exogenous melatonin to advance the circadian phase in DSPD patients have methodological flaws and provide limited and variable results. Melatonin is not approved by the Food and Drug Administration (FDA) for CRSD treatment, and its production is largely unregulated. Clearly, more studies on the long-term efficacy and safety of melatonin are required, especially with children and adolescents.

Lifestyle Changes
Coping with certain CRSD can be made easier for children by adjusting exposure to daylight, changing the timing of daily routines, and strategically scheduling naps. A well-organized and regular schedule of wake-up time, bedtime, meals, and activities is important to provide non-photic circadian cues.

Sleep Hygiene
Instructions on sleep hygiene help children to develop healthy sleeping habits and assist in diminishing the exacerbation of additional problems.

The following cases from our outpatient clinic are presented as examples of circadian problems in children and adolescents.

Example 1
MK was a 12-year-old female referred by an ADHD clinic. She was an average student with daytime difficulties in terms of attention and self-organization. MK had been diagnosed with ADHD combined type (DSM-IV) at the age of seven years, and had since been treated with stimulant medication which improved her ability to remain focused and alert. However, she was constantly tired during the day and had difficulty falling asleep before 12 a.m. to 1 a.m. There was parental concern about school functioning and the health effects of constant tiredness. She was extremely difficult to wake in the morning, and her mood was often bad, particularly in the mornings. As a result, mornings were very stressful for the family.

She was assessed using an Actiwatch coupled with a sleep diary for three weeks. The data confirmed a delayed bedtime (between 12 a.m. and 1 a.m. 80% of the time), and both parent and self reports indicated daytime sleepiness. The diagnosis was Delayed Sleep Phase Disorder.

The patient was advised to perform half-an-hour of bright light therapy (BLT) daily for one week between 6:00 and 7:00 a.m. BLT was recommended using a portable light box that emitted full-spectrum visible light (10,000 lux at a distance of 60 cm). Despite attempts over two weeks, she was not able to comply with the therapy and the sleep patterns remained unchanged. A therapist then assessed her motivation, discussed with her the treatment plan, explained circadian system physiology, the necessity of light therapy, and the expected benefits. She was then given the freedom to continue trying the therapy or not. She chose to continue but with no parental involvement. Daily updates and weekly follow-up sessions were scheduled. The patient consistently complied with the light therapy and scheduled bedtime. At the end of the two-week intervention, bedtime had advanced to 10.30 p.m., sleep latency had become significantly shorter, mornings became more manageable and daytime fatigue was significantly reduced. The mother reported a positive change in mood, and that mornings had become less stressful for the family. Follow up after three months confirmed the new schedule had been maintained.

Example 2
PL was a six-year-old boy brought to our clinic by his parents who were concerned by his daytime sleepiness. He was assessed for two weeks using Actiwatch coupled with a sleep diary. The data revealed an early bedtime (around 7.00 p.m. every night) and a very early wake up time (between 4 and 5 a.m. every morning). The parent and self reports showed a high degree of daytime sleepiness. The diagnosis was Advanced Sleep Phase Disorder.

BLT was recommended using a portable light box that emitted full-spectrum visible light (10,000 lux at a distance of 60 cm) daily for two weeks between 6 and 7 p.m. The patient was fully compliant. By the end of therapy the wakeup time had been delayed by two hours. PL was far more alert during the day, and was able to interact with his siblings and take part in evening family time, which was reinforcing as it provided positive interactions. Mood improved, as did the ability to interact socially.

CONCLUSION

In conclusion, the circadian system evolves continuously throughout development. Basic mechanisms within these systems are intimately connected to the individual's regulation of sleep and arousal, and should these mechanisms be disrupted or thrown off course, there may be considerable ramifications upon development, functioning, and the occurrence of psychiatric and/or behavioral disorders.

Consequently, the treatment of individuals presenting with sleep, psychiatric, and behavioral disorders must be chosen based upon an understanding of the interactions among the underlying systems, with an appreciation for the impact of these systems in the presentation and exacerbation of symptoms.

REFERENCES

1. Moore RY, Eichler VB. Loss of a circadian adrenal corticosterone rhythm following suprachiasmatic lesions in the rat. Brain Res 1972; 42(1):201–6.
2. Dunlap JC. Molecular bases for circadian clocks. Cell 1999; 96(2):271–90.
3. Czeisler CA, Duffy JF, Shanahan TL, et al. Stability, precision, and near-24-hour period of the human circadian pacemaker. Science 1999; 284(5423):2177–81.
4. Moore RY. A clock for the ages. Science 1999; 284(5423):2102–3.
5. Czeisler CA, Allan JS, Strogatz SH, et al. Bright light resets the human circadian pacemaker independent of the timing of the sleep-wake cycle. Science 1986; 233(4764):667–71.
6. Ebadi M, Govitrapong P. Neural pathways and neurotransmitters affecting melatonin synthesis. J Neural Transm Suppl 1986; 21:125–55.
7. Allada R, White NE, So WV, et al. A mutant Drosophila homolog of mammalian clock disrupts circadian rhythms and transcription of period and timeless. Cell 1998; 93(5):791–804.
8. Blau J, Young MW. Cycling vrille expression is required for a functional Drosophila clock. Cell 1999; 99(6):661–71.

9. Kloss B, Price JL, Saez L, et al. The Drosophila clock gene double-time encodes a protein closely related to human casein kinase Iepsilon. Cell 1998; 94(1):97–107.
10. Myers MP, Wager-Smith K, Wesley CS, et al. Positional cloning and sequence analysis of the Drosophila clock gene, timeless. Science 1995; 270(5237):805–8.
11. Rutila JE, Suri V Le M, et al. CYCLE is a second bHLH-PAS clock protein essential for circadian rhythmicity and transcription of Drosophila period and timeless. Cell 1998; 93(5):805–14.
12. Lu BS, Zee PC. Circadian rhythm sleep disorders. Chest 2006; 130(6):1915–23.
13. Reppert SM, Weaver DR. Coordination of circadian timing in mammals. Nature 2002; 418(6901):935–41.
14. Korf HW, Schomerus C, Stehle JH. The pineal organ, its hormone melatonin and the photoneuroendocrine system. Adv Anat Embryol Cell Biol 1998; 146:1–100.
15. Ross WA, Morgan PJ. The pars tuberalis as a target of the central clock. Cell Tissue Res 2002; 309(1):163–71.
16. Morgan PJ, Barrett H, Howell E, et al. Melatonin receptors: Localization, molecular pharmacology and physiological significance. Neurochem Int 1994; 24(2):101–46.
17. Arendt J. Melatonin: Characteristics, concerns, and prospects. J Biol Rhythms 2005; 20(4):291–303.
18. Lerchl A. Biological rhythms in the context of light at night (LAN). Neuro Endocrinol Lett 2002; Suppl 2:23–7.
19. Morin LP, Allen CN. The circadian visual system, 2005. Brain Res Rev 2006; 51(1):1–60.
20. Hannibal J. Neurotransmitters of the retino-hypothalamic tract. Cell Tissue Res 2002; 309(1):73–88.
21. Moore RY, Speh JC, Leak RK. Suprachiasmatic nucleus organization. Cell Tissue Res 2002; 309(1):89–98.
22. Chou TC, Scammell TE, Gooley JJ, et al. Critical role of dorsomedial hypothalamic nucleus in a wide range of behavioral circadian rhythms. J Neurosci 2003; 23(33):10691–702.
23. Moore RY, Danchenko RL. Paraventricular-subparaventricular hypothalamic lesions affect circadian functions. Chronobiol Int 2002; 19(2):345–60.
24. Buijs RM, van Eden CG, Goncharuk VD, et al. The biological clock tunes the organs of the body: Timing by hormones and the autonomic nervous system. J Endocrinol 2003; 177(1):17–26.
25. Gachon F, Nagoshi E, Brown SA, et al. The mammalian circadian timing system: From gene expression to physiology. Chromosoma 2004; 113(3):103–12.
26. Reppert SM, Weaver DR, Rivkees SA, et al. Putative melatonin receptors in a human biological clock. Science 1988; 242(4875):78–81.
27. Mirmiran M, Swaab DF, Kok JH, et al. Circadian rhythms and the suprachiasmatic nucleus in perinatal development, aging and Alzheimer's disease. Progr Brain Res 1992; 93:151–62.
28. Reppert SM, Schwartz WJ. Maternal coordination of the fetal biological clock in utero. Science 1983; 220(4600):969–71.
29. Sladek M, Sumova A, Kovacikova Z, et al. Insight into molecular core clock mechanism of embryonic and early postnatal rat suprachiasmatic nucleus. Proc Natl Acad Sci USA 2004; 101(16):6231–6.
30. Moore RY. Development of the suprachiasmatic nucleus. In: Klein DC, Moore RY, Reppert SM, eds. Suprachiasmatic Nucleus: The Mind's Clock. New York: Oxford University Press, 1991: pp. 391–404.
31. Reppert SM, Schwartz WJ. The suprachiasmatic nuclei of the fetal rat: Characterization of a functional circadian clock using 14C-labeled deoxyglucose. J Neurosci 1984; 4(7):1677–82.
32. Fuchs JL, Moore RY. Development of circadian rhythmicity and light responsiveness in the rat suprachiasmatic nucleus: A study using the 2-deoxy[1-14C]glucose method. Proc Natl Acad Sci USA 1980; 77(2):1204–8.

33. Ohta H, Honma S, Abe H, et al. Effects of nursing mothers on rPer1 and rPer2 circadian expressions in the neonatal rat suprachiasmatic nuclei vary with developmental stage. Eur J Neurosci 2002; 15(12):1953–60.
34. Damiola F, Le Minh N, Preitner N, et al. Restricted feeding uncouples circadian oscillators in peripheral tissues from the central pacemaker in the suprachiasmatic nucleus. Genes Dev 2000; 14(23):2950–61.
35. Wakamatsu H, Yoshinobu Y, Aida R, et al. Restricted feeding-induced anticipatory activity rhythm is associated with a phase-shift of the expression of MPer1 and MPer2 MRNA in the cerebral cortex and hippocampus but not in the suprachiasmatic nucleus of mice. Eur J Neurosci 2001; 13(6):1190–6.
36. Maywood ES, Mrosovsky N, Field MD, et al. Rapid down-regulation of mammalian period genes during behavioral resetting of the circadian clock. Proc Natl Acad Sci USA 1999; 96(26):15211–16.
37. Davis KF, Parker KP, Montgomery GL. Sleep in infants and young children: Part one: Normal sleep. J Pediatr Health Care 2004; 18(2):65–71.
38. Roffwarg HP, Muzio JN, Dement WC. Ontogenetic development of the human sleep-dream cycle. Science 1966; 152(3722):604–19.
39. Anders TF, Sadeh A, Appareddy V. Normal sleep in neonates and children. In: Ferber R, Kryger M, eds. Principles and Practice of Sleep Medicine in the Child. Philadelphia: W. B. Saunders Company, 1995: pp. 7–18.
40. Sheldon SH. Sleep in infants and children. In: Lee-Chiong TL, Sateia MJ, Carskadon MA, eds. Sleep Medicine, Philadelphia: Hanley & Belfus, Inc, 2002: pp. 99–103.
41. Weissbluth M. Naps in children: 6 months-7 years. Sleep 1995; 18(2):82–7.
42. Wolfson A. Sleeping patterns of children and adolescents: Developmental trends, disruptions, and adaptations. In: Dahl RE, ed. Sleep Disorders (Child and Adolescent Psychiatric Clinics of North America) 5(3), Philadelphia: WB Saunders, 1996: pp. 549–68.
43. Carskadon MA. Patterns of sleep and sleepiness in adolescents. Pediatrician 1990; 17(1):5–12.
44. Carskadon MA, Viera C, Acebo C. Association between puberty and delayed phase preference. Sleep 1993; 16(3):258–62.
45. Carskadon MA, Acebo C. Regulation of sleepiness in adolescents: Update, insights, and speculation. Sleep 2002; 25(6):606–14.
46. Dahl RE, Lewin DS. Pathways to adolescent health: Sleep regulation and behavior. J Adolesc Health 2002; 31(6 Suppl):175–84.
47. Carskadon MA. Sleep and circadian rhythms in children and adolescents: Relevance for athletic performance of young people. Clin Sports Med 2005; 24(2):319–28.
48. Saarenpaa-Heikkila OA, Rintahaka PJ, Laippala PJ, et al. Sleep habits and disorders in Finnish schoolchildren. J Sleep Res 1995; 4(3):173–82.
49. Andrade MM, Benedito-Silva AA, Domenice S, et al. Sleep characteristics of adolescents: A longitudinal study. J Adolesc Health 1993; 14(5):401–6.
50. Edgar DM, Dement WC, Fuller CA. Effect of SCN lesions on sleep in squirrel monkeys: Evidence for opponent processes in sleep-wake regulation. J Neurosci 1993; 13(3):1065–79.
51. Circadian rhythm sleep disorders. In: The International Classification of Sleep Disorders: Diagnostic & Coding Manual, 2nd edn Westchester, IL: American Academy of Sleep Medicine, 2005: pp. 117–28.
52. Diagnostic and statistical manual of mental disorders, 4th ed. Washington, D.C.: American Psychiatric Association, 1994.
53. Silber MH, Krahn LE, Morgenthaler TI. Circadian rhythm disorders. In: Silber MH, Krahn LE, Morgenthaler TI, eds. Sleep Medicine in Clinical Practice. London: Taylor & Francis, 2004: pp. 253–76.
54. Ferber R. Sleeplessness, night awakening, and night crying in the infant and toddler. Pediatr Rev 1987; 9(3):69–82.
55. Herman JH. Circadian rhythm disorders in infants, children, and adolescents. In: Lee-Chiong TL, ed. Sleep: A Comprehensive Handbook. New York: John Wiley & Sons, Inc., 2006: pp. 589–95.

56. Schrader H, Bovim G, Sand T. The prevalence of delayed and advanced sleep phase syndromes. J Sleep Res 1993; 2(1):51–5.
57. Ando K, Kripke DF, Ancoli-Israel S. Estimated prevalence of delayed and advanced sleep phase syndromes. Sleep Res 1995; 24, 509.
58. Kotagal S. Sleep disorders in childhood. Neurol Clin N Am 2003; 21(4):961–81.
59. Owens JA, Davis KF. Sleep in children with behavioural and psychiatric disorders. In: Lee-Chiong TL, ed. Sleep: A Comprehensive Handbook. New York: John Wiley & Sons, Inc., 2006: pp. 581–7.
60. Reite M. Sleep disorders presenting as psychiatric disorders. Psychiatr Clin North Am 1998; 21(3):591–607.
61. Jones S, Benca RM. Psychiatric disorders associated with circadian rhythm disorders. In: Lee-Chiong TL, ed. Sleep: A Comprehensive Handbook. New York: John Wiley & Sons, Inc., 2006: pp. 409–14.
62. Dahl RE, Lewin DS. Pathways to adolescent health: Sleep regulation and behaviour. J Adolesc Health 2002; 31(6 Suppl):175–84.
63. Geller B, DelBello MP. Bipolar Disorder in Childhood and Early Adolescence. New York: Guilford Press, 2003.
64. Harvey AG, Mullin BC, Hinshaw SP. Sleep and circadian rhythms in children and adolescents with bipolar disorder. Dev Psychopathol 2006; 18(4):1147–68.
65. Golan N, Shahar E, Ravid S, et al. Sleep disorders and daytime sleepiness in children with attention-deficit/hyperactive disorder. Sleep 2004; 27(2):261–6.
66. Lecendreux M, Konofal E, Bouvard M, et al. Sleep and alertness in children with ADHD. J Child Psychol Psychiatry 2000; 41(6):803–12.
67. Dagan Y, Sela H, Omer H, et al. High prevalence of personality disorders among circadian rhythm sleep disorder (CRSD) patients. J Psychosom Res 1996; 41(4):357–63.
68. Dagan Y, Stein D, Steinbock M, et al. Frequency of delayed sleep phase syndrome among hospitalized adolescent psychiatric patients. J Psychosom Res 1998; 45(1 Spec No):15–20.
69. Jan JE, Freeman RD. Melatonin therapy for circadian rhythm sleep disorders in children with multiple disabilities: What have we learned in the last decade? Dev Med Child Neurol 2004; 46(11):776–82.
70. Lindblom N, Heiskala H, Kaski M, et al. Neurologic impairments and sleep-wake behavior among the mentally retarded. J Sleep Res 2001; 10(4):309–18.
71. Stores G. Sleep studies in children with a mental handicap. J Child Psychol Psychiatry 1992; 33(8):1303–17.
72. Stores G. Children's sleep disorders: Modern approaches, developmental effects, and children at special risk. Dev Med Child Neurol 1999; 41(8):568–73.
73. Ancoli-Israel S, Cole R, Alessi C, et al. The role of actigraphy in the study of sleep and circadian rhythms. Sleep 2003; 26(3):342–92.
74. Dagan Y, Borodkin K. Behavioral and psychiatric consequences of sleep-wake schedule disorders. Dialogues Clin Neurosci 2005; 7(4):357–65.
75. Weitzman ED, Czeisler CA, Coleman RM, et al. Delayed sleep phase syndrome: A chronobiological disorder with sleep-onset insomnia. Arch Gen Psychiatry 1981; 38(7):737–46.
76. Wyatt JK. Delayed sleep phase syndrome: Pathophysiology and treatment options. Sleep 2004; 27(6):1195–203.
77. Chesson AL, Littner M, Davila D, et al. Practice parameters for the use of light therapy in the treatment of sleep disorders. Standards of Practice Committee, American Academy of Sleep Medicine. Sleep 1999; 22(5):641–60.
78. Lack LC, Wright HR, Kemp K, et al. The treatment of early-morning awakening insomnia with 2 evenings of bright light. Sleep 2005; 28(5):616–23.
79. Campbell SS, Dawson D, Anderson MW. Alleviation of sleep maintenance insomnia with timed exposure to bright light. J Am Geriatr Soc 1993; 41(8):829–36.
80. Murphy PJ, Campbell SS. Enhanced performance in elderly subjects following bright light treatment of sleep maintenance insomnia. J Sleep Res 1996; 5(3):165–72.

81. Lack LC, Wright HR. The effect of evening bright light in delaying the circadian rhythms and lengthening the sleep of early morning awakening insomniacs. Sleep 1993; 16(5):436–43.
82. McArthur AJ, Lewy AJ, Sack RL. Non-24-hour sleep-wake syndrome in a sighted man: Circadian rhythm studies and efficacy of melatonin treatment. Sleep 1996; 19(7):544–53.
83. Lack LC, Wright HR. Treating chronobiological components of chronic insomnia. Sleep Med 2007; 8(6):637–44.
84. Skene DJ, Arendt J. Human circadian rhythms: Physiological and therapeutic relevance of light and melatonin. Ann Clin Biochem 2006; 43(Pt 5):344–53.
85. Arendt J. Melatonin and human rhythms. Chronobiol Int 2006; 23(1–2):21–37.
86. Lewy AJ, Ahmed S, Sack RL. Phase shifting the human circadian clock using melatonin. Behav Brain Res 1996; 73(1–2):131–4.

7 School Start Time and Its Impact on Learning and Behavior

Edward B. O'Malley[a] and Mary B. O'Malley[b]

[a]Sleep Disorders Center, Norwalk Hospital, Norwalk, Connecticut, U.S.A. and NYU School of Medicine, New York, New York, U.S.A.
[b]Sleep Disorders Center, Norwalk Hospital, Norwalk, Connecticut, U.S.A. and NYU Department of Psychiatry, New York, New York, U.S.A.

INTRODUCTION

Following the U.S. baby boom in the 1960s, schools not only increased in number but educators also began to experiment with staggered class schedules to accommodate the influx of new students. As other social, economic, and politico–legal pressures converged, school start times, particularly for the older high school students, gradually migrated to earlier hours (1). By 1975 most U.S. high schools started as early as 8:00 a.m. and school systems throughout the Western world, under similar pressures, eventually followed suit (2). Consequently, increasing societal demands promoted by a 24/7 culture over the past three decades have contributed to even earlier school start times for both middle and high school students (3); (Fig. 1).

Based on early sleep research, it initially appeared that after birth the number of sleep hours needed per day would decline steadily during childhood development, and level off at about eight hours needed per night during puberty and through adulthood. Instead, the past twenty-five years of laboratory and field research have shown that the need for sleep in children does not decline from age 10 to 17 years of age, but remains at nine hours or more per night during the explosion of growth and other body changes of puberty. In addition, the work of Wolfson and colleagues (4) has shown that puberty brings on a biological delay in the circadian timing of sleep, making the preferred sleep onset time for most adolescents after 11 p.m. These adolescent biological sleep needs, as well as psychosocial pressures to remain awake later at night, clash with early school start times, leading to the net result that adolescents get significantly less than the optimal 9.2 hours of sleep per night, particularly during school nights (5–7). A 2006 poll conducted by the National Sleep Foundation on 1600 adolescents nationwide found that more than half (56%) of teenagers report getting less sleep than they need to feel rested during the school week (8). The often serious impact of this chronic under-sleeping is now evident in both high school and middle school students.

For all students one of the most salient—and correctable—social factors contributing to student sleep deprivation, is school start times. This chapter will review the developmental sleep needs of adolescents, the accumulated evidence documenting sleep deprivation imposed by earlier school start times, and its detrimental effect on learning and behavior. Finally, this chapter will discuss the positive impact on students' health that delaying school start times has demonstrated in several communities across the U.S.

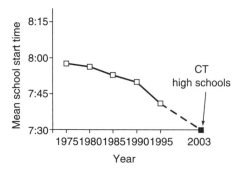

FIGURE 1   Average scheduled start times of high schools in Providence, Rhode Island school districts through 1995 (2), and in Fairfield County, Connecticut through 2003.

DEVELOPMENTAL SLEEP NEEDS IN ADOLESCENTS

The first longitudinal study of sleep need in adolescents took place at the Stanford Sleep Disorders Center "summer sleep camp" conducted by Drs. Mary Carskadon and William Dement, in the late 1970s. Pre-pubertal children aged 10–12 years were evaluated prospectively during consecutive summers over the course of four to six years. Biological age was determined by Tanner stage (assessment of appearance of secondary sex characteristics as indicator of pubertal stage) to insure uniformity of developmental groups. Notably, nocturnal sleep studies were designed to allow a maximum time in bed of up to 10 hours because prior research had established on average a maximum 10-hour sleep requirement for this age group. The chief hypothesis was that as children matured, sleep need would decrease until reaching a nadir of eight hours sleep, the adult requirement. Both diurnal and nocturnal sleep was assessed with polysomnography. In contrast to the expected result, not only did pubertal children require more sleep than predicted, but they demonstrated significant daytime sleepiness despite even 9–10 hours of sleep at night (5), consistent with a higher incidence of sleep deprivation. One manifestation of this was that a greater number of older adolescents than young adolescents had to be awakened as the 10-hour time in-bed limit was reached. Optimal sleep length in adolescents was shown to be 9.2 hours per night (9). No gender differences in sleep patterns were observed in these early studies.

Additional research over the past twenty-five years has reinforced and extended these initial findings. Laboratory studies confirmed the need for 9–10 hours in older adolescents (10). Comparative studies have identified some differences in sleep practices and challenges among adolescents from 11 European countries (11), but the underlying biological sleep need appears to be relatively constant among growing children everywhere.

Normal adolescent sleep is an essential physiologic component of healthy development. The huge changes in body development during adolescence are directly linked to the sleep process. Growth hormone is released in conjunction with slow-wave sleep during the night, and the development of secondary sex characteristics also depends upon the secretion of the gonadotrophic hormones during sleep (12). These critical physiological processes are highly conserved, but can be significantly affected in situations that alter adolescent sleep patterns such as sleep deprivation, illness, or the use of substances or certain medications. In addition, normal sleep appears to serve a vital role in learning new skills, both by fostering memory encoding and consolidation (13), and by facilitating the generation of insight that solves complex problems (14). Getting adequate dream (rapid eye movement [REM]) sleep is essential to perceptual, cognitive, and emotional processing. Selective REM sleep deprivation has been demonstrated to cause symptoms of irritability and moodiness, as well as problems with memory (15). The issue of under-sleeping in adolescents takes on added significance when one considers that waking up too early costs the sleeper mostly REM sleep which predominates during the last two to three hours of a night's sleep.

CIRCADIAN BIOLOGY OF SLEEP IN ADOLESCENCE

Many parents and teachers become frustrated that adolescents seem to create their own problem of not getting enough sleep by choosing a late bedtime, despite their complaints of sleepiness in the morning. However, there are multiple factors that contribute to later bedtimes, and it is increasingly clear that adolescents stay awake later largely for biological, not social, reasons. As with adults, the physiological factor that most powerfully regulates the timing of waking and sleeping in adolescents is the circadian rhythm, a hard-wired "clock" in the suprachiasmatic nucleus (SCN) of the brain (16). The SCN determines whether one is an "evening-type" or a "morning-type" by setting the timing of wakefulness relative to exposure to morning sunlight. In addition to determining the timing of wakefulness, the circadian rhythm system also *drives* alertness increasingly throughout the day, right up until the biological bedtime, when this drive for alertness is withdrawn (Fig. 2). This circadian-dependent wakefulness allows extended periods of waking despite rising levels of sleepiness as the day progresses (17). This underlying physiology is very clear from many lines of research in humans, and other animals with similar circadian biology (18).

In 1993, Carskadon and colleagues (19) demonstrated that more mature self-reported pubertal ratings in sixth-grade girls was associated with a delay in circadian sleep timing as evident in increasingly greater "eveningness" scores. Subsequent studies more precisely demonstrated that advancing Tanner stage of puberty evokes a delay in the secretion of melatonin by about an hour (2). These findings indicate that a change in the biological system regulating circadian timing appears to accompany puberty, which prompts later timing of sleep seen during adolescence. This puberty-linked delay in sleep timing has been confirmed in studies of children in Japan (20), Brazil (21) and Australia (22).

The circadian rhythm also underlies the common problem of "Sunday night insomnia." Sleeping-in on weekend mornings tends to shift the underlying circadian rhythm to even later timing, making it more difficult to reset the circadian clock for early school rise times on Monday morning (2). Thus, teens who regularly sleep in over the weekend will likely experience a harder time waking for school on Monday, and greater performance impairments during the morning as they struggle with alertness, especially early in the week.

The fact that teens' late bedtime is a reflection of their biology rather than a social choice is illustrated by data collected on the sleep habits of young recruits to the U.S. Navy (23). In 2000, the young men (predominantly ages 17–19) at the

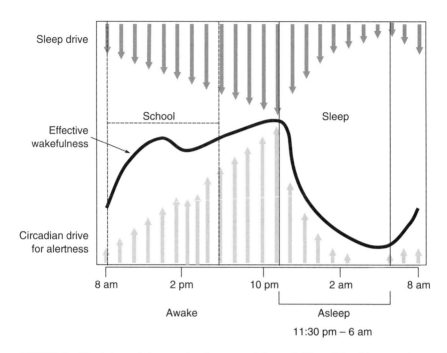

FIGURE 2 Physiology of sleep and wake in an adolescent. Sleep Drive (downward arrows) is the physiologic pressure to return to sleep that begins to build upon waking from sleep. This drive is satisfied by normal sleep, and reduced to near zero at the end of a full night's sleep. If less than a full night's sleep occurs, residual sleep drive (a.k.a., sleep debt) remains upon waking, and is carried forward along with the additional sleepiness that builds normally during wakefulness. The effect of the sleep drive is opposed by the increasing Circadian Drive for Alertness (upward arrows), which increases in intensity as the day progresses, with a short mid-afternoon lessening (the "siesta"). The onset timing of the Circadian Drive is cued by the brain's circadian rhythm pacemaker, the suprachiasmatic nucleus (SCN), a hard-wired pacemaker that determines whether one is an "evening-type" or 'morning-type'. Note that the Alerting Drive is maximally effective in the evening up until the biologic bedtime when the support for alertness is rapidly withdrawn, allowing night time sleep to occur. The cumulative effect of both these opposing drives manifests as one's Effective Wakefulness. In this example, biologic bedtime allows sleep onset by 11:30 p.m. and Sleep Drive is not fully satisfied (residual sleepiness remaining) by the early rise time of 6:00 a.m. Note also that the Effective Wakefulness in this teen is low at school start time of 8:00 a.m., rising rapidly to more effective levels by 10–11 a.m.. Adapted from Ref. (24).

Navy's academically and physically demanding training camp were scheduled to sleep from 10:00 p.m. to 4:00 a.m., allowing only six hours of sleep. To address visible signs of sleepiness among the men, in 2001 Navy officials added another hour of "rack time": from 9:00 p.m. to 4:00 a.m.. Though the young recruits were forced to retire at 9:00 p.m., they were not able to fall asleep despite lying quietly in their dark bunks because they simply felt "awake." Like other teens, these young men could not override their circadian-dependent sleep schedule even if commanded to do so. However, the following year, when sleep hours were shifted to 10:00 p.m. to 6:00 a.m., not only were the recruits able to fall asleep more easily but

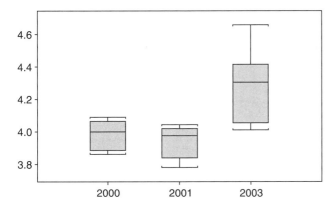

FIGURE 3 Grade averages for standardized test (ASVAB) scores of students at U.S. Naval training academy during years with schedule allowing six hours of night time sleep 3.97 (2000) and 3.94 (2001); and after scheduled night time sleep was increased to eight hours per night 4.28 (2003). (Attrites removed; p-value = 0.0004). Figure adapted from Ref. (25).

the added hours of sleep made a dramatic impact on their daytime performance. The average standardized test scores increased significantly when recruits were scheduled to allow eight hours of sleep at conducive times (Fig. 3). In addition, the number of "sick calls" decreased by 70%, and the rate of attrition decreased by half when the recruits were allowed more time for sleep.

The circadian biology of sleep would predict that among individual children, those who are predisposed to be "night owls" would be even more likely to suffer the consequences of sleepiness in a school system that imposes start times before 9 a.m. A recent, comprehensive survey of 6331 14–18-year-old students in Italy examined the role of individual circadian preferences on sleep symptoms and school performance utilizing the validated "Morningness/Eveningness Questionnaire" (26). As expected, students with the trait of "eveningness" were significantly more likely to report later bedtime and wake-up time, especially on weekends. As a result, this group also reported more irregular sleep–wake schedules, and subjectively poorer sleep than their "morning-type" counterparts. Moreover, evening types napped more frequently during school days, complained of daytime sleepiness, and had more behavioral and psychiatric comorbidities. This chronotype also reported greater use of caffeine-containing beverages and substances to promote sleep. No significant sex differences were reported in the eveningness scores of the students studied, consistent with the gender-neutral biology of circadian rhythm systems. This data confirmed earlier results from studies showing that students with an evening-type circadian preference had more difficulty adjusting to earlier start times and got less total sleep than their morning-type peers (27–29). These studies demonstrate the significant impact that underlying circadian rhythm biology can have on adolescent students, especially those whose individual biology is even less suited to early school start times.

In brief, there are two features of the circadian rhythm especially important to understand regarding sleep in teenagers: (1) the drowsy signal that cues bedtime is dependent on the dampening of circadian-dependent alertness; and (2) the physiology of puberty causes a shift in the circadian rhythm which delays the timing of this biological bedtime by about an hour. These two biological factors underlie the main difficulties faced by adolescents attending school before 9:00 a.m.: the general problem that one cannot easily fall asleep before their biological bedtime, and the additional problem that puberty creates a tendency for even later bedtimes.

ADOLESCENT SLEEP BEHAVIOR

As children move through puberty, common behavioral changes affecting sleep patterns have been observed. A recent large study compared the sleep habits of children in the U.S. and China, in grades 1–4 with the Children's Sleep Habits Questionnaire (CHSQ). U.S. children reported sleeping an age-appropriate amount of 10.15 hours per night, with average bedtime of 8:46 p.m. and rise time of 7:00 a.m. (30). Interestingly, children of the same age in China reported an hour less of sleep per night (9.25 hours), due to half-hour later bedtime and half-hour earlier rise time, and had higher rates of sleepiness symptoms such as "hard time getting out of bed," though on the whole were rather well-rested. The authors note that children in China routinely take 30 minutes to one-hour naps at lunch time which were not assessed as part of this study, but attributed the decreased night time sleep observed to cultural pressures (smaller living spaces, co-sleeping with parents) and earlier elementary school start time. This study also demonstrated that for both children in the U.S. and China, total sleep time decreased progressively as children matured due to later bedtimes.

Research surveys of adolescent sleep behavior have consistently shown that teens generally obtain significantly less sleep than younger children despite their continued need for 9–10 hours of sleep at night (5,6,31,32). Wolfson and Carskadon (6) reported after measuring total sleep time in over 3000 Rhode Island high school students ages 13–19, that the mean total sleep time on school nights for all the children was well below the 9.2 hours per night needed: sleep per night was only 7 hours 42 minutes among 13-year-olds, and decreased to 7 hours 4 minutes among the oldest children. The sleep loss was due to increasingly later bedtimes in older teens with rise times remaining constant (reflecting school start times). Surprisingly, 45% of 10th to 12th graders went to bed after midnight on school nights and 90% reported going to bed later than midnight on weekends. Weekend sleep time was greater, but average weekend total sleep decreased from 9 hours 20 minutes in the youngest children to 8 hours 38 minutes in the oldest teens. Notably, few differences were found between male and female high school students' sleep/wake patterns. Surprisingly, the sleep timing of the teens studied was consistent across a broad range of socioeconomic backgrounds among the participating schools, suggesting that their bedtime reflected factor(s) common to the group as a whole, such as their underlying biology.

On the other hand, surveys consistently demonstrate that teens are often busy with activities in the evenings. Recent studies have begun to clarify when, and to what extent these activities are responsible for postponing bedtime beyond an adolescent's biologically-driven sleep timing. Teens spend increasing amounts of time with out-of-school activities as they get older and face mounting academic pressure as well. Many students also choose to take on part-time jobs after school. Carskadon (33) demonstrated that 11th and 12th grade students who work 20 hours or more per week at part-time jobs report more problems getting adequate sleep, and problems being alert in school. Further, Wolfson (34) found that for every 10 hours per week of part-time work, a student lost an average of 14 minutes of sleep per night. These studies show that students who cut short their sleep due to work hours were significantly more likely to report drowsiness while driving, school tardiness, and substance abuse. A growing number of high school students enter the workforce during the school year, and the increasing pressures of consumerism make it likely that this trend will only continue.

In addition to scheduled hours for study, extracurricular events, and work, teens are increasingly surrounded by electronic devices and other activities that can interfere with getting to bed "on time." Though young children depend upon their caretakers to provide an appropriate environment, regular bedtimes, and other habits that promote good sleep, teens must begin to employ these habits for themselves. A few research studies have examined the impact of adolescents' sleep hygiene practices on their night sleep. In Canada, a survey of over 3000 high school students found that bedtime habits such as staying up late or drinking caffeinated beverages before bed were significantly associated with sleep debt and excessive daytime sleepiness (35). As sleepiness scores (Epworth Sleepiness Scale scores of > 10) increased in these teens, there was an increase in the proportion of students who felt their grades had dropped because of sleepiness, were late for school, were often extremely sleepy at school, and were involved in fewer extracurricular activities.

An even more detailed evaluation of sleep hygiene in teens has been contributed by LeBourgeois and colleagues in their comparative study of 12–17-year-old students from Hattiesburg, Mississippi and Rome, Italy (36). This study utilized adolescent-specific sleep assessment tools (the Adolescent Sleep Hygiene Scale, ASHS; and the Adolescent Sleep–Wake Scale, ASWS) to identify specific sleep habits and their effects on measures of sleep quality. Teens answered questions about their sleep behaviors in the past month, and rated the frequency of any problems with their sleep quality, where good sleep quality was defined as: one goes to bed easily at bedtime, transitions effortlessly from wakefulness to sleep, maintains undisturbed sleep, re-initiates sleep after nocturnal arousal, and transitions easily from sleep to wakefulness in the morning. Interestingly, the Italian adolescents reported significantly higher sleep quality and better sleep hygiene practices than the Americans. U.S. students were more likely to report problems with sleep due to physiological factors (e.g., being very active before bedtime, going to bed hungry), and cognitive factors (e.g., going to bed after playing video games). Notably, U.S. students had substantially higher rates of medical illnesses and use of medications than the Italian students, though it was not clear how much this contributed to their poorer sleep measures. Though the two populations had significant racial differences (Italian 99% Caucasian vs. U.S. 78% black students), the authors found that this did not appear to account for the variance in sleep quality. Rather, sleep measures corresponded most closely to individual reports of sleep hygiene practices. However, the authors add that better sleep hygiene observed in Italian teens may have been influenced by the cultural tendency for comparatively more parental supervision in the older students. Indeed, self-report data on bedtimes in U.S. children demonstrate that the percentage of students who report a "parent" is the reason for the time they went to bed on school nights decreased from 50% among 10–11-year-olds, to less than 5% among 14–18 year olds (37).

Adolescents often sleep later on weekend mornings to "catch up" on sleep, but also tend to choose even later bedtimes as well. This well-known behavioral pattern creates a weekday/weekend discrepancy in sleep timing that makes Sunday night bedtimes even more difficult. Petta et al. (38) demonstrated more than 20 years ago that children averaged 30–60 minutes more sleep on weekends as 10–14-year-olds and this difference increases to over two hours of "catch-up sleep" by age 18. This pattern of rising sleep debt during the week followed by weekend catch-up still leaves most teens sleep-deprived by an estimated 10 hours sleep per week.

A recent study of teens in Busan, Korea demonstrates a more extreme example of behaviorally-induced sleep deprivation (39). Using the School Sleep Habits Survey among children from grades five to 12, mean school night sleep time was found to be eight hours or more for 5th and 6th graders but dropped to an appalling 4.86 hours a night for 12th graders! The authors found that school night sleep time was "dramatically shortened" when students entered high school in 10th grade (mean school night sleep time 6.02 hours). Though the high school's earlier school start time contributed to the problem, the intense competition for college entrance exams coupled with other cultural factors appeared to be the main impetus for older students' sleep restriction. Mean bedtime hours for these Korean adolescents was 12:54 a.m. in 11th and 12th grade, and many students reported self-imposed added study time, along with part-time jobs as contributing factors. Though weekend sleeping-in was apparent, it was not nearly enough to make up for the serious under-sleeping found in these students.

Adolescents are developmentally challenged with learning to make good choices for themselves, (and hopefully to embrace parental guidelines, much as they may desire to rebel against them), and in the realm of sleep habits there are many choices that can interfere with a teen's sleep. Several recent studies have shown that adolescents have a general lack of knowledge about sleep and healthy sleep habits in the U.S. and abroad (40,41). However, an intervention-education program to teach healthy sleep habits to middle-school students has been shown to significantly improve their sleep patterns and increase total nighttime sleep (42,43). Arming teens with this self-knowledge is an essential component in addressing their sleep problems.

EARLY SCHOOL START TIMES AND ADOLESCENT SLEEP PROBLEMS

The idea that being better rested is more conducive to better learning is certainly a compelling, some would say "common sense" idea that many people can relate to directly from their personal experiences. That adolescents across the world are found to be increasingly sleepy in school is also virtually undisputed. However, the hypothesis that adolescent sleepiness is at least partially due to schools starting too early is less widely embraced, in part because accepting its premise has far-reaching implications for educators and communities that have evolved around earlier school start times. The relationship between school starting time and the sleep and wellness of adolescents has been examined in detail (37,44,45), and it is clear that teens' biology is simply not suited to optimal learning and health when school schedules are too early. Though what "too early" means is still not precisely proven; available data so far point to 8:30 a.m. being the earliest time for effective learning in older adolescents.

The first study to directly examine the effects of school start times on adolescents' sleep habits was a longitudinal field study conducted in a group of Rhode

Island students in the early 1990s (6). Students were studied prospectively in the spring of 9th grade, the following summer and the fall of their 10th grade, with a subgroup monitored again in the spring of 10th grade. During ninth grade they attended middle school that began at 8:25 a.m.; the following year in 10th grade they attended high school which began at 7:20 a.m. Students were assessed both in the home environment and in the laboratory for sleep amounts, sleep timing, and daytime alertness. This pivotal study demonstrated that both ninth and tenth graders went to sleep at similar times, but the tenth graders had significantly less sleep on school nights due to earlier rise times. The tenth graders showed significantly greater daytime sleepiness: mean sleep latency on four naps across the day of a Multiple Sleep Latency Test (MSLT) of 8.5 minutes compared with 11.4 minutes for 9th graders. The sleepiness was especially marked in the older students on the first test of the morning at 08:30 hours: sleep onset was 5.1 minutes—a pathological level of sleepiness similar to that seen in sleep disorders such as narcolepsy. Further, at least one REM sleep episode was observed in 48% of the tenth graders, consistent with underlying REM sleep deprivation from truncated sleep on school nights. Essentially, this was the first study to demonstrate that adolescents who transition to an hour earlier school start time experience a corresponding biological consequence: clinically significant sleepiness.

The problem of early start time-related sleepiness in high school students is evident in other Westernized countries as well. The "school duty schedule" was found to be the major determinant of sleepiness and earlier waking times for a group of Polish students age 10–14 who were under-sleeping during the school week, with delayed waking times on weekends (46). A large, longitudinal survey of Icelandic children (47) that examined individual sleep habits over a 5–10 year period found that significant daytime sleepiness and naps increased in adolescence, as progressively earlier wake-up times for school occurred. Similarly, a large survey study of 3235 high school students in Canada found 70% reported sleeping fewer than 8.5 hours per night, and the majority of students reported feeling "really sleepy" between 8:00 and 10:00 a.m., consistent with the expected timing of their underlying circadian clock, and the effects of sleep deprivation. As might be expected, even pre-adolescent fifth grade students reported significant sleep deprivation when an extremely early school start time of 7:00 a.m. was imposed in Israel (48).

We found that self-reported sleep amounts in adolescents has continued to worsen as high school start times have gotten even earlier since the last survey in our region by Carskadon and colleagues in 1998 (49) (Fig. 1). Other chapters in this text offer a detailed discussion of the psychological and behavioral effects of sleep deprivation in adolescents, but is important to review here some of the data illustrating the consequences of sleep deprivation in the context of early high school start times. There is ample evidence that excessive sleepiness due to chronic under-sleeping impairs cognitive functioning (50). As sleepiness rises, critical higher cortical processes are essentially turned off as the brain prepares for sleep. Sleepiness in children as well as adults makes it harder to sustain attention and stay on task, interferes with memory, decreases creativity, the ability to multitask and make effective choices, and increases impulsivity and irritability (44,51–53). Further, installing new memories—i.e., learning—clearly benefits from, if not depends upon, intervals of normal sleep (13). Given this, it should be no surprise that adolescents who are found to be sleep-deprived also report more attentional difficulties, poorer academic performance, and less interest or involvement in extracurricular activities (29). Wolfson and Carskadon's study of over 3000 high school students (3) found that students who were struggling or failing academically (i.e., they reported obtaining more Cs, Ds, Fs) also reported being more sleepy, having later bedtimes and more irregular sleep/wake schedules than students with better grades (As and Bs). Students who report being sleep-deprived due to later bedtimes are much more likely to fall asleep in school, particularly in the morning classes, compared with their peers enrolled in schools with later start times (50). More total sleep, earlier and consistent weekday bedtimes, and later weekday rise times are consistently found to correlate with better grades in school (7,32,48,55).

In addition to the impact of sleep deprivation on school performance, adolescents who obtain less than six hours of sleep per night report significantly more feelings of depression, anxiety and high-risk behavior (56). The emotional lability and social stresses that all adolescents experience are further aggravated as a result of sleep deprivation. The detrimental effects of sleep deprivation on judgment and insight are especially concerning when one considers the high incidence of alcohol and substance use among adolescents. Indeed, substance use is greater among teenagers with sleep difficulties (57,58). For example, Giannotti and colleagues (26) found that the more sleep-deprived "evening-type" Italian high school students experienced significantly greater problems with attention, poor school achievement, more injuries and were emotionally upset more than the morning-type students. These students also reported greater consumption of caffeine-containing beverages and substances to promote sleep. Sleep deprivation, and poor sleep quality also increase the likelihood of interpersonal problems and psychiatric illness (58,59). While many students are able to function well in school with shorter amounts of sleep, they may pay a price in other ways such as emotional instability, argumentativeness, and disturbed social interactions. One unintended consequence of the earlier school schedule is the amount of unstructured time some teens are faced with after school in the afternoons. This "self-care" time lends itself to greater risk taking, and has been correlated with increased substance use and depressed mood (60). Indeed, juvenile crimes are four times more likely to occur in the hours after school than at other times during the day or night (44).

Perhaps the most dramatic and potentially devastating consequence of sleep-deprivation in teens is car accidents. Students who drive themselves to school early in the morning are at even greater risk of a fall-asleep at the wheel car accident because of the combined effects of their greater cumulative sleep-deprivation, and the challenge of operating a vehicle before their circadian-dependent alertness is fully engaged. These factors, compounded by their lack of driving experience, are cited as the reason that the peak age of sleep-related car crashes is 20 years, and the peak time of accidents is between 7:00 and 8:00 a.m. (61). In sum, early school start times clearly contribute to sleep-deprivation in growing teens, making them even more vulnerable to all the challenges of adolescence, and increases the likelihood of accidents, psychological problems, and impaired learning in school.

BENEFIT OF DELAYED SCHOOL START TIMES ON ADOLESCENT SLEEP AND BEHAVIOR

There are so many negative consequences associated with sleep deprivation in adolescents that school leaders in many areas are beginning to consider the practical measures that would improve total sleep time for their students to promote their health and learning. Though research has not yet identified an ideal school schedule, the wealth of evidence reviewed in this chapter and elsewhere strongly suggests that students have a better opportunity to be rested and ready to learn by delaying school start time to 8:30 a.m. or later.

Initial data documenting statistical improvements in academic performance, mood and attendance after a delayed start time in the Edina, Minnesota school district prompted the first large-scale longitudinal study of the effects of delayed school start time in Minneapolis-St. Paul, Minnesota (44,45). The School Start Time Study was a comprehensive investigation of the impact of a district-wide delay in high school start time for the 1996–1997 school year. Outcomes were collected from over 18,000 students beginning two years prior until three years after high schools changed their start time from 7:15 a.m. to 8:40 a.m. This was a landmark study not only because it documented the impact of such a potentially important determinant of students' educational experience, but also because the study included elements that reflected the changes to the community as a whole. This study demonstrated multiple benefits to the students as a result of the delayed schedule: increased daily attendance and reduced tardiness, increased rates of continuous attendance and graduation, and overall improvement in student academic performance. Surveys of teachers demonstrated a qualitative leap in the school morale as a result of the later schedule, with comments like "there is an alertness in the students coming into school that I haven't seen in many, many years." Administrators reported the school seemed "calmer" and were impressed with the attendance changes. Parents cited some of the challenges, like "eats dinner later because of sports, no time for a job," but also "less stressful mornings," "breakfast never missed," and "the later start time is very beneficial, both relative to grades and to energy level." Many parents also commented "fix the middle schools too!" The vast majority of the students approved of the change in start time.

In addition to evaluating the students in the Minneapolis-St. Paul districts, the School Start Time Study also surveyed secondary schools in neighboring districts with school start times between 7:20 a.m. and 8:40 a.m. This study demonstrated that for all six grade levels (7–12), there was a significant increase in the reported academic grades with progressively later start times. Academic performance was poorest across the board at schools starting before 7:30 a.m., and the most rapid increase in performance was seen between 7:30 a.m. and 8:00 a.m. for 7th and 8th grade students. Whereas 11th and 12th grade students showed only modest improvement academically as start times were compared between 7:20 a.m. and 8:00 a.m., but academic grades rose dramatically when start times were 8:15 a.m. and later. These data are consistent with the known underlying circadian phase biology of adolescents, though the author is careful to point out this does not prove a causal relationship between start times and grades.

In 1999, the Fayette County Kentucky school district delayed their high school start time by one hour to 8:30 a.m. Dr. Fred Danner compared accident rate data for the 17- and 18-year-old age groups before and after the school start time delay. He found that following the school start time delay, teen crash rates in that district dropped by 15.6% while crash rates throughout the rest of the state *increased* by 8.9% during the same time period. He is quick to point out that other factors besides additional sleep time may have accounted for the dramatic difference in accidents in this age group (e.g., increased school bus ridership and fewer teens driving to

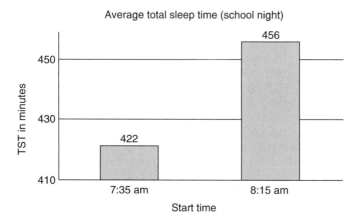

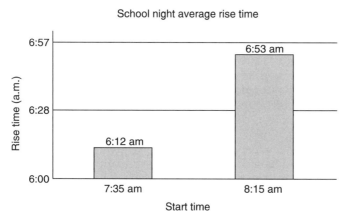

FIGURE 4 Sleep changes in high school students after a 40-minute delay in school start time. Students attending Wilton High School (Wilton, CT) were surveyed with the Condensed Sleep Habits Questionnaire in 2001 and 2002 (N = 297) when school start time was 7:35 a.m. (mean ± S.D., 422 ± 60 minutes), and again in 2004 (N = 977) after the school start time was delayed 40 minutes (mean ± S.D., 456 ± 55 minutes; p>0.0005) Average total school night sleep time (top graph) increased by 34 minutes after the schedule change allowed students to delay their school day rise times (bottom graph) by an average of 41 minutes later (before mean ± S.D., 6:12 a.m. ± 24 min; after mean ± S.D., 6:53 a.m. ± 28 minutes).

school). However such a sizable reduction in accident rate in this highly vulnerable population is remarkable, and that it follows the delayed high school start time is consistent with the expected outcome of less sleep deprivation among teen drivers.

Recently, our laboratory performed a study of high school students in Wilton, Connecticut before and after their high school chose to delay its start time by 40 minutes to 8:15 a.m. (Fig. 4). Our goal was to evaluate whether teens actually took advantage of this schedule adjustment to get more sleep, or whether they simply used the extra time for more late-night activities, as some feared would happen. We found that student bedtimes were essentially unchanged compared with before the schedule change, but later rise times were reported such that they obtained nearly all of this time as additional sleep. Rather than extending their waketime activities at night, students got to "sleep in" before school. As a result, students benefited from a significant increase in their overall weekly sleep amounts after the school start time was delayed. Student self-report measures of daytime sleepiness dropped significantly after the schedule change but at least one third of students reported still having "problem sleepiness" some of the time. Because of the overwhelmingly positive response among students, teachers and parents to the schedule change, other communities surrounding this high school are considering similar schedule changes to promote healthy sleep for their students.

As the magnitude of the problem is often unrecognized, and school schedule adjustments at least initially are met with resistance for practical reasons, studies like ours will help provide necessary data that these changes are effective. Indeed, it is likely that a longer delay in start time than was adopted in Wilton could have an even greater benefit for students, given the number of teens who reported continuing to experience significant sleepiness. However, it is reassuring that the new schedule did result in increased sleep and the impact was so widely apparent. It is almost assumed that insufficient sleep is the normal right of passage for high school and college students, but is this problem of insufficient sleep the beginning of problems with sleep in adults? Could insomnia, anxiety and depression, psychosomatic disorders and the widespread use of stimulants in adults have their genesis in the poor sleep patterns that develop in adolescence? The answers to these questions await further research.

REFERENCES

1. Drobnich D. A National Sleep Foundation's Conference Summary: The National Summit to Prevent Drowsy Driving and a New Call to Action. Ind Health 2005; 43:197–200.
2. Carskadon, MA, Acebo, C, Richardson, BS, Tate, BA, Seifer, R. Long nights protocol: Access to circadian parameters in adolescents. Journal of Biological Rhythms 1997; 12:278–89.
3. Wolfson AR, Carskadon MA. Understanding adolescents' sleep patterns and school performance: a critical appraisal. Sleep Med Rev 2003; 7:491–506.
4. Wolfson AR, Carskadon M. Sleep schedules and daytime functioning in adolescents. Child Dev 1998; 69(4):875–87.
5. Carskadon MA. The second decade. In Guilleminault. C. (ed.), Sleeping and Waking Disorders: Indications and tecdhniques. Menlo Park. Addison-Wesley, 1982.
6. Wolfson AR, Carskadon M. Sleep schedules and daytime functioning in adolescents. Child Development 1998; 69(4):875.
7. Manber R, Bootzin RR, Acebo C, Carskadon MA. The effects of regularizing sleep-wake schedules on daytime sleepiness. Sleep, 1996; 19:432–41.
8. www.sleepfoundation.org/site/c.huIXKjM0IxF/b.2419167/k.14D6/2006_Sleep_in_America_Poll.htm.
9. Carskadon, MA, Harvey, K, Duke, P, Anders, TF, Dement, WC. Pubertal changes in daytime sleepiness. Sleep 1980; 2:453–60.
10. Mercer PW, Merritt SL, Cowell JM. Differences in reported sleep need among adolescents. J Adolesc Health 1998; 23:259–63.
11. Tynjala J, Kannas, L, Valimaa R. How young Europeans sleep. Health Educ Res 1993;8:69–80.
12. Wu RC, Butler GE, Kelnar CJ, Huhtaniemi I, Veldhuis JD. Ontogeny of pulsatile gonadotropin releasing hormone secretion from midchildhood, through puberty, to adulthood in the human male: A study using deconvolution analysis and an ultrasensitive immunofluorometric assay. J Clin Endocrinol Metab 1996; 81(5):1798–805.

13. Stickgold, R. Sleep-dependent memory consolidation. Nature 2005; 437:1272–8.
14. Wagner U, Gais S, Haider H, Verleger R, Born J. Sleep inspires insight. Nature 2004; 427:352–5.
15. Wagner U Gais S, Born J. Emotional memory formation is enhanced across sleep intervals with high amounts of rapid eye movement sleep. Learn Mem 2001; 8: 112–19.
16. Moore RY. Organization and function of a central nervous system circadian oscillator: The suprachiasmatic hypothalamic nucleus. Fed Proc 1983; 42:2783–9.
17. Borbely AA. A two process model of sleep regulation. Hum Neurobiol 1982; 1:195–204.
18. Czeisler CA, Wright KP Jr. Influence of light on circadian rhythmicity in humans. In: Turek FW, Zee PC (eds) Regulation of Sleep and Circadian Rhythms. New York, NY: Marcel Dekker Inc, 1999: pp. 149–180.
19. Carskadon MA, Vieira C, Acebo C. Association between puberty and delayed phase preference. Sleep. 1993; 16:258–62.
20. Ishihara K, Honma Y, Miyake S. Investigation of the children's version of morningness–eveningness questionnaire with primary and junior high school pupils in Japan Percept Mot Skills 1990; 71(pr. 2):1353–4.
21. Andrade MMM, Menna-Bareeto L, Benedito Silva AA, Domenice S, Arnhold IPJ. Sleep characteristics following change in adolescent maturity status. Sleep Res 1993; 22:521.
22. Bearpark HM. Sleep/wake disturbances in Sydney adolescents: A survey of prevalence and correlates. Sydney: Master's thesis, Macquarie University, 1986.
23. Miller L, Dyche J, Andrews C, Lucus T. The impact of additional sleep on test scores at US Navy boot camp. Sleep 2004; 27:A164.
24. Edgar DM. In: Shiraki K et al. (eds). Physiological Basis of Occupational Health: Stressful Environments, Amsterdam: Academic Publishing, 1996; Vol 11: pp.253–265.
25. Miller L, Dyche J, Andrews C, Lucus T. The impact of additional sleep on test scores at US Navy boot camp. Sleep 2004; 27:A164.
26. Giannotti F, Cortesi F, Sebastiani T, Ottaviano S. Circadian preference, sleep and daytime behaviour in adolescence. J Sleep Res 2002; 11(3):191–9.
27. Achenbach, TM. The Child Behavior Checklist. University of Vermont, Department of Psychiatry, 1991.
28. Brown C, Tzischinsky O, Wolfson A, Acebo C, Wicks J, Darley C, Carskadon MA. Circadian phase preference and adjustment to the high school transition. Sleep Research 1995; 24:90.
29. Wolfson, AR, Tzischinsky, O, Brown, C, Darley, C, Acebo, C, Carskadon, M. Sleep, behavior and stress at the transition to senior high school. Sleep Research 1995; 24:115.
30. Liu X, Liu L, Owens JA, Kaplan DL. Sleep patterns and sleep problems among schoolchildren in the United States and China. Pediatrics 2005; 115(1):241–9.
31. Carskadon, MA. Patterns of sleep and sleepiness in adolescents. Pediatrician 1990; 17:5–12.
32. Allen, R. Social factors associated with the amount of school week sleep lag for seniors in an early starting suburban high school. Sleep Research, 1992; 21:114.
33. Carskadon, MA. Adolescent sleepiness: Increased risk in a high-risk population. Alcohol, Drugs and Driving 1990; 5–6:317–28.
34. Wolfson, A. (2002). Bridging the gap between research and practice: What will adolescents' sleep/wake patterns look like in the 21st century? In Carskadon MA (ed.), Adolescent Sleep Patterns: Biological, Social, and Psychological Influences. Cambridge, UK: Cambridge University Press, 2002,pp. 198–219.
35. Gibson ES, Powles AC, Thabane L, O'Brien S, Molnar DS, Trajanovic N, Ogilvie R, Shapiro C, Yan M, Chilcott-Tanser L, "Sleepiness" is serious in adolescence: Two surveys of 3235 Canadian students. BMC Public Health 2006; 6:116.
36. LeBourgeois MK, Giannotti F, Cortesi F, Wolfson AR, Harsh J. The relationship between reported sleep quality and sleep hygiene in Italian and American adolescents. Pediatrics 2005; 115(1):257–65.

37. Carskadon MA. Factors influencing sleep patterns. In: Carskadon MA (ed.), Adolescent Sleep Patterns: Biological, Social, and Psychological Influences. Cambridge, UK: Cambridge University Press, 2002, pp.4–26.
38. Petta D, Carskadon M, Dement WC. Sleep habits in children aged 7–13 years. Sleep Research 1984; 13:86.
39. Yang, C-K, Kim JK, Patel SR Lee J-H. Age-related changes in sleep/wake patterns among Korean teenagers. Pediatrics 2005; 115(1): 250–6.
40. Grunstein R, Grunstein RR. Knowledge about sleep and driving in Australian adolescents [abstract]. Sleep 2001; 24:A111.
41. Cortesi F, Giannoti F, Sebastiani T, Burni O, Ottaviano S. Knowdege of sleep in Italian high school students: Pilot-test of a school-based sleep educational program. J Adolesc Health 2004; 34:344–51.
42. Rossi CM, Campbell AL, Vo OT, Charron T, Marco CA, Wolfson AR. Middle school sleep-smart program: A pilot evaluation [abstract]. Sleep 2002; 25:A279.
43. Vo OT, LeChasseur K, Wolfson AR, Marco CA. Sleepy pre-teens: Second pilot of the sleep-smart program: A pilot evaluation [abstract]. Sleep 2003; 26:A411.
44. Wahlstrom K. Changing times: Findings from the first longitudinal study of later high school start times. NASSP Bulletin 2002; 86:633.
45. Wahlstrom K. Áccomodating the sleep patterns of adolescents within current educational structures: An uncharted path, In: M Carskadon, (ed.) Adolescent Sleep Patterns: Biological, Social, and Psychological Influences. Cambridge, UK: Cambridge University Press, 2002.
46. Szymczak JT, Jasinska M, Pawlak E, Zwierzykowska M. Annual and weekly changes in the sleep-wake rhythm of school children. Sleep 1993; 16(5):433–5.
47. Thorleifsdottir B, Björnsson JK, Benediktsdottir B, Gislason T, Kristbjarnarson H. Sleep and sleep habits from childhood to young adulthood over a 10-year period. J Psychosom Res 2002 Jul; 53(1):529–37.
48. Epstein R, Chillag N, Lavie P. Starting times of school: Effects on daytime functioning of fifth-grade children in Israel. Sleep 1998; 21: 250–6.
49. Carskadon MA, Wolfson AR, Acebo C, Tzischinsky O, Seifer R. Adolescent sleep patterns, circadian timing, and sleepiness at a transition to early school days. Sleep 1998; 21:871–81.
50. Van Dongen HP, Maislin G, Mullington JM, Dinges DF. The cumulative cost of additional wakefulness: Dose-response effects on neurobehavioral functions and sleep physiology from chronic sleep restriction and total sleep deprivation. Sleep 2003; 26:117–26.
51. Maayan LA, Roby G, Casey BJ, et al. Sleep deprivation in adolescents: Effects on emotional and cognitive processing [abstract 226.G]. Sleep Suppl 1998;21:250.
52. Randazzo AC, Muehlbach MJ, Schweitzer PK, Walsh JK. Cognitive function following acute sleep restriction in children ages 10–14. Sleep 1998; 21:861–8.
53. Fallone G, Acebo C, Arnedt JT, Seifer R, Carskadon MA. Effects of acute sleep restriction on behavior, sustained attention, and response inhibition in children. Percept Mot Skills 2001;93:213–29.
54. Dahl RE. The regulation of sleep and arousal: Development and psychopathology. Dev Psychopathol 1996; 8:3–27.
55. Link SC, Ancoli-Israel S. Sleep and the teenager. Sleep Res 1995: 24a:184.
56. O'Brien and Mindell JA. Sleep and risk-taking behavior in adolescents. Behav Sleep Med 2005; 3(3):113–33.
57. Manni R, Ratti MR, Marchioni E, et al. Poor sleep in adolescents: A study of 869 17-year-old Italian secondary school students. J Sleep Res 1997; 6:44–9.
58. Patten CA, Choi WS, Gillin JC, Pierce JP. Depressive symptoms and cigarette smoking predict development and persistence of sleep problems in US adolescents. Pediatrics 2000; 106(2). Available at: www.pediatrics.org/cgi/content/full/106/2/e23.

59. Roberts RE, Roberts CR, Chen IG. Impact of insomnia on future functioning of adolescents. J Psychosom Res 2002; 53:561–9.
60. Richardson JL, Radziszewska B, Dent CW, Flay BR. Relationship between after-school care of adolescents and substance use, risk taking, depressed mood, and academic achievement. Pediatrics 1993; 92(1):32–8.
61. Pack AI, Pack AM, Rodgman D, Cucchiara A, Dinges DF, Schwab CW. Characteristics of crashes attributed to the the driver having fallen asleep. Accident Analysis and Prevention 1995; 27:769–75.

8 Evaluation of Sleep Disorders in Children and Adolescents

Lynn A. D'Andrea

Department of Pediatrics, Medical College of Wisconsin and Children's Hospital of Wisconsin, Milwaukee, Wisconsin, U.S.A.

INTRODUCTION

Sleep problems are extremely common during childhood, from infancy to adolescence. Unfortunately, despite the prevalence of sleep problems, childhood sleep disorders are often under-recognized and undiagnosed, despite being either preventable or treatable. According to information gathered from the National Sleep Foundation's *Sleep in America* polls (1,2), two-thirds of young children experience at least one sleep problem at least a few nights per week, and greater than half of all adolescents report feeling sleepy during the day. But greater than half of all parents surveyed reported that their child's physician did not ask about their child's sleep; and the older the child, the less likely the discussion. Table 1 shows the recommended amount of sleep that children should be getting and the actual amount of sleep that children achieve (1–3).

Children experience the same broad range of sleep disorders encountered in adults, including sleep apnea, insomnia, parasomnias, delayed sleep phase disorder (DSPD), narcolepsy, and restless leg syndrome, but the clinical presentation, evaluation, and management may differ (Table 2). Although snoring and sleep apnea are common indications for referral to a sleep specialist, many children also have a behavioral or non-respiratory sleep disorder either as a second comorbid diagnosis or as a primary sleep disorder. This chapter reviews a variety of diagnostic techniques available to assist the primary care practitioner and other health care personnel in the evaluation of a child with a suspected sleep disorder.

CLINICAL ASSESSMENT
Sleep History and Physical Examination

Parents may present with a specific complaint such as "My child snores." But often the concern is more general such as "My child is tired during the day" or "My child can't fall asleep or stay asleep at night." The assessment must include a logical, but comprehensive evaluation to determine the cause(s) of the sleep disorder and any comorbid conditions.

It is imperative to get a sense of a child's general sleep and wake patterns (8) (Table 3). It is important to ask about differences in patterns on weekdays versus weekends, or vacations and summer time when the child is out of school. Answers to these questions will guide the necessary follow-up.

A careful sleep history includes information about other primary sleep disorders. Most children with obstructive sleep apnea have symptoms of snoring and labored breathing during sleep (15–18). Parents may describe paradoxical breathing

TABLE 1   Recommended Amount of Sleep that Children Should Receive Versus the Actual Amount of Achieved Sleep They Report

Age group	Recommendation (hours)	Amount reported (hours)
Infants (3–11 months)	14–15	12.8
Toddlers (12–35 months)	12–14	11.7
Preschoolers (3–6 years)	11–13	10.4
School age (1st–5th grade)	10–11	9.5
Adolescents (6th–12th grade)	8.25–9.25	7

Source: Adapted from Refs (1–3).

efforts or obstructed or gasping noises in their child during sleep. It is believed that obstructive sleep apnea occurs in 1–3% of all children (4–6). All children should be screened for sleep-disordered breathing (SDB) during their yearly well-child examination (19). The first, and most direct, question to ask is "Does your child snore?"

As noted above, non-respiratory or behavioral sleep disorders are also quite common in children. Restless leg syndrome is being increasingly recognized

TABLE 2   Prevalence of Pediatric Sleep Disorders

Sleep disorder	Prevalence
Sleep-related breathing disorder	
Obstructive sleep apnea	1–3% (4–6)
Parasomnias	
Confusional arousals	5–15% (7)
Sleepwalking	3–4% of children have frequent episodes, 15–40% of children will have at least one episode (8)
Sleep terrors	3% (8)
Sleep enuresis	15–25% of children 5 years, decreasing to 1–3% of adolescents (9)
Nightmares	24% for children 2 to 5 years, increasing to 41% for children 6 to 10 years (8)
Sleep-related movement disorders	
Restless leg syndrome	Unknown, 17% of children report "restless legs at night" (10)
Periodic limb movement disorder	8–12% (11)
Sleep-related rhythmic movements	Up to 66% in infants 9 months, decreasing to 8% of children 4 years (12)
Bruxism	Up to 20% of children < 11 years (13)
Circadian rhythm disorders	
Delayed sleep phase type	5–10% of adolescents (8)
Insomnia	
Behavioral insomnia of childhood	10–30% (1,14)
Insomnia in adolescents	12–33% (8)
Hypersomnia	
Narcolepsy	0.03–0.16%, one-third of adults report onset of symptoms before 15 years (8)

TABLE 3 Questions for a Comprehensive History of Sleep–Wake Patterns

General questions	More specific questions
Does your child have a bedtime routine?	Is the routine consistent?
Does your child have problems going to bed?	
Does your child have problems falling asleep?	Does your child complain of leg pains? Is your child a "worrier" or does he/she have racing thoughts that keep him or her awake? Does your child watch television while trying to fall asleep?
Does your child wake up during the night?	Does your child require parental intervention to re-initiate sleep? Does your child seek out something to eat or drink during the awakening?
Does your child have problems waking up in the morning?	How does your child feel upon awakening—tired or refreshed?
Is your child sleepy during the day?	Does your child fall asleep in the classroom, or the school bus, or parent's car? Does your child have habitual napping after school?
Does your child maintain a similar weekday and weekend schedule in regard to sleep?	
What about vacation or summer schedules?	Is the schedule shifted to a later sleep time and wake time? On that schedule does your child wake spontaneously?

in children. Presenting symptoms may include leg pains or "growing pains," or a "pins and needles" or "creepy-crawly" feeling in the legs, but may also present more subtly as difficulty falling asleep with the child getting back out of bed several times to move around. Additional sleep concerns that need to be asked about include parasomnias such as nightmares, night terrors, and sleepwalking. An older child may have issues with enuresis that need to be addressed.

A comprehensive sleep history includes information about a child's sleep environment. This includes questions as to whether the child has his or her own bed and bedroom; whether the room is dark, quiet, and conducive to sleep; and if the room is at the appropriate temperature. It is important to know if the child falls asleep in his/her bed or is transferred there after sleep onset. This may also be at the appropriate part of the history to ask about other substances used that may enhance sleep (e.g., lavender, chamomile) or hinder sleep (e.g., caffeine, alcohol). In addition, certain medications may be associated with sleep abnormalities. Finally, a comprehensive history includes information about other medical conditions, mental health issues, developmental concerns, as well as a family history of any sleep disorders.

The physical examination may provide additional information in determining which children are at risk for having obstructive sleep apnea. Although most children have relatively normal examinations when they are awake, there are

TABLE 4 Findings on Physical Examination and the Implications for Sleep-Disordered Breathing

Features on physical examination	Implications
Inability to breathe comfortably through nose with mouth closed or hyponasal voice	Suggestive of adenoidal hypertrophy or inflammation (e.g., allergic rhinitis) (20)
Tonsillar hypertrophy	Relation between tonsil size and presence of sleep apnea remains controversial (21–23)
Length of soft palate	A long soft palate is a risk factor for obstructive sleep apnea
Size of tongue	Mallampati classification designed as a guideline for ease or
Size of pharyngeal space	difficulty of tracheal intubation, but has become associated with risk factors for the development of obstructive sleep apnea (24)
Position of teeth and jaw	Abnormal positioning of the jaw structures may be a risk factor for development of obstructive sleep apnea. Class II occlusion ("overbite" of the maxillary teeth or "underbite" of the mandibular teeth) may be associated with a retrognathic mandible. Class III occlusion is associated with protrusion of the mandible secondary to a deficiency of the maxilla. Both types of occlusion may be associated with a smaller pharyngeal space
Weight	Obesity is a risk factor for development of obstructive sleep apnea (25–27)
Blood pressure	Hypertension may be an indicator of chronic obstructive sleep apnea (28). Associated findings may include pulmonary hypertension, corpulmonale, or even congestive heart failure (29,30)
Pectus excavatum	May be an indication of chronic upper airway obstruction and increased work of breathing
Neurological examination including cranial nerve function and neuromuscular strength	Nocturnal stridor secondary to a central nervous system abnormality (e.g., a brainstem malformation) may be mistakenly diagnosed as snoring. Pharyngeal hypotonia or neuromuscular weakness may may be associated with sleep-disordered breathing

certain anatomical features that may put children at an increased risk of having obstructive symptoms during sleep (Table 4).

Adenotonsillar hypertrophy is often cited as the most common risk factor for obstructive sleep apnea, although a number of studies have shown that there is no relation between the size of the tonsils and adenoids and the presence of sleep apnea (21–23). Rather the size of the oropharyngeal area should also be considered. Relatively small tonsils that are positioned in a crowded space may be more obstructive than relatively large tonsils that are positioned in a larger, more open space. Of note, adenotonsillar hypertrophy tends to be a more important risk factor for the development of sleep apnea in younger children, but is typically less of an issue in adolescents as the lymphoid tissue regresses.

Most adults with obstructive sleep apnea are overweight. Children with obstructive sleep apnea may also be overweight; however, most are of normal weight and height. A subset of children may present with failure to gain weight.

The etiology of this is not clear, but may be related to decreased nutritional intake secondary to difficulty swallowing, increased energy expenditure during sleep (25), or disruption of release of growth factors during sleep (26,27). Excess weight may be a contributing factor to the development of sleep apnea in younger children, but becomes a primary factor in adolescents.

Questionnaires

There are several validated questionnaires available to help the physician screen for the most common sleep problems in children. Chervin (31) validated the Pediatric Sleep Questionnaire to investigate the presence of childhood sleep-disordered breathing with snoring, sleepiness, and behavioral problems in children 2–18 years of age. The 22-question survey is a parent-report screening instrument with questions that focus on snoring, daytime sleepiness, and behavior. The questionnaire demonstrated a sensitivity of 0.81 to 0.85 and a specificity of 0.87, with correct predictive classification for 85% to 86% of studied children. The Pediatric Sleep Questionnaire is used primarily for research purposes.

Owens et al. (32) developed the Children's Sleep Habits Questionnaire (CSHQ) to screen for the most common medical and behavioral sleep problems in children 4–12 years of age. The CSHQ is a parent-report screening instrument. It is not intended to diagnose specific sleep disorders, but rather to identify the need for possible further evaluation in certain children. The CSHQ yields a total score and eight subscale scores, reflecting key sleep domains that encompass the most common sleep disorders in this age group (i.e., bedtime resistance, sleep onset delay, sleep duration, sleep anxiety, night wakings, parasomnias, SDB, and daytime sleepiness). Reliability and validity data have been collected on a sample of 495 elementary school children and on a clinical sample from a pediatric sleep clinic. The CSHQ is also used primarily for research purposes. There are no established normative values for the total or subscale scores. The instrument has been found to be most helpful in assessing sleep before and after intervention.

Sleep Diaries

Sleep diaries provide useful information for children with the chief complaint of excessive daytime sleepiness. The child and family are asked to record a child's sleep and wake patterns during a 24-hour period. The diary is typically kept during a two-week period. It may be helpful to obtain information that compares a school week to a vacation week. The sleep diary can provide important clues to inadequate sleep hygiene, insomnia, or circadian rhythm disorders.

Laboratory Evaluation

A hemoglobin suggestive of polycythemia or a blood gas suggestive of a compensatory metabolic alkalosis may support the diagnosis of SDB, but are rarely seen except for children with severe disease. Anemia, abnormal thyroid function tests, or evidence of an ongoing Epstein-Barr infection may occasionally be seen in a child who presents with excessive daytime sleepiness or fatigue. A drug screen should be obtained for a child with excessive daytime sleepiness if there is a concern about substance abuse as a contributing factor. The DQB1 *0602 human leukocyte antigen is found in many people with narcolepsy, but is not specific for that disease (33,34). Similarly, cerebrospinal fluid hypocretin levels are significantly decreased in people with narcolepsy plus cataplexy, but similar levels are seen in people with narcolepsy without cataplexy or idiopathic hypersomnia; cerebral spinal fluid (CSF) hypocretin levels are primarily used for research purposes. A low ferritin level is the most common cause of restless leg syndrome in children. Children found to have severe SDB with significant hypoxemia may have right ventricular hypertrophy evident on an electrocardiogram or right ventricular dysfunction with pulmonary hypertension evident on an echocardiogram (29).

Radiographic Evaluation

Radiographic evaluation of the airway is unnecessary in most children. A lateral soft tissue radiograph of the neck obtained while the child is awake and upright can identify tonsil and adenoid tissue, but does not reliably predict the presence or severity of obstruction when the child is asleep and supine (21,22,35–38). A lateral soft tissue radiograph of the neck may be helpful in a child to determine if there has been regrowth of the adenoidal tissue in a child who has undergone a previous adenoidectomy.

Magnetic resonance imaging of the pediatric upper airway is still in the research stage, but holds promise as a means to assess airway dimensions and structural relationships. Arens et al. (39–41) have shown that children with obstructive sleep apnea in comparison to controls have smaller airway volumes and longer soft palates that can cause airway restriction.

Actigraphy

An actigraph is a small portable device (similar to a large wristwatch) that is worn by the child while awake and asleep. The device senses physical motion and stores information to be downloaded at a later time. The number of movements per minute is calculated into an "activity count." Actigraphy provides an objective measure of a child's sleep–wake pattern (42). It is a useful, non-invasive method for assessing specific sleep disorders such as insomnia or circadian rhythm disorders. Preliminary results from adult studies suggest that obstructive sleep apnea may have a particular pattern including a higher movement index during sleep (43), but similar information is not yet available for children.

NOCTURNAL MONITORING
Polysomnography (Nocturnal)

Polysomnography is used to evaluate respiratory as well as non-respiratory or behavioral sleep disorders. The American Thoracic Society published a Consensus Statement on Standards and Indications for Cardiopulmonary Sleep Studies in Children (44). Several studies have suggested that obstructive sleep apnea cannot be reliably diagnosed by history alone (15–18). Overnight polysomnography is the gold standard for the diagnosis of obstructive sleep apnea in children. Polysomnography can be used to confirm the suspected diagnosis of obstructive sleep apnea, to assess the severity of the obstructive symptoms, and to monitor the efficacy of treatment. Polysomnography is also used to diagnose or monitor

TABLE 5   Polysomnographic Monitoring

Physiologic variables	Sensors
Sleep state	Electroencephalogram
	Electro-oculogram
	Surface electromyogram (chin)
Breathing efforts	Strain gauges or uncalibrated respiratory inductance plethysmography to monitor chest and abdominal wall motion
Gas exchange	Arterial oxygen saturation by pulse oximetry
	End-tidal CO_2 monitoring by mass spectometry
Oronasal airflow	Thermistors or thermocouples
	Nasal pressure monitoring
Snoring	Microphone placed over the neck
	Audiotaping
Cardiac rhythm	Electrocardiogram
Muscle activity and movements	Surface electromyogram (legs)
	Videotaping

children with underlying illnesses that predispose them to the development of nocturnal hypoventilation. Finally, polysomnography can be used to assess sleep architecture and non-respiratory-related sleep disorders (e.g., narcolepsy, periodic limb movement disorder, parasomnias, or nocturnal seizures).

Several physiologic functions related to sleep and breathing are monitored during polysomnography (Table 5). Unique or specialized monitoring may be required for pediatric patients. In polysomnography performed in children, oronasal airflow is usually monitored with a thermistor. Expiratory end-tidal CO_2 may be monitored from a nasal cannula as a measure of hypoventilation, and, probably as a surrogate of nasal airflow. With this method, hypopneas or hypoventilation is detected when the expired end-tidal CO_2 curve shows loss of a clear-cut plateau or when the curve becomes smaller or dome-shaped (45). A recent study has shown that as in adults (46–49), events detected in children by esophageal pressure monitoring were also detected by nasal pressure monitoring (50). Obstructive events, in particular hypopneas, detected by esophageal pressure monitoring are not detected by end-tidal CO_2 monitoring (51). Thus, nasal pressure may become more commonplace for pediatric studies as an accurate, non-invasive means to detect obstructive events (52). End-tidal CO_2 monitoring should be performed in children who require assessment for alveolar hypoventilation. Transcutaneous carbon dioxide monitoring can be used for children who do not tolerate a nasal cannula (53).

Surface electromyography (EMG) using both legs should be considered in all polysomnographic studies of children who are at least of school age. In adults, restless leg syndrome (RLS) and period leg movements during sleep (PLMS) are associated with excessive daytime sleepiness. More recent studies have shown that RLS and PLMS may also be associated with behavioral changes in children.

Most pediatric sleep studies consist of a limited electroencephalogram montage in order to determine wake and sleep, and to distinguish the various sleep stages. A full electroencephalogram (EEG) should be considered in those children in whom the possibility of nocturnal seizures is being considered. Obstructive sleep apnea may precipitate nocturnal seizures in a child with an underlying seizure disorder (54).

TABLE 6   Polysomnographic Measurements of Pediatric Sleep-Disordered Breathing

Parameter	Recommended normal value
Snoring	None
Nasal airflow	Continuous
Respiratory efforts	In-phase and unlabored during NREM and REM sleep
Obstructive apnea index, #/hour	≤ 1 (any length)
Obstructive apnea/hypopnea index, #/hour	≤ 1.5
Desaturation index (4%), #/hour	≤ 1.4
Minimum SpO2, %	$\geq 92\%$
Duration of hypoventilation ($ETCO_2$>45 mmHg), %total sleep time	$\leq 60\%$
Duration of hypoventilation ($ETCO_2$>50 mmHg), %total sleep time	$\leq 8\%$
Maximum ETCO2, mmHg	≤ 53 mmHg

Source: Adapted from Refs. (55,57).

Videotaping the child while in the sleep laboratory may be a helpful adjunct in the diagnosis of both respiratory and non-respiratory sleep disorders. Videotaping with an audio component can provide additional visual and auditory assessment of the child's work of breathing. Videotaping is also helpful in the diagnosis of various parasomnias including bruxism, night terrors, or headbanging. It may also provide useful information in a child with nocturnal seizures.

INTERPRETATION OF PEDIATRIC POLYSOMNOGRAPHIC STUDIES

Pediatric polysomnographic studies must be interpreted by a sleep specialist familiar with pediatric sleep disorders and pediatric standards (44,55,56) (Table 6). Findings that are considered abnormal include snoring with paradoxical or labored respiratory efforts, and decreased or absent nasal airflow with a switch to mouth breathing. Children less than three years of age may have paradoxical respiratory efforts during rapid eye movement (REM) sleep as a normal physiologic finding. This finding is suggestive of increased upper airway resistance, however, if it occurs during non-REM sleep or if it persists in children older than three years of age. An apnea index (i.e., the number of apneas per hour of sleep) greater than one is rare among normal children (55) although the clinical significance of this finding is not yet clear. An apnea/hypopnea index greater than 1.5 is rare among normal children (57). In addition, children may have shorter apneas than adults (<10 seconds). These short events can be associated with physiologic phenomena (i.e., paradoxical respiratory efforts, oxygen desaturations, arousals) and therefore are thought to be significant. This is in part because of a faster respiratory rate in younger children leading to more missed breaths during even a short apnea event.

Finally, children may demonstrate a pattern of obstructive hypoventilation with partial upper airway obstruction, cyclic oxygen desaturations, and hypercapnia rather than discrete obstructive events (56). Cortical arousals after apnea events are not as common or as visible in the EEG of children compared to adult EEGs (58). However, arousals associated with spontaneous movements are frequent (59).

Interpretation of pediatric polysomnographic studies also includes non-respiratory measurements such as time of sleep onset (e.g., midnight for a three-year-old child or 7 p.m. for an adolescent may be unusual), sleep latency, sleep efficiency, number of arousals or awakenings with associations (e.g., a two-year-old who wakes three times during the study to feed), number of leg movements, and a careful description of movements or behaviors.

"SCREENING" STUDIES FOR PEDIATRIC SLEEP DISORDERS

In part, because polysomnography is expensive and labor-intensive, and facilities with expertise in evaluating pediatric patients may not be readily available, various "screening" studies have been suggested as a means to diagnose SDB in children. These tests are limited, however, because often they cannot determine the cause or severity of the sleep-disordered breathing and give no information about sleep disruption.

Audiotaping and Videotaping

Overnight audiotaping can be suggestive of obstructive sleep apnea, but is not able to reliably distinguish primary snoring from snoring associated with sleep apnea. Among seven trained observers listening to a 15-minute audiotape, median sensitivity for the prediction of sleep apnea was 71% (range 43–86%) and median specificity was 80% (range 67–80%) based on detection of a "struggle sound" (60). Videotaping of a child sleeping is easy and inexpensive and can be used to verify the history of snoring, but the reliability of this method has not been validated. Children with positive findings on audiotaping or videotaping should have further evaluation to confirm the diagnosis and assess the severity of their symptoms.

Overnight Oximetry Studies

Overnight oximetry studies can be used to document hypoxemia during sleep (61). Brouillette (62) compared oximetry studies to simultaneous full polysomnography studies in 349 children with suspected obstructive sleep apnea. Children at risk for other causes of hypoxemia were excluded. Compared with polysomnography, oximetry studies had a positive predictive value of 97% and a negative predictive value of 47%. This suggests that a positive oximetry study can be used to identify children with symptoms of sleep apnea who need further evaluation, but that a negative study cannot rule out sleep apnea. Finally, a normal oximetry study can be an underestimation of the severity of the symptoms if the child did not sleep during the study.

Nap Studies

Nap studies generally are not thought to provide an effective screening evaluation for children with suspected obstructive sleep apnea. Marcus compared nap studies with overnight polysomnography in children with sleep apnea (63). Nap studies had a sensitivity of 74% and positive predictive value of 100%. Thus nap studies may underestimate the severity of the SDB. However, the presence of SDB detected by nap studies was always confirmed by overnight polysomnography. The authors recently repeated the study with a larger group of children (64). It was again seen that individual parameters (e.g., short obstructive apneas, hypopneas, hypoxemia, snoring, paradoxical breathing) were not sensitive in predicting abnormal overnight polysomnograms. When nap study parameters were abnormal, however, the chance of SDB was high. Both groups caution that overnight polysomnography should be performed if nap polysomnography is inconclusive.

Home or Unattended Portable Studies

The efficacy of home studies or unattended portable studies has not been fully evaluated in children. Portable studies typically include some measurement of oxygen saturation, electrocardiogram, respiratory effort (often only one channel rather than two), and oronasal airflow. Sleep staging is generally not included. Only one study has compared results from children studied by home testing versus laboratory testing (65). Study duration, apnea/hypopnea index, oxygen desaturation index, and respiratory and spontaneous movement/arousal indices during sleep were similar for home and laboratory studies. The American Academy of Pediatrics guidelines (19) caution that the equipment used in this study was relatively sophisticated and not easily reproducible in all settings.

The American Academy of Sleep Medicine (formerly known as the American Sleep Disorders Association) in a position paper addressed the issue of unattended studies for adults (66). Based on a review of the available literature including existing published standards of practice and consensus opinion, the committee concluded that unattended portable recording may be effective for the diagnosis of severe SDB when used by a qualified sleep specialist as part of a comprehensive sleep consultation. This has not been fully evaluated in children.

ASSESSMENT OF DAYTIME SLEEPINESS

The most common cause of daytime sleepiness is an inadequate amount of sleep at night. Children with obstructive sleep apnea may have symptoms of daytime sleepiness related to fragmented nighttime sleep. Children with non-respiratory or behavioral sleep disorders (e.g., narcolepsy, periodic leg movement disorder, circadian rhythm disorder) may also present with symptoms of daytime sleepiness. The tests listed below are often done after an overnight sleep study that provides contextual information about the amount and quality of the previous nocturnal sleep period. This is important in the interpretation of the daytime sleepiness test results.

Multiple Sleep Latency Test

Sleepiness is commonly assessed by measuring the length of time required to fall asleep when asked to do so. The Multiple Sleep Latency Test (MSLT) is a series of four to five nap opportunities presented at two-hour intervals and beginning two hours after the first morning awakening (67). Patients undergoing an MSLT are instructed to allow themselves to fall asleep or to not resist falling asleep. Sleep latency (i.e., the time from lights out to sleep onset) is measured. In children, sleep latency greater than 10–12 minutes is considered normal (68,69). Pathological sleepiness is defined as a mean sleep latency of less than 5–6 minutes. Latencies falling between the normal and the pathological values are considered a diagnostic gray zone.

There are limitations in interpreting MSLT studies in children. It has not been validated in children younger than six years. It is difficult to interpret sleep latency when some daytime napping is still appropriate. It is also difficult to take into account the natural wakefulness of mid-childhood that may overwhelm an underlying sleep tendency. Normal values will vary with age and Tanner stage of sexual development (70).

CONCLUSION
In summary, pediatric sleep disorders are common and relatively easily treatable once they have been diagnosed. Sleep disorders include both respiratory and non-respiratory or behavioral sleep disorders. Often a child may have more than one sleep disorder, or have other comorbid medical or developmental conditions that affect or exacerbate the sleep disorder. Evaluation of a child who presents with a sleep complaint must consist of a logical, but comprehensive investigation, often using a multidisciplinary approach. Because of the impact of sleep on children's physical, psychological, academic, and overall functioning, the impact of an increased recognition, evaluation, and management of pediatric sleep disorders will likely have a significant impact on the general health and well-being of children.

REFERENCES
1. National Sleep Foundation. Sleep in America Poll 2004. Washington, DC: National Sleep Foundation, 2004.
2. National Sleep Foundation. Sleep in America Poll 2006. Washington, DC: National Sleep Foundation, 2006.
3. Anders TF, Sadeh A, Appareddy V. Normal sleep in neonates and children. In: Ferber R, Kryger M, eds Principles and Practice of Sleep Medicine in the Child., 1st edn Philadelphia PA: W.B. Saunders, 1995: pp. 7–18.
4. Ali NJ, Pitson DJ, Stradling JR. Snoring, sleep disturbance, and behavior in 4–5 year olds. Arch Dis Child 1993; 68(2):360–6.
5. Gislason T, Benediktsdottir B. Snoring, apneic episodes, and nocturnal hypoxemia among children 6 months to 6 years. Chest 1995; 107(4):963–6.
6. Redline S, Tishler PV, Schluchter M, Aylor J, Clark K, Graham G. Risk factors for sleep-disordered breathing in children. Associations with obesity, race, and respiratory problems. Am J Respir Crit Care Med 1999; 159:1527–32.
7. Rosen GM, Mahowald MW. Disorders of arousal in children. In: Sheldon SH, Ferber R, Kryger MH, eds Principles and Practice of Pediatric Sleep Medicine, 1st edn Elsevier Saunders, 2005: pp. 293–304.
8. Mindell JA, Owens JA, eds. A Clinical Guide to Pediatric Sleep: Diagnosis and management of sleep problems. 1st edn Philadelphia PA: Lippincott Williams and Wilkins, 2003.
9. Thiedke CC. Nocturnal enuresis. Am Fam Physician 2003; 67:1499–506.
10. Chervin RD, Archbold KH, Dillon JE, Pituch KJ, Panahi P, Dahl RE, Guilleminault C. Associations between symptoms of inattention, hyperactivity, restless legs, and periodic leg movements. Sleep 2002; 25(2):213–18.
11. Crabtree VM, Ivanenko A, O'Brien LM, Gozal D. Periodic limb movement disorder in children. J Sleep Res 2003; 12:73–81.
12. Klackenberg G. Rhythmic movements in infancy and early childhood. Acta Paediatr Scand 1971; suppl 224:74–83.
13. Kato T, Thie NM, Montplaisir JY, Lavigne GJ. Bruxism and orofacial movements during sleep. Dent Clin North Am 2001; 45:657–84.

14. Stern MA, Mendelsohn J, Obermeyer WH, Amromin J, Benca R. Sleep and behavior problems in school-aged children. Pediatrics 2001; 107:4. URL:http://www.pediatric.org/cgi/content/full/107/4/e60.
15. Carroll JL, McColley SA, Marcus CL, Curtis S, Loughlin GM. Inability of clinical history to distinguish primary snoring from obstructive sleep apnea syndrome in children. Chest 1995; 108(3):610–18.
16. Wang RC, Elkins TP, Keech D, Wauquier A, Hubbard D. Accuracy of clinical evaluation in pediatric obstructive sleep apnea. Otolaryngol Head Neck Surg 1998; 118(1):69–73.
17. Goldstein NA, Sculerati N, Walslebe JA, Bhatia N, Freidman DM, Rapoport DM. Clinical diagnosis of pediatric obstructive sleep apnea validated by polysomnography. Otolaryngol Head Neck Surg 1994; 111(5):611–17.
18. Nieminen P, Tolonen U, Lopponen H. Snoring and obstructive sleep apnea in children: A 6-month follow-up study. Arch Otolaryngol Head Neck Surg 2000; 126:481–6.
19. American Academy of Pediatrics. Clinical practice guideline: Diagnosis and management of childhood obstructive sleep apnea syndrome. Pediatrics 2002; 109(4):704–12.
20. Paradise JL, Bernard BS, Colborn DK, Janosky J. Assessment of adenoidal obstruction in children: Clinical signs versus roentgenographic findings. Pediatrics 1998; 101(6):979–86.
21. Mahboubi S, Marsh RR, Potsic WP, Pasquariello PS. The lateral neck radiograph in adenotonsillar hyperplasia. Int J Pediatr Otorhinolaryngol 1985; 10(1):67–73.
22. Laurikainen E, Erkinjuntti M, Alihanka J, Rikalainen H, Suonpaa J. Radiological parameters of the bony nasopharynx and the adenotonsillar size compared with sleep apnea episodes in children. Int J Pediatr Otorhinolaryngol 1987; 12:303–10.
23. Brooks LJ, Stephens BM, Bacevice AM. Adenoid size is related to severity but not the number of episodes of obstructive apnea in children. J Pediatr 1998; 132(4):682–6.
24. Mallampati SR, Gatt SP, Gugino LD, Desai SP, Waraksa B, Freiberger D, Liu PL. A clinical sign to predict difficult tracheal intubation: A prospective study. Can Anaesth Soc J 1985; 32(4):429–34.
25. Marcus CL, Carroll JL, Koerner CB, Hamer A, Lutz J, Loughlin GM. Determinants of growth in children with the obstructive sleep apnea syndrome. J Pediatr 1994; 125(4):556–62.
26. Bar A, Tarasiuk A, Segev Y, Phillip M, Tal A. The effect of adenotonsillectomy on serum insulin-like growth factor-I and growth in children with obstructive sleep apnea syndrome. J Pediatr 1999; 135(1):76–80.
27. Nieminen P, Lopponen T, Tolonen U, Lanning P, Knip M, Lopponen H. Growth and biochemical markers of growth in children with snoring and obstructive sleep apnea. Pediatrics 2002;109(4). URL: http://www.pediatrics.org/cgi/content/full/109/4/e55.
28. Marcus CL, Greene MG, Carroll JL. Blood pressure in children with obstructive sleep apnea. Am J Respir Crit Care Med 1998; 157:1098–103.
29. Amin RS, Kimball TR, Bean JA, Jeffries JL, Willging JP, Cotton RT, et al. Left ventricular hypertrophy and abnormal ventricular geometry in children and adolescents with obstructive sleep apnea. Am J Respir Crit Care Med 2002; 165:1395–9.
30. Chowdary YC, Patel JP. Recurrent pulmonary edema: An uncommon presenting feature of childhood obstructive sleep apnea hypoventilation syndrome in an otherwise healthy child. Clin Pediatr 2001; 40:287–90.
31. Chervin R, Hedger K, Dillon JE, Pituch KJ. Pediatric sleep questionnaire (PSQ): Validity and reliability of scales for sleep-disordered breathing, snoring, sleepiness, and behavioral problems. Sleep Medicine 2000; 1:21–32.
32. Owens JA, Spirito A, McGuinn M. The Children's Sleep Habits Questionnaire (CSHQ): Psychometric properties of a survey instrument for school-aged children. Sleep 2000; 23(8):1–9.
33. Mignot E, Hayduk R, Black J, Grumet FC, Guilleminault C. HLA DQB1*0602 is associated with cataplexy in 509 narcoleptic patients. Sleep 1997; 20:1012–20.
34. Mignot E. Genetic and familial aspects of narcolepsy. Neurology 1998; 50(suppl 1):S16–S22.

35. Kawashima S, Peltomaki T, Sakata H, Mori K, Happonen R-P, Ronning O. Craniofacial morphology in preschool children with sleep-related breathing disorder and hypertrophy of tonsils. Acta Paediatr 2002; 91:71–7.
36. Kawashima S, Peltomaki T, Laine J, Ronning O. Cephalometric evaluation of facial types in preschool children without sleep-related breathing disorder. Internat J Pediatr Otorhinolaryngol 2002; 63(2):119–27.
37. Ferrario VF, Sforza C, Poggio CE, Schmitz JH. Craniofacial growth: A three-dimensional soft-tissue study from 6 years to adulthood. J Craniofac Genet Dev Biol 1998; 18:138–49.
38. Kulnis R, Nelson S, Strohl K, Hans M. Cephalometric assessment of snoring and non-snoring children. Chest 2000; 118(3):596–603.
39. Arens R, McDonough JM, Corbin AM, Hernandez ME, Maislin G, Schwab RJ, Pack AI. Linear dimensions of the upper airway structure during development: Assessment of magnetic resonance imaging. Am J Respir Crit Care Med 2002; 165:117–22.
40. Arens R, McDonough JM, Costarino AT, Mahboubi S, Tayag-Kier CE, Maislin G, et al. Magnetic resonance imaging of the upper airway structure of children with obstructive sleep apnea syndrome. Am J Respir Crit Care Med 2001; 164:698–703.
41. Arens R, McDonough JM, Corbin AM, Rubin NK, Carroll ME, Pack AI et al. Upper airway size analysis by magnetic resonance imaging of children with obstructive sleep apnea syndrome. Am J Respir Crit Care Med 2003; 167(1):65–70.
42. Mortenthaler T, Alessi C, Friedman L, Owens J et al. Practice parameters for the use of actigraphy in the assessment of sleep and sleep disorders: An update for 2007. Sleep 2007; 30:519–29.
43. Aubert-Tulkens G, Culee C, Harmant-Van Rijckevorsel K, Rodenstein DO. Ambulatory evaluation of sleep disturbances and therapeutic effects in sleep apnea syndrome by wrist activity monitoring. Am Rev Respir Dis 1987; 136:851–6.
44. American Thoracic Society. Standards and indications for cardiopulmonary sleep studies in children. Am J Respir Crit Care 1996; 153:866–78.
45. Kryger MH. Monitoring respiratory and cardiac function. In: Kryger MH, Roth T, Dement WC, eds Principles and Practice of Sleep Medicine. 3rd edn Philadelphia;WB. Saunders Company, 2000: pp. 1217–30.
46. Hosselet JJ, Norman RG, Ayappa I, Rapoport DM. Detection of flow limitation with a nasal cannula/pressure transducer system. Am J Respir Crit Care Med 1998; 157:1461–7.
47. Thurnheer R, Xie X, Bloch KE. Accuracy of nasal cannula pressure recordings for assessment of ventilation during sleep. Am J Respir Crit Care Med 2001; 164:1914–19.
48. Heitman SJ, Atkar RS, Hajduk EA, Wanner RA, Flemons WW. Validation of nasal pressure for the identification of apneas/hypopneas during sleep. Am J Respir Crit Care Med 2002; 166:386–91.
49. American Academy of Sleep Medicine Task Force. Sleep-related breathing disorders in adults: Recommendations for syndrome definition and measurement techniques in clinical research. Sleep 1999; 22(5):667–89.
50. Serebrisky D, Cordero R, Mandeli J, Kattan M, Lamm C. Assessment of inspiratory flow limitation in children with sleep-disordered breathing by a nasal cannula pressure transducer system. Pediatr Pulmonol 2002; 33:380–7.
51. Guilleminault C, Pelayo R, Leger D, Clerk KA, Bocian RCZ. Recognition of sleep-disordered breathing in children. Pediatrics 1996; 98(5):871–82.
52. Trang H, Leske V, Gaultier C. Use of nasal cannula for detecting sleep apneas and hypopneas in infants and children. Am J Respir Crit Care Med 2002; 166:464–8.
53. Moriellli A, Desjardins D, Brouillette RT. Transcutaneous and end-tidal carbon dioxide pressures should be measured during pediatric polysomnography. Am Rev Respir Dis 1993;148:1599–604.
54. Malow, BA, Levy K, Maturen K, Bowes R. Obstructive sleep apnea is common in medically refractory epilepsy patients. Neurology 2000; 55(7):1002–7.

55. Marcus CL, Omlin KJ, Basinki DJ, Bailey SL, Rachal AB, Von Pechmann WS, et al. Normal polysomnographic values for children and adolescents. Am Rev Respir Dis 1992; 146:1235–9.
56. Rosen CL, D'Andrea L, Haddad GG. Adult criteria for obstructive sleep apnea do not identify children with serious obstruction. Am Rev Respir Dis 1992; 146:1231–4.
57. Witmans MB, Keens TG, Ward SLD, Marcus CL. Obstructive hypopneas in children and adolescents: Normal values. Am J Resp Crit Care Med 2003; 168:1540.
58. McNamara F, Issa FG, Sullivan CE. Arousal pattern following central and obstructive breathing abnormalities in infants and children. J Appl Physiol 1996; 81:2651–7.
59. Mograss MA, Ducharme FM, Brouillette RT. Movement/arousals. Description, classification, and relationship to sleep apnea in children. Am J Respir Crit Care Med 1994; 150:1690–6.
60. Lamm C, Mandeli J, Kattan M. Evaluation of home audiotapes as an abbreviated test for obstructive sleep apnea syndrome (OSAS) in children. Pediatr Pulmonol 1999; 27:267–72.
61. Urschitz MS, Wolff J, von Einem V, Urschitz-Duprat PM, Schlaud M, Poets CF. Reference values for nocturnal home pulse oximetry during sleep in primary school children. Chest 2003; 123(1):96–101.
62. Brouillette RT, Morielli A, Leimanis A, Water KA, Luciano R, Ducharme FM. Nocturnal pulse oximetry as an abbreviated testing modality for pediatric obstructive sleep apnea. Pediatrics 2000;105(2):405–12.
63. Marcus CL, Keens TG, Ward SLD. Comparison of nap and overnight polysomnography in children. Pediatr Pulmonol 1992; 13:16–21.
64. Saeed MM, Keens TG, Stabile MW, Bolokowicz J, Davidson Ward SL. Should children with suspected obstructive sleep apnea syndrome and normal nap studies have overnight sleep studies? Chest 2000; 118:360–5.
65. Jacob SV, Morielli A, Mograss MA, Ducharme FM, Schloss MD, Brouillette RT. Home testing for pediatric obstructive sleep apnea syndrome secondary to adenotonsillar hypertrophy. Pediatr Pulmonol 1995; 20:241–52.
66. American Sleep Disorders Association. Indications for the clinical use of unattended portable recordings for the diagnosis of sleep-related breathing disorders. ASDA News 1999; 6(1):19–22.
67. Carskadon MA, Dement WC, Mitler MM et al. Guidelines for the multiple sleep latency test (MLST): A standard measure of sleepiness. Sleep 1986; 9:519–24.
68. Littner MR, Kushida C, Wise M, Davila DG et al. Practice parameters for clinic use of the multiple sleep latency test and the maintenance of wakefulness test. Sleep 2005; 28:113–21.
69. Hoban TF, Chervin RD. Assessment of sleepiness in children. Sem in Pediatr Neurol 2001; 8:216–28.
70. Carskadon MA, Harvey K, Duke P, Anders TF, Litt IF, Dement WC. Pubertal changes in daytime sleepiness. Sleep 1980; 2:453–60.

9 Assessment of Sleep Problems in a School Setting or Private Practice

Marsha Luginbuehl[a] and Kathy L. Bradley-Klug[b]

[a]Child Uplift, Inc., Fairview, Wyoming, U.S.A.
[b]University of South Florida, Tampa, Florida, U.S.A.

INTRODUCTION

One out of every three elementary school age children suffers serious sleep problems (1). While some of these may disappear during childhood, 12–15% of all students may have a sleep problem impacting their daytime functioning that will not disappear without treatment (2). These sleep problems can impact the social, emotional, neurocognitive, and academic performance of these children. Because sleep problems are not typically considered a possible cause for school-related issues such as poor academic performance or behavioral concerns, many children with sleep problems may never be identified or may be mislabeled.

The focus of this chapter is to provide clinical professionals with an overview of the most current research regarding the link between sleep problems and educational outcomes for children and adolescents. Screening of sleep disorders is discussed within the context of a prevention to intervention continuum. The chapter will introduce clinical professionals to new instruments available for assessing children with suspected sleep disorders as part of their problem-solving evaluation process. Finally, the importance of collaboration between school-based, community, and medical professionals is discussed with regard to identifying children with sleep problems and providing them with interventions that will allow them to experience positive educational outcomes.

LINK BETWEEN SLEEP, LEARNING, AND BEHAVIOR

Sleep problems in children can result in poor cognitive and academic performance (3) in addition to associated poor performance on tasks measuring working memory (4). For example, Gozal found a relationship between first-grade children identified with sleep-disordered breathing and their poor academic performance (5). Sleep deprivation alone limits overall cognitive efficiency (6). Specifically, inadequate sleep may lead to excessive daytime sleepiness which impacts one's overall functioning.

The impact of sleep problems may also be manifested by a child in the form of overactivity, irritability or depressive tendencies, oppositional behavior, and/ or poor impulse control. Research has shown that a relationship exists between Sleep Disordered Breathing (SDB), Periodic Limb Movement Disorder (PLMD), and symptoms of Attention-Deficit/Hyperactivity Disorder (ADHD) (7). Additionally, a relationship has been shown between sleep disorders and challenging behavior/conduct disorder (8). Specifically, Chervin found that bullying and other aggressive types of behaviors were generally two to three times more frequent among children at high risk for SDB than among other children. Researchers have also found that children with sleep problems experience reduced quality of life which also impacts psychological well-being (9).

A meta-analysis was conducted on 17 research studies published between 1966 and 2001 exploring the effects of obstructive sleep apnea syndrome (OSAS) or SDB on children (10). This study reported that the children with OSAS or SDB had significantly more problems than children in control groups without these sleep disorders in the areas of cognition, behavior (irritability, hyperactivity, etc.), academic performance, and daytime sleepiness. Furthermore, results of this meta-analysis indicated that there were significant improvements in those areas post-treatment of the OSAS or SDB.

RECENT SLEEP SCREENING RESULTS IN THE SCHOOLS AND PRIVATE PRACTICES

Recent educational screening research provides prevalence rates of sleep problems in pediatric populations and reports further evidence of the impact of these problems on educational outcomes. Luginbuehl screened 595 students from across school and clinical settings for sleep problems using the Sleep Disorders Inventory for Students (SDIS) (11). Parents were asked to rate their child's behaviors, and report information on their child's grade point average (GPA), educational placement, and any formally identified diagnoses. Significant relationships were found between sleep problems, lower GPA, and problem behaviors. Students with multiple sleep problems or a diagnosed sleep disorder had a much higher rate of placement in special education than peers without sleep problems/disorders. These students also had significantly higher rates of diagnoses such as depression, bi-polar disorder, conduct disorder, oppositional defiant disorder, and ADHD, than students without sleep problems. Forty-nine percent of students with a medically diagnosed sleep disorder were receiving special education services compared to the national average of approximately 12–14%. Students' GPAs and behaviors improved significantly post-treatment.

Witte investigated the relationship between children who were at risk for sleep problems and their subsequent development in pre-academic and behavior skills (12). Eighty-six at-risk preschool children ranging in age from three to five years were screened as part of a school district Child Find effort. Data were collected on the children's sleep using the SDIS-C (11), pre-academic skills, and internalizing and externalizing behaviors. Results demonstrated that 33% of the sample of children was rated as high risk in at least one category of sleep disorder on the SDIS-C. Additionally, another 10% of the sample scored in the cautionary range for a sleep disorder. There was a significant inverse relationship found between scores on the SDIS-C and pre-academic performance, indicating that children at risk for a sleep disorder had fewer of the skills required for success in kindergarten (i.e., skills in language, motor, and conceptual knowledge). Children with high SDIS-C scores also had significantly higher externalizing and internalizing scores than their at-risk peers.

Ax investigated the prevalence of sleep problems/disorders in 216 second- and third-grade students attending a school district in the northeast (13). This study also investigated the relationship between students with and without symptoms of sleep disorders on the following variables: classroom behavior, academic achievement in reading and math, quality of life, and life satisfaction. Symptoms of sleep disorders measured by parent completion of the SDIS-C occurred in almost one-fifth (17%) of the sample. Results supported an overall difference in school behavior and reading between students with and without symptoms of sleep disorders. Students with symptoms of sleep disorders performed significantly worse in reading achievement and exhibited significantly more internalizing and externalizing behaviors than students without symptoms of sleep disorders. There were no significant differences found between children with and without symptoms of sleep disorders on measures of quality of life and life satisfaction.

Similarly, a study conducted with a clinic-referred sample of 104 children ages two to five years found that a significant number of young children are at risk for at least one type of sleep disorder (14). In this study, 31% of the children were found to be at high-risk for at least one type of sleep disorder and an additional 10% were found to be at cautionary risk for at least one sleep disorder. Young children displaying symptoms of a sleep disorder also were reported by parents as demonstrating higher rates of externalizing and internalizing behaviors.

Clearly, the research has established a relationship between sleep problems and difficulties with learning and behavior. Furthermore, studies have demonstrated significant improvements in students' cognition, learning, and behaviors after sleep disorders are treated and corrected. The high incidence rate and negative effects of sleep problems/disorders on children's behaviors and academic performance warrants the use of a thorough screening process to identify and correct sleep problems before they significantly impair children's daytime functioning. Implementation of a comprehensive screening process in all schools and pediatric practices could ensure that the majority of children with sleep disorders are identified early and receive appropriate treatment.

COMPREHENSIVE CARE FOR CHILDREN WITH SLEEP PROBLEMS: PROGRAMMING ACROSS THE PREVENTION–INTERVENTION CONTINUUM

Treatment of children with health issues has changed over the past 10 years. Historically, in the school setting targeted children were those who were already identified and school personnel took on the roles of problem solving and intervention implementation (15). A more contemporary approach focuses on prevention and intervention, incorporating a public health model that includes all children. The emphasis is on building resources to help all children and solving problems before they become critical (16). This more contemporary approach results in an expanded model that addresses a continuum of need.

Applying this more contemporary approach to pediatric sleep disorders requires school personnel and professionals in private practice to take a more proactive role in the prevention and intervention of sleep problems. The Institute of Medicine (IOM) categorical framework of prevention can be applied to sleep disorders (Table 1) (17). For example, at the level of *universal prevention*, strategies are applied to all populations in an effort to prevent the development of sleep problems. Within this level of prevention, school personnel may decide to screen for sleep problems in all children entering kindergarten. Those children who appear at risk for sleep problems would be targeted for further assessment and intervention development. At the *selective prevention* level, a subset of children who may be at higher risk

TABLE 1   Levels of Prevention Related to Sleep Problems

Level of prevention	Recommended for screening
Universal	• All students entering kindergarten • Children referred for well child visits
Selective	• Children referred to Child Find Screenings • Students with learning problems • Students with behavior problems • Students described as lethargic, tired, or unmotivated to work • Students with DSM-IV-R diagnoses
Indicated	• Middle and high school students with frequent tardies or truancies • All students with identified drug or alcohol problems

for a sleep disorder due to membership in a particular group (i.e., students with identified learning and behavior problems) would be targeted for screening. Finally, the *indicated prevention* level is for students who may or may not meet diagnostic criteria for a sleep disorder but who are displaying characteristics of a sleep disorder such as falling asleep in class, frequent tardies or truancies, and experimentation with drugs or alcohol. This focus on prevention serves to screen for sleep problems and disorders, and target students before the disorder significantly and negatively impacts the development of academic and behavior skills.

Clearly, screening and assessment for sleep disorders is necessary within the school setting, pediatric, and mental health private practices. The following section will review screening and assessment tools developed for research or screening children and adolescents for sleep disorders. Each instrument is reviewed with respect to its intended use, psychometric properties, strengths, limitations, and implications for screening. The purpose of this chapter is not to recommend a particular instrument, but to offer the reader an objective overview of these measures and provide more than one inventory choice, depending on the child's presenting problems.

Phase I Screening

It is critical that all pediatric professionals recognize the major warning signs of a possible pediatric sleep disorder and ask parents the right questions to identify these problems. It is not enough to ask parents if their child has trouble sleeping because more than half the parents who have a child with a sleep disorder will answer this question "No" (11). Inquiries about a child exhibiting excessive daytime sleepiness (EDS), difficulty falling asleep, or frequent nighttime awakenings are more specific and may identify about 25–30% of the children with sleep problems/disorders. However, these questions alone are still insufficient. Young children with sleep disorders like OSA rarely exhibit EDS until they reach adolescence (18) or have a more serious sleep disorder or early onset narcolepsy (19). Due to the high incidence rate of sleep problems/disorders in children with learning, behavior, or emotional problems, professionals should ask parents of these children some poignant questions regarding their child's sleep habits. In Phase I, the professional only needs to ask 5–10 questions to pinpoint some of the characteristics of the major pediatric sleep disorders that impair children's daytime performance: (1) Obstructive Sleep Apnea Syndrome (OSAS), (2) Periodic Limb Movement Disorder (PLMD); (3) Restless Legs Syndrome (RLS); (4) Behavioral Insomnia of Childhood (BIC); (5) Delayed Sleep Phase Syndrome (DSPS); and (6) Narcolepsy. By asking these initial questions, the professional will rule out a sleep disorder in approximately 60% of the children/youth they screen. If parents respond in the affirmative to some of these initial questions, then the professional should proceed to Phase II, which would involve a more in-depth sleep screening inventory.

BEARS
Owens and Dalzell recommended that pediatric professionals begin by screening all children between 2 and 12 years with a simple 5-question screening tool referred to as the BEARS(20). Mindell and Owens stated that it could also be used to screen adolescents through 18 years (1). This initial screener inquires about (1) **B**edtime problems, (2) **E**xcessive daytime sleepiness, (3) **A**wakenings during the night, (4) **R**egularity of evening sleep time and morning awakenings, and (5) **S**leep-related breathing problems or snoring (20). Owens and Dalzell also reported that almost twice as many children's sleep problems were identified when the BEARS was used as a brief screener in a clinical setting than when it was left up to the pediatricians to ask questions on their own about sleep. However, less than a third of these pediatricians rated themselves as self-confident enough about sleep disorders to know how to evaluate a pediatric sleep disorder even if parents answered any of these questions in the affirmative, and only one quarter of them reported that they knew enough to treat sleep disorders. It is even less likely that school professionals or psychologists know what to do or how to assess and treat sleep problems. Therefore, a Phase I screener like the BEARS would merely alert professionals, if parents answer "yes" to any of these questions, that they need to proceed to screening with a more comprehensive inventory that can provide them with more accurate assessment information and treatment possibilities.

Strengths of the BEARS
This measure is a quick, simple screener for pediatricians and other pediatric professionals to use universally for all children from 2 through 18 years to determine if a child needs to be administered a more comprehensive sleep disorders screening inventory (Phase II). Professionals can easily remember these brief questions using the "BEARS" acronym.

Limitations of the BEARS
This measure was designed to be used by pediatricians and other medical professionals in Well Clinic Checks. However, it appears that any professional could use it due to its simplicity. It does not ask information about excessive leg movements or other movements in sleep and may miss children who have PLMD, RLS, or other parasomnias. No validity or reliability studies were reported on the BEARS in the literature. The BEARS is designed as a Phase I screener to give professionals enough information to determine if they should give a more extensive sleep screening measure.

TISS

The Ten Item Sleep Screener (TISS) is another Phase I screener for pediatric and school professionals to use. It takes a small sampling of 10 questions from the more comprehensive SDIS (11) and can be easily integrated into all pediatric and adolescent screenings. Questions on the TISS include the following about the child or adolescent: (1) Snore lightly or loudly at night? (2) Exhibit excessive daytime sleepiness? (3) Have difficulty falling asleep at night? (4) Roll, kick, or move around frequently in sleep? (5) Wake up frequently in the night? (6) Difficult to awaken in the morning? (7) Gasp, choke, or snort in sleep? (8) Stop breathing during sleep? (9) Get enough sleep at night compared to peers of the same age? and (10) Have a difficult temperament (irritable or easily frustrated)?

Strengths of the TISS

This quick and simple to administer screener is designed for use by all school and pediatric professionals working with children and adolescents. It provides one or two questions on most of the major pediatric sleep disorders, including OSAS, PLMD, RLS, DSPS, and Narcolepsy. The results can assist in determining the necessity of Phase II screening.

Limitations of the TISS

No validity or reliability studies have been conducted on the TISS. It is only designed as a Phase I screener, but does not give enough information to know with confidence if a child should be referred to a pediatric sleep specialist.

If parents answer "Yes" to any of the BEARS or the TISS questions, then the professional should proceed to Phase II screening. Phase II is a more in-depth sleep screening capable of predicting more accurately if a child has a sleep disorder and needs to be referred to a pediatric sleep specialist.

Phase II Screening

This more comprehensive screening should enable the school or pediatric professional to determine with confidence one of three things about a child/youth's sleep: (1) The child's sleep is normal or typical for a child of the same age; (2) the child/adolescent has significant sleep problems and/or a strong probability of a major sleep disorder and needs to be referred to a pediatrician or a pediatric sleep specialist; or (3) the child has significant sleep problems that probably can be corrected by a psychologist, psychiatrist, pediatrician, or school professional working together with the parent and child/youth. For example, if a child appears to have BIC or an adolescent appears to have DSPS, both of which can often be improved by teaching good sleep habits/hygiene, then the professional can give the parents and child/adolescent a list of recommendations and work with them to decrease or correct their sleep problems.

However, if there is a good probability that the child or adolescent has OSAS, PLMD, RLS, or Narcolepsy, then a referral to a pediatric sleep specialist is warranted to ensure the proper identification, treatment, and correction of these sleep disorders. The following section reviews three measures that professionals may consider using for Phase II screening. When considering the quality of screening instruments, it is important to note that desirable validity, internal consistency (reliability), and test–retest reliability coefficients range from 0.70 to 0.79, good coefficients range from 0.80 to 0.89, and high coefficients are 0.90+ (22).

Children's Sleep Habits Questionnaire—Abbreviated Form (CSHQ) (see Appendix A)
Developer: Judith A. Owens, MD (21).

Setting: At three elementary schools and a Pediatric Sleep Disorders Clinic at Rhode Island Hospital, all in southeastern New England.

Participants: 623 students in total: 469 children ages 4 through 10 years without sleep disorders (community sample) and 154 children diagnosed with a sleep disorder (clinical sample).

Demographics: The community and clinical samples did not differ by gender, but the community sample was significantly older and had a higher socioeconomic status (SES) than the clinical sample; both samples were predominantly White, middle-income English-speaking suburban families that did not reflect the 2000 U.S. census demographics.

Questionnaire Qualities: The CSHQ is a 33-item parent questionnaire for children from 4 to 10 years of age, which is rated on a three-point scale ("usually," meaning behavior occurred 5–7 times per week; "sometimes," or 2–4 times per week; "rarely," or 0–1 time per week). It is available in English. The CHSQ yields a Total Score and eight sleep domain scale scores: (1) Bedtime Resistance, (2) Sleep Duration, (3) Parasomnias, (4) Sleep-disordered Breathing, (5) Night Awakenings, (6) Daytime Sleepiness, (7) Sleep Anxiety, and (8) Sleep Onset Delay. The developer of this questionnaire reported that the CHSQ's primary purpose is for research by pediatric sleep specialists, not for screenings by clinicians. She also stated that there is a longer, more comprehensive CSHQ version, but it has not been validated.

Sleep Problems Measured and Results: Using the CSHQ, it was possible to distinguish between the community sample and children with sleep disorders on each subscale and by using the total score. The CSHQ had an overall sensitivity of 0.80, meaning that 80% of the clinical group with sleep problems/disorders would have been correctly identified by this measure. Children in the clinical sample diagnosed with a sleep problem/disorder scored significantly higher on that specific sleep scale than other scales of the CSHQ. Internal consistency for the total CSHQ was 0.68 for the community sample and 0.78 for the clinical sample. The eight subscales varied in their psychometric qualities based on the reported validity and reliability coefficients. Six of the eight sleep scales had internal consistency coefficients below 0.70 for the community sample, and three scales were below 0.70 for the clinical sample. Internal consistency was not reported for the Sleep Onset Delay Scale because it consisted of only one item. Seven of the eight sleep scales had test–retest reliability coefficients below 0.70. A few of the scales fell below the adequate range on some of the reliability coefficients (Table 2).

Strengths
The CSHQ was developed by a leading pediatric sleep specialist. The rating scale is well-defined, which helps to prevent misinterpretation by parents. The cut-off score for referring children for further evaluation is clearly delineated. It can be used to

TABLE 2 Summary of the Empirical Features of the Children's Sleep Habits Questionnaire (CSHQ)

Inventory and subscales	Sample size	Age range	Content validation	Hit rate	Sensitivity	Specificity	EFA	CFA	Mann-Whitney U	Internal consistency	Test retest	Computer score/report
CSHQ total	623	4–10 yr	No	?	0.80	0.72	No	No	p<0.001	0.68	?	No
Bedtime resistance	Comm. 382	4–10 yr	No	?	Not reported	Not reported	No	No	p<0.001	0.70	N=56	No
	Clinical 128	4–10 yr	No				No	No		0.83	0.68	
Sleep onset delay	Comm. 403	4–10 yr	No	?	Not reported	Not reported	No	No	p<0.001	None	N=60	No
	Clinical 128	4–10 yr	No				No	No		None	0.62	
Sleep duration	Comm. 398	4–10 yr	No	?	Not reported	Not reported	No	No	p<0.001	0.69	N=60	No
	Clinical 122	4–10 yr	No				No	No		0.80	0.40	
Sleep anxiety	Comm. 374	4–10 yr	No	?	Not reported	Not reported	No	No	p<0.001	0.63	N=56	No
	Clinical 119	4–10 yr	No				No	No		0.68	0.79	
Night wakings	Comm. 384	4–10 yr	No	?	Not reported	Not reported	No	No	p<0.001	0.54	N=56	No
	Clinical 120	4–10 yr	No				No	No		0.44	0.63	
Parasomnias	Comm. 371	4–10 yr	No	?	Not reported	Not reported	No	No	p<0.001	0.36	N=57	No
	Clinical 117	4–10 yr	No				No	No		0.56	0.62	
Sleep disorder breathing	Comm. 382	4–10 yr	No	?	Not reported	Not reported	No	No	p<0.001	0.51	N=58	No
	Clinical 117	4–10 yr	No				No	No		0.93	0.69	
Daytime sleepiness	Comm. 381	4–10 yr	No	?	Not reported	Not reported	No	No	p<0.001	0.65	N=56	No
	Clinical 119	4–10 yr	No				No	No		0.70	0.65	

Note 1. CSHQ=Children's Sleep Habits Questionnaire; EFA=Exploratory Factor Analysis; CFA=Confirmatory Factor Analysis

Note 2. Adequate validity and reliability coefficients are 0.70–0.79; Good coefficients are 0.80–0.89; High coefficients are 0.90+

predict that a child has some of the pediatric sleep disorders such as SDB and various nighttime behavioral problems. It has adequate internal consistency reliability on the Bedtime Resistance subscale for both the community and clinical samples and adequate internal consistency for the clinical sample for Sleep Duration, SDB, and Daytime Sleepiness, but not for the community sample. This is the only pediatric sleep inventory to date that screens for sleep anxiety, which many young children experience. Therefore, if parents are mentioning these specific sleep problems to the professional, the CSHQ may be a helpful tool to use. The abbreviated and comprehensive versions of the CSHQ can be downloaded from Dr. Owens' website. There are also a variety of other sleep surveys on the website for parents and the child/adolescent, as well as sleep logs and sleep diaries that can be helpful in gathering information about a child's sleep problems. The website also has many journal articles posted on pediatric sleep problems.

Limitations
The CSHQ was normed and validated in only one sleep clinic and three schools in the nation. There were significant differences in age and SES between the community and clinical samples, which may have confounded the results. The CSHQ participant demographics do not reflect the 2000 U.S. census demographics, which poses concerns about nationwide use of the CSHQ with children from differing race, ethnic backgrounds, or regions of the country. All of the subscales, except Bedtime Resistance, had an internal consistency alpha coefficient score < 0.70 for the community sample, which is somewhat problematic if a professional wants to screen community populations. Therefore, as recommended by the developer, the CSHQ might be more appropriate for use by sleep specialists in clinical or research settings with predominantly White, English-speaking patients.

Only one subscale (Sleep Anxiety) had a test–retest reliability coefficient of > 0.70. The Sleep Onset Delay Scale consists of only one item, which is less than the recommended minimum of three items (22). The Sleep-Disordered Breathing scale has the minimum requirement of three items. However, this small amount of items may explain why the internal consistency for the community sample and test–retest reliability coefficients are lower than desirable for this scale. Although the CSHQ gives valuable and comprehensive information about a variety of sleep problems that young children may experience, it was not designed for use with adolescents or use by most pediatric professionals in clinical practice or school settings.

For Further Information: see Owens, Spirito, and McGuinn (21) or website: www.kidzzzsleep.org

Pediatric Sleep Questionnaire (PSQ)
(see Appendix B)
Developer: Ronald Chervin, M.D. (23–25).

Participants: In the initial validation, participants included 162 children from 2 through 18 years of age: 108 were patients at two general pediatric clinics without sleep disorders (quasi-community sample) and 54 children were diagnosed with a Sleep-Related Breathing Disorder (SRBD) (clinical sample). Validation of a Periodic Limb Movement Disorder (PLMD) scale was conducted on a sample of 113 children from 2.8 to 18.0 years between 1996 and 2000; 29 children had PLMD and 84 did not (24). A further validation of the 22-item SRBD scale was completed on 105 children between 5.0 to 12.9 years of age.

Demographics: Specific demographic characteristics for the community and clinical samples were not available.

Questionnaire Qualities: The PSQ was initially a 22-item parent questionnaire for children from 2 through 18 years, and rated on a simple three-point scale ("yes," "no," or "don't know") for all items except the inattention/hyperactivity items that are rated on a four-point Likert scale. The PSQ provides an overall Total Score and five sleep scales: (1) Sleep-Related Breathing Disorder (SRBD), (2) Snoring, (3) Sleepiness, (4) Behavior, and (5) PLMD. The questionnaire is in English.

Sleep Problems Measured and Results: Exploratory factor analysis was used in the first validation study to determine the need for the four specific sleep scales on this measure. Using these PSQ scales and a total score, the PSQ distinguished the children with a diagnosis of SRBD 85% of the time (sensitivity of 0.85) for Group A and 81% for Group B. It had a specificity of 0.87 for both groups (n=54). The subscales had fairly good internal consistency reliability coefficients ranging from 0.66 to 0.89, as well as test–retest reliability ranging from .66 to .92; the Sleepiness Scale had slightly lower than desirable reliability. In the second validation of the PSQ for SRBD, it had an overall hit rate of 74%, a sensitivity of 0.78, and a specificity of 0.72. The PSQ SRBD scale also had moderate to low correlations ($p<0.001$ to 0.06) with polysomnographic measures. The overall predictive validity hit rate for the PLMD scale was 62%, the sensitivity was 79%, and the specificity was 56%. Internal consistency reliability was 0.71 and test–retest reliability was 0.62 (see Table 3 for a summary of the PSQ psychometric qualities).

Strengths: The PSQ was developed by a leading pediatric sleep specialist. It has good structural validity and the ability to predict SRBD (sensitivity), as well as distinguish the community sample from the clinical sample. It has fair predictive validity for PLMD. It has good internal consistency reliability for the SRBD, Snoring, and Behavior scales. The scoring cut-off for recommended referral is clearly delineated for SRBD. The PSQ: SRBD scale has been validated in numerous other sleep research studies and has proven its screening benefits in that capacity.

Limitations: It does not appear that the PSQ has been normed and validated on samples that reflect the 2000 U.S. census demographics, resulting in some concern about its use for children of different races and ethnic backgrounds. Furthermore, it was reported that the sample sizes of young children and older adolescents were too small in the validation studies to accurately determine differences in age groups, which suggests that more validation studies need to be conducted specifically on young children and adolescents from varying ethnic and SES levels. The sleepiness scale had somewhat weak internal consistency and the sleepiness and PLMD scales had slightly lower than desirable test–retest reliability. However, the PSQ gives valuable information about SRBD and PLMD and can identify many of the children with these disorders. If pediatricians, psychologists, psychiatrists, and other professionals are going to take the time to screen children or adolescents for sleep problems/disorders, then it would be beneficial to add items to the PSQ for other major pediatric sleep disorders negatively impacting daytime performance such as BIC, DSPS, and Narcolepsy.

Table 3 Summary of the Empirical Features of the Pediatric Sleep Questionnaire (PSQ)

Inventory and subscales	Sample size	Age range	Content validation	Hit rate	Sensitivity	Specificity	EFA	CFA	Mann-Whitney U	Internal consistency	Test retest	Computer score/report
PSQ Total	162	2–18 yr	Not reported	Not reported	Grp A=0.85 Grp B=0.81	Grp A=0.87 Grp B=0.87	Yes Good	No	Logistic Regress	No report	No report	No
Sleep related breathing	Grp A=116 Grp B=154	2–18 yr	Not reported	Not reported	0.85	0.87	Good	No	0.92 <0.0001	Grp A=0.89 Grp B=.88	N=21 0.75	No
Snoring	Grp A=116 Grp B=154	2–18 yr	Not reported	Not reported	Not reported	Not reported	Good	No	0.85 <0.0001	Grp A=0.86 Grp B=0.86	N=21 0.92	No
Sleepiness	Grp A=116 Grp B=154	2–18 yr	Not reported	Not reported	Not reported	Not reported	Good	No	0.77 0.0016	Grp A=0.66 Grp B=0.77	N=21 0.66	No
Behavior	Grp A=116 Grp B=154	2–18 yr	Not reported	Not reported	Not reported	Not reported	Good	No	0.79 0.0017	Grp A=0.84 Grp B=0.83	N=21 0.83	No
PLMD	N=113	2.8–18 yr	Not reported	0.62	0.79	0.56	None	None		0.71	0.62	No

Note 1. PSQ=Pediatric Sleep Questionnaire; EFA=Exploratory Factor Analysis; CFA=Confirmatory Factor Analysis
Note 2. Adequate validity and reliability coefficients are 0.70–0.79; Good coefficients are 0.80–0.89; High coefficients are 0.90+

Contact Information: Ronald D. Chervin, M.D., M.S. Michael S. Aldrich, Sleep Disorders Laboratory, C734 Med Inn Building, 1500 E. Medical Center Drive, Ann Arbor, MI 48109, U.S.A.

Sleep Disorders Inventory for Students (SDIS)
(see Appendix C)

Developer: Marsha Luginbuehl, Ph.D.; assisted by W. McDowell Anderson, M.D., George Batsche, Ed.D., Selim R. Benbadis, M.D., Kathy L. Bradley-Klug, Ph.D., John Ferron, Ph.D., Trevor Stokes, Ph.D., University of South Florida (11).

Setting: The SDIS was validated and standardized on children and adolescents from 45 schools, two psychology private practices, and seven pediatric sleep centers nationwide, six of which were American Academy of Sleep Medicine (AASM) accredited.

Participants: There were 821 total children; 602 were in the school/community sample and had not undergone a sleep evaluation of any kind; 219 were in the clinical sample and were undergoing a comprehensive sleep evaluation at a sleep center or had already been diagnosed with a sleep disorder at a pediatric sleep center.

Demographics: The main study sample of 595 children and their families closely reflected the 2000 U.S. Census demographics for ethnicity, SES, parents' education, and primary language.

Questionnaire Qualities: The SDIS has two inventories: (1) the SDIS-Children's Form (SDIS-C) for children from 2 through 10 years and (2) the SDIS-Adolescent Form (SDIS-A) for youth from 11 through 18 years. The SDIS-C has 25 items measuring four sleep scales and the SDIS-A has 30 items measuring five sleep scales. The SDIS-C has the following scales: Obstructive Sleep Apnea Syndrome (OSAS), Periodic Limb Movement Disorder (PLMD), Delayed Sleep Phase Syndrome (DSPS), and Excessive Daytime Sleepiness (EDS). The SDIS-A has the same scales plus some Restless Legs Syndrome questions added to the PLMD scale and a narcolepsy scale. Both inventories have five items measuring five parasomnias, as well as 11 general health questions written in a "yes" or "no" format. Both inventories also yield a total Sleep Disturbance Index and are available in English and Spanish. The items are written on a well-defined seven-point Likert scale to provide more sensitivity, and the reading level for items ranges from third to fifth grade. The inventories also have computer scoring that produces a comprehensive report and graph with standard T-scores, percentiles, and three sleep classifications ("Normal Sleep," "Caution" range, and "High Risk" of a sleep disorder).

Sleep Problems Measured and Results: The SDIS has high content validity of 0.94, construct or structural validity indicating good exploratory factor analysis factor loadings for the scales and good fit indices for the SDIS-C and SDIS-A confirmatory factor analyses. Predictive validity for the SDIS-C was 0.86 and 0.96 for the SDIS-A; Sensitivity for the SDIS-C was 0.82 and 0.81 for the SDIS-A; Specificity for the SDIS-C was 0.91 and 0.95 for the SDIS-A; internal consistency for the total SDIS-C was 0.91 and 0.92 for the total SDIS-A; test–retest reliability for the total SDIS-C was 0.97 and 0.86 for the SDIS-A.

    The subscales of the SDIS-C and SDIS-A have good predictive validity coefficients ranging from 0.72 to 1.0; sensitivity ranges from a low of 0.50 and 0.55 for the

PLMD/RLS scales to a high of 1.0 for two other scales; specificity ranges from 0.62 to 0.98; and internal consistency ranges from 0.71 to 0.92. Test–retest reliability was calculated for the overall SDIS-C and SDIS-A (see Table 4 for a summary of the SDIS qualities).

Strengths: The SDIS was developed with the assistance of many leading pediatric sleep specialists. It was validated on a relatively large sample, and the main study samples closely reflected the 2000 U.S. census demographics. It uses a broad, well-defined rating scale, which enables professionals to determine the severity of the various sleep problems. Both the SDIS-C and SDIS-A have good predictive validity, structural validity, and sensitivity for all subscales except the PLMD/RLS scales. However, PLMD is difficult to accurately diagnose using a one-night sleep study because nighttime inconsistencies of leg movements are frequently noted in children with PLMD, and the PLMD scale sensitivity might be higher if the hospital cases were measured with actigraphy over 4–5 nights. Similar problems were noted when validating the PLMD scale on the PSQ. The PLMD scales have good specificity. Both SDIS inventories have good internal consistency and test–retest reliability, and are available in both English and Spanish. Computer scoring provides a graph and report with recommendations and interventions when any sleep scale or parasomnia is rated higher than normal. Finally, the SDIS-C and SDIS-A were validated on community, school, private practice, and hospital populations with the purpose of using these inventories for any pediatric population in any setting, even if the professionals conducting the screenings had limited knowledge about sleep disorders. Furthermore, if professionals do not want to do a comprehensive screening for pediatric sleep disorders, but parents have mentioned some sleep concerns in Phase I questioning, the professional can refer these parents to the SDIS website: www.Sleepdisorderhelp.com where the parents can click onto the "Screening by Parents" to quickly screen their child on line with the SDIS and immediately download the results with a graph and report. This on-line report provides parents with a website where they can obtain the names and addresses of sleep clinics in their local area. This website also provides a great deal of information about the major pediatric sleep disorders and related problems, and how they negatively impact a child's daytime performance and health.

Limitations: It would be beneficial for more hospital validation studies to be conducted on larger populations of children and adolescents, including larger samples of narcolepsy, DSPS, PLMD/RLS, and Spanish-speaking families. However, no differences were noted between responses of the Spanish-speaking and English-speaking parents in the initial validation study. When a child has severe OSAS, it negatively impacts and escalates all of the SDIS sleep scales, making it appear that the child has four or five sleep disorders. In this case, the report states that the child rarely has all of these sleep disorders, but it is most likely that s/he has OSAS, which should be ruled out first because severe OSAS escalates all scales.

For Further Information: see Luginbuehl (11) or contact: Child Uplift, Inc., PO Box 146; Fairview, WY 83110; Phone: 307-886-9096; Email: Childuplift@aol.com or contact: www.Sleepdisorderhelp.com or Harcourt Assessment, Inc. at www.PsychCorp.com, the national distributor of the SDIS.

TABLE 4 Summary of the Empirical Features of the Sleep Disorders Inventory for Students (SDIS)

Inventory/ subscales	Sample size	Age range	Content validation	Hit rate	Sensitivity	Specificity	EFA	CFA	Internal consistency	Test retest	Computer score/report
SDIS Total	821	2–18 yr	0.94				Good	Good	0.91	0.97	Yes
SDIS-Child	412	2–10 yr		86%	0.82	0.91	Good	>0.90 Fit	0.90	Not done	Yes
OSAS	412	2–10 yr		72%	0.91	0.62	Good	>0.90 Fit	0.85	Not done	Yes
PLMD	412	2–10 yr		77%	0.50	0.93	Good	>0.90 Fit	0.76	Not done	Yes
BIC/DSPS	412	2–10 yr		100%	1.0	0.98	Good	>0.90 Fit	0.84	Not done	Yes
EDS	412	2–10 yr		80% NARC	N/A	N/A	Good	>0.90 Fit	0.92	Not done	Yes
SDIS-Adol.	180	11–18 yr		96%	0.81	0.95	None	>0.90 Fit	0.88	0.86	Yes
OSAS	180	11–18 yr		100%	1.0	0.92	None	>0.90 Fit	0.85	Not done	Yes
PLMD/RLS	180	11–18 yr		78%	0.55	0.91	None	>0.90 Fit	0.71	Not done	Yes
DSPS	180	11–18 yr		100%	1.0	0.98	None	>0.90 Fit	0.92	Not done	Yes
NARC	180	11–18 yr		100%	0.88	0.97	None	>0.90 Fit	0.92	Not done	Yes
EDS	180	11–18 yr		80% NARC	N/A	N/A	None	>0.90 Fit	0.83	Not done	Yes

Note 1. EFA=Exploratory Factor Analysis, CFA=Confirmatory Factor Analysis, OSAS=Obstructive Sleep Apnea Syndrome, PLMD= Periodic Limb Movement Disorder, DSPS=Delayed Sleep Phase Syndrome, EDS=Excessive Daytime Sleepiness, RLS=Restless Legs Syndrome, NARC=Narcolepsy

CONCLUSIONS

Having tools to screen for sleep disorders is vital, but is only one part of the process in working with children to prevent and monitor the development of sleep problems. In order to provide the most appropriate services for children and families with sleep problems, professionals must engage in a structured problem-solving process that incorporates collaboration and communication among professionals (26). Problem identification is the most important step of the problem-solving process, followed by problem analysis, which involves a comprehensive assessment of the child's needs and factors within the ecology. For many children, problem identification and analysis involves a comprehensive assessment that should include data collection with a sleep-screening inventory and a discussion with parents about the child's sleep hygiene. If the screening and data collection indicate a high risk of a sleep disorder, then interdisciplinary collaboration between professionals becomes crucial. This includes communication among all of the individuals involved, including the child, family, pediatrician and/or sleep specialist, school psychologist, teachers, school nurse, and other professionals in the community working with the student. These professionals should discuss with the parents the importance of follow through with a visit to the pediatrician to pursue a comprehensive sleep evaluation. This process often requires follow-up with the parents a month or two later to inquire about the status of the referral. Parents must be educated as to the serious health and educational consequences if the child's sleep disorder is not corrected.

Screening for sleep problems/disorders at the universal, selective, and indicated levels may prevent students from experiencing the collateral academic and/or behavioral problems often associated with these disorders. Correct identification and treatment of the sleep disorder may significantly improve a child's learning and behaviors post treatment. When considering the negative impact sleep disorders have on learning, behaviors, health, career, and safety throughout a lifetime, pediatric professionals in our society cannot afford to neglect early and regular screening of children for these disorders.

REFERENCES

1. Mindell JA, Owens JA. A Clinical Guide to Pediatric Sleep: Diagnosis and Management of Sleep Problems. Philadelphia: Lippincott Williams & Wilkins, 2003.
2. National Institute of Health. Wake Up America: A national sleep alert, Vol. 1. Washington, DC: Government Printing Office, 2001:1–76.
3. Montgomery-Downs HE, Crabtree VM, Gozal D. Cognition, sleep and respiration in at risk children treated for obstructive sleep apnea. European Respiratory Journal 2005; 25:336–42.
4. Steenari M. Working memory and sleep in 6- to 13-year old children. Journal of the American Academy of Child and Adolescent Psychiatry 2003; 42:85–92.
5. Gozal D. Sleep-disordered breathing and school performance in children. Pediatrics 1998; 102:616–20.
6. Mitru G, Millrood D, Mateika J. The impact of sleep on learning and behavior in adolescents. Teachers College Record 2002; 104:704–26.
7. Chervin RD, Dillon J, Bassetti C, et al. Symptoms of sleep disorders, inattention, and hyperactivity in children. Sleep 1997; 20(12):1185–92.
8. Chervin RD, Archbold KH, Dillon JE, et al. Inattention, hyperactivity, and symptoms of sleep-disordered breathing. Pediatrics 2002; 109:449–56.

9. Crabtree V, Ivanenko A, O'Brien L, et al. Periodic limb movement disorder of sleep in children. Journal of Sleep Research 2003; 12:73–81.
10. Ebert CS, Drake AF. The impact of sleep-disordered breathing on cognition and behavior in children: A review and meta-synthesis of the literature. Otolaryngology-Head and Neck Surgery 2004; 131:814–26.
11. Luginbuehl ML. The initial development and validation study of the Sleep Disorders Inventory for Students. Dissertation Abstracts International Section A: Humanities & Social Sciences 2004; 64(12-A):4376.
12. Witte R. The relationship between sleep disorders, behaviors, and pre-academic skills in pre-kindergarteners. Unpublished educational specialist thesis, Tampa, Florida: University of South Florida, 2007.
13. Ax EA. Effect of Sleep Disorders on School Behavior, Academic Performance and Quality of Life. Unpublished doctoral dissertation, Tampa, Florida: University of South Florida, 2006.
14. Popkave KM. The relationship between parent identified sleep problems, internalizing behaviors, externalizing behaviors, and adaptive functioning in a pediatric population. Unpublished educational specialist thesis, Tampa, Florida: University of South Florida, 2007.
15. Power TJ, DuPaul GJ, Shapiro ES, et al. Pediatric school psychology: The emergence of a subspecialty. School Psychology Review 1995; 24:244–57.
16. Power TJ, DuPaul GJ, Shapiro ES, et al. Promoting Children's Health: Integrating school, family, and community. New York: Guilford Press 2003.
17. Institute of Medicine. Reducing Risks For Mental Disorders: Frontiers for Preventive Intervention Research. Washington, DC: National Academy Press 1994.
18. Carroll, JL, Loughlin, GM. Obstructive Sleep Apnea Syndrome in infants and children: Clinical features and pathophysiology. In Ferber, R. & Kryger, M. (eds.), Principles and Practices of Sleep Medicine in the Child. Philadelphia: W.B. Saunders Company, 1995: pp. 163–91.
19. Rosen RC, Zozula R, Jahn EG, Carson JL. Low rates of recognition of sleep disorders in primary care: Comparison of a community-based versus clinical academic setting. Sleep Medicine, 2001; 2(1):47–55.
20. Owens JA, Dalzell V. Use of the 'BEARS' sleep screening tool in a pediatric residents' continuity clinic: A pilot study. Sleep Medicine 2005; 6:63–9.
21. Owens JA, Spirito A, McGuinn M. The Children's Sleep Habits Questionnaire (CSHQ): Psychometric properties of a survey instrument for school-aged children. Sleep 2000; 23(8):1043–51.
22. Crocker L, Algina J. Introduction to Classical Modern Test Theory. New York: Holt, Rinehart and Winston.
23. Chervin RC, Hedger K, Dillon JE, et al. Pediatric Sleep Questionnaire (PSQ): Validity and reliability of scales for sleep-disordered breathing, snoring, sleepiness, and behavioral problems. Sleep Medicine 2000; 1:21–32.
24. Chervin RD, Hedger KM. Clinical prediction of periodic leg movements during sleep in children. Sleep Medicine 2001; 2:501–10.
25. Chervin RD, Weatherly RA, Garetz SL, et al. Pediatric Sleep Questionnaire. Arch Otolaryngol. Head Neck Surgery 2007; 133:216–22.
26. Bradley-Klug KL, Grier EC, Ax EE. Chronic illness. In Bear, GG, Minke, KM eds. Children's needs III: Development, prevention, and intervention. Bethesda, MD: National Association of School Psychologists, 2006: pp. 857–69.

Appendix A

Children's Sleep Habits Questionnaire—Abbreviated Form (CSHQ)

The following statements are about your child's sleep habits and possible difficulties with sleep. Think about the past week in your child's life when answering the questions. If last week was unusual for a specific reason (such as your child had an ear infection and did not sleep well or the TV set was broken), choose the most recent typical week. Answer USUALLY if something occurs **5 or more times** in a week; answer SOMETIMES if it occurs **2–4 times** in a week; answer RARELY if something occurs **never or 1 time** during a week. Also, please indicate whether or not the sleep habit is a problem by circling "Yes," "No," or "Not applicable (N/A)."

Bedtime

Write in child's bedtime: _____

	3 Usually (5–7)	2 Sometimes (2–4)	1 Rarely (0–1)	Problem?
1) Child goes to bed at the same time at night **(R)**	☐	☐	☐	Yes No N/A
2) Child falls asleep within 20 minutes after going to bed **(R)**	☐	☐	☐	Yes No N/A
3) Child falls asleep alone in own bed **(R)**	☐	☐	☐	Yes No N/A
4) Child falls asleep in parent's or sibling's bed	☐	☐	☐	Yes No N/A
5) Child needs parent in the room to fall asleep	☐	☐	☐	Yes No N/A
6) Child struggles at bedtime (cries, refuses to stay in bed, etc.)	☐	☐	☐	Yes No N/A
7) Child is afraid of sleeping in the dark	☐	☐	☐	Yes No N/A
8) Child is afraid of sleep alone	☐	☐	☐	Yes No N/A

Sleep Behavior

Child's usual amount of sleep each day: _____ hours and _____ minutes (combining nighttime sleep and naps)

Sleep Behavior (continued)

	3 Usually (5–7)	2 Sometimes (2–4)	1 Rarely (0–1)	Problem?
9) Child sleeps too little	☐	☐	☐	Yes No N/A
10) Child sleeps the right amount **(R)**	☐	☐	☐	Yes No N/A
11) Child sleeps about the same amount each day **(R)**	☐	☐	☐	Yes No N/A
12) Child wets the bed at night	☐	☐	☐	Yes No N/A
13) Child talks during sleep	☐	☐	☐	Yes No N/A
14) Child is restless and moves a lot during sleep	☐	☐	☐	Yes No N/A
15) Child sleepwalks during the night	☐	☐	☐	Yes No N/A
16) Child moves to someone else's bed during the night (parent, brother, sister, etc.)	☐	☐	☐	Yes No N/A
17) Child grinds teeth during sleep (your dentist may have told you this)	☐	☐	☐	Yes No N/A
18) Child snores loudly	☐	☐	☐	Yes No N/A
19) Child seems to stop breathing during sleep	☐	☐	☐	Yes No N/A
20) Child snorts and/or gasps during sleep	☐	☐	☐	Yes No N/A
21) Child has trouble sleeping away from home (visiting relatives, vacation)	☐	☐	☐	Yes No N/A
22) Child awakens during night screaming, sweating, and inconsolable	☐	☐	☐	Yes No N/A
23) Child awakens alarmed by a frightening dream	☐	☐	☐	Yes No N/A

Waking During the Night

	3 Usually (5–7)	2 Sometimes (2–4)	1 Rarely (0–1)	Problem?
24) Child awakes once during the night	☐	☐	☐	Yes No N/A
25) Child awakes more than once during the night	☐	☐	☐	Yes No N/A

Write the number of minutes a night waking usually lasts: _____

Morning Waking/Daytime Sleepiness

Write in the time of day child usually wakes in the morning: _____

	3 Usually (5–7)	2 Sometimes (2–4)	1 Rarely (0–1)	Problem?
26) Child wakes up by him/herself **(R)**	☐	☐	☐	Yes No N/A
27) Child wakes up in negative mood	☐	☐	☐	Yes No N/A
28) Adults or siblings wake up child	☐	☐	☐	Yes No N/A
29) Child has difficulty getting out of bed in the morning	☐	☐	☐	Yes No N/A
30) Child takes a long time to become alert in the morning	☐	☐	☐	Yes No N/A
31) Child seems tired	☐	☐	☐	Yes No N/A

Child has appeared very sleepy or fallen asleep during the following (check all that apply):

	3 Not Sleepy	2 Very Sleepy	1 Falls Asleep
32) Watching TV	☐	☐	☐
33) Riding in car	☐	☐	☐

Appendix B

PEDIATRIC SLEEP QUESTIONNAIRE

Version 991207

Child's Name: _____,_____ _____.
                        (Last)   (First)   (M.I.)

Name of Person Answering Questions:_____.
                    Relation to Child:_____.
Your phone number, days: _____, and evenings:_____.
                        Area Code   Number   Area Code   Number

Relative's name and number in case we cannot reach you: _____.
                                                        _____.
                                                        Area Code   Number

Instructions:

Please answer the questions on the following pages regarding the behavior of your child during sleep and wakefulness. The questions apply to how your child acts in general, not necessarily during the past few days since these may not have been typical if your child has not been well. If you are not sure how to answer any question, please feel free to ask your husband or wife, child, or physician for help. You should circle the correct response or *print* your answers neatly in the space provided. A "Y" means "yes," "N" means "no," and "DK" means "don't know." When you see the word "usually" it means "more than half the time" or "on more than half the nights."

GENERAL INFORMATION ABOUT YOUR CHILD:

	Office use only
	GI1
Today's Date: _____. Month Day Year	GI2
Where are you completing this questionnaire? _____.	GI3
Date of Child's Birth: _____. Month Day Year	GI4
Sex: Male or Female? _____.	GI5
Current Height (feet/inches): _____.	GI6
Current Weight (pounds): _____.	GI7
Grade in school (if applicable): _____.	GI8
Racial/Ethnic Background of your Child (please circle):	GI9

    1.) American-Indian   2.) Asian-American
    3.) African-American   4.) Hispanic
    5.) White/not Hispanic   6.) Other or unknown

A. Nighttime and sleep behavior: WHILE SLEEPING, DOES YOUR CHILD …		Office use only
… ever snore?	Y N DK	A1
… snore more than half the time?	Y N DK	A2
… always snore?	Y N DK	A3
… snore loudly?	Y N DK	A4
… have "heavy" or loud breathing?	Y N DK	A5
… have trouble breathing, or struggle to breathe?	Y N DK	A6
HAVE YOU EVER …		
… seen your child stop breathing during the night? If so, please describe what has happened:	Y N DK	A7
… been concerned about your child's breathing during sleep?	Y N DK	A8
… had to shake your sleeping child to get him or her to breathe, or wake up and breathe?	Y N DK	A9
… seen your child wake up with a snorting sound?	Y N DK	A11
DOES YOUR CHILD …		
… have restless sleep?	Y N DK	A12
… describe restlessness of the legs when in bed?	Y N DK	A13
… have "growing pains" (unexplained leg pains)?	Y N DK	A13a
… have "growing pains" that are worst in bed?	Y N DK	A13b
WHILE YOUR CHILD SLEEPS, HAVE YOU SEEN …		
… brief kicks of one leg or both legs?	Y N DK	A14
… repeated kicks or jerks of the legs at regular intervals (i.e., about every 20 to 40 seconds)?	Y N DK	A14a
AT NIGHT, DOES YOUR CHILD USUALLY …		
… become sweaty, or do the pajamas usually become wet with perspiration?	Y N DK	A15
… get out of bed (for any reason)?	Y N DK	A16
… get out of bed to urinate?	Y N DK	A17
If so, how many times each night, on average?	_____ times	A17a
Does your child usually sleep with the mouth open?	Y N DK	A21
Is your child's nose usually congested or "stuffed" at night?	Y N DK	A22
Do any allergies affect your child's ability to breathe through the nose?	Y N DK	A23
DOES YOUR CHILD …		
… tend to breathe through the mouth during the day?	Y N DK	A24
… have a dry mouth on waking up in the morning?	Y N DK	A25
… complain of an upset stomach at night?	Y N DK	A27

… get a burning feeling in the throat at night?	Y N DK	A29
… grind his or her teeth at night?	Y N DK	A30
… occasionally wet the bed?	Y N DK	A32
Has your child ever walked during sleep ("sleep walking")?	Y N DK	A33
Have you ever heard your child talk during sleep ("sleep talking")?	Y N DK	A34
Does your child have nightmares once a week or more on average?	Y N DK	A35
Has your child ever woken up screaming during the night?	Y N DK	A36
Has your child ever been moving or behaving, at night, in a way that made you think your child was neither completely awake nor asleep? If so, please describe what has happened:	Y N DK	A37
Does your child have difficulty falling asleep at night?	Y N DK	A40
How long does it take your child to fall asleep at night? (a guess is O.K.)	_____ minutes	A41
At bedtime does your child usually have difficult "routines" or "rituals," argue a lot, or otherwise behave badly?	Y N DK	A42
DOES YOUR CHILD … … bang his or her head or rock his or her body when going to sleep?	Y N DK	A43
… wake up more than twice a night on average?	Y N DK	A44
… have trouble falling back asleep if he or she wakes up at night?	Y N DK	A45
… wake up early in the morning and have difficulty going back to sleep?	Y N DK	A46
Does the time at which your child *goes to bed* change a lot from day to day?	Y N DK	A47
Does the time at which your child *gets up from bed* change a lot from day to day?	Y N DK	A48
WHAT TIME DOES YOUR CHILD USUALLY … … go to bed during the week?		A49
… go to bed on the weekend or vacation?		A50
… get out of bed on weekday mornings?		A51
… get out of bed on weekend or vacation mornings?		A52

B. Daytime behavior and other possible problems: DOES YOUR CHILD …		Office Use Only
… wake up feeling *un*refreshed in the morning?	Y N DK	B1
… have a problem with sleepiness during the day?	Y N DK	B2
… complain that he or she feels sleepy during the day?	Y N DK	B3
Has a teacher or other supervisor commented that your child appears sleepy during the day?	Y N DK	B4
Does your child usually take a nap during the day?	Y N DK	B5
Is it hard to wake your child up in the morning?	Y N DK	B6
Does your child wake up with headaches in the morning?	Y N DK	B7
Does your child get a headache at least once a month, on average?	Y N DK	B8
Did your child stop growing at a normal rate at any time since birth?	Y N DK	B9
If so, please describe what happened:		
Does your child still have tonsils?	Y N DK	B10
If not, when and why were they removed?:		
HAS YOUR CHILD EVER …		
… had a condition causing difficulty with breathing? If so, please describe:	Y N DK	B11
… had surgery?	Y N DK	B12
If so, did any difficulties with breathing occur before, during, or after surgery?	Y N DK	B12a
… become suddenly weak in the legs, or anywhere else, after laughing or being surprised by something?	Y N DK	B13
… felt unable to move for a short period, in bed, though awake and able to look around?	Y N DK	B15
Has your child felt an irresistible urge to take a nap at times, forcing him or her to stop what he or she is doing inorder to sleep?	Y N DK	B16
Has your child ever sensed that he or she was dreaming (seeing images or hearing sounds) while still awake?	Y N DK	B17
Does your child drink caffeinated beverages on a typical day (cola, tea, coffee)?	Y N DK	B18
If so, how many cups or cans per day?	_____ cups	B18a
Does your child use any recreational drugs?	Y N DK	B19
If so, which ones and how often?:		
Does your child use cigarettes, smokeless tobacco, snuff, or other tobacco products? If so, which ones and how often?:	Y N DK	B20
Is your child overweight?	Y N DK	B22
If so, at what age did this first develop?	_____ years	B22a
Has a doctor ever told you that your child has a high-arched palate (roof of the mouth)?	Y N DK	B23

Has your child ever taken Ritalin (methylphenidate) for behavioral problems?	Y N DK	B24
Has a health professional ever said that your child has attention-deficit disorder (ADD) or attention-deficit/hyperactivity disorder (ADHD)?	Y N DK	B25

C. Other Information

1. If you are currently at a clinic with your child to see a physician, what is the problem that brought you?

2. If your child has long-term medical problems, please list the three you think are most significant.

_____.
_____.
_____.

3. Please list any medications your child currently takes:

Medicine	**Size (mg) or amount per dose**	**Taken when?**
_____	_____	_____
Effect:_____.		
_____	_____	_____
Effect:_____.		
_____	_____	_____
Effect:_____.		
_____	_____	_____
Effect:_____.		

4. Please list any medication your child has taken in the past if the purpose of the medication was to improve his or her behavior, attention, or sleep:

Medicine	**Size (mg) or amount per dose**	**Taken how often?**	**Dates Taken**
_____	_____	_____	_____
Effect:_____.			
_____	_____	_____	_____
Effect:_____.			
_____	_____	_____	_____
Effect:_____.			
_____	_____	_____	_____
Effect:_____.			

5. Please list any sleep disorders diagnosed or suspected by a physician in your child. For each problem, please list the date it started and whether or not it is still present.

6. Please list any psychological, psychiatric, emotional, or behavioral problems diagnosed or suspected by a physician in your child. For each problem, please list the date it started and whether or not it is still present.

7. Please list any sleep or behavior disorders diagnosed or suspected in *your child's* brothers, sisters, or parents:

Relative   **Condition**
_____   _____
_____   _____
_____   _____

D. Additional Comments:
   Please use the space below to print any additional comments you feel are important. Please also use this space to describe details regarding any of the above questions.

Instructions: Please indicate, by checking the appropriate box, how much each statement applies to this child:

This child often …	Does not apply 0	Applies just a little 1	Applies quite a bit 2	Definitely applies most of the time 3
… does not seem to listen when spoken to directly.				
… has difficulty organizing tasks and activities.				
… is easily distracted by extraneous stimuli.				
… fidgets with hands or feet or squirms in seat.				
… is "on the go" or often acts as if "driven by a motor."				
… interrupts or intrudes on others (e.g., butts into conversations or games).				

THANK YOU

Appendix C

SLEEP DISORDERS INVENTORY FOR STUDENTS— CHILDREN'S FORM (SDIS—C)

Ages 2 through 10 years

© 2004 Marsha Luginbuehl, Ph.D., Child Uplift, Inc.

Student's Name: _____ Parent/Guardian: _____

Address: _____

            Street / Apt #   City   State   Zip

Date of Birth: _/_/_   Today's Date: _/_/_   Age: _____

School: _____ Grade: ____ Sex: M / F Home Phone: (___)_____

Thank you for agreeing to complete this inventory. It is important that you answer *every question* to the best of your abilities based on your child's behaviors *only over the past 6–12 months*. If possible, rate your child's behaviors when s/he is not taking medication. If you are not sure how to mark some questions, observe your child sleep on two different nights for two hours, beginning approximately 1–2 hours after s/he falls asleep, and again for 60 minutes around 5:00 a.m.

Please rate your child/teen's behaviors based on the following rating scale:

1 = **NEVER:** The student *never* exhibited this behavior immediately before evaluation.

2 = **RARELY:** The student exhibited the behavior maybe **once every month or two**.

3 = **OCCASIONALLY:** Student exhibited the behavior **3-to-4 times per month**.

4 = **SOMETIMES:** The student exhibited the behavior **several times per week**.

5 = **OFTEN:** Student exhibited this behavior on a **daily basis** before the evaluation.

6 = **ALMOST ALWAYS:** Student exhibited behavior **multiple times per day or night**.

7 = **ALWAYS:** Student exhibited this behavior *multiple times per hour daily or nightly*.

1 = Never 2 = Rarely 3 = Occasionally 4 = Sometimes 5 = Often 6 = Almost Always 7= Always

Behaviors   Ratings

1. Child stops breathing for 5 or more seconds while sleeping   1 2 3 4 5 6 7
2. Breathes through the mouth while awake   1 2 3 4 5 6 7

3. Breathes through the mouth while asleep   1 2 3 4 5 6 7
4. Appears sleepy more often in daytime than other children
    of the same age   1 2 3 4 5 6 7
5. Makes repeated leg or arm jerking movements during sleep.   1 2 3 4 5 6 7
6. Child has raspy breathing or snores lightly at night   1 2 3 4 5 6 7
7. Snores *loudly* at night   1 2 3 4 5 6 7
8. Shows confusion or disorientation when awakened   1 2 3 4 5 6 7
9. Child rolls or moves around the bed when sleeping   1 2 3 4 5 6 7
10. Gasps, snorts, or chokes for breath during sleep   1 2 3 4 5 6 7
11. Sweats a lot while asleep   1 2 3 4 5 6 7
12. Is irritable   1 2 3 4 5 6 7
13. Child is very tired during the morning in school between 8:00
    and 12:00, but alert in the afternoon and evening   1 2 3 4 5 6 7
    (Check with teachers if unsure)
14. Sleeps in strange positions such as cocking the head backwards
    or sleeping while sitting upright on pillows or kneeling   1 2 3 4 5 6 7
15. Exhibits heavy breathing without exercising   1 2 3 4 5 6 7
16. Wakes up during the night   1 2 3 4 5 6 7
17. Seems tired after getting plenty of sleep   1 2 3 4 5 6 7
18. Takes more than 30 minutes to fall asleep once child is in bed
    and attempts to sleep   1 2 3 4 5 6 7
19. Student's attempts to change bedtime from a post-midnight to
    a pre-midnight pattern on school nights are unsuccessful
    because the student is unable to fall asleep earlier   1 2 3 4 5 6 7
20. Falls asleep more during the daytime than other children
    of the same age   1 2 3 4 5 6 7
21. Has a high activity level and has difficulty sitting still   1 2 3 4 5 6 7
22. Student is often touchy or loses temper   1 2 3 4 5 6 7
23. Actively defies or refuses to comply with adults' requests   1 2 3 4 5 6 7
24. Has difficulty falling asleep on *school nights* before
    (circle one answer below):
    (1) No Difficulty (2) 10:00 p.m. (3) 11:00 p.m. (4) 12:00 a.m.
    (5) 1:30 p.m. (6) 3 a.m. (7) 4 a.m.
25. Has difficulty falling asleep on weekend nights before
    (circle one answer below):
    (1) No Difficulty (2) 10:00 p.m. (3) 11:00 p.m. (4) 12 a.m.
    (5) 1:30 a.m. (6) 3 a.m. (7) 4 a.m.
26. Does child grind teeth while sleeping?   1 2 3 4 5 6 7
27. Does child sleep-walk?   1 2 3 4 5 6 7
28. Does child talk in sleep?   1 2 3 4 5 6 7
29. Does child awaken with night terrors (wild-eyed, crying or
    screaming; unresponsive to parent comforting and cannot
    remember the night terror the following morning)?   1 2 3 4 5 6 7
30. Does child have bed-wetting episodes?   1 2 3 4 5 6 7

SLEEP DISORDERS INVENTORY FOR STUDENTS—ADOLESCENT FORM (SDIS—A)

(Ages 11 through 18 years)

© 2004, Marsha Luginbuehl, Ph.D., Child Uplift, Inc.

(SDIS—A asks for the same demographic information and has the same rating scale as seen on the SDIS—C so it will not be repeated again.)

1 = Never 2 = Rarely 3 = Occasionally 4 = Sometimes 5 = Often 6= Almost Always 7 = Always

Behaviors	Ratings
1. Student stops breathing for 5 or more seconds while sleeping.	1 2 3 4 5 6 7
2. Breathes through the mouth while asleep	1 2 3 4 5 6 7
3. Appears sleepy more often in daytime than other of the same age	1 2 3 4 5 6 7
4. When student is awakened on school days by parent or alarm clock, s/he arises within 5 to 10 minutes and begins the daily routine	1 2 3 4 5 6 7
5. Is unable to talk or move for seconds to minutes when awakened by parent	1 2 3 4 5 6 7
6. Makes repeated leg or arm jerking movements during sleep	1 2 3 4 5 6 7
7. Student has raspy breathing or snores lightly at night	1 2 3 4 5 6 7
8. Snores *loudly* at night	1 2 3 4 5 6 7
9. Shows confusion or disorientation when awakened	1 2 3 4 5 6 7
10. Stays up *past 1:00 a.m. on school nights* (playing video/computer games, watching T.V., talking on the phone, or partying with friends)	1 2 3 4 5 6 7
11. Gasps, snorts, or chokes for breath during sleep	1 2 3 4 5 6 7
12. Is irritable	1 2 3 4 5 6 7
13. Student reports an urge to move legs or an uncomfortable crawling feeling in legs or arms when resting or laying down to sleep	1 2 3 4 5 6 7
14. Student is very tired during the morning in school between 8:00 and 12:00, but alert in the afternoon and evening (Check with teachers if unsure)	1 2 3 4 5 6 7
15. Sleeps in strange positions such as cocking the head backwards or sleeping while sitting upright on pillows or kneeling	1 2 3 4 5 6 7
16. Has attacks of extreme muscular weakness or loss of muscle function (such as limpness in the neck, knees, or limbs, inability to speak clearly, and/or falling down) that occurs *only when laughing, surprised, fearful, or angry*	1 2 3 4 5 6 7
17. Wakes up during the night	1 2 3 4 5 6 7
18. Seems tired after getting plenty of sleep	1 2 3 4 5 6 7
19. Student has complained of vivid, often frightening dreams or hallucinations when *drifting into sleep or awakening*	1 2 3 4 5 6 7
20. Skips or is late for early classes due to difficulty waking up (Check report card for attendance if unsure)	1 2 3 4 5 6 7

21. Takes more than 30 minutes to fall asleep once student is in
    bed and attempts to sleep   1 2 3 4 5 6 7
22. Falls asleep while talking to others or while standing up   1 2 3 4 5 6 7

**1 = Never 2 = Rarely 3 = Occasionally 4 = Sometimes 5 = Often 6 = Almost Always
7 = Always**

Behaviors   Ratings
23. Student's attempts to change bedtime from a post-midnight
    to a pre-midnight pattern on school nights are unsuccessful
    because the student is unable to fall asleep earlier   1 2 3 4 5 6 7
24. Performs some strange automatic behaviors (i.e., like putting
    a jacket in the refrigerator), and does not remember doing them 1 2 3 4 5 6 7
25. Falls asleep more during the daytime than other students of
    the same age   1 2 3 4 5 6 7
26. Student is often touchy or loses temper   1 2 3 4 5 6 7
27. Actively defies or refuses to comply with adults' requests   1 2 3 4 5 6 7
28. Has difficulty falling asleep on *school nights* before
    (circle one answer below):
    (1) No Difficulty (2) 10:00 p.m. (3) 11:00 p.m. (4) 12:00 a.m.
    (5) 1:30 p.m. (6) 3 a.m. (7) 4 a.m.
29. Has difficulty falling asleep on *weekend nights* before
    (circle one answer below):
    (1) No Difficulty (2) 10:00 p.m. (3) 11:00 p.m. (4) 12 p.m.
    (5) 1:30 a.m. (6) 3 a.m. (7) 4 a.m.
30. Circle the average amount of time your child takes
    daytime naps: (1) No Naps (2) Naps 2-3 times a wk.
    (3) 30 min. per day (4) 1 hr/day (5) 1 ½ hrs/day
    (6) 2 hrs/day (7) 3+ hrs/day
31. Does adolescent grind teeth while sleeping?   1 2 3 4 5 6 7
32. Does adolescent sleep-walk?   1 2 3 4 5 6 7
33. Does s/he talk in sleep?   1 2 3 4 5 6 7
34. Does s/he awaken with night terrors (wild-eyed, crying or
    screaming; unresponsive to parent comforting and cannot
    remember the night terror the following morning)?   1 2 3 4 5 6 7
35. Does s/he have bed-wetting episodes?   1 2 3 4 5 6 7

BOTH THE SDIS—C AND SDIS—A ASK THE FOLLOWING HEALTH QUESTIONS:

Please circle either "Yes" or "No" for the following questions:

1. Was your adolescent underweight as an infant or
   preschool-aged child?   Yes / No
   If yes, circle one: a) mildly underweight
   b) moderately c) severely
2. Is your adolescent underweight now?   Yes / No
   If yes, circle one: a) mildly underweight
   b) moderately c) severely

3. Is your adolescent overweight now?   Yes / No
    If yes, circle one: a) mildly overweight
    b) moderately c) severely
4. Was adolescent under normal height as an infant or   Yes / No
    preschool-aged child?
    If yes, circle one: a) mildly under height
    b) moderately c) severely
5. Is adolescent under normal height for his/her age now?   Yes / No
    If yes, circle one: a) mildly under height
    b) moderately c) severely
6. Does your adolescent have multiple ear infections per year?   Yes / No
7. Does your adolescent have multiple respiratory infections
    per year?   Yes / No
8. Has a physician ever reported that your child has large tonsils?   Yes / No
9. Have your adolescent's tonsils been removed?   Yes / No
10. Has a physician ever reported that your adolescent has
    enlarged adenoids?   Yes / No
11. Have your adolescent's adenoids been removed?   Yes / N0

Child Uplift, Inc.

To purchase the SDIS, submit your requests to: www.SleepDisorderHelp.com

or write to the following address:

Child Uplift, Inc., P.O. Box 146, Fairview, WY 82119

Bus: (307) 886-9096; Fax (307) 886-9093

10 Impact of Sleep Loss on Children and Adolescents

Valerie McLaughlin Crabtree[a] and Lisa A. Witcher[b]

[a]*Division of Behavioral Medicine, St. Jude Children's Research Hospital, Memphis, Tennessee, U.S.A.*
[b]*Division of Pediatric Sleep Medicine and Kosair Children's Hospital Research Institute, Department of Pediatrics, University of Louisville, Louisville, Kentucky, U.S.A.*

INTRODUCTION

Recent National Sleep Foundation (NSF) polls demonstrate that both school-aged children and adolescents are obtaining less than the recommended amounts of sleep for optimal daytime functioning. In 2004, the NSF Sleep in America poll (1) reported that most school-aged children were sleeping 9.5 hours per night in comparison to the recommended 10–11 hours per night. Actigraphically documented sleep in children ages 4–8 revealed even less sleep, with an average of 8 hours, 17 minutes total sleep time (2). This chronic insufficient sleep may be even more prevalent in boys, particularly minority boys (3–5). Insufficient sleep appears to be an increasing problem as children age. Sadeh and colleagues (4), in an actigraphic study of 140 children second through sixth grade, found a significant decline in total sleep time as children aged, from approximately 8 hours, 36 minutes in second grade (mean age = 7.9 years) to approximately 7 hours, 41 minutes in sixth grade (mean age = 11.8 years).

Adolescents are at particular risk of sleep loss due to the natural delaying of the circadian rhythm that accompanies adolescent development (6). In 2006, the NSF Sleep in America poll (7) reported that adolescents were sleeping, on average, 6.9 hours per night in comparison to the recommended 9 hours in this age group. Similarly, in a large sample of Canadian adolescents, more than 70% reported sleeping less than 8.5 hours per night, and 41% had Epworth Sleepiness Scale scores above 10, reflecting significant daytime sleepiness (8). In a large survey of high-school students, self-reported school-night total sleep time continually declined across high school, from 7 hours, 42 minutes at ages 13–14 (notably similar to the sleep time of the 11.8-year-old children in Sadeh et al.'s (4) study) to 7 hours, 4 minutes at ages 17–19 (9). This decline was related primarily to the increasingly delayed bedtime across the age groups with relatively similar rise times. The sleep loss accrued during adolescence is compounded by the tendency of many adolescents to maintain even later bedtimes and rise times on weekends (10). Self-reported weekend-night total sleep time declined from 9 hours, 27 minutes at ages 13–14 to 8 hours, 38 minutes at ages 17–19 (9). Children and adolescents in our society, therefore, clearly are obtaining insufficient sleep on a chronic basis.

Partial sleep deprivation has been consistently found to impair cognitive performance and, to an even greater extent, mood in adults (11). However, the impact of chronic partial sleep restriction in children and adolescents is not entirely clear. While it is widely assumed that sleep loss can induce irritability and behavioral disturbances in children, little empirical evidence exists to demonstrate a causal link between the two. Studies that have focused on examining the impact of sleep loss on daytime functioning in children and adolescents have typically utilized one of

139

three methodologies: (1) naturalistic, questionnaire-based studies to relate typical sleep duration to daytime functioning; (2) laboratory-based restriction of sleep during one night followed by objective neurobehavioral assessments; or (3) partial restriction of sleep over 3–7 nights followed by objective and/or subjective neurobehavioral assessments. Certainly, one night of in-laboratory sleep restriction can be expected to have different impact on a child's daytime functioning than a more chronic course of mild sleep restriction. This chapter will examine the distinctions between these paradigms of assessing the impact of reduced sleep on children's and adolescents' functioning and will describe the impact of different forms of sleep loss on behavioral, cognitive, and affective functioning.

IMPACT OF SLEEP LOSS ON CHILDREN'S BEHAVIOR

Studies investigating the impact of sleep loss on behavior in children and adolescents have relied on naturalistic, survey methods or on chronic partial sleep restriction. No large-scale studies have specifically measured behavior in children following one night of significant sleep restriction.

Naturalistic Studies

Naturalistic studies have documented some associations between sleep duration and daytime behavior in children and adolescents. Specifically, adolescents who report obtaining less sleep and feeling sleepier on the Epworth Sleepiness Scale are also more likely to report being late to school, feeling sleepy in class, having poor grades because of sleepiness, and having impairment in social functioning (8). In younger children, those who were classified as "poor sleepers," defined as at least three awakenings per night and sleep efficiency of less than 90% over the course of five nights, had significantly higher parent-rated delinquent behavior, thought problems, and total behavior problems (12).

Chronic Partial Sleep Restriction

After one week of extending sleep by one hour or remaining on their typical sleep schedule, young children exhibited parent-reported improvements in hyperactivity and anxiety. Those whose sleep was extended also had parent-reported improvements in an index of attention-deficit/hyperactivity disorder (ADHD) and psychiatric symptoms. In contrast, children whose sleep was restricted by one hour each night over the course of one week exhibited no parent-reported differences in behavior (13).

Adolescents whose sleep was restricted to 6.5 hours in bed versus extended to 10 hours in bed over the course of five nights had both self- and parent-reported increased sleepiness, oppositionality, and irritability (14). Dahl and Lewin (15) have speculated that the consequences of insufficient sleep in children and adolescents impair their emotional regulation and may either contribute to and/or exacerbate developmental psychopathology.

IMPACT OF SLEEP LOSS ON CHILDREN'S COGNITION

The majority of studies that have focused on impaired daytime functioning in children and adolescents following sleep loss have assessed subsequent cognitive impairments.

A substantial amount of data from naturalistic, chronic partial sleep restriction, and acute sleep restriction paradigms suggests that reduction of total sleep time significantly affects cognition and learning in children and adolescents.

Naturalistic Studies

The majority of naturalistic studies examining relationships between sleep duration and cognitive functioning have focused on adolescents. Sadeh and colleagues (4) assessed daytime function of second through sixth grade students in relation to their actigraphically recorded sleep over five nights. They found significantly reduced sustained attention and psychomotor vigilance in children who obtained less sleep than their same age peers. Interestingly, this relationship was much greater for the second grade children than for the older age groups.

In their review examining the effects of sleep loss on adolescents from middle school through the first year of college, Wolfson and Carskadon (16) concluded that across studies, adolescents with reduced total sleep time, irregular sleep schedules, and increased sleep onset latencies tended to have poorer academic achievement. Adolescents with lower grades (mostly Cs, Ds, and Fs) reported lower school-night total sleep time, later school- and weekend-night bedtimes, and later weekend-morning rise times than students with higher grades (mostly As and Bs). Some of the contribution in poor grades may be attributed to the increased likelihood of arriving late to school because of oversleeping reported by adolescents sleeping less than 6 hours, 45 minutes on school nights (9). Furthermore, 21% of poor sleepers had school failures and were behind in grade level by one or more years. In fact, the best predictors of school failure were adolescents' fatigue (difficulty rising in the morning and requiring a daytime nap) and parents' education levels (17).

Chronic Partial Sleep Restriction

After one week of one hour sleep restriction, young children demonstrated a lack of expected practice effects on a standardized measure of visual attention, reflecting a potential lack of expected learning for a task. In contrast, those children whose sleep was extended or who remained on their typical sleep schedule showed expected practice effects (13). This difference in ability was highlighted by decreased brainwaves as measured by event-related potentials (ERPs) in these subjects. Those children whose sleep was restricted had ERP amplitudes on a directional Stroop task that were reduced from their baseline week (18). This difference appeared to reflect an increase in cognitive effort during processing of stimuli (19).

By extending 9- to 12-year-old children's sleep by at least 30 minutes over a period of three nights, Sadeh and colleagues (20) demonstrated reduced reaction time on a measure of continuous performance, reflecting improved sustained attention and vigilance, and improvement in short-term memory. Those children who had their sleep restricted, and those who remained on their typical sleep schedule, exhibited no change in reaction time or short-term memory. On a measure of simple reaction time, children who had their sleep restricted and those who remained on their typical sleep schedule, showed decreased performance after three nights; whereas children whose sleep times had been extended showed no change. Fallone and colleagues (21) restricted children's sleep over the course of one week and demonstrated decreased teacher-reported academic performance, attention, processing speed, and memory in comparison to both the baseline and optimized sleep weeks. However, while children were in both the restricted and optimized weeks, teachers reported greater total school-related problems than during the baseline condition (21).

In the only study examining chronic partial sleep restriction in adolescents, Beebe and colleagues (14) found decreased parent- and self-reported attention and poorer metacognition in adolescents while within the five-night sleep restriction condition in comparison to both the baseline and sleep extension conditions.

Acute Sleep Restriction

Acute significant restriction during one night of sleep in the laboratory has resulted in impaired attention, verbal creativity, abstract thinking, and concept formation in children and adolescents (22,23). This level of impairment reflects impaired executive functioning, as each of the areas of impairment were tied to frontal lobe functioning (23).

Notably, after one night of sleep deprivation, Carskadon and colleagues (24) discovered significant individual variability in cognitive performance among adolescents. Decrements observed in memory, in particular, were typically associated with brief sleep episodes occurring during the testing protocol. For subjects who did not fall asleep while the test was administered, performance was virtually identical to that of the baseline condition, indicating individual susceptibility to sleep loss in adolescents.

IMPACT OF SLEEP LOSS ON CHILDREN'S MOOD

A large amount of data on the relationship between impaired mood and sleep loss exists from the naturalistic studies. Recent data are also emerging from chronic partial sleep restriction studies indicating that there may be a causal link between loss of sleep and impaired mood in adolescents, though there are no clear data regarding this relationship in younger children. No large-scale studies have specifically examined mood in children and adolescents following one night of significant sleep restriction.

Naturalistic Studies

Oginska and Pokorski (25), in a large survey across age groups, reported that adolescents had a much greater discrepancy between self-reported perceived need for sleep and actual sleep time than did adults. In fact, adolescents in their sample reported obtaining 106 minutes less sleep per weeknight than they required to feel refreshed and well-rested. Furthermore, almost half of the adolescent sample reported feeling fatigued upon awakening. When daytime functioning was assessed in these adolescents, apathy was strongly associated with sleep loss. Finally, the authors reported that the discrepancy between perceived need for sleep and actual sleep time predicted daytime impairments significantly better than did total sleep time as measured independently (25). Similarly, 87% of adolescents in Wolfson and Carskadon's (9) study reported that they obtained less sleep than they needed. Those adolescents with self-reported total sleep times of less than 6 hours,

45 minutes reported significantly more depressive symptoms than adolescents who reported sleeping more than 8 hours, 15 minutes.

In Meijer et al.'s (26) study of Dutch children and adolescents ages 9–14, those who reported higher quality sleep and feeling more rested also reported feeling more receptive of their teachers, more positive self-images, higher motivation to achieve in school, and better control over their aggression. Interestingly, however, the self-reported length of time in bed did not significantly predict academic functioning.

In addition to typical mood impairments observed in children and adolescents with restricted sleep, sleep loss can exacerbate clinically significant mood symptoms. Dahl and Lewin (15) delineate the link between sleep loss and depression in adolescents. They indicate a bidirectional relationship between sleep habits and daytime functioning, whereby behavioral and/or emotional disturbances can precede sleep disturbance, while sleep disruption may trigger or exacerbate daytime behavioral and emotional distress. Both insomnia and hypersomnia are noted in children and adolescents with major depressive disorder, and hypersomnia becomes more prevalent as children enter adolescence. Because of this bidirectional relationship, it is often difficult for clinicians to clearly delineate between depressive symptoms and delayed circadian rhythms in adolescents.

Among children and adolescents with mood disorders, those with self-reported sleep disturbance have been reported to have more prolific and severe depressive symptoms and more comorbid anxiety disorders than those children with mood disorders who do not have sleep disturbance. Within the group of children with depression and sleep disturbance, those with both insomnia and hypersomnia were more likely on a structured clinical interview to report a long history of psychiatric illness, more severe depression, anhedonia, weight loss, psychomotor retardation, and fatigue than those with either insomnia or hypersomnia alone (27).

Chronic Partial Sleep Restriction

In Beebe and colleagues' (14) study, adolescents' affect was impacted by sleep restriction to a much greater extent than was behavior. Specifically, adolescents who were sleep restricted exhibited poorer emotional regulation, impulse control, and flexibility. In fact, the authors speculated that the irritability that is traditionally associated with adolescents may, in fact, be attributed to the chronic sleep deprivation present during this developmental period (7).

IMPLICATIONS FOR DELAYED SCHOOL START TIMES

As the evidence for the impact of restricted sleep on children and adolescents' daytime functioning accumulates, policy issues such as school start times become crucial to address. In their review of studies addressing school start times on adolescents' functioning, Wolfson and Carskadon (16) reported that delayed sleep onset coupled with early school start times are associated with excessive daytime sleepiness, falling asleep in class, inattention, and decreased school performance. When adolescent students were monitored by actigraphy while transitioning from ninth grade in a later-starting school (8.25 a.m.), to tenth grade in an earlier-starting school (7.20 a.m.), no differences were found in schoolnight bedtimes.

Rise times advanced, however, while total sleep time significantly decreased from 7 hours, 9 minutes to 6 hours, 50 minutes, clearly below the recommended 9 hours of sleep in this age group. When assessed with Multiple Sleep Latency Tests (MSLT), significant decreases were seen in mean sleep onset latency time across naps after entering tenth grade in comparison to ninth grade. This difference was strikingly apparent during the first nap attempt given at 8.30 a.m., in which the mean sleep onset latency was 5.1 minutes during the tenth grade academic year. Additionally, 12.5% of ninth-graders had at least one rapid eye movement (REM) onset, while 48% of tenth graders had one and 16% had two REM onset periods, indicative of clinically significant hypersomnia (28).

In the 1997–1998 academic year, school start times were delayed for high schools in the Minneapolis Public Schools from 7.15 a.m. to 8.40 a.m. Students did not have later bedtimes than those with earlier start times but did, however, have later rise times, resulting in increased total sleep time of almost one hour per night. Furthermore, attendance rates and continuous enrollment improved, while those students in the later starting schools reported significantly fewer symptoms of depression and excessive daytime sleepiness than those in the earlier starting schools. Of note, while it had previously been a concern that students would be less available to participate in after-school extra-curricular activities if the school start time was delayed, teacher reports indicated that the number of students participating in after-school activities did not change (29).

CONCLUSIONS

While naturalistic studies have postulated a relationship between shortened sleep time and poorer cognition, behavior, and mood in children and adolescents, experimental designs inducing sleep extension versus restriction paradigms have begun to establish a causal link between reduced total sleep time and impaired daytime functioning. An overview of these studies is presented in Table 1. Specifically, experimental manipulation of sleep times has indicated that children and adolescents with restricted sleep are at greater risk for increased oppositionality and irritability, as well as reduced attention, executive functioning, processing speed, memory, behavioral/emotional regulation, motivation, and academic achievement. Interestingly, while clinical lore suggests that sleepy children may be more hyperactive, there is little evidence to support this. Studies that have assessed both parent- and teacher-reported hyperactivity in children and adolescents who are sleep restricted have found no consistent reports of increased hyperactivity, but rather, sleep loss is more commonly associated with inattention.

Certainly, this causal link between sleep loss and impaired functioning in children and adolescents provides the impetus for consideration of delaying school start times, particularly for adolescents, who are experiencing a natural delay in circadian rhythm. Students in schools who have delayed their start times have not delayed their bedtimes significantly but have been provided with the opportunity to obtain more sleep by sleeping later in the morning. This then provides a pathway whereby these students are better rested at school, have better attendance, and report better mood. Such policy changes may have a major impact on the health and education of adolescents.

TABLE 1   Synopsis of Studies Investigating Relationships Between Sleep Loss and Daytime Functioning in Children and Adolescents

Study	Sample size	Age	Methods	Findings
Beebe et al. (14)	20	13–16	1 baseline week 1 week restriction: 6.5 hours 1 week extension:10 hours (naturalistic setting)	SD: increase in homeostatic sleep drive; greater problems with sleepiness, attention, oppositionality/irritability, behavior regulation, metacognition
Carskadon et al. (24)	12	11–14	1 adaptation day, 2 BSLN days, 1 SD day, and 2 REC days(sleep lab)	SD: related to decrease in performance
Crabtree et al. (13)	74	4–8	1 baseline week; 1 week of 1 hour sleep restriction vs. extension vs. control	SE and control: reduced hyperactivity; Improved visual attention; No change in psychomotor skills SR: no change in hyperactivity, visual attention, or psychomotor skills
Fallone et al. (22)	82	8–15	5 nights baseline (naturalistic), random assignment to one overnight 10 hour sleep or 4 hour sleep condition in laboratory	SR: associated with shorter daytime sleep latency, increased subjective sleepiness, increased inattentive behaviors; not associated with hyperactive-impulsive behavior or impaired performance on response inhibition or sustained attention tests
Fallone et al. (21)	74	6–12	Naturalistic setting, BSLN week, optimized week, restricted week	SR: increased academic problems, attention problems, slower processing speed, impaired memory function and daytime sleepiness; no evidence of increase in hyperactivity
Kahn et al. (17)	972	8–10	Parent report of good sleepers vs. poor sleepers	Poor sleepers demonstrate more school problems; show higher incidence of somnambulism, somniloquia, and night fears; fatigue and parent education best predictors for school failure

Continued

TABLE 1 Synopsis of Studies Investigating Relationships Between Sleep Loss and Daytime Functioning in Children and Adolescents (*continued*)

Study	Sample size	Age	Methods	Findings
Liu et al. (27)	553	7–14	Psychiatric evaluation using the ISCA-D	Children with both hypersomnia and insomnia were most severely depressed; children with and without different sleep disturbances manifest features of clinical depression
Meijer et al. (26)	449	9–14	Questionnaires	Good sleep quality: direct positive relationship with school satisfaction factors and achievement
Oginska and Pokorski (25)	432 (adolescent group=191) (university students=115) (young employees=126)	Adolescent 14–16; Student 20–27; Employees 30–45	Self-report questionnaire	Adolescents: reported feeling tired on awakening, nervousness, general weakness; no difference was observed in fatigue, mood, or cognitive symptoms
Randazzo et al. (23)	16	10–14	3 BSLN nights, 1 night in selected group SR (5 hr in bed); 1 group (11 hr in bed); 1 CRL group; laboratory setting	SR: verbal creativity and abstract thinking are impaired
Sadeh et al. (20)	77	9–12	2 BSLN nights, 1 group extended by 1 hr; 1 group restricted by 1 hr	SR: lead to improved sleep quality, increase in night awakenings, reduction of sleep percent, reduced alertness; neurobehavioral functioning impaired
Spilsbury et al. (5)	755	8–11	Sleep questionnaire and journal	Ethnic minority children likely to sleep less than others
Wahlstrom (29)	18,000	14–18	Self-report questionnaires	Later school start times: improved attendance, slight improvement in grades, increased TST

TABLE 1 Synopsis of Studies Investigating Relationships Between Sleep Loss and Daytime Functioning in Children and Adolescents (*continued*)

Study	Sample size	Age	Methods	Findings
Wolfson and Carskadon (16)	3120	13–19	School Sleep Habits Survey completed	Short-sleepers: poor grades, daytime sleepiness, depressive mood, sleep/wake behavior problems

BSLN = Baseline; REC = Recovery; SD = Sleep Deprivation; SE = Sleep Extension; SR = Sleep Restriction; ISCA-D = Interview Schedule for Children and Adolescents—Diagnostic Version; TST = Total Sleep Time.

REFERENCES

1. http://www.kintera.org/atf/cf/%7BF6BF2668-A1B4-4FE8-8D1AA5D39340D9CB%7D/2004SleepPollFinalReport.pdf (accessed April 2007)
2. Crabtree VM, Dayyat E, Molfese DL, et al. Objective quantification of sleep duration in healthy children. Sleep 2007; Abstract Supplement, 30:A74.
3. Crabtree VM, Korhonen JB, Montgomery-Downs HE, et al. Cultural influences on bedtime behavior of young children. Sleep Med 2005; 6:319–24.
4. Sadeh A, Raviv A, Gruber R. Sleep patterns and sleep disruptions in school-age children. Develop Psychol 2000; 36:291–301.
5. Spilsbury JC, Storfer-Isser A, Drotar D, et al. Sleep behavior in an urban US sample of school-aged children. Arch Pediatr Adolesc Med 2004; 158:988–94.
6. Carskadon MA, Acebo C, Jenni OG. Regulation of adolescent sleep: Implications for behavior. Ann N Y Acad Sci 2004; 1021:276–91.
7. http://www.sleepfoundation.org/atf/cf/%7BF6BF2668-A1B4-4FE8-8D1A-A5D39340D9CB%7D/2006_summary_of_findings.pdf (accessed April 2006)
8. Gibson ES, Powles ACP, Thabane L, et al. "Sleepiness" is serious in adolescence: Two surveys of 3235 Canadian students. BMC Public Health 2006; 6.
9. Wolfson AR, Carskadon MA. Sleep schedules and daytime functioning in adolescents. Child Dev 1998; 69:875–87.
10. Carskadon MA, Acebo C. Regulation of sleepiness in adolescents: Update, insights, and speculation. Sleep 2002; 25:606.
11. Pilcher JJ, Huffcutt AI. Effects of sleep deprivation on performance: A meta-analysis. Sleep 1996; 19:318–26.
12. Sadeh A, Gruber R, Raviv A. Sleep, neurobehavioral functioning, and behavior problems in school-age children. Child Dev 2002; 73:405–17.
13. Crabtree VM, Dayyat E, Millis BG, et al. Effect of sleep restriction on children's cognitive and behavioral functioning. Presented at the 3rd Annual Pediatric Sleep Medicine Meeting, March 2007, Amelia Island, Florida.
14. Beebe DW, Fallone G, Godiwala N, Flanigan M, et al. Feasibility and behavioral effects of an at-home multi-night sleep restriction protocol for adolescents. (manuscript under review).
15. Dahl RE, Lewin DS. Pathways to adolescent health: Sleep regulation and behavior. J Adol Health 2002; 31:175–84.
16. Wolfson AR, Carskadon MA. Understanding adolescents' sleep patterns and school performance: A critical appraisal. Sleep Med Rev 2003; 7:491–506.
17. Kahn A, Van de Merckt C, Rebuffat E, et al. Sleep problems in healthy preadolescents. Pediatrics 1989; 84:542–6.
18. Wu J, Dykman R, Molfese D. Sleep restriction decreased ERP brainwaves in directional stroop task. Sleep 2007; Abstract Supplement, 30:A141.
19. Barnes M, Warren C, Millis B, et al. Sleep restriction and event-related potentials: Developmental implications. Sleep 2007; Abstract Supplement, 30:A145.

20. Sadeh A, Gruber R, Raviv A. The effects of sleep restriction and extension on school-age children: What a difference an hour makes. Child Dev 2003; 74, 444–55.
21. Fallone G, Acebo C, Seifer R, et al. Experimental restriction of sleep opportunity in children: Effects on teacher ratings. Sleep 2005; 28, 1561–7.
22. Fallone G, Acebo C, Arnett JT, et al. Effects of acute sleep restriction on behavior, sustained attention, and response inhibition in children. Perceptual & Motor Skills 2001; 93:213–29.
23. Randazzo AC, Muehlbach MJ, Schweitzer PK, et al. Cognitive function following acute sleep restriction in children ages 10–14. Sleep 1998; 21:861–8.
24. Carskadon MA, Harvey K, Dement WC. Sleep loss in young adolescents. Sleep 1981; 4:299–312.
25. Oginska H, Pokorski J. Fatigue and mood correlates of sleep length in three age-social groups: School children, students, and employees. Chronobiol Int 2006; 23:1317–28.
26. Meijer AM, Habekothe HT, van den Wittenboer GLH. Time in bed, quality of sleep and school functioning of children. J Sleep Res 2000; 9:145–53.
27. Liu X, Buysse DJ, Gentzler AL, et al. Insomnia and hypersomnia associated with depressive phenomenology and comorbidity in childhood depression. Sleep 2007; 30:83–90.
28. Carskadon MA, Wolfson AR, Acebo C, et al. Adolescent sleep patterns, circadian timing, and sleepiness at a transition to early school days. Sleep 1998; 21:871–81.
29. Wahlstrom K. Changing times: Findings from the first longitudinal study of later high school start times. NASSP Bulletin 2002; 86:3–21.

Neurocognitive and Behavioral Consequences of Sleep-Disordered Breathing in Children

Louise M. O'Brien

Sleep Disorders Center, Departments of Neurology and Oral and Maxillofacial Surgery, University of Michigan, Ann Arbor, Michigan, U.S.A.

INTRODUCTION

It is becoming increasingly clear that neurocognitive deficits and behavioral problems are among the most common morbidities associated with sleep-disordered breathing (SDB) in children. While there has been an explosion of interest in the relationship between pediatric SDB and neurocognitive and behavioral problems, one of the first reports of impaired intellectual function in children with adenotonsillar hypertrophy was in 1889 when Hill reported on "some causes of backwardness and stupidity in children" (1). However, it was almost a century later when a subsequent report of a small group of children with SDB was published in the 1970s (2). Since then, a multitude of studies have been published in this field. Recent data suggest that some of the cognitive and behavioral deficits observed in children with SDB may be reversible, thus providing strong evidence for early recognition and appropriate treatment of pediatric SDB. This chapter will review the current state of knowledge of behavior and cognition in pediatric SDB and provide evidence for SDB as an important contributor to neurocognitive and behavioral problems.

PREVALENCE OF SDB IN CHILDREN

SDB is a term used to describe a range of sleep-related breathing problems, from habitual snoring at one end of the spectrum to obstructive sleep apnea (OSA) at the other. OSA is a frequent condition and is estimated to affect between 1% and 3% of young children, often in association with adenotonillar hypertrophy as well as craniofacial abnormalities and disorders affecting upper airway patency (3). OSA is characterized by repeated events of partial or complete upper airway obstruction during sleep, resulting in disruption of normal ventilation, hypoxemia, and sleep (Fig 1). Clinical history and physical examination are not sufficient to make a diagnosis of OSA, nor to differentiate between OSA and primary snoring (4), and as such, the gold standard for diagnosis is overnight polysomnography.

Snoring is the hallmark symptom of SDB although many snoring children may have primary snoring, i.e., habitual snoring without alterations in sleep architecture, alveolar ventilation, and oxygenation. Habitual snoring is a much more frequent occurrence than OSA, and affects up to approximately 12% of children (3). Recent studies have suggested that it is not just OSA that impacts neurocognition and behavior, but also primary snoring (5–7), and therefore this chapter will consider the whole spectrum of SDB and its associated neurobehavioral morbidities. Despite the wealth of data on the adverse effects of SDB and neurobehavioral function, the majority of children with symptoms of SDB likely go unrecognized (8–11) despite the fact that screening tools exist and could easily be incorporated

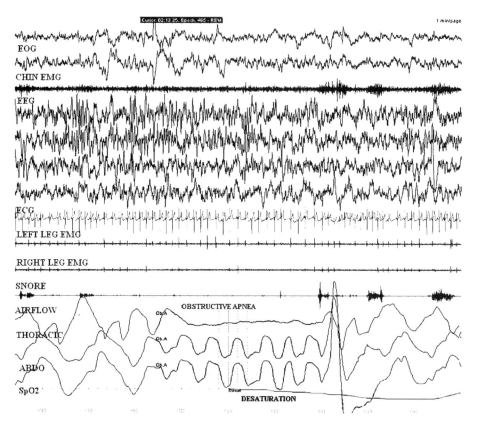

FIGURE 1   An example of an obstructive apnea with an associated desaturation.
EOG—electrooculogram; Chin EMG—chin electromyogram; EEG—electroencephalogram; ECG—
electrocardiogram; Left leg EMG—left tibial EMG; Right leg EMG—right tibial EMG; Snore—snore
vibrations; Airflow—nasal/oral airflow; Thoracic—chest wall movement; Abdo—abdominal
movement; SpO2—oxyhemoglobin saturation

into primary care (12,13). This is a critical issue since children with SDB are heavy
consumers of healthcare resources (14,15) even from their first year of life, which is
mostly related to respiratory diseases (16).

BEHAVIORAL IMPACT OF SDB

SDB has been associated with a number of behavioral morbidities, particularly hyperactivity, inattention, aggression, and mood disturbances (for a comprehensive review
see 17). These behaviors are summarized in Table 1 and briefly discussed below.

Hyperactivity

Hyperactivity is the most commonly reported behavioral morbidity associated with
SDB. Even in the 1970s and 1980s, Guilleminault and colleagues (18,19) reported
that behavioral problems such as hyperactivity were a daytime symptom of SDB.

TABLE 1 Summary of Evidence for and Association Between SDB and Daytime Behavior

SDB Based on Parental Report	
Hyperactivity	7,18–27
Inattention	18,19,22,26,41
Aggression	7,20,23,24
Mood disorders	7,42
SDB Based on Laboratory Findings	
Hyperactivity	6,28–31
Inattention	5,6,27,30,37–40
Aggression	31
Mood Disorders	6,28,31,43

Since then there has been a multitude of published studies supporting this associa-tion, including studies where sleep was measured by both subjective, parental reports of SDB symptoms (7,20–27) and more objective testing in the laboratory (28–31). Even primary snoring has been shown in several investigations to be associ-ated with hyperactive/impulsive behavior (6,7,32) when assessed by well-validated tools such as the Conners' Parent Rating Scales (33), the Child Behavior Checklist (34), or the Behavioral Assessment Scale for Children (35).

Inattention

Attention can be measured both subjectively by parent-report questionnaires as mentioned above and objectively by continuous performance tests (36), although the majority of studies have utilized subjective assessments. Use of continuous performances tests has the advantage that different aspects of attention can be distinguished, for example, selective or sustained attention. A number of studies have demonstrated negative associations between SDB and attention, but the evi-dence is not as consistent as that relating to hyperactive behaviors (5,6,22,26,27,30,37–40; see Table 1), perhaps due in part to differing aspects of atten-tion being measured. In studies that have utilized continuous performance tests, children with SDB appear to be unable to sustain attention or vigilance over time (5,30,41). Since attention is an important component of more complex cognitive abilities and is critical for normal development, insults affecting attention have the potential to affect higher cognitive functioning.

Aggression

Aggressive behavior has not been well studied in relation to SDB. Nonetheless, there are several large, parent-report studies which suggest that pediatric SDB is associated with aggressive behaviors (7,20,23,24). In a study of 872 children aged 2–14 years old at two general pediatric clinics, Chervin et al. (23) demonstrated that children at high risk for SDB were found to be two to three times more likely to bully others, and to be quarrelsome and cruel, in comparison to other children, even after adjustment for comorbid hyperactivity or use of stimulants. Furthermore, a dose–response relationship was found between the SDB score and the conduct problem index. In a cross-sectional community-based study, 829 children aged between 9 and 11 years old underwent overnight polysomnography (31). Those with SDB were almost five times more likely to have aggressive behaviors, even after adjustment for potential covariates such as race, prematurity, and obesity. Furthermore, a dose–response relationship was found between degrees of snoring and aggressiveness. Although aggressive behaviors are likely to arise from a number of social, environmental, and biological factors, these emerging data also suggest that occult SDB may indeed play a role.

Mood Disturbances

Emotional problems in children with SDB have been reported in a few studies using parent-report questionnaires. While results are conflicting, several studies have hinted at an association between SDB and anxiety/depression and impaired emotional functioning when using well-validated behavioral screens such as the Conners Parent Report Scale or the Child Behavior Checklist (6,7,28,31,42). However, few studies have focused on anxiety/depression other than using the latter screens. Of interest, a recent study utilizing a screen specifically for depression—the Children's Depression Inventory—found that snoring children were more likely to report depressive symptoms than nonsnoring children, particularly anhedonia (43). This relationship was independent of obesity, a known risk factor for both depressive symptoms and SDB, as the normal weight snoring children had comparable depressive symptoms to the obese snoring children, while the nonsnoring, non-obese children had significantly lower scores. Notably, the children with primary snoring had depressive scores similar to children with OSA. These data add to a growing body of evidence that primary snoring may not be as benign as previously believed, and may adversely affect psychosocial functioning.

IS THERE AN ASSOCIATION BETWEEN SDB AND ADHD?

Attention-deficit/hyperactivity disorder (ADHD) is one of the most frequently encountered pediatric neurobehavioral disorders. Since both ADHD and SDB are relatively common in children, it is not unreasonable to hypothesize that they may frequently coexist, most likely with a bidirectional relationship. However, sleep disturbances were so widely assumed to be part of the clinical phenotype of ADHD that they were included as one of the previous Diagnostic and Statistical Manual of Mental Disorders—III (DSM-III) diagnostic criteria for ADHD (44), although neither of the more recent diagnostic manuals have included sleep disturbance as a criterion (45,46). Thus, it is not surprising that studies using earlier diagnostic criteria found a significant association between ADHD and sleep problems. Nonetheless, more recent studies suggest that parents of children with ADHD do report sleep disturbances much more often than parents of non-ADHD children (47,48) and children with SDB often present with behavioral problems that are remarkably similar to those observed in children with ADHD (20,21,49). Chervin et al. (21) found that about one third of children with ADHD snore more than half the time, compared with only 9–11% of control children. However, LeBourgeios et al. (50) did not find that snoring was more common in children with ADHD than in children without ADHD, but did find that snoring was common among children with the hyperactive/impulsive subtype. These findings support others where snoring was found to be common in children with elevated hyperactive scores but not in children who were at high risk of a diagnosis of ADHD (29).

Results of polysomnographic studies in children with ADHD have been much less consistent with regard to a relationship between SDB and ADHD. The majority of studies focused on sleep architecture rather than SDB, and in those studies where sleep-related breathing disorders were considered, the results are inconsistent. However, current studies suggest that SDB is indeed more common in ADHD particularly when the threshold used to define SDB is lower than that traditionally used (51,52). A limitation to a number of studies of sleep and ADHD is that very few used thorough, structured interviews by child psychiatrists to determine a diagnosis of ADHD. In one study that did, formal diagnoses of ADHD were found in 28% of children scheduled for adenotonsillectomy, typically because of suspicion for SDB (39), which is considerably higher than would be normally expected. A review of the literature which included only studies with rigorous diagnoses of ADHD and objective sleep evaluations determined that children with ADHD are indeed more likely to have SDB, albeit in mild form (53).

COGNITIVE IMPACT OF SDB
In addition to behavioral problems, cognitive problems have also been reported in children with SDB. As early as 1889 Hill reported on "some causes of backwardness and stupidity in children" (1), and in 1892 Osler noted that children with tonsillar hypertrophy were "stupid looking" and slow to respond to questions (54). Although a cognitive impact of SDB has been demonstrated in several studies (Table 2), the relationship is less consistent than the behavioral manifestations previously discussed. In part, factors such as socioeconomic status, the child's age, and whether or not the child was born prematurely (55,56) may play an important role in any such relationship between SDB and cognition (for a review, see 17).

Intelligence
A number of studies have demonstrated that standardized IQ scores are lower in children with SDB compared to controls (5,6,32,38,57–60), although typically still within the normal range. In the study by Gottlieb et al. (57), children with SDB performed less well than control children on measures of general intelligence, but on closer examination of these affluent and highly educated families, children with SDB still had relatively high IQ scores. This highlights the need to be aware of selection bias in such studies and also to take account of confounding variables (55,56)

TABLE 2 Summary of Evidence for an Association Between SDB and Cognitive Dysfunction

SDB Based on Parental Report	
Cognitive impairment	37,57,59,60
Academic problems	7,55,69–71
SDB Based on Laboratory Findings	
Cognitive impairment	5,6,28,30,32,38,57–62,67
Academic problems	61,68,72

as a higher socioeconomic status may afford some protection from the neurocognitive impact of SDB. Not all studies have supported an overall IQ difference between children with and without SDB (28,61), although deficits in particular domains have been reported, such as verbal IQ scale, in association with SDB severity (28).

Memory
In children, the relationships between SDB and memory are not well defined. Only a few studies have reported memory deficits (5,32,61,62) while other studies have failed to find memory impairment even in samples with a range of SDB severity (6,37,38). Such inconsistencies are likely due to the fact that different age groups and different aspects of memory are measured (e.g., declarative memory, verbal memory, or working memory). For example, Kaemingk et al. (61) reported significant differences between 6–12-year-old children with SDB and a matched control group using a test of learning of and memory for words, but Gottlieb et al. (57) did not show any differences in memory as measured by the NEPSY (63) in a group of five-year-olds with and without SDB.

Executive Function
Executive function is crucial for normal psychological and social development and for goal-directed and flexible functioning. The executive functions allow individuals to adaptively use basic skills such as core language skills and visual-perceptual ability in a complex and continually changing external environment (64). The prefrontal cortex—which likely plays a critical role in integrative regulation of arousal, sleep, affect, and attention (65)—has been implicated in the executive dysfunction observed after sleep disruption (66). Despite the fact that executive function is complex and isolation of particular executive functions from other cognitive abilities is inherently difficult, executive dysfunction has been found in a number of children with SDB (28,30,37,57,58,67). Nonetheless, even in severe SDB, some executive functions may be impaired while others appear not to be; for example, in the recent study by Halbower et al. (58), children with severe SDB had deficits in word fluency but not in problem solving and planning.

Academic Achievement
SDB has been associated in a number of studies with schooling and learning problems (7,55,68–72). Learning is a complex process which requires the brain to store and retain information that can be recalled in the future. In a large school-based survey of 1129 nine-year-old children, analysis of school grades revealed an increasing prevalence of poor academic performance with increasing snoring frequency, which was significant for mathematics, science, and spelling, even after adjustment for potential confounders (71). Among 114 habitual snorers, 52% performed poorly at school (i.e., had grade 4 or worse in at least one of the three school subjects under study) in comparison with 31% of the nonsnorers (7). Another study of first-graders in the bottom 10% of their class found a 6–9 fold increase in sleep-associated gas exchange abnormalities (68). Furthermore, in a large survey of 1600 middle-school children (800 poor achievers matched to 800 high achievers), those who were poor achievers were much more likely to have snored during the preschool years than

those who were high achievers (13% vs. 5%) (69). In addition, the low achievers were three times more likely to have required adenotonsillectomy for snoring. While intermittent hypoxia is believed to underlie such learning problems (for a review see 73), attention problems may also contribute since impaired attention may impact the ability to rehearse, encode, store, and retrieve information (5).

DOES SDB CAUSE NEUROCOGNITIVE OR BEHAVIORAL MORBIDITY?

While the vast majority of studies provide cross-sectional evidence for some type of relationship between SDB and neurocognitive or behavioral outcome, there are no clinical trials to date which explicitly prove that SDB causes the above-mentioned morbidities. The study by Gozal and Pope (69) in which poor-achieving middle school children were significantly more likely to snore during their preschool years than were high achieving children gives some preliminary evidence that symptoms of SDB may occur prior to neurocognitive deficits. Furthermore, some children with SDB who do not meet criteria for ADHD before adenotonsillectomy do meet criteria one year later, again suggesting that damage to the brain earlier in life may only emerge as a visible phenotype years later (39). The strongest evidence in support of a causal relationship can be found in a recent longitudinal study which showed that snoring and other symptoms of SDB precede the development or exacerbation of behavioral problems (74). Chervin and colleagues showed that habitual snoring at baseline increased the risk for hyperactivity at a four-year follow-up by more than four-fold. These findings were particularly strong for boys under the age of eight years and were independent of hyperactivity at baseline and stimulant use at follow-up. Of note, the findings remained similar even after accounting for SDB symptoms at follow-up, again suggesting that damage done four years earlier may not be evident until years later.

Treatment studies may also provide evidence of causality. There are now a number of studies whereby children have had behavior and cognition assessed both before and after adenotonsillectomy, the first line treatment for SDB. Results show that treating SDB is associated with cognitive and behavioral improvement (39–41,75–79). In poorly performing children with SDB, school grades were obtained and children whose parents elected surgical intervention showed significantly improved school grades one year later, while those whose parents pursued no treatment showed no improvement of school grades (68). More recently, Chervin et al. (39) found that 78 children who were scheduled to undergo adenotonsillectomy were much more likely to be hyperactive than controls, whereas no group differences retained significance one year after surgery. Huang et al. (80) studied 66 children with ADHD with polysomnography and all were found to have mild SDB. Parents were able to select treatment; either treatment of the ADHD with stimulants, treatment of the mild SDB with adenotonsillectomy, or no treatment. Before and after the intervention, all children completed parent report behavior screens and an objective assessment of attention. After comprehensive follow-up six months later, children in both treatment groups improved compared to the no treatment group, although it was the children who had adenotonsillectomy who improved across more domains (both parentally reported as well as objectively assessed) than did the children whose parents elected stimulant medication as the treatment. While several studies report that after treatment, children with SDB have cognitive scores which improve to control levels (77), other studies suggest that not all of the cognitive abilities may improve to baseline levels (78). Thus, it is still unclear whether there is a window of vulnerability for the pediatric brain and whether any neurocognitve and behavioral morbidities associated with SDB are completely reversible.

Possible Mechanisms

It is believed that the mechanism by which SDB is associated with neurocognitive and behavioral morbidity includes intermittent hypoxia and sleep fragmentation. Both of the latter may alter the neurochemical substrate of the prefrontal cortex and manifest as deficits in executive functioning (66).

Intermittent Hypoxia

Hypoxiemia is associated with neurobehavioral problems in children with other disease states as well as those with SDB (for a comprehensive review see 73). Although mild desaturations can be associated with adverse effects, hypoxia is unlikely to be the sole cause of neurobehavioral deficits observed in SDB because children with primary snoring and other sleep disorders that involve no hypoxemia can show similar neurocognitive and/or behavioral problems (6,7). In rodent models, intermittent hypoxia during sleep, in the absence of significant sleep fragmentation, induces neuronal cell loss and impairs spatial memory (81), with developing rats potentially being more vulnerable (82,83). Intriguingly, the window of vulnerability in developing rats corresponds to a period of development in humans of early childhood when the prevalence of SDB is at its peak.

Sleep Fragmentation

Sleep fragmentation, such as that caused by multiple respiratory-related arousals from sleep, results in daytime performance deficits similar to those seen after sleep deprivation (84). Such findings are supported by animal models in which sleep deprivation and restriction impair hippocampal-dependent learning processes (85), and sleep fragmentation impedes spatial learning in rats (86). Sensitive measures of sleep state now suggest that sleep continuity in children with SDB is not preserved and that the degree of fragmentation may be associated with neurobehavioral outcome (87,88). One novel technique is able to determine alterations in the electroencephalogram (EEG) that are not visible to the naked eye and suggests that the respiratory cycle-related EEG changes attenuate after adenotonsillectomy to an extent predictive of improvement in objective tests for daytime sleepiness (89). Such EEG changes may even correlate more robustly with neurobehavioral outcome than does the traditional measure of SDB (the apnea/hypopnea index). Of note, a recent review (89) concluded that sleep deprivation, sleep disruption, and intermittent hypoxia independently may be sufficient to cause daytime neurobehavioral effects in vulnerable children, and that the combination of two or more of these factors may result in particular impairment of daytime functioning.

Recently, Halbower and colleagues (58) provided novel data from a brain imaging study and showed that neuronal metabolites in children with severe SDB were altered in the hippocampus and the right frontal cortex —areas of the brain that are implicated in cognition and executive function. Children with SDB scored worse on tests of intelligence and some executive functions compared to control children who were matched for age, gender, ethnicity, and socioeconomic status. It is possible that intermittent hypoxia and sleep fragmentation may disrupt cellular processes and trigger inflammatory responses and oxidative stress that may play a role in the pathogenesis of neurocognitive and behavioral deficits (90,91). However, not all children with SDB will develop such morbidities, suggesting that genetic and environmental factors may also play a role (92).

CONCLUSION

In summary, there is a growing body of literature from cross-sectional, longitudinal, and treatment intervention studies suggesting robust associations between SDB and neurocognitive and behavioral morbidities. Childhood is a time of intense brain development and so from a physiological standpoint it is logical that insults during this period may have significant consequences which may or may not be reversible. Nonetheless, the pediatric brain is also plastic, and so adaptive or compensatory mechanisms may occur more easily at certain stages of brain development than at others. This may go some way towards explaining some of the inconsistencies observed across studies. Definitive evidence such as that obtained from a randomized controlled clinical trial has yet to prove that SDB causes neurocognitive or behavioral morbidity but, despite this, clinicians need to be aware of the accumulating evidence of the public health impact of untreated SDB.

REFERENCES

1. Hill W. On some causes of backwardness and stupidity in children: And the relief of the symptoms in some instances by nasopharyngeal scarifications. BMJ 1889; II:711–12.
2. Guilleminault C, Eldridge FL, Simmons FB, et al. Sleep apnea in eight children. Pediatrics 1976; 58:23–31.
3. American Academy of Pediatrics Section on Pediatric Pulmonology. Clinical Practice Guideline: Diagnosis and management of childhood obstructive sleep apnea syndrome. Pediatrics 2002: 109:704–12.
4. Carroll JL, McColley SA, Marcus CL, et al. Inability of clinical history to distinguish primary snoring from obstructive sleep apnea syndrome in children. Chest 1995; 108:610–18.
5. Blunden S, Lushington K, Kennedy D, et al. Behavior and neurocognitive performance in children aged 5–10 years who snore compared to controls. J Clin Exp Neuropsychol 2000; 22(5):554–68.
6. O'Brien LM, Mervis CB, Holbrook CR, et al. Neurobehavioral implications of habitual snoring in children. Pediatrics 2004; 114:44–9.
7. Urschitz MS, Eitner S, Guenther A, et al. Habitual snoring, intermittent hypoxia, and impaired behavior in primary school children. Pediatrics 2004; 114(4):1041–48.
8. Richards W, Ferdman RM. Prolonged morbidity due to delays in the diagnosis and treatment of obstructive sleep apnea in children. Clinical Pediatrics 2000:9:103–8.
9. Chervin RD, Archbold KH, Panahi P, et al. Sleep problems seldom addressed at two general pediatric clinics. Pediatrics 2001 Jun; 107(6):1375–80.
10. Blunden S, Lushington K, Lorenzen B, et al. Are sleep problems under-recognised in general practice? Arch Dis Child 2004 Aug; 89(8):708–12.
11. Uong EC, Jeffe DB, Gozal D, et al. Development of a measure of knowledge and attitudes about obstructive sleep apnea in children (OSAKA-KIDS). Arch Pediatr Adolesc Med 2005 Feb; 159(2):181–6.

12. Owens JA, Dalzell V. Use of the 'BEARS' sleep screening tool in a pediatric residents' continuity clinic: A pilot study. Sleep Med 2005 Jan; 6(1):63–9.
13. Chervin RD, Weatherly RA, Garetz SL, et al. Pediatric sleep questionnaire: Prediction of sleep apnea and outcomes. Arch Otolaryngol Head Neck Surg 2007 Mar; 133(3):216–22.
14. Reuveni H, Simon T, Tal A, et al. Health care services utilization in children with obstructive sleep apnea syndrome. Pediatrics 2002 Jul; 110:68–72.
15. Tarasiuk A, Simon T, Tal A, et al.Adenotonsillectomy in children with obstructive sleep apnea syndrome reduces health care utilization. Pediatrics 2004 Feb; 113(2):351–6.
16. Tarasiuk A, Greenberg-Dotan S, Simon-Tuval T, et al. Elevated morbidity and health care use in children with obstructive sleep apnea syndrome. Am J Respir Crit Care Med 2007 Jan 1; 175(1):55–61.
17. Beebe DW. Neurobehavioral morbidity associated with disordered breathing during sleep in children: A comprehensive review. Sleep 2006 Sep 1; 29(9):1115–34.
18. Guilleminault C, Korobkin R, Winkle R. A review of 50 children with obstructive sleep apnea syndrome. Lung 1981; 159:275–87.
19. Guilleminault C, Winkle R, Korobkin R, et al. Children and nocturnal snoring: Evaluation of the effects of sleep related respiratory resistive load and daytime functioning. Eur J Pediatr 1982; 139:165–71.
20. Ali NJ, Pitson D, Stradling JR. Snoring, sleep disturbance and behaviour in 4–5 year olds. Arch Dis Child 1993; 68:360–66.
21. Chervin R, Dillon J, Bassetti C, et al. Symptoms of sleep disorders, inattention, and hyperactivity in children. Sleep 1997; 20:1185–1192.
22. Chervin RD, Archbold KH, Dillon JE, et al. Inattention, hyperactivity, and symptoms of sleep-disordered breathing. Pediatrics 2002; 109(3):449–56.
23. Chervin RD, Dillon JE, Archbold KH, et al. Conduct problems and symptoms of sleep disorders in children. J Am Acad Child Adolesc Psychiatry 2003; 42(2):201–8.
24. Gottlieb DJ, Vezina RM, Chase C, et al. Symptoms of sleep-disordered breathing in 5-year-old children are associated with sleepiness and problem behaviors. Pediatrics 2003; 112(4):870–7.
25. Melendres MC, Lutz JM, Rubin ED, et al. Daytime sleepiness and hyperactivity in children with suspected sleep-disordered breathing. Pediatrics 2004; 114(3):768–75.
26. Arman AR, Ersu R, Save D, et al. Symptoms of inattention and hyperactivity in children with habitual snoring: Evidence from a community-based study in Istanbul. Child Care Health Dev 2005; 31(6).
27. Mulvaney SA, Goodwin JL, Morgan WJ, et al. Behavior problems associated with sleep disordered breathing in school-aged children: The Tucson children's assessment of sleep apnea study. J Pediatr Psychol 2006; 31(3):322–30.
28. Lewin DS, Rosen RC, England SJ, et al. Preliminary evidence of behavioral and cognitive sequelae of obstructive sleep apnea in children. Sleep Med 2002; 3(1):5–13.
29. O'Brien LM, Holbrook CR, Mervis CB, et al. Sleep and neurobehavioral characteristics in 5–7 year old children with parentally reported symptoms of ADHD. Pediatrics 2003; 111:554–63.
30. Beebe DW, Wells CT, Jeffries J, et al. Neuropsychological effects of pediatric obstructive sleep apnea. J Int Neuropsychol Soc 2004; 10(7):962–75.
31. Rosen CL, Storfer-Isser A, Taylor HG, et al. Increased behavioral morbidity in school-aged children with sleep-disordered breathing. Pediatrics 2004; 114(6):1640–8.
32. Kennedy JD, Blunden S, Hirte C, et al. Reduced neurocognition in children who snore. Pediatr Pulmonol 2004; 37(4):330–7.
33. Conners CK. Conners' Rating Scales-Revised: Technical Manual. North Tonawanda, NY: Multi-health Systems Publishing, 1997.
34. Achenbach TM. Manual for the Revised Child Behavior Checklist. Burlington, VT: University of Vermont, Department of Psychiatry, 1991.
35. Reynolds CR, Kamphaus RW. BASC-Behavioral Assessment System for Children manual. Circle Pines, MN. Am Guid Serv 1992.

36. Conners CK. Conners' Continuous Performance Test II. Technical Guide and Software Manual. Toronto, ON, Canada: Multi-Heatlh Systems Inc, 2000.
37. Blunden S, Lushington K, Lorenzen B, et al. Neuropsychological and psychosocial function in children with a history of snoring or behavioral sleep problems. J Pediatr 2005; 146(6):780–6.
38. O'Brien LM, Mervis CB, Holbrook CR, et al. Neurobehavioral correlates of OSA in children. J Sleep Res 2004; 13:165–72.
39. Chervin RD, Ruzicka DL, Giordani BJ, et al. Sleep-disordered breathing, behavior, and cognition in children before and after adenotonsillectomy. Pediatrics 2006; 117(4):e769–78.
40. Galland BC, Dawes PJ, Tripp EG, et al. Changes in behavior and attentional capacity after adenotonsillectomy. Pediatr Res 2006; 59(5):711–16.
41. Avior G, Fishman G, Leor A, et al. The effect of tonsillectomy and adenoidectomy on inattention and impulsivity as measured by the Test of Variables of Attention (TOVA) in children with obstructive sleep apnea syndrome. Otolaryngol Head Neck Surg 2004; 131(4):367–71.
42. Stein MA, Mendelsohn J, Obermyer WH, et al. Sleep and behavior problems in school-aged children. Pediatrics 2001; 107:e60.
43. Crabtree VM, Varni JW, Gozal D. Health-related quality of life and depressive symptoms in children with suspected sleep-disordered breathing. Sleep 2004; 27:1131–8.
44. American Psychiatric Association. Diagnostic and Statistical Manual of Mental Disorders, 3rd edn Washington DC: American Psychiatric Association, 1980.
45. American Psychiatric Association. Diagnostic and Statistical Manual of Mental Disorders, 3rd edn revised, Washington DC: American Psychiatric Association, 1987.
46. American Psychiatric Association. Diagnostic and Statistical Manual of Mental Disorders, 4th edn Washington DC: American Psychiatric Association, 1994.
47. Owens J, Maxim R, Nobile C, et al. Parental and self-report of sleep in children with attention deficit/hyperactivity disorder. Arch Pediatr Adolesc Med 2000; 154:549–55.
48. Corkum P, Tannock R, Moldofsky H, et al. Actigraphy and parental ratings of sleep in children with attention deficit/hyperactivity disorder (ADHD). Sleep 2001; 24:303–12.
49. Stein MA. Unravelling sleep problems in treated and untreated children with ADHD. J Child Adolesc Psychopharmacol 1999; 9:157–68.
50. LeBourgeios MK, Avis K, Mixon M, et al. Snoring, sleep quality, and sleepiness across attention-deficit/hyperactivity disorder subtypes. Sleep 2004; 27(3):520–5.
51. Golan N, Shahar E, Ravid S, et al. Sleep disorders and daytime sleepiness in children with attention-deficit/hyperactive disorder. Sleep 2004; 27(2):261–6.
52. Huang YS, Chen NH, Li HY, et al. Sleep disorders in Taiwanese children with attention deficit/hyperactivity disorder. J Sleep Res 2004; 13(3):269–77.
53. Cortese S, Konofal E, Yateman N, et al. Sleep and alertness in children with attention-deficit/hyperactivity disorder: A systematic review of the literature. Sleep 2006; 29(4):504–11.
54. Osler W. The Principles and Practice of Medicine. 1st edn New York: D. Appleton and Company, 1892.
55. Chervin RD, Clarke DF, Huffman JL, et al. School performance, race, and other correlates of sleep-disordered breathing in children. Sleep Med 2003; 4(1):21–7.
56. Emancipator JL, Storfer-Isser A, Taylor HG, et al. Variation of cognition and achievement with sleep-disordered breathing in full-term and preterm children. Arch Pediatr Adolesc Med 2006; 160(2):203–10.
57. Gottlieb DJ, Chase C, Vezina RM, et al. Sleep-disordered breathing symptoms are associated with poorer cognitive function in 5-year-old children. J Pediatr 2004; 145(4):458–64.
58. Halbower AC, Degaonkar M, Barker PB, et al. Childhood obstructive sleep apnea associates with neuropsychological deficits and neuronal brain injury. PLoS Med 2006 Aug; 3(8):e301.

59. Suratt PM, Peruggia M, D'Andrea L, et al. Cognitive function and behavior of children with adenotonsillar hypertrophy suspected of having obstructive sleep-disordered breathing. Pediatrics 2006 Sep; 118(3):e771–81.
60. Suratt PM, Barth JT, Diamond R, et al. Reduced time in bed and obstructive sleep-disordered breathing in children are associated with cognitive impairment. Pediatrics 2007 Feb; 119(2):320–9.
61. Kaemingk KL, Pasvogel AE, Goodwin JL, et al. Learning in children and sleep disordered breathing: Findings of the Tucson Children's Assessment of Sleep Apnea (tuCASA) prospective cohort study. J Int Neuropsychol Soc 2003; 9(7):1016–26.
62. Rhodes SK, Shimoda KC, Waid LR, et al. Neurocognitive deficits in morbidly obese children with obstructive sleep apnea. J Pediatr 1995; 127(5):741–4.
63. Korkman M, Kirk U, Kemp S. NEPSY: A developmental neuropsychological assessment manual. San Antonio, TX: Harcourt Brace, 1998.
64. Goldberg E. The Executive Brain: Frontal Lobes and the Civilized Mind. Oxford: Oxford University Press, 2001.
65. Dahl RE. The impact of inadequate sleep on children's daytime cognitive function. Semin Pediatr Neurol 1996; 3(1):44–50.
66. Beebe DW, Gozal D. Obstructive sleep apnea and the prefrontal cortex: Towards a comprehensive model linking nocturnal upper airway obstruction to daytime cognitive and behavioral deficits. J Sleep Res 2002; 11(1):1–16.
67. Archbold KH, Giordani B, Ruzicka DL, et al. Cognitive executive dysfunction in children with mild sleep-disordered breathing. Biol Res Nurs 2004; 5(3):168–76.
68. Gozal D. Sleep-disordered breathing and school performance in children. Pediatrics 1998; 102:616–20.
69. Gozal D, Pope Jr DW. Snoring during early childhood and academic performance at ages 13–14 years. Pediatrics 2001; 107:1394–9.
70. Goodwin JL, Kaemingk KL, Fregosi RF, et al. Clinical outcomes associated with sleep-disordered breathing in Caucasian and Hispanic children: The Tucson Children's Assessment of Sleep Apnea study (TuCASA). Sleep 2003; 26(5):587–91.
71. Urschitz MS, Guenther A, Eggebrecht E, et al. Snoring, intermittent hypoxia and academic performance in primary school children. Am J Respir Crit Care Med 2003; 168(4):464–8.
72. Urschitz MS, Wolff J, Sokollik C, et al. Nocturnal arterial oxygen saturation and academic performance in a community sample of children. Pediatrics 2005; 115(2):e204–09.
73. Bass JL, Corwin M, Gozal D, et al. The effect of chronic or intermittent hypoxia on cognition in childhood: A review of the evidence. Pediatrics 2004; 114(3):805–16.
74. Chervin RD, Ruzicka DL, Archbold KH, et al. Snoring predicts hyperactivity four years later. Sleep 2005; 28(7):885–90.
75. Stradling JR, Thomas G, Warley ARH, et al. Effect of adenotonsillectomy on nocturnal hypoxaemia, sleep disturbance, and symptoms in snoring children. Lancet 1990; 335:249–53.
76. Ali NJ, Pitson D, Stradling JR. Sleep disordered breathing: Effects of adenotonsillectomy on behaviour and psychological functioning. Eur J Pediatr 1996; 155(1):56–62.
77. Friedman BC, Hendeles-Amitai A, Kozminsky E, et al. Adenotonsillectomy improves neurocognitive function in children with obstructive sleep apnea syndrome. Sleep 2003; 26(8):999–1005.
78. Montgomery-Downs HE, Crabtree VM, Gozal D. Cognition, sleep and respiration in at-risk children treated for obstructive sleep apnoea. Eur Resp J 2005; 25(2):336–42.
79. Roemmich JN, Barkley JE, D'Andrea L, et al. Increases in overweight after adenotonsillectomy in overweight children with obstructive sleep-disordered breathing are associated with decreases in motor activity and hyperactivity. Pediatrics 2006; 117(2):e200–08.
80. Huang YS, Guilleminault C, Li HY, et al. Attention-deficit/hyperactivity disorder with obstructive sleep apnea: A treatment outcome study. Sleep Med 2007; 8:18–30.

81. Gozal D, Daniel JM, Dohanich GP. Behavioral and anatomical correlates of chronic episodic hypoxia during sleep in the rat. J Neurosci 2001; 21:2442–50.
82. Gozal E, Row BW, Schurr A, et al. Developmental differences in cortical and hippocampal vulnerability to intermittent hypoxia in the rat. Neurosci Lett 2001; 305:197–201.
83. Row BW, Kheirandish L, Neville JJ, et al. Impaired spatial learning and hyperactivity in developing rats exposed to intermittent hypoxia. Pediatr Res 2002; 52: 449–53.
84. Martin SE, Engleman HM, Deary IJ, et al. The effect of sleep fragmentation on daytime function. Am J Respir Crit Care Med 1996; 153(4 Pt 1):1328–32.
85. Hairston IS, Little MT, Scanlon MD, et al. Sleep restriction suppresses neurogenesis induced by hippocampus-dependent learning. J Neurophysiol 2005; 94(6):4224–33.
86. Tartar JL, Ward CP, McKenna JT, et al. Hippocampal synaptic plasticity and spatial learning are impaired in a rat model of sleep fragmentation. Eur J Neurosci 2006; 23(10):2739–48.
87. O'Brien LM, Tauman R, Gozal D. Sleep pressure correlates of cognitive and behavioral morbidity in snoring children. Sleep 2004; 27:279–82.
88. Chervin RD, Burns JW, Subotic NS, et al. Correlates of respiratory cycle-related EEG changes in children with sleep-disordered breathing. Sleep 2004; 27(1):116–21.
89. Blunden SL, Beebe DW. The contribution of intermittent hypoxia, sleep debt and sleep disruption to daytime performance deficits in children: Consideration of respiratory and non-respiratory sleep disorders. Sleep Med Rev 2006; 10(2):109–18.
90. Lavie L. Obstructive sleep apnoea syndrome: An oxidative stress disorder. Sleep Med Rev 2003; 7(1):35–51.
91. Tauman R, Ivanenko A, O'Brien LM, et al. Plasma C-reactive protein in children with sleep–disordered breathing. Pediatrics 2004; 113:e564–9.
92. Gozal D, Kheirandish L. Oxidant stress and inflammation in the snoring child: Confluent pathways to upper airway pathogenesis and end-organ morbidity. Sleep Med Rev 2006; 10(2):83–96.

12 Narcolepsy and Idiopathic Hypersomnia in Childhood

Suresh Kotagal

Center for Sleep Medicine and Departments of Neurology and Pediatrics, Mayo Clinic, Rochester, Minnesota, U.S.A.

INTRODUCTION

In 1880, Gelineau coined the term *narcolepsie* to describe a pathological condition that was characterized by recurrent, brief attacks of sleepiness (1). He recognized that the disorder was accompanied by falls or *astasias* which were subsequently defined as cataplexy. Narcolepsy is a lifelong disorder of rapid eye movement (REM) in which there are attacks of *irresistible daytime sleep, cataplexy* (sudden loss of muscle tone and weakness in response to emotional triggers such as laughter, fright, or rage that can lead to head dropping or falls), *hypnagogic hallucinations* (vivid dreams at sleep onset), and *sleep paralysis* (momentary inability to move as one is falling asleep). Commenting about what he felt was a possible psychiatric basis for the disease, Adie in 1926 (2) wrote that true narcolepsy "is a functional disorder of the nervous system, probably an undue fatigability of the nerve cells in individuals with a peculiar kind of nervous activity that allows excessive responses to emotional stimuli and favors the spread of inhibitions." By 1963, however, the organic basis for narcolepsy had been firmly established by Rechtschaffen and colleagues following their description of the pathognomonic sleep onset REM periods on polysomnography (3).

The incidence of narcolepsy in the United States is estimated at 1.37 per 100,000 persons per year—1.72/100,000 for men and 1.05/100,000 for women (4). It is highest in the second decade, followed by a gradual decline from thereon. The prevalence rate has been reported as 56 per 100,000 in the United States (4), in Japan as 1 in 600 (5), and in Israel as 1 in 500,000 (6). While narcolepsy is often diagnosed in the third and fourth decades, a meta-analysis of 235 subjects derived from three studies found that 34% of all subjects had onset of symptoms prior to the age of 15 years. In this subgroup, 16% had onset prior to age 10 years, and 4.5% prior to age five years (Figure 1) (7). With the emergence of pediatric sleep medicine as a discipline, it is likely that narcolepsy will be diagnosed in greater numbers during childhood and adolesence. Males and females are afflicted equally. Cataplexy, one of the most reliable clinical features of narcolepsy, is present only in 50–70% of all subjects. Some epidemiologic studies have required the presence of cataplexy as a prerequisite to making the diagnosis (6) whereas other studies (5,8) have not made this a stipulation. This lack of uniformity in clinical diagnostic criteria might explain some of the variation in prevalence rates.

PATHOPHYSIOLOGY
Narcolepsy in Animals

Miniature horses, quarter horses, Brahman bulls, cats, and about 15 breeds of dogs with narcolepsy have been described (9). An autosomal recessive pattern of inheritance

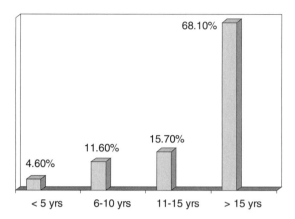

FIGURE 1   Age of onset of narcolepsy, based upon a meta-analysis of 235 cases (7).

has been described in Doberman Pinschers and Labrador retrievers (9). Feline narcolepsy has proven a useful model for the study of cataplexy, and has advanced understanding of its pathophysiology—cataplectic behavior can be induced in narcoleptic cats by the injection into the pontine reticular formation of carbachol, an acetylcholine-like substance (10). Microscopic examination of the brain stem however fails to disclose any abnormalities. In 1999, mutations in the preprohypocretin receptor gene were documented in canine narcolepsy (11). This also directed attention to the possible role of hypocretin (synonymous with orexin) in the pathogenesis of human narcolepsy (12). Hypocretin is a peptide that is secreted by neurons located in the dorsolateral hypothalamus. The hypocretin neurons have widespread projections to neurons in the ventral forebrain and the brain stem. Their activation promotes arousal, locomotion, and appetite control. Hypocretin "knock out" mice models display features that resemble human narcolepsy (13), with excessive sleep, decreased mobility, hypophagia, and obesity.

Human Narcolepsy
The presence of the histocompatibility antigens DQB1*0602 in close to 100% of human narcolepsy patients, as compared to about 25% prevalence in the general population points to a genetic susceptibility for narcolepsy (14). Monozygotic twins have been reported however to remain discordant by many years for developing symptoms of narcolepsy (15). This suggests a possible role for acquired conditions as triggers for narcolepsy. Life stresses such as bereavement or systemic infection have been identified as precipitants for narcolepsy in a large proportion of subjects. Human narcolepsy is best explained on the basis of a *two-threshold hypothesis*— genetic susceptibility combined with environmental factors is probably essential for narcolepsy to become clinically manifest.

Unlike canine narcolepsy, abnormalities of the hypocretin receptors *per se* are rare in human narcolepsy. Humans with narcolepsy-cataplexy show a marked reduction of levels of hypocretin-1 within the cerebrospinal fluid (16). Owing to the strong association of human narcolepsy with HLA DQB1 *0602, an immune-mediated

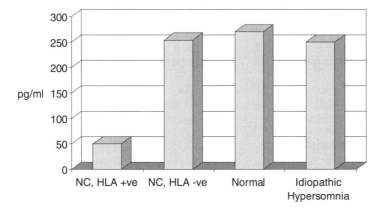

FIGURE 2 Cerebrospinal fluid levels of hypocretin in subjects with narcolepsy-cataplexy (n=5, column 1), narcolepsy without cataplexy (n=5, column 2), normal controls (n=15, column 3), and idiopathic hypersomnia (n=12, column 4). Data derived from: Kanbayashi T, Inoue Y, Chiba S, et al. Cerebrospinal fluid hypocretin-1 (orexin A) concentrations in narcolepsy with and without cataplexy and idiopathic hypersomnia. J Sleep Res 2002; 11(1): 91–3.

injury to the hypocretin secreting neurons has been suggested (18). Narcolepsy without cataplexy and idiopathic hypersomnia show normal levels of cerebral spinal fluid (CSF) hypocretin-1 (Figure 2). The deficiency of hypocretin leads to unstable sleep–wake regulation, especially at the REM sleep–wakefulness interface, and this phenomenon underlies many of the clinical features of narcolepsy. There is an increased propensity for intrusion of fragments of REM sleep on to wakefulness—this is manifested in the form of cataplexy, sleep paralysis, or hypnagogic hallucinations (17,18). The converse may also be true, in that activity of the wakefulness promoting hypocretin system intrudes on the activity of the "sleep switch," i.e., the ventrolateral preoptic nuclei (19). Over a 24-hour period, narcolepsy patients tend to fall asleep more often, though not necessarily for a longer period of time.

While the majority of narcolepsy is *idiopathic,* structural lesions involving the diencephalon/brain stem may on rare occasions be associated with the development of symptomatic narcolepsy. This is due to disruption of secretion of hypocretin-1 by the lesion. Third ventricular gliomas, craniopharyngomas, sarcoidosis, viral encephalitis, and head injury have been implicated (20). Cataplexy has also been observed in Niemann Pick Type C disease, Norrie disease, Coffin Lowry syndrome, and Mobius syndrome (20).

CLINICAL FEATURES

In some children, all major symptoms are present right at the very onset. In others, however, the full tetrad set of symptoms may evolve gradually over a period of years. One must acknowledge however that it is at times difficult to reliably ascertain cataplexy, hypnagogic hallucinations, and sleep paralysis in young children. There may be a lag period of 5–10 years between the onset of sleepiness and establishing a definitive diagnosis of narcolepsy. In part, this is due to insufficient awareness of childhood narcolepsy amongst healthcare professionals.

Pollack et al. studied the circadian sleep–wake rhythms in subjects with narcolepsy who were isolated from their environmental cues (21). They found that the major sleep episode was still about six hours long, and occurred about once every 24 hours, thus indicating that the circadian clock was functioning normally. They confirmed that patients with narcolepsy tended to sleep *more often*, but *not longer* than people without narcolepsy. While significant daytime sleepiness may have onset even prior to age 4–5 years, it is difficult to establish a firm diagnosis of narcolepsy in preschool age children simply because physiological napping is quite common in this age group (CSF hypocretin testing may enable diagnosis at this early age, however). Daytime sleepiness related to unequivocal narcolepsy is more often seen by 6–7 years of age—Lenn has reported a six-year-old boy with narcolepsy who would fall asleep 5–10 times a day (22). Wittig et al. have described a seven-year-old boy who tended to fall asleep while watching television for longer than a half hour, at the dinner table, and while seated in his mother's lap at a doctor's office (23). The naps in children with narcolepsy may be longer than those in adults. They are often 30–90 minutes in length, and not consistently followed by a refreshed feeling (24). The attacks of sleepiness occur most often during sedentary activities such as sitting at a desk in the classroom. The daytime sleepiness is frequently associated with automatic behaviors of which the subject is unaware, and with impairments of memory and concentration. A loss of "affect control" from sleepiness also impairs prefrontal cortical inhibitory function, with consequent mood swing problems (25). Children with daytime sleepiness are at times mistaken as being "lazy" and thus become the target of negative and hurtful comments from their peers and teachers.

Cataplexy

The second but most reliable feature of narcolepsy, consists of a sudden loss of muscle tone in the extensor muscles of the neck, trunk and lower extremities in response to emotional triggers such as laughter, fright, rage, or surprise. This symptom may be difficult to elicit by history in young children. This author recalls a six-year-old girl with proven narcolepsy who denied any episodic muscle weakness, but would repeatedly become weak and fall when she jumped on a trampoline. Consciousness and respiration remain fully preserved during cataplexy events, which can last 1–30 minutes. Cataplexy results from intrusion of REM sleep onto wakefulness. It is accompanied by generalized muscle atonia and loss of tendon reflexes. At the cellular level, there is hyperpolarization of the spinal motor neurons. Challamel et al. (7) found cataplexy in 80% of children with idiopathic narcolepsy and in 95% of children with symptomatic narcolepsy.

Hypnagogic Hallucinations and Sleep Paralysis

These are seen in close to 50–60% of subjects. Like cataplexy, they represent sleep–wake dissociation with intrusion of fragments of REM sleep onto wakefulness. Nighttime sleep is also disturbed in narcolepsy, with frequent awakenings which may or may not be associated with periodic limb movements in sleep.

Neuropsychological and Behavioral Manifestations
These are also common in childhood narcolepsy, but have not been adequately studied. It is not unusual for children to present with inattentiveness or mild depression. Adult subjects with narcolepsy have selective cognitive deficits in response latency, word recall and estimation of frequency (26,27). Stores et al. recently surveyed 42 children with narcolepsy aged 4–18 years (28). They also surveyed 18 children with daytime sleepiness that did not meet diagnostic criteria for narcolepsy and age- and gender-matched controls. They found that as compared to the controls, children both with narcolepsy and non-narcolepsy sleepiness showed significantly higher levels of depression, behavioral problems, and impairments in the quality of life. The narcolepsy subjects were indistinguishable from the non-narcoleptic sleepy children on the testing measures. This suggests that sleepiness per se, rather than narcolepsy underlies the psychological problems.

DIAGNOSIS
The diagnosis of narcolepsy is established on the basis of the characteristic sleep–wake history combined with the *nocturnal polysomnogram* and *multiple sleep latency test* (MSLT) (29). During the nocturnal polysomnogram, multiple physiological parameters like the electroencephalogram (EEG), eye movements, chin electromyogram, nasal airflow, respiratory effort, end tidal carbon dioxide, and oxygen saturation are recorded simultaneously on a computerized system. By utilizing wrist actigraphy or sleep logs for 2–3 weeks immediately prior to the sleep studies, one can ensure that the patient has been receiving adequate sleep at home and that a circadian rhythm sleep disorder such as delayed sleep phase syndrome (DSPS) has been excluded. The nocturnal polysomnogram helps exclude sleep pathologies like obstructive sleep apnea, periodic limb movement disorder (PLMD) and idiopathic hypersomnia which can also lead to daytime sleepiness and thus mimic narcolepsy. In one study, children with narcolepsy showed a shortened nocturnal REM latency (time from initial sleep onset to the first epoch of REM sleep) of 24.5 min (SD 50.9, n=8) as compared to controls with non-narcolepsy sleep disorders (mean of 143 min, SD 50.9, n=12) (30). Patients with depression may show abbreviation of the nocturnal REM latency, but not to levels below 70 minutes (31).

On the morning after the nocturnal polysomnogram, the patient undergoes an MSLT. This provides quantitative and qualitative information about the transition from wakefulness into sleep (29). It consists of four or five nap opportunities provided at two hourly intervals in a darkened, quiet room (e.g., at 1000, 1200, 1400, and 1600 hours). Eye movements, chin electromyogram, electrocardiogram, and the EEG are monitored simultaneously. The nap opportunity is terminated after 20 minutes if the patient does not fall asleep or at 15 minutes after sleep onset. For each nap, the time from "lights out" to sleep onset constitutes the sleep latency. A mean sleep latency is also calculated from all the four or five provided nap opportunities. The time interval between "lights out" and sleep onset observed on the EEG during the MSLT is termed the *sleep latency;* a mean sleep latency is derived by adding the sleep latencies of all naps and dividing the sum by the number of naps. The mean sleep latency is closely linked to the Tanner stage of sexual development and shows a progressive decrease concurrent with advancing sexual maturation. In narcolepsy, the mean sleep latency is markedly shortened to less than five minutes, whereas in control pre-adolescent children it ranges from 19 to 23 minutes (32,33). The MSLT also helps in evaluating the transition from wakefulness into sleep—the physiological transition is from wakefulness into non-REM sleep, whereas patients with narcolepsy show sleep onset REM periods during at least two of the four nap opportunities. This diagnostic feature of two or more sleep onset REM periods (SOREMPs) is not consistently present in the early stages of narcolepsy in all children and young adults but appears gradually over time, thus sometimes serial sleep studies are needed to establish a definitive diagnosis (34).

Assay of CSF hypocretin-1 levels is helpful in diagnosis whenever the patient is receiving multiple psychotropic medications which cannot be stopped for the purpose of obtaining nocturnal polysomnography or MSLT without compromising patient safety. The scenario of depression that is being treated with a selective serotonin reuptake inhibitor and suspicion of coexisting narcolepsy is commonly encountered in adolescents. Levels of CSF hypocretin-1 are not compromised by age, gender, time of collection of the sample, or medications. Patients with narcolepsy–cataplexy usually have levels below 110 pg/ml, whereas narcolepsy without cataplexy and idiopathic hypersomnia remain in the normal range (>200 pg/ml range) (35). The diagnostic sensitivity of low CSF hypocretin-1 (<100 pg/ml) is 84% (35). Arii et al. studied CSF hypocretin-1 levels in 132 patients with pediatric neurological disorders (36). Hypocretin levels were severely reduced (<110 pg/ml) in 6/6 patients with narcolepsy–cataplexy, but in only 7/126 (5.5%) of the control group, which included intracranial tumors, head trauma, acute infectious polyneuritis and acute disseminated encephalomyelitis.

Formal neuropsychological assessment is helpful in determining comorbidities like learning disability, attention deficit disorder, and depression, but it is prudent to delay this evaluation until the control of sleepiness has been optimized.

Differential Diagnosis

Idiopathic hypersomnia should be considered in the differential diagnosis of narcolepsy. It is discussed in the next section. Depression may present with mood swings, apathy, and sleepiness, but the hypnagogic halucinations and sleep paralysis that are characteristic of narcolepsy are lacking. The MSLT in depression may document moderate daytime sleepiness, but it is of a lesser severity than in narcolepsy. Subjects with depression can manifest an occasional SOREMP, but once again the two or more SOREMPs typical of narcolepsy are infrequent. The DSPS is common circadian rhythm sleep disorder in adolescent males. Parents may have concerns about the inability of their teen to rise in time to attend school; the clinical features of narcolepsy are lacking. Wrist actigraphy and sleep logs for 2–3 weeks can assist in making the diagnosis. Inadequate sleep hygiene can also be established by sleep history, sleep logs for 2–3 weeks, and wrist actigraphy. In periodic hypersomnia (Kleine Levin syndrome), there is usually a history of 10–14-day periods of sleepiness, hyperphagia, hypersexual behavior, and mood disturbance that alternate with weeks to months of normal sleep–wake function. Incomplete forms of periodic hypersomnia that are lacking some of the clinical features are common. One must always be alert to substance abuse as a cause of daytime sleepiness. At our institution, it is a routine practice to obtain a urine drug screen during the MSLT if the naps opportunities are suggesting pathologic sleepiness.

MANAGEMENT
General Measures
Narcolepsy is a lifelong disorder with considerable impact upon the quality of life. Extensive counseling is required to ensure that both pharmacological and nonpharmacological management issues are appreciated and adhered to by the patient and family. This includes repeated discussions about maintaining regularity in sleep–wake schedules, avoiding alcohol and illicit substances, avoiding driving whenever possible, and appreciating the role of regular exercise and mobility in countering sleepiness. One to two planned naps per day of 25–30 minutes may help enhance daytime alertness and improve psychomotor performance. Writing a letter to the school authorities in support of a planned nap opportunity at school is reasonable. Some teenagers may require intensive and individualized pychological counseling. Upon learning of the diagnosis of narcolepsy, the parents may also show denial and feelings of guilt which need attention. It is difficult for the child to adapt to the diagnosis of narcolepsy if the parent is unable to come to grips with it. Vocational guidance is important in helping the young person with narcolepsy make appropriate career choices. Because of the increased risk of accidents related to sleepiness, patients should be cautioned against driving long distances and working near sharp, moving machinery. *The Narcolepsy Network* (telephone 973-276-0115; email narnet@aol.com*)* is a useful private, nonprofit resource for patients, families and health professionals

Psychostimulants
Daytime sleepiness is countered pharmacologically by using *preparations of methyphenidate*, or various formulations of *amphetamine* (37). The side effects of these agents include loss of appetite, nervousness, tics, headache, and insomnia. *Modafinil* (PROVIGIL) is also effective in enhancing alertness and improving psychomotor performance (38). Its side effects include headache, nervousness, anxiety, and nausea. In order to maintain optimum alertness, the stimulant medication may need to be administered in 2–3 divided doses. Evidence about the therapeutic efficacy of methylphenidate/amphetamines in narcolepsy consists of three level II and four level V studies (39). The practice parameters published by the American Academy of Sleep Medicine state that the benefit to risk ratio of stimulants has not been well documented because published trials have been composed of small numbers of patients (39). If daytime sleepiness is not controlled despite adequate doses of psychostimulants, an open mind should be kept about comorbidities such as inadequate sleep hygiene, restless legs syndrome, obstructive sleep apnea, and depression that can exacerbate daytime sleepiness.

Cataplexy
Mild cataplexy may not require therapy. Since cholinergic pathways in the brain stem mediate cataplexy, drugs with anticholinergic properties such as *protryptiline* and *clompiramine* have been used for its control. Potential side effects include dryness of the mouth, constipation, weight gain, and drowsiness. Selective serotonin reuptake inhibitors like fluoxetine, sertraline, and venlafaxine are also helpful in managing cataplexy, especially when there is a superimposed element of depression. Common side effects with these agents include dizziness, headache, and nervousness.

Gamma hydroxybutyrate (sodium oxybate, XYREM) has been approved by the Food and Drug Administration for treating cataplexy in adults (40). It seems to work by stabilizing nocturnal sleep architecture, which in turn might indirectly lessen REM sleep intrusions onto wakefulness, the basis for the daytime features of narcolepsy–cataplexy. In an off-label, retrospective study of eight children with severe narcolepsy–cataplexy, Murali and Kotagal found that seven of eight showed significant improvement in their cataplexy, and that all had improvement in daytime sleepiness as well (41). The mean age at initiation of treatment was 13.75 years (range 9–16 years). The dose ranged from 3 to 7 grams nightly in two divided doses. Suicidal ideation, dissociative episodes, tremor, and constipation were observed in one subject each. Depression may be a contraindication to the use of sodium oxybate, given the tendency for its worsening during treatment with this drug.

As dysregulation of the immune system may play a role in the pathogenesis of narcolepsy–cataplexy, Dauvilliers et al. have reported upon treatment of four hypocretin deficient subjects using intravenous immunoglobulin, shortly after the diagnosis of narcolepsy–cataplexy was established (42). There was significant and sustained improvement in cataplexy, which minimized the need for other medications to treat cataplexy. They acknowledge the limitations of their study, which include small sample size, open label design, and lack of adequate history of the natural history of narcolepsy–cataplexy in older adults (one of their subjects was 57 years old).

IDIOPATHIC HYPERSOMNIA
Definition
The International Classification of Sleep Disorders defines idiopathic hypersomnia as a disorder associated with nonimperative sleepiness, long unrefreshing naps, difficulty reaching full awakening after sleep, sleep drunkenness, as well as absence of sleep onset REM periods on the MSLT (43). In contrast to narcolepsy, where the mean sleep latency on the MSLT is frequently less than five minutes, in idiopathic hypersomnia the mean sleep latency is generally in the 5–10 minute range. Nocturnal polysomnograms show normal sleep quantity and quality as well. Levels of CSF hypocretin remain in the normal range. The upper airway resistance syndrome can mimic idiopathic hypersomnia.

Clinical Features
Basetti and Aldrich have reviewed a series of 42 subjects with idiopathic hypersomnia who were followed up at the University of Michigan (44). The mean age at onset of symptoms was 19 years (range from 6 to 43). Almost half described restless sleep with frequent arousals. Habitual dreaming was present in about 40%. Habitual snoring was common, occurring in 45 % of subjects, but was not any more frequent than in narcoleptics. They categorized idiopathic hypersomnia into three forms:

a. the classic form in which sleepiness was not overwhelming, and there was a tendency to take long naps; night sleep was prolonged and there was difficulty with morning awakening
b. the narcolepsy-like idiopathic hypersomnia, with overwhelming daytime sleepiness, a tendency to take short and refreshing daytime naps; sleep attacks could occur even during standing
c. the "mixed" form in which the naps were brief but not refreshing.

Bassetti and Aldrich remarked that there was a substantial overlap between narcolepsy and idiopathic hypersomnia. This has been substantiated by others as well (30). This author has described six children with daytime sleepiness who upon initial presentation met the diagnostic criteria for idiopathic hypersomnia, but who, upon longitudinal follow up and repeat nocturnal polysomnography and MSLT evaluation, met the diagnostic criteria for narcolepsy. It is possible, therefore, that in some children, idiopathic hypersomnia is a transitional phase en route to the development of full blown narcolepsy.

FUTURE DIRECTIONS OF INQUIRY

Is idiopathic hypersomnia a transitional stage in the course of evolution of childhood narcolepsy (34) or is it a free-standing disorder that is unrelated to narcolepsy? Early recognition of the symptoms of narcolepsy will likely become an important management issue, especially if large scale, prospective studies also confirm a favorable response to treatment with intravenous immunoglobulin at the onset of symptoms, mimicking the favorable short-term results (42). The psychosocial and neuropsychological impairments resulting from childhood narcolepsy warrant further study. The long-term outcome of patients who develop narcolepsy during childhood is a potential area for investigation. Many clinicians suspect that patients go through a "honey moon" period in which symptom severity often diminishes for a few months. This presumed phenomenon needs verification. Some of the drugs used to treat childhood narcolepsy–cataplexy are prescribed on an "off-label" basis. Formal pharmacokinetic, safety and efficacy studies are needed for drugs like sodium oxybate.

REFERENCES

1. Gelineau J. De la narcolepsie. Gaz Hosp (Paris) 1880; 53: 626–28.
2. Adie WJ. Idiopathic narcolepsy: A disease sui generis; with remarks on the mechanism of sleep. Brain 1926; 49:257–306.
3. Rechtschaffen A, Wolpert EA, Dement WC, et al. Nocturnal sleep of narcoleptics. Electroencephalogr Clin Neurophysiol 1963; 15:599–609.
4. Silber MH, Krahn LE, Olson EJ, et al. The epidemiology of narcolepsy in Olmstead County, Minnesota: A population based survey. Sleep 2002; 25(2):197–202.
5. Honda Y. Clinical features of narcolepsy: Japanese experiences. In: Honda Y, Juji T, eds HLA in Narcolepsy. Berlin: Springer–Verlag, 1988: pp. 24–57.
6. Lavie P, Peled R. Narcolepsy is a rare disease in Israel. Sleep 1987; 10(6):608–9.
7. Challamel MJ, Mazzola ME, Nevsimalova S, et al. Narcolepsy in children. Sleep 1994; 17(8 suppl):S17–S20.
8. Matsuki K, Honda Y, Juji T. Diagnostic criteria for narcolepsy and HLA DR2 frequencies. Tissue Antigens 1987; 30(4):155–60.
9. Foutz AS, Mitler MM, Cavalli-Sforza LL, et al. Genetic factors in canine narcolepsy. Sleep 1979; 1(4):413–21.
10. Mitler MM, Dement WC. Cataplectic-like behavior in cats after microinjection of carbachol in the pontine reticular reticular formation. Brain Res 1974; 68(2):335–43.
11. Lin L, Faraco J, Li R, et al. The sleep disorder, canine narcolepsy, is caused by a mutation in the hypocretin (orexin) receptor 2 gene. Cell 1999; 98(3):365–76.
12. Nishino S, Ripley B, Overeem S, et al. Hypocretin (orexin) deficiency in human narcolepsy. Lancet 2000; 355(9197):39–40.
13. Chemelli RM, Willie JT, Sinton CM, et al. Narcolepsy in orexin knockout mice: Molecular genetics of sleep regulation. Cell 1999; 98(4):409–12.

14. Mignot E, Young T, Lin L, et al. Nocturnal sleep and daytime sleepiness in normal subjects with HLA-DQB1*0602. Sleep 1999; 2 (3):347–52.
15. Honda M, Honda Y, Uchida S, et al. Monozygotic twins incompletely concordant for narcolepsy. Biol Psychiatry 2001; 49(11) 943–7.
16. Nishino S. The hypocretin/orexin system in health and disease. Biol Psychiatry 2003; 54(2):87–95.
17. Thannickal TC, Moore RY, Nienhuis R, et al. Reduced number of hypocretin neurons in human narcolepsy. Neuron 2000; 27(3):469–74.
18. Silber MH, Rye DB. Solving the mysteries of narcolepsy: The hypocretin story. Neurology 2001; 56(12):1616–18.
19. Saper CB, Cano S, Scammell TE. Homeostatic, circadian, and emotional regulation of sleep. J Comp Neurol 2005; 493(1):92–8.
20. Nishino S, Kanbayashi T. Symptomatic narcolepsy, cataplexy and hypersomnia and their implications in the hypothalamic hypocretin/orexin system. Sleep Medicine Reviews 2005; 9(4):269–310.
21. Pollack CP. The rhythms of narcolepsy. Narcolepsy Network 1995; 8:1–7.
22. Lenn NJ. HLA- DR2 in childhood narcolepsy. Pediatr Neurol 1986; 2(5):314–15.
23. Wittig R, Zorick F, Roehrs T, et al. Narcolepsy in a 7 year old. J Pediatr 1983; 102(5):725–7.
24. Kotagal S, Hartse KM, Walsh JK. Characteristics of narcolepsy in pre-teen aged children. Pediatrics 1990; 85(2):205–9.
25. Dahl R. Affect regulation, brain development, and behavioral/emotional health in adolescence. CNS Spectr 2001; 6(1):60–72.
26. Rogers AE, Rosenberg RS. Tests of memory in narcoleptics. Sleep 1990; 13(1):42–52.
27. Henry GK, Satz P, Heilbronner RL. Evidence of a perceptual encoding deficit in narcolepsy. Sleep 1993; 16(2):123–7.
28. Stores G, Montgomery P, Wiggs L. The psychosocial problems of children with narcolepsy and those with excessive daytime sleepiness of uncertain origin. Pediatrics 2006; 118(4):e1116–23.
29. Review by the MSLT and MWT Task Force of the Standards of Practice Committee of the American Academy of Sleep Medicine. Sleep 2005; 28(1):123–44.
30. Kotagal S. A developmental perspective on narcolepsy. In Loughlin GM, Carroll JL, Marcus CL, eds. Sleep and Breathing: A Developmental Approach. New York: Marcel Dekker, 2000: pp. 347–62.
31. Dahl RE, Ryan ND, Perel J, et al. Cholinergic REM induction test with arecholine in depressed children. Psychiatry Res 1994; 51(3):269–82.
32. Gozal D, Wang M, Pope DW. Objective sleepiness measures in pediatric obstructive sleep apnea. Pediatrics 2001; 108(3):693–7.
33. Carskadon MA, Dement WC, Mitler MM, et al. Guidelines for the multiple sleep latency test (MSLT): A standard measure of sleepiness. Sleep 1986; 9(4):519–24.
34. Kotagal S, Swink TD. Excessive daytime sleepiness in a 13 year old. Semin Pediatr Neurol 1996; 3 (3): 170–2.
35. Nishino S, Ripley B, Overeem S, et al. Low cerebrospinal fluid hypocretin (Orexin) and altered energy homeostasis in human narcolepsy. Ann Neurol 2001; 50(3):381–8.
36. Arii J, Kanbayashi T, Tanabe Y, et al. CSF hypocretin-1 (orexin A) levels in childhood narcolepsy and neurological disorders. Neurology 2004; 63(12):2440–2.
37. Mitler MM: Evaluation of treatment with stimulants in narcolepsy. Sleep 1994; 17 (suppl 1):103–6.
38. Ivanenko A, Tauman R, Gozal D. Modafinil in the treatment of excessive daytime sleepiness in children. Sleep Med 2003 Nov; 4(6):579–82.
39. Littner M, Johnson SF, McCall WV, et al. Practice parameters for the treatment of narcolepsy: An update for 2000. Sleep 2001; 24(4):451–66.
40. US Xyrem Multicenter Study Group. A randomized, double-blind, placebo-controlled multicenter trial comparing the effects of three doses of orally administered sodium oxybate with placebo for the treatment of narcolepsy. Sleep 2002; 25(1):42–9.

41. Murali H, Kotagal S. Off-label treatment of severe childhood narcolepsy-cataplexy with sodium oxybate. Sleep 2006; 29(8):1025–9.
42. Dauvilliers Y, Carlander B, Rivier F, et al. Successful management of cataplexy with intravenous immunoglobulin at narcolepsy onset. Ann Neurol 2004; 56(6):905–8.
43. American Academy of Sleep Medicine. International classification of sleep disorders, 2nd edn, pocket version: Diagnostic and Coding Manual. Westchester, Illinois: American Academy of Sleep Medicine, 2006: pp. 66–9.
44. Bassetti C, Aldrich MS. Idiopathic hypersomnia: A series of 42 patients. Brain 1997; 120(8):23–1435.

13 Kleine–Levin Syndrome

Giora Pillar[a] and Sarit Ravid[b]

[a]Pediatric Sleep Clinic, [b]Pediatric Neurology, Meyer Children's Hospital, Rambam Medical Center and Technion Faculty of Medicine, Haifa, Israel

INTRODUCTION

The Kleine–Levin syndrome (KLS) was initially named by Critchley, who reviewed previous case reports by Willi Kleine (1) and Max Levin (2,3), and described 11 additional cases in young adults (4,5). The hallmark of the syndrome is periodic extreme hypersomnia. At that time, excessive daytime somnolence had been mainly attributed to either narcolepsy or the Pickwickian syndrome/obstructive sleep apnea (6). These were known as chronic somnolence states, while the major novel description by Kleine, Levine, and Critchley was the periodic nature of this new syndrome, as well as the association to attacks of hyperphagia. Since these initial reports, there were quite a number of case reports published, some on a fairly large group of patients, but population-based studies have not been performed. The largest summary work so far on this topic was carried out by Arnulf et al. (7), who systematically reviewed previous publications on KLS, added them into one database, and analyzed 186 recognized cases. Two relatively large studies on KLS (descriptions of 34 and 30 patients) were not included, due to potential overlap with other publications and lack of sufficient individual data (8,9). In all cases attacks were associated with hypersomnolence (100%) (7). Additional characteristics of attacks consisted of cognitive changes (96%), eating disturbances (80%), depressed mood (48%), hypersexuality (43%), and compulsions (29%). It is generally accepted that this is a rare disease, but probably under-diagnosed. However, the frequency may be somewhat higher in specific communities/ethnics. The incidence of reported cases in Israel is relatively high, as it may be more prevalent among Jews (9,10). A significantly increased Jewish predisposition of KLS was observed in the U.S. as well, where 15% of KLS patients were Jews versus 2% Jewish in the general population (7). While KLS affects approximately one in a million people in the U.S., the 34 patients reported in Israel in 2001 (approximately six million population) yield a prevalence that is approximately sixfold (9).

KLS has been reported to occur after trauma (11), viral infections such as Epstein–Barr virus (EBV) (12), or encephalitis (13), but is commonly idiopathic. The median age of onset appears to be 15 years, with 81% of cases diagnosed during the second decade of life (7,9). The syndrome lasts an average of eight years, with a clear tendency of spontaneous alleviation with time, and eventually spontaneous remission, yielding an excellent prognosis. The complete remission may occur somewhat later (i.e., there is a longer period of disease) in women and in patients with less frequent episodes during the first year. Attacks may last between several days (usually over three) and several weeks, but typically last around 5–10 days, recurring every several months (median 3.5). Attacks are commonly precipitated by

175

infections (38.2%), head trauma (9%), alcohol consumption (5.4%), or others (such as sleep deprivation, stress etc.).

Between the episodes of sleepiness, the patients are typically completely normal, both physically and mentally. They are not sleepy and their behavior is normal. Investigational studies between episodes such as polysomnography (PSG), Multiple Sleep Latency Test (MSLT), computed tomography of the brain, full-montage electroencephalogram (EEG), etc. reveal normal findings. During an attack, PSG may reveal longer albeit fragmented sleep, with reduced slow-wave and rapid eye movement (REM) sleep; the most consistent finding during an episode is hypoperfusion to the thalamic/hypothalamic regions evident by Single-Photon Emission-Computed Tomography (SPECT) (14–20).

Since this is a rare disorder, and the literature relies mostly on sporadic case reports with a few larger-scale studies, there is still much mystery and many unexplained features of this syndrome (more than meets the eye). There are a relatively large variety of clinical characteristics, precipitating factors, and investigational findings, suggesting there may be more than one pathophysiological and etiological explanation for this disorder.

CLINICAL CHARACTERISTICS

The Kleine–Levin syndrome, also known as recurrent hypersomnia or periodic hypersomnia, is an episodic disorder. In between the episodes the affected individuals are classically completely asymptomatic and healthy. When this is not the case, and there are neurological and/or psychiatric symptoms prior to the first episode or persist between episodes, the term "secondary KLS" has been used (7). The episodes are always characterized by severe hypersomnolence, frequently with additional symptoms including cognitive changes, hyperphagia, depressed mood, sexual disinhibition, and behavioral changes in some of the cases. Sometimes the manifestation is monosymptomatic, with only sleepiness and without any of the other associated features.

Hypersomnia

Hypersomnia is the most important and key symptom of KLS, and essential to this diagnosis. During a symptomatic KLS episode, affected individuals experience a very strong drive to sleep, and typically sleep around 18 hours per day. This is a severe sleepiness state, described in various case reports as a continuous somnolent state with refusal to go to school, see friends or talk to people (21). One 13-year-old female slept for 20 hours per day (22), waking up almost solely to eat or void. When these adolescents are forced to go to school, they frequently fall asleep in the class or in other school areas (23). One report described a male adolescent who was found sleeping under a neighbor's porch (24), and in one extreme episode the affected adult patient fell asleep on the pavement on the street (25).

During the course of an episode sleepiness usually remains stable, changing gradually to fatigue and may even slightly overshoot in the form of short-term mild insomnia at the termination of the episode (7,26).

Quite a number of objective sleep monitorings were performed on KLS patients during a sleep attack, and in between episodes. Data from our lab on

34 patients demonstrated increased total sleep time despite decreased sleep efficiency. Slow-wave sleep was also reduced (9). On average, patients slept for 9.5±3.5 hours, with approximately 75% sleep efficiency and 13% slow-wave sleep. Others reported similar PSG findings when studying patients during episodes (27–30). REM sleep in our group was relatively preserved (18.5±6.8%), but others reported reduced REM sleep (27). During asymptomatic periods (in between attacks), most studies revealed normal sleep architecture (10,27,29).

Daytime MSLTs for KLS patients during episodes always reveal short sleep onsets (29–31), and occasionally also sleep onset REMs (7,29–31).

Hyperphagia

During episodes, in approximately 70–80% of cases, there is a unique feature of hyperphagia, described in some case reports as binge eating, almost attacking the refrigerator (32), and eating an unusual combination of foods such as salted apples or water melon rings with cucumbers (16,21,33–36). During an episode, patients may gain 3 kg in their weight, and in severe cases it can even exceed 10 kg (7). Some of the reports pointed out that excessive drinking accompanied the excessive eating, commonly sweet drinks such as juice or chocolate syrup (37).

Cognitive, Mood and Behavioral Changes, Hypersexuality

During the symptomatic period, approximately 40–50% of individuals with KLS may experience behavioral changes, the most distinctive of which is hypersexuality. They commonly experience a significant increase in sexual activity and behavior (masturbation even in front of others, inappropriate sexual acts and language) (7,9,38–40). In addition, KLS episodes are frequently associated with cognitive mood and behavioral changes. Patients are confused, unable to focus, experience speech disturbances, feel disconnected and disabled. One 13-year-old female described her episodes as "a persistent sense of unreality …" (22). Ferguson described a case of a 10-year-old child who was suspected of having depression before the diagnosis of KLS was made (41). Fontenelle et al. (42) reported on a patient with academic decline, neuropsychological sequelae and personality alterations during the symptomatic episodes. Loss of memory and additional cognitive changes were also reported (17,43). While most cases reported full recovery in between episodes, one report of four KLS cases found short-term memory dysfunction even between episodes, which correlated to temporal lobe hypoperfusion in SPECT studies (44). Poor emotional control, irritability, confusion, depressed mood, and extreme swings in mood (bi-polar) were also commonly reported during attacks (34,36,45,46).

PATHOPHYSIOLOGY

The pathophysiology of KLS is unknown. Due to nonprogressive mood and behavioral changes, it used to be thought that KLS may be a primary psychiatric disorder (46–50). However, reports on association with infections, findings in post mortem and brain imaging, led to a more organic theory (7,12,17,18,51–54). The combination of sleepiness and changes in eating habits is suggestive of a hypothalamic dysfunction, which indeed is supported by several reports (55,56), but not by all (28). Several organic pathological findings were reported in cases of KLS. SPECT may show hypoperfusion of the thalamus or hypothalamus during the symptomatic period of KLS (14,57). The findings completely disappeared during the asymptomatic period (at least one month after the attack ended) (14). Hypoperfusion in other regions were also noted in some but not all subjects. They persisted during the asymptomatic period in two cases over the temporal lobe (2/7 cases), frontal lobe (1/7 cases), and basal ganglia (1/7 cases). The most prominent persistent hypoperfusion was seen in the subject with longest clinical evolution. In all cases EEG (awake and asleep), computed tomography (CT) scan, and magnetic resonance imaging (MRI) were normal. The authors concluded that hypoperfusion of the thalamus is a consistent finding during the symptomatic period, but perfusion abnormalities may persist even during the asymptomatic period. The longer the duration of the syndrome, the more extended the hypoperfusion regions during the asymptomatic period (14). Additional SPECT studies reported various central nervous hypoperfusion regions as well, but most commonly involving the hypothalamus (15–20).

Further evidence that the brain region affected in KLS is the thalamus and/or hypothalamus comes from various case studies including autopsies, blood and CSF analyses. Carpenter et al. (51) reported a typical 39-year-old KLS patient who died during a symptomatic period. Autopsy disclosed recent and old lesions in the medial thalamus involving intralaminar, medial, and some dorsal nuclei, as well as the pulvinar.

Several cases studied the hypothesis that KLS arises from hypothalamic or other brain neurotransmitter/neurohormonal dysfunction and analyzed blood or CSF contents usually during an episode. Blood samples were obtained and assayed for hypothalamic hormones such as thyroid-stimulating hormone (TSH), cortisol, prolactin, growth hormone (GH), luteinizing hormone (LH), and follicle-stimulating hormone (FSH), and for neurotransmitter predominantly serotonergic and dopaminergic. Some studies reported hypothalamic hormone changes supporting hypothalamic dysfunction hypothesis (55,58,59), potentially due to decreased dopaminergic tone during symptomatic episodes (27). Decreased hypothalamic dopaminergic tone along with reduced slow-wave sleep may lead to the observed reduction in GH during KLS episodes (43,60). Other sporadic reports suggested different pathophysiological processes in KLS. One case of the sudden death of a 17-year-old patient with KLS revealed increased premortem CSF levels of 5-hydroxytryptamine (5-HT) and 5-hydroxyindoleacetic acid (5-HIAA), suggestive of involvement of the serotonergic system (52). The same adolescent had depigmentation of the locus ceruleus in his PM, suggestive of norepinephric involvement (52). Fluctuations of acetylcholine have been theoretically proposed as well (61).

Some researchers have raised the theory that KLS is an autoimmune disease. Dauvilliers et al. (8) reported that the human leukocyte antigen (HLA) DQB1*0201 allele was significantly increased in patients with KLS. This finding along with the young age at onset, the recurrence of symptoms, and the frequent infectious precipitating factors, led the researchers to conclude that KLS has an autoimmune etiology. Manni et al. (62) reported on two KLS patients sharing the same HLA haplotype (HLA-DR1, DQ1).

In summary, the pathophysiology of KLS is still unknown, but most evidence suggests hypothalamic abnormalities.

DIAGNOSIS AND DIFFERENTIAL DIAGNOSIS

The diagnosis of KLS is usually made clinically, and further laboratory testing is not obligatory. The combination of episodes of excessive sleepiness (classically over 18 hours of sleep per 24 hours, with episodes lasting over three days) without any other explanation (i.e., narcolepsy, obstructive sleep apnea (OSA), epilepsy, depression, psychosis) is usually sufficient to make the diagnosis. Existence of associated features like hyperphagia, hypersexuality, irritability, aggression, disorientation, and confusion even further support the diagnosis. Nevertheless, due to the rarity of the syndrome the diagnosis is commonly delayed, by an average of 3.8 years (9). Thus, the key point is to keep this diagnosis in mind and to consider it in the right clinical settings. In uncertain cases PSG and MSLT are required, which may reveal several findings. During an episode, the patients' PSG demonstrate long sleep albeit with low sleep efficiency, sleep fragmentation (57) and somewhat reduced stages 3, 4, and REM sleep (27,57). MSLT reveals short sleep latencies, potentially with one or more SOREMs.

The differential diagnosis in most cases is not difficult. Theoretically, during an episode, all other causes of hypersomnia may be considered as differential diagnosis of KLS. Indeed, during the first episode it may be hard to determine this diagnosis. Narcolepsy, the primary diagnosis of hypersomnolence, may also exhibit some fluctuations with periods of exacerbation and relief. However, in none of the KLS cases reported, cataplexy or sleep paralysis were noted. In addition, the long periods of normal alertness in between episodes makes the differential diagnosis of narcolepsy, idiopathic hypersomnia, post-traumatic hypersomnia, and sleep apnea unlikely. Snoring, dry mouth upon awakening, witnessed apneas as well as obesity and hypertension are not seen in KLS. Menstrual-cycle induced hypersomnia may be in some circumstances confused with KLS, although by history it is always associated with the period, and is not associated with hyperphagia or other KLS-related features. Depression, especially atypical, may mimic KLS (50). Major depression is commonly associated with sleep disturbances and frequently with excessive daytime sleepiness. Atypical depression and more importantly seasonal (winter) depression may be periodic and even associated with weight gain. However, these patients are frequently complaining of fatigue rather than sleepiness, and symptoms of depression are more obvious than ones of sleepiness (41). Anti-depressive medications which have modest effect on KLS, commonly substantially alleviate depression. When the psychiatric symptomatology dominates, schizophrenia and conversion disorders may be difficult to distinguish from KLS (63). Both may consist of sleepiness, indiscriminate hypersexuality, irritability, and impulsive behaviors (40). Careful history, course, therapeutic intervention, and perhaps PSG, MSLT, and SPECT may help in making the diagnosis in these cases. Finally, epileptic discharges with seizures, particularly if prolonged, and more prominently in psychomotor retarded patients, may be associated with (periodic) post-ictal hypersomnia. When this diagnosis is considered, EEG is indicated and can be distinguished from KLS (60).

TREATMENT

There is no specific treatment for KLS. Therapy should be individualized and be primarily supportive (including safety and protective measures). When the precipitating factor is recognized (i.e., stress, fever, alcohol, etc.), treatment should be directed to reduce its occurrence. Stimulants may potentially alleviate sleepiness, although there are insufficient data to support their use. Stimulants such as methylphenidate and pemoline administered to patients in our lab even in high doses were not beneficial (9). It is plausible that they were given too late in the course of the attack, and if given very early on, these, as well as the new wake promoting agents such as modafinil, may shorten the hypersomniac period duration.

Tricyclic antidepressants, Flumazenil and Amantadine given to single patients were ineffective (9). Many other medications have been tried either during the acute symptomatic period or as a preventive medicine. Perhaps the most commonly suggested medication for KLS is lithium (39,57,63–66). Lithium has been proposed for prophylactic use (67). It has been shown to shorten relapses in five adolescents. Episodes of hypersomnia under lithium therapy were shorter and monosymptomatic with lack of behavioural symptoms. The risk of a relapsing episode under maintenance of lithium was calculated to drop by 7% per month, and the duration of episodes dropped to 19% (68). Lithium has also been proposed in combination with carbamazepine (67). Other sole medications or other combinations of antiepileptic medications such as Carbamazepine (69) or Valproic acid (39,70) were proposed, but it remains unclear whether any of them can alter the natural history of this disorder (i.e., shorten episodes or decrease their frequency). One study demonstrated hypoperfusion to the pineal gland (by SPECT) (15), which may explain the proposed treatment with Melatonin (71). Light therapy was also suggested (72).

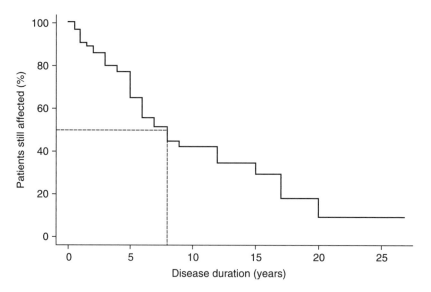

FIGURE 1 Duration of KLS (n=110 patients). Taken from Arnulf et al. with permission (7). On the X axis is the total duration of the disease (years) and on the Y axis is the cumulative decreasing percentage of patients still presenting with KLS episodes. The median duration of the disease (dashed line) is eight years.

CONCLUSION

In summary, treatment should be focused on reduced precipitating factors when recognized, and administration of stimulants early on when an episode begins. In patients with frequent episodes it seems indicated to attempt Lithium preventive treatment.

COURSE AND PROGNOSIS

KLS is commonly presented during adolescence. Attacks are commonly precipitated by physical or emotional stimuli such as febrile illness, infection, head trauma, stress, alcohol, sleep deprivation, and others. With increasing age there is a spontaneous decrease in the frequency, duration, and severity of attacks, until they completely cease at mid to late adulthood (73). The median duration of the disease after diagnosis was reported to be four years in 65 cases where the data were available (7), and in 15 patients from our laboratory (9). A nice Kaplan–Meier analysis to express the natural history of the diseases was presented by Arnulf et al. (7) (Fig. 1). Less than five patients over the age of 40 with KLS are reported worldwide. Thus, with or without treatment, it appears that KLS has an excellent prognosis.

REFERENCES

1. Klein W. Periodische schlafsucht. Monats Psychiatr Neurol 1925; 57:285–320.
2. Levine M. Narcolepsy (Gelineau's syndrome) and other varieties of morbid somnolence. Arch Neurol Psychiat 1929; 22:1172–200.
3. Levine M. Periodic somnolence and morbid hunger: A new syndrome. Brain 1936; 59:494–504.
4. Critchley M. Periodic hypersomnia and megaphagia in adolescent males. Brain 1962; 85:627–56.
5. Critchley M, Hoffman H. The syndrome of periodic somnolence and morbid hunger (Kleine–Levin syndrome). BMJ 1942; 1:137–9.
6. Lavie P. Nothing new under the moon. Historical accounts of sleep apnea syndrome. Arch Intern Med 1984; 144(10):2025–8.
7. Arnulf I, Zeitzer JM, File J, Farber N, Mignot E. Kleine–Levin syndrome: A systematic review of 186 cases in the literature. Brain 2005; 128(Pt 12):2763–76.
8. Dauvilliers Y, Mayer G, Lecendreux M, et al. Kleine–Levin syndrome: An autoimmune hypothesis based on clinical and genetic analyses. Neurology 2002; 59(11):1739–45.
9. Gadoth N, Kesler A, Vainstein G, Peled R, Lavie P. Clinical and polysomnographic characteristics of 34 patients with Kleine–Levin syndrome. J Sleep Res 2001; 10(4):337–41.
10. Kesler Λ, Gadoth N, Vainstein G, Peled R, Lavie P. Kleine Levin syndrome (KLS) in young females. Sleep 2000; 23(4):563–7.
11. Will RG, Young JP, Thomas DJ. Kleine–Levin syndrome: Report of two cases with onset of symptoms precipitated by head trauma. Br J Psychiatry 1988; 152:410–2.
12. Salter MS, White PD. A variant of the Kleine–Levin syndrome precipitated by both Epstein-Barr and varicella-zoster virus infections. Biol Psychiatry 1993; 33(5):388–90.
13. Sethi S, Bhargava SC. Kleine–Levin syndrome following acute non-specific encephalitis. Indian J Pediatr 2002; 69(5):451.
14. Huang YS, Guilleminault C, Kao PF, Liu FY. SPECT findings in the Kleine–Levin syndrome. Sleep 2005; 28(8):955–60.
15. Lu ML, Liu HC, Chen CH, Sung SM. Kleine–Levin syndrome and psychosis: Observation from an unusual case. Neuropsychiatry Neuropsychol Behav Neurol 2000; 13(2):140–2.
16. Hong SB, Joo EY, Tae WS, Lee J, Han SJ, Lee HW. Episodic diencephalic hypoperfusion in Kleine–Levin syndrome. Sleep 2006; 29(8):1091–3.

17. Landtblom AM, Dige N, Schwerdt K, Safstrom P, Granerus G. A case of Kleine–Levin syndrome examined with SPECT and neuropsychological testing. Acta Neurol Scand 2002; 105(4):318–21.
18. Nose I, Ookawa T, Tanaka J, et al. Decreased blood flow of the left thalamus during somnolent episodes in a case of recurrent hypersomnia. Psychiatry Clin Neurosci 2002; 56(3):277–8.
19. Peraita-Adrados R. Kleine–Levin syndrome: Diagnostic contribution made by brain SPECT. Rev Neurol 2003; 36(6):599; author reply 600.
20. Portilla P, Durand E, Chalvon A, et al. SPECT-identified hypoperfusion of the left temporomesial structures in a Kleine–Levin syndrome. Rev Neurol (Paris) 2002; 158(5 Pt 1):593–5.
21. Mukaddes NM, Alyanak B, Kora ME, Polvan O. The psychiatric symptomatology in Kleine–Levin syndrome. Child Psychiatry Hum Dev 1999; 29(3):253–8.
22. Katz JD, Ropper AH. Familial Kleine–Levin syndrome: Two siblings with unusually long hypersomnic spells. Arch Neurol 2002; 59(12):1959–61.
23. Frank Y, Braham J, Cohen BE. The Kleine–Levin syndrome. Case report and review of the literature. Am J Dis Child 1974; 127(3):412–3.
24. Powers PS, Gunderman R. Kleine–Levin syndrome associated with fire setting. Am J Dis Child 1978; 132(8):786–9.
25. Prabhakaran N, Murthy GK, Mallya UL. A case of Kleine–Levin syndrome in India. Br J Psychiatry 1970; 117(540):517–19.
26. Russell J, Grunstein R. Kleine–Levin syndrome: A case report. Aust N Z J Psychiatry 1992; 26(1):119–23.
27. Chesson AL Jr., Levine SN, Kong LS, Lee SC. Neuroendocrine evaluation in Kleine–Levin syndrome: Evidence of reduced dopaminergic tone during periods of hypersomnolence. Sleep 1991; 14(3):226–32.
28. Mayer G, Leonhard E, Krieg J, Meier-Ewert K. Endocrinological and polysomnographic findings in Kleine–Levin syndrome: No evidence for hypothalamic and circadian dysfunction. Sleep 1998; 21(3):278–84.
29. Reimao R, Shimizu MH. Kleine–Levin syndrome. Clinical course, polysomnography and multiple sleep latency test. Case report. Arq Neuropsiquiatr 1998; 56(3B):650–4.
30. Rosenow F, Kotagal P, Cohen BH, Green C, Wyllie E. Multiple sleep latency test and polysomnography in diagnosing Kleine–Levin syndrome and periodic hypersomnia. J Clin Neurophysiol 2000; 17(5):519–22.
31. Reynolds CF, Kupfer DJ, Christiansen CL, et al. Multiple Sleep Latency Test findings in Kleine–Levin syndrome. J Nerv Ment Dis 1984; 172(1):41–4.
32. Gilligan BS. Periodic megaphagia and hypersomnia—an example of the Kleine–Levin syndrome in an adolescent girl. Proc Aust Assoc Neurol 1973; 9:67–72.
33. Gallinek A. The Kleine–Levin syndrome: Hypersomnia, bulimia, and abnormal mental states. World Neurol 1962; 3:235–43.
34. Gau SF, Soong WT, Liu HM, et al. Kleine–Levin syndrome in a boy with Prader–Willi syndrome. Sleep 1996; 19(1):13–17.
35. Gilbert GJ. Periodic Hypersomnia and Bulimia. The Kleine–Levin syndrome. Neurology 1964; 14:844–50.
36. Malomo IO, Lawal RA, Orija OB. Kleine–Levin syndrome: Case report. East Afr Med J 1998; 75(1):55–6.
37. Garland H, Sumner D, Fourman P. The Kleine–Levin syndrome. Some further observations. Neurology 1965; 15(12):1161–7.
38. Hauri PJ. Recurrent hyper- and hyposomnia: A new diagnostic entity? Polysomnographic findings and a 30-year follow-up. Sleep Med 2002; 3(1):15–20.
39. Mapari UU, Khealani BA, Ali S, Syed NA. Kleine–Levin syndrome. J Coll Physicians Surg Pak 2005; 15(1):46–7.
40. Masi G, Favilla L, Millepiedi S. The Kleine–Levin syndrome as a neuropsychiatric disorder: A case report. Psychiatry 2000; 63(1):93–100.

41. Ferguson BG. Kleine–Levin syndrome: A case report. J Child Psychol Psychiatry 1986; 27(2):275–8.
42. Fontenelle L, Mendlowicz MV, Gillin JC, Mattos P, Versiani M. Neuropsychological sequelae in Kleine–Levin syndrome: Case report. Arq Neuropsiquiatr 2000; 58(2B):531–4.
43. Fukunishi I, Hosokawa K. A female case with the Kleine–Levin syndrome and its physiopathologic aspects. Jpn J Psychiatry Neurol 1989; 43(1):45–9.
44. Landtblom AM, Dige N, Schwerdt K, Safstrom P, Granerus G. Short-term memory dysfunction in Kleine–Levin syndrome. Acta Neurol Scand 2003; 108(5):363–7.
45. Gillberg C. Kleine–Levin syndrome: Unrecognized diagnosis in adolescent psychiatry. J Am Acad Child Adolesc Psychiatry 1987; 26(5):793–4.
46. Jeffries JJ, Lefebvre A. Depression and mania associated with Kleine–Levin–Critchley syndrome. Can Psychiatr Assoc J 1973; 18(5):439–44.
47. Haberland C, Weissman S. The Kleine–Levin syndrome. A case study with a psychopathologic approach. Acta Psychiatr Scand 1968; 44(1):1–10.
48. Markman RA. Kleine–Levin syndrome: Report of a case. Am J Psychiatry 1967; 123(8):1025–6.
49. Miller DL. Kleine–Levin syndrome: An atypical case? Psychiatr Q 1970; 44(1):26–35.
50. Reynolds CF 3rd, Black RS, Coble P, Holzer B, Kupfer DJ. Similarities in EEG sleep findings for Kleine–Levin syndrome and unipolar depression. Am J Psychiatry 1980; 137(1):116–18.
51. Carpenter S, Yassa R, Ochs R. A pathologic basis for Kleine–Levin syndrome. Arch Neurol 1982; 39(1):25–8.
52. Koerber RK, Torkelson R, Haven G, Donaldson J, Cohen SM, Case M. Increased cerebrospinal fluid 5-hydroxytryptamine and 5–hydroxyindoleacetic acid in Kleine–Levin syndrome. Neurology 1984; 34(12):1597–600.
53. Green LN, Cracco RQ. Kleine–Levin syndrome. A case with EEG evidence of periodic brain dysfunction. Arch Neurol 1970; 22(2):166–75.
54. Vollmer R, Toifl K, Kothbauer P, Riederer P. EEG- and biochemical findings in Kleine–Levin-syndrome. A case report (author's transl). Nervenarzt 1981; 52(4):211–18.
55. Gadoth N, Dickerman Z, Bechar M, Laron Z, Lavie P. Episodic hormone secretion during sleep in Kleine–Levin syndrome: Evidence for hypothalamic dysfunction. Brain Dev 1987; 9(3):309–15.
56. Boris NW, Hagino OR, Steiner GP. Case study: Hypersomnolence and precocious puberty in a child with pica and chronic lead intoxication. J Am Acad Child Adolesc Psychiatry 1996; 35(8):1050–4.
57. Arias M, Crespo Iglesias JM, Perez J, Requena-Caballero I, Sesar-Ignacio A, Peleteiro-Fernandez M. Kleine–Levin syndrome: Contribution of brain SPECT in diagnosis. Rev Neurol 2002; 35(6):531–3.
58. Fernandez JM, Lara I, Gila L, O'Neill of Tyrone A, Tovar J, Gimeno A. Disturbed hypothalamic-pituitary axis in idiopathic recurring hypersomnia syndrome. Acta Neurol Scand 1990; 82(6):361–3.
59. Malhotra S, Das MK, Gupta N, Muralidharan R. A clinical study of Kleine–Levin syndrome with evidence for hypothalamic-pituitary axis dysfunction. Biol Psychiatry 1997; 42(4):299–301.
60. Grigg-Damberger M. Neurologic disorders masquerading as pediatric sleep problems. Pediatr Clin North Am 2004; 51(1):89–115.
61. Brown DW. Abnormal fluctuations of acetylcholine and serotonin. Med Hypotheses 1993; 40(5):309–10.
62. Manni R, Martinetti M, Ratti MT, Tartara A. Electrophysiological and immunogenetic findings in recurrent monosymptomatic-type hypersomnia: A study of two unrelated Italian cases. Acta Neurol Scand 1993; 88(4):293–5.
63. Pike M, Stores G. Kleine–Levin syndrome: A cause of diagnostic confusion. Arch Dis Child 1994; 71(4):355–7.

64. Goldberg MA. The treatment of Kleine–Levin syndrome with lithium. Can J Psychiatry 1983; 28(6):491–3.
65. Hart EJ. Kleine–Levin syndrome: normal CSF monoamines and response to lithium therapy. Neurology 1985; 35(9):1395–6.
66. Muratori F, Bertini N, Masi G. Efficacy of lithium treatment in Kleine–Levin syndrome. Eur Psychiatry 2002; 17(4):232–3.
67. Billiard M, Carlander B. Wake disorders. I. Primary wake disorders. Rev Neurol (Paris) 1998; 154(2):111–19.
68. Poppe M, Friebel D, Reuner U, Todt H, Koch R, Heubner G. The Kleine–Levin syndrome – effects of treatment with lithium. Neuropediatrics 2003; 34(3):113–19.
69. Mukaddes NM, Kora ME, Bilge S. Carbamazepine for Kleine–Levin syndrome. J Am Acad Child Adolesc Psychiatry 1999; 38(7):791–2.
70. Crumley FE. Valproic acid for Kleine–Levin syndrome. J Am Acad Child Adolesc Psychiatry 1997; 36(7):868–9.
71. Kornreich C, Fossion P, Hoffmann G, Baleriaux M, Pelc I. Treatment of Kleine–Levin syndrome: Melatonin on the starting block. J Clin Psychiatry 2000; 61(3):215.
72. Crumley FE. Light therapy for Kleine–Levin syndrome. J Am Acad Child Adolesc Psychiatry 1998; 37(12):1245.
73. Papacostas SS, Hadjivasilis V. The Kleine–Levin syndrome. Report of a case and review of the literature. Eur Psychiatry 2000; 15(4):231–5.

14 Sleep Problems in Children with ADHD, Impact of Treatment and Comorbidities

Samuele Cortese[a] and Michel Lecendreux[b]

[a]*Child and Adolescent Psychopathology Unit, Robert Debré Hospital, Paris VII University, Paris, France and Child Neuropsychiatry Unit, G.B. Rossi Hospital, Department of Mother-Child and Biology-Genetics, Verona University, Verona, Italy* [b]*Pediatric Sleep Disorders Center and Child and Adolescent Psychopathology Unit, Robert Debré Hospital, Paris VII University, Paris, France*

INTRODUCTION

In clinical practice, parent-reported sleep problems in children diagnosed with Attention-Deficit/Hyperactivity Disorder (ADHD) are quite frequent. According to a review of the literature by Corkum et al. (1), the estimate of the prevalence of sleep problems in children with ADHD is between 25% and 50%, compared with 7% of normal controls. This represents approximately a fivefold increase in the rate of sleep problems in children with ADHD. From a clinical standpoint, sleep disturbances associated with ADHD are of relevance, since they represent a significant source of distress for the child and/or the family. Moreover, sleep alterations may worsen or, in some cases, mimic daytime ADHD symptoms (i.e., inattention, impulsivity, and hyperactivity).

In the last two decades, the relevance of sleep issues in children diagnosed with ADHD has prompted an increasing series of studies to better understand the nature, as well as the management, of sleep problems in these patients. Results from these studies, both subjective (i.e., based on questionnaires filled out by parents or children) and, in particular, objective (i.e., based on polysomnography, actigraphy, or infrared video analysis), have been inconsistent. It has been correctly pointed out that sleep problems reported by patients with ADHD are likely to be multifactorial (2), meaning that they may be ascribed to ADHD itself and/or to other factors associated with ADHD. It is possible that the discrepancies reported in the studies are accounted for, at least in part, by the fact that not all the studies excluded or controlled for these confounding factors.

In this chapter, we focus on two important factors that may impact on sleep and, therefore, should be considered in the clinical management of sleep disorders in children with ADHD: psychiatric comorbidities, and medications used to treat ADHD or comorbid disorders.

In the first part of this chapter, we briefly review literature on sleep alterations associated with the most relevant psychiatric disorders comorbid with ADHD, as well as with psychotropic drugs used to treat this disorder, to show that these conditions do impact on sleep. In the second part, we present the results of a meta-analysis of the literature on sleep alterations in ADHD subjects, controlling for comorbid psychiatric disorders, and medications, in order to understand to what extent psychiatric comorbid disorders and psychotropic drugs may specifically impact on sleep in children with ADHD. Finally, in the third part, we discuss the clinical relevance of psychiatric comorbid disorders and pharmacological treatment in the management of sleep disorders in pediatric patients with ADHD.

SLEEP ALTERATIONS ASSOCIATED WITH COMORBID PSYCHIATRIC DISORDERS AND ADHD MEDICATIONS
Comorbid Psychiatric Disorders
Psychiatric comorbidity is present in as many as two-thirds of clinically referred children with ADHD, including up to 50% for oppositional disorder, 30% to 50% for conduct disorder, 15% to 20% for mood disorders, 20% to 25% for anxiety disorders, and 10% to 25% for learning disorders. Moreover, Tourette syndrome and, in adolescents, substance abuse may also be comorbid with ADHD (3). Finally, although the validity of an early-onset form of bipolar disorder (BPD) is still debated, there is some evidence to support the notion that a subgroup of children with ADHD may present with comorbid BPD (4,5). In the following sections, we briefly present available data from literature on sleep alterations associated with most of these comorbidities. A more detailed description of sleep alterations associated with childhood depression, anxiety, and substance abuse is provided, respectively, in Chapters 20, 23, and 26 of this book.

Major Depressive Disorder
Subjective sleep disturbances are a frequent complaint in children and adolescents with Major Depressive Disorder (MDD). In one large review of depressive symptomatology in childhood, Ryan et al. (6) found that more than 90% of children and adolescents with MDD reported sleep problems, including insomnia, hypersomnia, sleep continuity problems (waking at night), daytime sleepiness, and circadian reversal. These problems parallel those reported by adults with MDD. On the other hand, as correctly pointed out in a comprehensive review of the literature by Ivanenko et al. (7), the findings from objective studies are still equivocal. While some researchers have found longer sleep latency and shorter rapid eye movement (REM) latency in depressed children and adolescents, as in adults with MDD, others have reported few significant differences from healthy controls. Sleep abnormalities have been found more consistently in adolescents with MDD than in younger children. As suggested by Bertocci et al. (8), it is possible that some of the electroencephalogram (EEG) sleep changes associated with depression in adults emerge gradually across adolescence and early adulthood or that these changes are not detected by traditional EEG measures. Alternatively, sleep may be physiologically normal in depressed children, but these patients might have a disturbed perception of their sleep.

Anxiety Disorders
Research on sleep problems and disturbances in children with anxiety disorders is still limited, both in community and clinical samples. Most of the available studies are limited to children with Generalized Anxiety Disorders (GAD) and used broad and nonspecific subjective indexes of sleep disturbance. In a recently published study examining several sleep-related problems in a large sample of children with various anxiety disorders (i.e., GAD, separation anxiety, and social anxiety), Alfano et al. (9)

reported that 88% of subjects had at least one sleep-related problem, and 55% experienced three or more sleep-related problems. Total sleep-related problems were positively associated with anxiety severity and interference in family functioning.

Bipolar Disorder

Evidence on sleep problems associated with BPD is still very limited, in part because the definition of pediatric BPD is still under discussion. Geller et al. (10) reported that 40% of children with mania presented with dramatically decreased need for sleep. In a longitudinal study comparing polysomnographic data in adolescents with MDD and normal control, Rao et al. (11) found that subjects who had a unipolar depression at follow up showed reduced REM latency, higher REM density, and more REM sleep, compared with depressed adolescents who converted to bipolar disorder, and controls who remained free from psychopathology. Depressed subjects who would later switch to BPD had more stage 1 sleep and diminished stage 4 sleep. In a recent study by Mehl et al. (4), children with a profile at risk for pediatric BPD reported poorer sleep efficiency and more awakenings after sleep onset, less REM sleep, and longer periods of slow-wave than matched controls. Moreover, on questionnaires filled out by their parents, the children with a profile at risk for pediatric BPD reported significantly more sleep problems, including difficulty initiating sleep, restless sleep, nightmares, and morning headaches, than did controls.

Tourette Syndrome

Since most of the studies on sleep alterations in patients with Tourette syndrome (TS) included mixed samples of both adults and children, evidence on sleep disturbances specific to childhood TS is limited. Available data suggest longer sleep period time, longer sleep latency, reduced sleep efficiency, and prolonged wakefulness after sleep onset; more time awake and less sleep stage 2, increased epochs with short arousal-related movements (12), increased frequency of sleepwalking, night terrors, trouble getting to sleep, early awakening, and inability to take afternoon naps as a young child. Moreover, Voderholzer et al. (13) found a significantly high number of Periodic Limb Movement in Sleep disorders in children with TS, although their small sample size limits the validity of their conclusions.

Oppositional Defiant Disorder

Oppositional Defiant Disorder (ODD) may be associated with limit-setting disorder, characterized by noncompliant behavior in response to parental requests to get ready for bed, bedtime resistance, and delayed sleep onset (2).

Substance Abuse

Although evidence on the effect of substance abuse on sleep in children and adolescents is limited, available data suggest a dose-dependent relationship between sleep problems and use of illicit drugs, alcohol, and cigarettes (7). It is possible that nicotine, illicit drugs, and alcohol directly impact on sleep. Alternatively, it has been hypothesized that their effect be mediated by comorbid psychiatric disorders (substance abuse is often associated with psychiatric comorbidity, perhaps as an effort to self-medicate).

Medications Used to Treat ADHD and Comorbid Conditions
Medications for ADHD

Stimulants (methylphenidate [MPH] and amphetamines) are the first line Food and Drug Administration (FDA)-approved treatment for ADHD, followed by the non-stimulant atomoxetine (ATX) (14). Bupropion, tricyclic antidepressants, alpha-agonists, and modafinil are also used.

Subjective and objective studies on the effect of stimulants on sleep have produced mixed results (15). While some investigators have reported polysomnographically determined lengthened total sleep time, increased sleep-stage shifts, increased number of REM periods, elevated indexes of REM activity and REM-period fragmentation, parent-reported longer latencies to sleep onset, or higher rates of insomnia in ADHD children treated with stimulants versus controls, others did not confirm these findings. It is difficult to combine the results of these studies because of different stimulant formulations, dose, and dose-scheduling. Moreover, some of the studies compared children with ADHD on medication with non-medicated healthy controls. Therefore, it is unclear whether sleep disturbances resulted from the children having ADHD or from their being treated with methylphenidate. However, clinical experience suggests that stimulants may negatively impact on sleep, either due to a direct effect or due to a secondary "rebound" effect as the medications wear off. The vulnerability to these negative effects is likely to be related to individual factors. As correctly pointed out by Brown and McMullen (16), while some patients with ADHD are able to get to sleep easily within just a few hours of taking a dose of stimulant, others need an interval of 6–8 hours.

As for ATX, in a recent randomized, double-blind, cross-over study comparing the effect of MPH (given thrice daily) and ATX (given twice daily) on the sleep of children with ADHD, Sangal et al. (15) found that MPH increased sleep onset latency (SOL) significantly more than did ATX, considering both actigraphic and polysomnographic data. Moreover, both child diaries and parent reports indicated a better quality of sleep (getting ready in the morning, getting ready for bed, falling asleep) with atomoxetine, compared with methylphenidate. Both medications decreased nighttime awakenings, but the decrease was greater for MPH. Clearly, these results need to be replicated.

Medications Used to Treat Comorbid Conditions
Antidepressants

Selective serotonin reuptake inhibitors (SSRIs) may increase SOL, cause daytime sedation, and suppress REM sleep. Citalopram, a new SSRI, has been reported to have fewer negative effects on sleep continuity (2).

Tricyclic antidepressants (TCA) have been associated with decreased SOL and decreased arousals during sleep stage transitions. They may also increase daytime sleepiness (in particular, amitriptyline, doxepin, and trimipramine) (2).

Venlafaxine may cause sleep onset difficulties and problems maintaining sleep. The new agents nefazodone and mirtazapine may cause significantly less insomnia than other SSRIs, although their use may be associated with daytime sleepiness (2).

Antipsychotics

Antipsychotics, used to treat aggression associated with ADHD when stimulants alone are not effective, as well as comorbid tics or bipolar disorder, may have a sedative effect, decrease SOL, increase sleep continuity, and suppress REM sleep (2).

Anticonvulsants

They are used to treat comorbid BPD. Most of these agents may have sedative effects, decreasing sleep-onset latency and causing excessive daytime sleepiness (2).

In conclusion, although research findings are quite mixed, results from several studies support the notion that psychiatric comorbid disorders and medications used to treat ADHD or comorbid disorders may negatively impact on sleep.

TO WHAT EXTENT MIGHT COMORBID PSYCHIATRIC DISORDERS AND PSYCHOTROPIC MEDICATIONS IMPACT ON SLEEP IN CHILDREN WITH ADHD?

In order to answer this question, our group conducted a systematic review of the literature on sleep problems and sleep disturbances in children with ADHD, controlling for psychiatric comorbidities and effect of psychotropic medications (17). We analyzed the most frequently studied parameters from both subjective and objective studies. In particular, we considered the following nine parameters from subjective studies: *bedtime resistance, sleep onset difficulties, night awakenings, restless sleep, sleep duration, difficulty with morning awakenings, excessive daytime sleepiness, parasomnias,* and *sleep disordered breathing (SDB)*; and eleven parameters from objective studies: *sleep-onset latency (SOL), number of sleep stage changes, % of sleep stage 1 (ST 1%), % of sleep stage 2 (ST 2%), % of slow wave sleep (SWS%), Rapid Eyes Movement (REM) sleep latency, % of REM (REM %), sleep efficiency (SE, i.e., the ratio of total sleep time to nocturnal time in bed), proportion of subjects who fell asleep at MSLT, number of movements in sleep,* and *apnea/hypopnea index (AHI, i.e., the number of apneas and hypopneas per hour of total sleep time).*

Results of our meta-analysis showed that the proportion of subjects who fell asleep at the MSLT, the number of objectively recorded movements in sleep, and the AHI, were significantly higher in children with ADHD than in controls. Findings from subjective studies, although limited, confirmed excessive daytime sleepiness, high motricity in sleep, and significant SDB, in children with ADHD. We found no significant differences in other objective parameters (SOL, number of stage changes, ST 1%, ST 2%, SWS %, REM %, REM latency, and SE), indicating that the sleep architecture may not be significantly altered in children with ADHD. Limited evidence from subjective studies suggested no significant differences in sleep onset difficulties and bedtime resistance between children with ADHD and controls, after controlling for psychiatry comorbidity and medication status. The data from subjective studies on sleep duration, night and morning awakenings, and parasomnias were very limited. We concluded that, while excessive daytime sleepiness, high nocturnal motricity, and significant SDB might be significantly associated with ADHD per se, other sleep problems (including initial insomnia) reported in previous studies on sleep in ADHD might be accounted for more by psychiatric comorbid disorders and medication effects than by ADHD itself. Interestingly, a study by Miano et al. (published after our review) analyzing Cyclic Alternating Pattern (CAP) rates in ADHD children supported the hypothesis of the existence of a hypoarousal state in children with ADHD (18), in line with our findings on excessive daytime sleepiness in these children. However, given the limited number of studies retained in our meta-analysis, as well as their small sample sizes, our conclusions should be considered with caution and one cannot exclude that future studies might contribute to a change in our conclusions. Indeed, in a recent large study (conducted after the publication of our meta-analysis), Mick et al. (19) found that children and adolescents with ADHD presented with significant insomnia; the increased risk for insomnia was not accounted for by comorbid psychopathology or pharmacotherapy for ADHD.

Although further research is needed to better understand which, and to what extent, sleep problems found in ADHD patients are accounted for by factors associated with ADHD, it is safe to state that comorbid psychiatric conditions and ADHD pharmacotherapy may, at least, aggravate sleep problems found in patients with ADHD.

IMPLICATIONS FOR THE MANAGEMENT OF SLEEP PROBLEMS IN CHILDREN WITH ADHD

Since, as concluded in the previous section, comorbid disorders and pharmacotherapy of ADHD (and its comorbidities) may impact on sleep, they should be taken into account in the clinical management of sleep problems in children with ADHD. We discuss this issue in the next sections.

Comorbid Disorders

On the basis of the above mentioned data, as well as clinical experience, we suggest that we should systematically look for and treat the most common psychiatric comorbid disorders in patients with ADHD who complain of sleep problems. Since comorbid disorders may evolve over time, we believe that it is important to periodically screen for these conditions at each consultation. The management of comorbid disorders should then promptly be addressed and should include appropriate nonpharmacological (behavioral or cognitive behavioral therapies) and/or pharmacological treatment. In the case of comorbid mood or anxiety disorders, antidepressants with activating properties, leading to increased SOL, should, if possible, be avoided or given in the morning. In our clinical experience, we usually find that symptoms of anxiety or mood disorders not fulfilling the full DSM-IV criteria (e.g., anxiety about school performance and mild mood changes in relation to difficulties associated with ADHD) may significantly account for impairing sleep problems. Therefore, we believe that these symptoms should be appropriately treated (e.g., with relaxation techniques).

Medications Used to Treat ADHD

If medications used to treat ADHD are thought to play a significant role in the etiopathology of sleep problems in a given patient, the clinician may consider various management strategies.

In the case of a direct stimulant effect on sleep, the following options may be considered:

1) simply wait (generally insomnia caused by stimulants attenuates after 1–2 months)
2) adjustment in dose or dosing schedules (e.g., avoid evening stimulant dose)
3) switching to another stimulant formulation (in our clinical experience, different formulations of the same stimulant may differently impact on sleep)
4) switching to another stimulant (there are some data suggesting that amphetamines may more significantly impact on sleep than stimulants)

5) switching to a non-stimulant (e.g., atomoxetine, buproprion)
6) add antihistamines, trazodone, mirtazapine, or melatonin (see Chapter 16 in this book)
7) use clonidine.

If, on the other hand, the impact on sleep is caused by a "rebound effect" (rebound hyperactivity leading to sleep onset difficulties), in our, as well as in others' (20), clinical experience, giving a low dose of MPH in the late afternoon or evening could be helpful. Doses in late evening could also be considered if the rebound effect persists. As noted more than 30 years ago by Kinsbourne, *"if a hyperactive child wakes during the night, giving him a stimulant should help him go back to sleep"* (21).

Since changes in medication type, dose, and dosing schedules are frequent over the course of management of children with ADHD, we suggest a periodic assessment of the impact on sleep of medications.

CONCLUSIONS

Psychiatric comorbid disorders and medication used to treat ADHD and/or its comorbidities may significantly impact on sleep. We suggest systematic and periodic screening for psychiatric-associated conditions and medication effects in children with ADHD complaining of sleep problems. This may lead to better management and, ultimately, a better quality of life for children with ADHD and their families.

REFERENCES

1. Corkum P, Tannock R, and Moldofsky H. Sleep disturbances in children with Attention-Deficit/Hyperactivity Disorder. J Am Acad Child Adolesc Psychiatry 1998; 37(6):637–46.
2. Mindell JA, Owens JA. A Clinical Guide To Pediatric Sleep: Diagnosis and Management of Sleep Problems. Lipincott Williams & Wilkins, 2003.
3. Dulcan M. Practice parameters for the assessment and treatment of children, adolescents, and adults with attention-deficit/hyperactivity disorder. American Academy of Child and Adolescent Psychiatry. J Am Acad Child Adolesc Psychiatry 1997; 36:85S–121S.
4. Mehl RC, O'Brien LM, Jones JH, et al. Correlates of sleep and pediatric bipolar disorder. Sleep 2006; 29:193–7.
5. Kunwar A, Dewan M, Faraone SV. Treating common psychiatric disorders associated with attention-deficit/hyperactivity disorder. Expert Opin Pharmacother 2007; 8(5):555–62.
6. Ryan ND, Puig-Antich J, Ambrosini P, et al. The clinical picture of major depression in children and adolescents. Arch Gen Psychiatry 1987; 44:854–61.
7. Ivanenko A, Crabtree VM, Gozal D. Sleep and depression in children and adolescents. Sleep Med Rev 2005; 9:115–29.
8. Bertocci MA, Dahl RE, Williamson DE, et al. Subjective sleep complaints in pediatric depression: A controlled study and comparison with EEG measures of sleep and waking. J Am Acad Child Adolesc Psychiatry 2005; 44:1158–66.
9. Alfano CA, Ginsburg GS, Kingery JN. Sleep-related problems among children and adolescents with anxiety disorders. J Am Acad Child Adolesc Psychiatry 2007; 46:224–32.
10. Geller B, Zimerman B, Williams M, et al. Phenomenology of prepubertal and early adolescent bipolar disorder: Examples of elated mood, grandiose behaviors, decreased need for sleep, racing thoughts and hypersexuality. J Child Adolesc Psychopharmacol 2002; 12:3–9.
11. Rao U, Dahl RE, Ryan ND, et al. Heterogeneity in EEG sleep findings in adolescent depression: Unipolar versus bipolar clinical course. J Affect Disord 2002; 70:273–80.

12. Kostanecka-Endress T, Banaschewski T, Kinkelbur J, et al. Disturbed sleep in children with Tourette syndrome: A polysomnographic study. J Psychosom Res 2003; 55:23–9.
13. Voderholzer U, Muller N, Haag C, et al. Periodic limb movements during sleep are a frequent finding in patients with Gilles de la Tourette's syndrome. J Neurol 1997; 244:521–6.
14. Pliszka SR, Crismon ML, Hughes CW, et al. The Texas Children's Medication Algorithm Project: Revision of the algorithm for pharmacotherapy of attention-deficit/hyperactivity disorder. J Am Acad Child Adolesc Psychiatry 2006; 45:642–57.
15. Sangal RB, Owens J, Allen AJ, et al. Effects of atomoxetine and methylphenidate on sleep in children with ADHD. Sleep 2006; 29:1573–85.
16. Brown TE, McMullen WJ Jr. Attention deficit disorders and sleep/arousal disturbance. Ann N Y Acad Sci 2001; 931:271–86.
17. Cortese S, Konofal E, Yateman N, et al. Sleep and alertness in children with attention-deficit-hyperactivity disorder: A systematic review of the literature. Sleep 2006; 29(4):504–11.
18. Miano S, Donfrancesco R, Bruni O, et al. NREM sleep instability is reduced in children with attention-deficit/hyperactivity disorder. Sleep 2006; 29(6):797–803.
19. Mick E, Surman C, Biederman J. Predictors of insomnia in children and adolescents with ADHD. Presented at the 54th meeting of the American Academy of Child and Adolescent Psychiatry, San Diego (CA). 2006.
20. Kent JD, Blader JC, Koplewicz HS, et al. Effects of late-afternoon methylphenidate administration on behavior and sleep in attention-deficit hyperactivity disorder. Pediatrics 1995; 96:320–5.
21. Kinsbourne M. Stimulants for insomnia. N Engl J Med 1973; 288:1129.

15 Restless Legs Syndrome and Periodic Limb Movement Disorders: Association with ADHD

Jeannine L. Gingras[a] and Jane F. Gaultney[b]

[a]Department of Psychology, University of North Carolina and United Sleep Medicine Centers, Charlotte, North Carolina, U.S.A.
[b]Department of Psychology, University of North Carolina, Charlotte, North Carolina, U.S.A.

INTRODUCTION

Restless Legs Syndrome (RLS) and Periodic Limb Movement Disorder (PLMD) are treatable neurologic disorders that affect 5% to 10% of adults (1). These disorders have been previously under-recognized in the pediatric population although 20–35% of adults with RLS report symptoms beginning in childhood (2,3). The true prevalence of these disorders in childhood is unknown. Recent diagnostic criteria for both pediatric RLS and PLMD have been established, thus increasing recognition of these disorders in children. Major advances in childhood RLS and PLMD include: (1) retrospective reports and case presentations of RLS and PLMD in children; (2) 2003 consensus definition for RLS in children; (3) 2005 definition of PLMD in children; and, (4) recent reports of the clinical characterization of childhood RLS and PLMD. These milestones introduced RLS and PLMD as important childhood disorders and led to standardized diagnostic criteria and the clinical characterization for RLS and PLMD in children that previously were unavailable. Such standardization will allow a higher degree of accuracy in clinical diagnosis and homogeneity within research study groups.

This chapter will review current diagnostic criteria for RLS and PLMD, their prevalence, clinical presentation and daytime sequelae; specifically, their association with ADHD. Additionally, the neurophysiology and treatment of these disorders will be discussed. Finally, practical approaches to the clinical diagnosis and treatment of the disorders will be presented.

RESTLESS LEG SYNDROME (RLS) IN CHILDREN

Restless Leg Syndrome (RLS) is a neurologic, sensorimotor disorder first described in the adult population by Ekbom in the 1940s (4). The International Restless Syndrome Study Group proposed four minimal clinical diagnostic criteria for Adult RLS (5,6). RLS is characterized by the following four essential diagnostic criteria: (1) an uncontrollable urge to move the legs (and sometimes arms) usually accompanied by uncomfortable or unpleasant sensations (paresthesias and dysesthesias); (2) the urge to move or uncomfortable sensations are worst at rest or with inactivity; (3) the urge to move or uncomfortable sensations are temporarily relieved by movement or stretching the legs, and; (4) the urge to move the legs or uncomfortable sensations usually occur in the evening or at night. The ICSD-2 (7) added a fifth criterion: the "condition is not better explained by another current sleep disorder, medical or neurologic disorder, mental disorder, medication use, or substance use disorder."

RLS is considered the most frequent movement disorder in adults but remains largely under-diagnosed and under-treated (1,8,9). This fact may also hold true in children (10).

Two forms have been reported in the adult literature: RLS is considered Primary when RLS symptoms cannot be attributed to other conditions. Primary RLS is typically associated with a strong family history of RLS, suggesting a genetic pre-disposition (7,11). RLS is considered Secondary when RLS symptoms are associated with other disorders such as iron deficiency anemia, pregnancy, or end-stage renal disease. RLS is also associated with type 2 diabetes in adults (12) although this does not appear true in children with insulin dependent diabetes (13). Medications such as Serotonin Receptor Uptake Inhibitors (SSRIs), antiemetics and antihistamines, caffeine, and alcohol can cause or exacerbate symptoms (7). Currently this distinc-tion of Primary and Secondary RLS is being questioned. In childhood, most RLS is familial and unassociated with other disorders, thus is considered Primary.

RLS has a significant motor counterpart in sleep in the form of recurrent jerk-ing movements of the legs termed "periodic limb movements in sleep" (PLMS). It is estimated that between 80% and 90% of adults with RLS have associated periodic limb movements during sleep (PLMS) and about 15% will have periodic limb movements during quiet wakefulness (PLMW), (7,3,14). This association appears to be true in children although there are no studies specifically addressing these issues in children. Population-based studies in adults using the four essential diagnos-tic criteria have found a prevalence of 5–10% in the United States and Western Europe (1). Many adults with RLS retrospectively recalled that their symptoms began in childhood; about 25–35 % reported symptoms before age 20 and 8–14% before age 10 (2,3). In 2003, consensus criteria for the diagnosis of RLS in children and ado-lescents were published and are summarized in Table 1 (6). The consensus group developed criteria for "Definite RLS" useful for the clinician evaluating children and two other categories, "Probable" and "Possible" RLS (Table 2) most suitable for research purposes and included here for completeness.

The current RLS criteria do not include a frequency criterion; however, in most studies, moderate to severe RLS is defined as symptoms that occur at least or greater than two times per week (10). A severity scale has been developed for adults with RLS but has not yet been validated in children (15).

Prevalence of RLS in Children

The first reported prevalence of RLS in the pediatric population was derived from retrospective data obtained from a pediatric sleep center and was reported at 5.9% (16). This is somewhat higher than the adult predicted prevalence of 1.25–2.55% calculated from the adult prevalence of 5–10% and considering that about 25% of adults recall symptom onset between 10 and 20 years of age (10). The higher preva-lence in the Mayo Clinic report of 5.9% may be due to referral bias. To date, the most comprehensive prevalence study for RLS in childhood is that reported by Picchietti et al. (10). This large-scale, population-based study obtained internet survey responses from 10,523 families with children aged 8–17 years. Both the parents and children participated. The survey consisted of questions about RLS and about the sleep, mood and behavioral sequelae of RLS, among other inquiries. Criteria for *def-inite* RLS were met by 1.9% of children aged 8–11 years (children) and 2.0% of ado-lescents aged 12–17 years (adolescents); 25% of the children and 50% of the

TABLE 1 NIH Workshop Diagnostic Criteria for RLS in Children (ages 2–18 yrs)

Definite RLS in children (ages 2–18 yrs)

1. The child meets all four essential adult criteria for RLS and relates a description, in the child's own words, consistent with leg discomfort.
   1. An urge to move the legs, usually accompanied or caused by uncomfortable and unpleasant sensations in the legs. (Sometimes the urge to move is present without the uncomfortable sensations and sometimes the arms or other body parts are involved in addition to the legs.)
   2. The urge to move or unpleasant sensations begin or worsen during periods of rest or inactivity such as lying or sitting.
   3. The urge to move or unpleasant sensations are partially or totally relieved by movement, such as walking or stretching, at least as long as the activity continues.
   4. The urge to move or unpleasant sensations are worse in the evening or night than during the day or only occur in the evening or night. (When symptoms are very severe, the worsening at night may not be noticeable but must have been previously present.)

OR

2. The child meets all 4 essential criteria for RLS and 2/3 criteria supportive of the diagnosis are present
   i. sleep disturbance for age,
   ii. a biologic parent or sibling has definite RLS,
   iii. the child has a PLMS index of > 5/hr on polysomnography.

Terms such as "oowies," "tickle," "spiders," "boo-boos," "want to run," and "a lot of energy in my legs" may be used by the child to describe symptoms. Age appropriate descriptors are encouraged.

For pediatric and adult RLS: The condition is not better explained by another current sleep disorder, medical or neurological disorder, mental disorder, medication use, or substance use disorder.

---

adolescents met criteria for moderate to severe RLS (symptoms occurring = to or >2 times/week). The authors point out that this prevalence exceeds that of non-febrile seizure disorders and types 1 and 2 diabetes combined. Additionally, parents reported recall of onset of RLS symptoms in the 8–11-year-olds at < 5 years of age in 15% and onset between five and seven years of age in 63% of the adolescent population, suggesting that RLS can have an earlier onset than the sample studied in

TABLE 2 NIH Workshop Research Criteria for RLS (Ages 0–18 yrs)

Probable RLS in children:

i. the child meets all 4 essential criteria for RLS, except #4; "worse in the evening or at night," *and*
ii. the child has a biologic parent or sibling with definite RLS.

OR*

i. the child is observed to have behavior manifestations of lower-extremety discomfort when sitting or lying, accompanied by motor movement of the affected limbs; the discomfort has characteristics 2, 3, and 4 of the essential criteria, *and*
ii the child has a biologic parent or sibling with definite RLS.

* This last category is intended for young children or cognitively impaired children, who do not have sufficient language to describe the sensory component of RLS.

Possible RLS in children:

i. the child has periodic limb movement disorder (PLMD), *and*
ii. the child has a biologic parent or sibling with definite RLS but the child does not meet definite or probable childhood RLS definitions (as above).

---

this survey. This is consistent with clinical experience. In fact, Walters et al. reported RLS symptoms in an 18-month-old infant (17).

Clinical Presentation of RLS in Children

Sleep complaints are common in children with RLS. Picchietti et al. (10) reported that children and adolescents with definite RLS are more likely to have a history of difficulty falling asleep or staying asleep at night, compared to those children who did not meet the criteria. Daytime sleepiness was reported in 21% of the 8–11-year-olds and 33% of the 12–17-year-olds. There is a strong relationship between RLS and daytime behavioral and mood disorders (see RLS, PLMD and attention-deficit/hyperactive disorder [ADHD]). Many parents describe daytime restlessness by: "my child moves constantly," "fidgets," "cannot sit still," "has a limb in constant motion." There does not appear to be a strong gender association in children (10) in contrast to a female to male gender ratio of 4:1 in adulthood (1,11). Many children with RLS have a positive family history of RLS in an immediate family member (10).

RLS is a clinical diagnosis that requires the child describe the sensory symptoms and that these symptoms fulfill the essential criteria for Pediatric RLS; symptoms meeting the established criteria confer a diagnosis of "definite" RLS. Importantly, children need to describe symptoms in their own words. Often the symptoms are difficult to describe even in the adult population and many children may report vague descriptors such as their legs have a "funny feeling," "warm feeling," "tingling or tickling"; some children use the word "pain." Children as young as three years of age have been able to articulate classic paresthesias and dyesthesias of RLS. In a clinical practice of sleep medicine (JLG), a three-year-old described his leg sensations as "jiggle-bugs in my legs"; a five-year-old girl described her sensations as "baby snakes crawling in my legs." Other children's descriptors of RLS derived from clinical experience (JLG) are listed in Table 3. Picchietti et al. report similar and additional descriptors (10), as do Mindell and Owens (18).

Often the discomfort described by the child is interpreted by the parent as growing pains. This association was first reported by Ekbom in 1975 (19). In children, Rajaram et al. reported that 10 out of 11 children reporting growing pains met the essential criteria for RLS (20). This topic is reviewed by Walters (21). Thus, in children with RLS, it is not uncommon to obtain a history of growing pains; often parents treat the symptoms with anti-inflammatory agents.

Thus, children who present with complaints of difficulty falling or staying asleep, nonrestorative sleep after an appropriate amount of sleep; children who report growing pains, and children with daytime sleepiness, ADHD-like behaviors and restlessness, should be screened for RLS. In all cases, the characteristics of worse at night, at rest and temporarily relieved by movement must be present. A screening questionnaire for RLS can be found in "A Clinical Guide to Pediatric Sleep" (22).

RLS symptoms are worse at night thus most children experience the sensations when lying down to fall asleep; some are awakened with the feelings and some report the sensations in the morning upon awakening, the latter being atypical in adults with RLS. Many children ask their parents to rub or massage their legs (or arms). Hot or cold baths may help temporarily relieve the leg sensations, as can cold or warm compresses. Some parents report having to "lie on his legs" in order to help the child fall asleep. Other children wrap their sheets around their legs to get relief when trying to fall asleep. Often the symptoms are precipitated with long

TABLE 3   RLS Descriptors

"an electric current"
"coca cola bubbles running through my veins"
"maggots, spiders, baby snakes crawling in my legs"
"jiggle bugs in my legs"
"pain, pulling, aching, itching, throbbing in legs"
"creepy feelings"
"scrambling in my legs"
"needles prickling my skin"
"water running down my legs"
"a wave in my legs"
"skin inside out"
"my legs have a toothache"
"my legs have a headache"
"something is inside my legs"

Restlessness
"the gotta moves"
"heebie jeebies"
"bounding energy in my legs"
" my legs need to exercise"
" my legs just gotta move"
"need to shake something off my legs"

Parent's report
Constantly asks to have legs rubbed, massaged
Cries out in middle of night that legs hurt
Unable to keep a sheet on the bed
Frequently treat with anti-inflamatory agents

---

periods of inactivity such as long car rides and plane flights or prolonged periods of sitting such as in school. Polysomnograms are not necessary for a diagnosis of RLS unless the symptoms are not classic or the patient fails first line therapy (see Therapy) and supportive diagnostic criteria are needed.

Supportive Diagnostic Criteria for RLS
Supportive diagnostic criteria for RLS include a family history of RLS, PLMS, and PLMW (see PLMS), or a favorable response to treatment with a dopaminergic agent (7,23).

Differential Diagnosis of RLS on Children
Care should be taken to exclude other causes of leg pain such as neuropathies/ radiculopathies, orthopedic conditions such as Osgood–Schlater and chondromalacia patella, rheumatologic disorders such as juvenile rheumatoid arthritis, vascular disorders, akathisia, and Nocturnal Leg Cramps. Typically the paresthesias associated with neuropathies and the pain associated with orthopedic and rheumatologic disorders are present throughout the day, at rest and with activity and not necessarily associated with a desire to move the limbs or relieved by moving the limbs. Symptoms also can be unilateral, often worsened with movement, and do not have

a circadian component. Vascular disorders such as an intermittent claudication are rare in childhood, and often worse during leg movements and improved at rest. Akathisia is an inner sense of restlessness that is accompanied by a desire to move that is similar to RLS, but akathisia is usually found in association with neuroleptic use. Nocturnal Leg Cramps are painful spasms of the calf or foot often described as a "hardening" of a muscle requiring excessive stretching to be relieved. Other causes of "uncomfortable leg sensations" include excessive exercise from muscle overuse and atopic dermatitis, and pruritus; in the former there is a history of excessive exercise and muscle overuse; in the latter sensations occur "on the skin" versus the sensation of "deep inside" as experienced in RLS (18,24).

Symptoms of RLS can be exacerbated by anemia, specific medications such as antihistamines, antiemetics, depressant medication (especially the SSRIs), psychotrophic medications, caffeine and alcohol (7,18).

PERIODIC LIMB MOVEMENTS IN SLEEP (PLMS)

Periodic Limb Movements during Sleep (PLMS) is a polysomnographic diagnosis characterized by repetitive, stereotyped, rhythmic leg movements lasting between 0.5 and 5 seconds in duration (recently modified to 10 s, [25]) with a 25% increase in amplitude from toe dorsiflexion during calibration (suggested change to an 8 µV increase above resting electromyogram (EMG) [25]), occurring in sequence of four or more movements with an intermovement interval of 5–90 seconds (26) (Fig. 1). Some allow scoring of PLMS if the intermovement interval is between 5 and 120 seconds as initially suggested by Coleman (27). Movements typically are bilateral, but may predominate in one leg or alternate between legs. Limb movements can also be seen in quiet wakefulness, called Periodic Limb Movements during Wake (PLMW) but are not typically scored on traditional polysomnography (28,29). This practice has been questioned and scoring of PLMW has been suggested to become standard scoring (30).

Clinically, PLMS are a sleep-related phenomenon characterized by dorsiflexion of the ankle, dorsiflexion of the toes, and a partial flexion of the knee and sometimes the hip, although all the motor components need not be present. Occasionally, the movements can be seen in the arms as flexion at the elbow.

PLMS were first described in 1953 by Symonds (31) who interpreted the movements as a form of epilepsy. The first polysomnography (PSG) characterization of PLMS was reported in 1972 by Lugaresi et al. (32); scoring criteria were subsequently proposed by Coleman in the early 1980s (27,33) and recently modified (25,34). Unless severe, PLMS occur predominantly in non-rapid eye movement (NREM) sleep (Fig. 2) in the first third of the night; severe PLMS can occur during REM.

PLMS are not scored if aperiodic or if induced by environmental factors such as noise or a technician changing leads, or by respiratory events such as increased upper airway resistance or apnea (Fig. 3). Thus, it is important to use sensitive respiratory monitoring devices.

If seen only in REM, other conditions such as increased upper airway resistance or REM-related phasic twitching should be considered. PLMS are often associated with other disorders such as narcolepsy, SDB, and RSBD, and RLS (35). In adults, PLMS may be seen in individuals without sleep complaints (36) although the general consensus is that PLMS associated with and without arousals impact

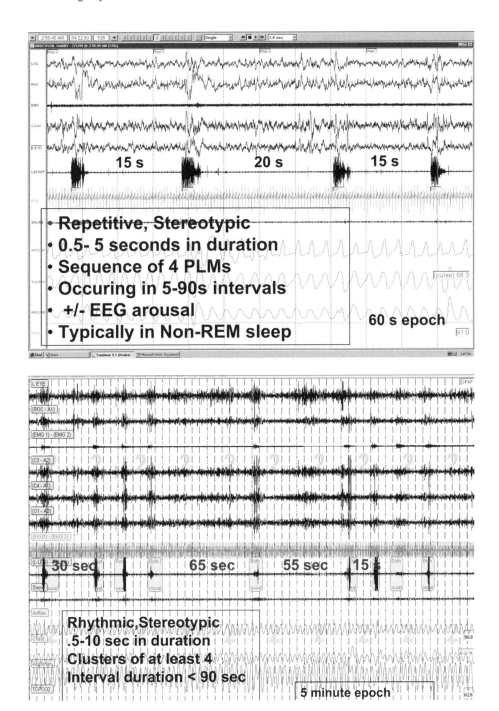

FIGURE 1   Epochs from polysomnogram demonstrating PLMS.

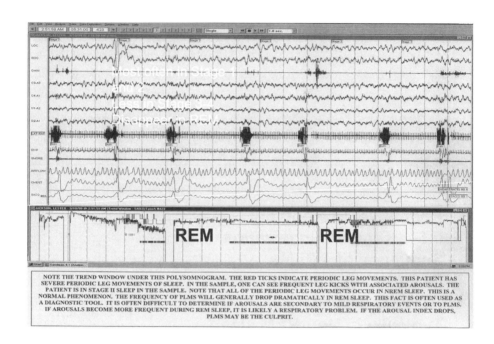

NOTE THE TREND WINDOW UNDER THIS POLYSOMNOGRAM. THE RED TICKS INDICATE PERIODIC LEG MOVEMENTS. THIS PATIENT HAS SEVERE PERIODIC LEG MOVEMENTS OF SLEEP. IN THE SAMPLE, ONE CAN SEE FREQUENT LEG KICKS WITH ASSOCIATED AROUSALS. THE PATIENT IS IN STAGE II SLEEP IN THE SAMPLE. NOTE THAT ALL OF THE PERIODIC LEG MOVEMENTS OCCUR IN NREM SLEEP. THIS IS A NORMAL PHENOMENON. THE FREQUENCY OF PLMS WILL GENERALLY DROP DRAMATICALLY IN REM SLEEP. THIS FACT IS OFTEN USED AS A DIAGNOSTIC TOOL. IT IS OFTEN DIFFICULT TO DETERMINE IF AROUSALS ARE SECONDARY TO MILD RESPIRATORY EVENTS OR TO PLMS. IF AROUSALS BECOME MORE FREQUENT DURING REM SLEEP, IT IS LIKELY A RESPIRATORY PROBLEM. IF THE AROUSAL INDEX DROPS, PLMS MAY BE THE CULPRIT.

FIGURE 2   Polysomnogram demonstrating PLMS in NREM.

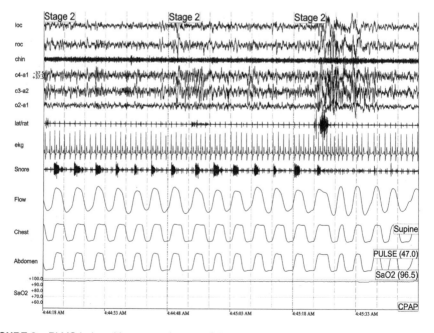

FIGURE 3   PLMS induced by upper airway resistance.

sleep quality and daytime functioning (37,38). This topic has recently been eloquently debated in a Pro and Con format (38,39) and in a recent editorial (40).

There may be some unique features of the PLMS in children. For instance, children may not necessarily meet the sequence criterion and many limb movements in children occur in clusters. Also, there may be a longer intermovement interval, and there is considerable night-to-night variability in the number of PLMS (see PLMD).

The severity of PLMS is reported as an index, calculated as the total number of PLMS/Total Sleep Time and reported as the Periodic Limb Movement Index (PLMI). Limb movements greater than 15/hr is considered abnormal in adults (35). In children, PLMS are rare (28,41), thus a PLMI greater than 5/hr is considered abnormal (35). The PLMI is further characterized as those PLMS associated with cortical arousals (PLMsAr). Recently, PLMS were found to be more prevalent in Caucasian children than in African-American children (42). PLMS are also seen in higher frequency in children with Asperger's syndrome (43), in children with William's Syndrome (44), and in childhood fibromyalgia (45).

Importantly, PLMS alone on PSG do not define a disorder (Periodic Limb Movement Disorder, see below) but simply report a phenomenon. A diagnosis of PLMD requires not only the presence of PLMS on PSG but also an associated sleep disturbance uncountable by another disorder of sleep (35). Earlier reports often used PLMS and PLMD interchangeably because of lack of nosology distinguishing the two, and many studies defined a PLMD group solely based on PLMI on PSG of greater than 5/hr (46–48). Thus, early characterization of PLMD may have been confounded by inappropriately assigning children with PLMS but not PLMD to a PLMD study group. This has been a serious limitation of earlier studies (Rev, RLS, PLMD, and ADHD). In 2005, diagnostic criteria for PLMD were published and PLMD now has specific clinical diagnostic criteria (35) with an associated clinical ICD-9 code (327.51). Research can now be conducted with standardized diagnoses resulting in more homogeneity in research study groups.

Thus, an important question is raised: "When do PLMS on PSG become PLMD?"

PERIODIC LIMB MOVEMENT DISORDER IN CHILDREN (PLMD)
PLMS on PSG become PLMD when the following criteria are met (35).

1. PLMS on PSG greater than 5/hr (PLMI >5/hr)
2. Associated with a clinical sleep disturbance
3. The sleep disturbance is not accountable by any other sleep disorder such as narcolepsy, SDB or medication effect.

PLMD Clinical Characterization
Previous characterization information about PLMD was derived primarily from analyses of PLMD groups defined solely by PLMS >5/hr on PSG (46–48) thus potentially introducing confounds. For instance, children with PLMD (defined by ICSD-2 criteria) were shown to have greater daytime behavior and attention problems than did children with SDB. These group differences were not apparent when analyzing data using PLMS on PSG alone to define the study groups (49), as many children with SDB and other sleep disorders have PLMS on PSG but do not fulfill

the ICSD-2 criteria for PLMD. Inconsistencies in published data about daytime mood and behavior consequences in children with PLMD may be explained, in part, by the practice of identifying PLMD based solely on a PLMI cutoff of 5/hr on PSG. Nonetheless, these studies have provided important information, underscoring PLMD as a serious and important pediatric sleep disorder.

To date, the only published data about the clinical characterization of children with PLMD based on the ICSD-2 criteria are published in an abstract form. These data were derived from a retrospective review of information from 442 children referred to a pediatric sleep practice over a period of two years and presented at the Sleep 2006 meeting (50). One hundred and four children fulfilled the ICSD-2 criteria for PLMD and no other sleep disorder, and 60 children had PLMD comorbidity with Sleep-Disordered Breathing (SDB). The characteristics of these children were compared to each other and to 179 children diagnosed with SDB only. The mean age of the children did not differ between groups and was 8.14 years (=/− 4.16 yrs) for the PLMD only group. Sixty percent of children with PLMD were male compared to a 1:1 male to female ratio reported in children with RLS (10). PLMD also showed ethnic differences: 84% of the children with PLMD were Caucasian, 13% were African-American and 3% were Asian. In this cohort, the prevalence for PLMD was 37% inclusive of children with a dual diagnosis, and 24% when considering those children with PLMD only.

By definition, children with PLMD have associated sleep disturbances. Figure 4 graphically shows the nocturnal complaints in children with PLMD alone, SDB alone, and children with dual diagnoses.

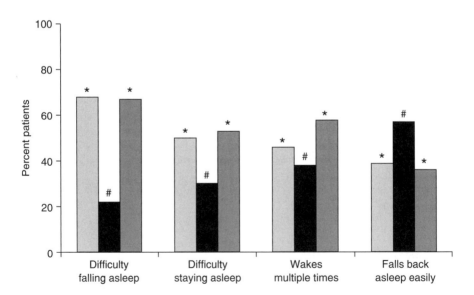

FIGURE 4 Nocturnal complaints in children with PLMD. Percent patients with nocturnal complaints in the following groups: PLMD (light gray), SDB (black), and PLMD +SDB (medium gray), respectively. Bars marked with the same symbol are equivalent, while bars marked with different symbols are significantly different from each other for each variable in each panel ($p < 0.05$). The data presented are collected from either questionnaire data or chart review.

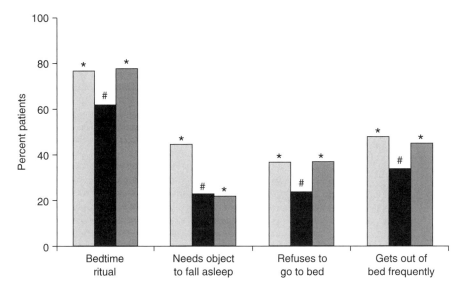

FIGURE 5 Bedtime resistance behaviors. Percent patients with nocturnal complaints in the following groups: PLMD (light gray), SDB (black), and PLMD +SDB (medium gray), respectively. Bars marked with the same symbol are equivalent, while bars marked with different symbols are significantly different from each other for each variable in each panel ($p < 0.05$). The data presented are collected from either questionnaire data or chart review.

Typically, children with PLMD report more difficulty falling asleep, staying asleep, greater number of awakenings after sleep onset and greater difficulty falling back to sleep after a nocturnal awakening. Earlier studies report similar findings (46–48). Importantly, children will often state that they "want to fall asleep but just cannot." This is in contrast to children with insomnia due to circadian rhythm disorder who clearly state they are not tired when put to bed. Children with PLMD also demonstrated more bedtime resistance behaviors (Fig. 5) and daytime psychopathology (Fig. 6), (see RLS, PLMD and ADHD).

Many parents and children with PLMD report being unrefreshed in the morning after an adequate amount of sleep. Sleep was always described as restless with "constant" motion; many parents report excessive kicking in sleep to the point that "no family member wants to share a bed with the child" or "cannot keep a sheet on the bed." Some parents report that children sleep with their legs wedged under them or in a cocoon with the sheets wrapped around the child's leg. Parents often describe their child as being a "light sleeper" and report a long history of poor sleep. Many parents state their child gave up naps unusually early. Table 4 lists typical descriptors reported by parents of children with PLMD. It must be noted, however, that up to 40% of parents are unaware of limb movements in their children who are subsequently diagnosed with PLMD (47,50).

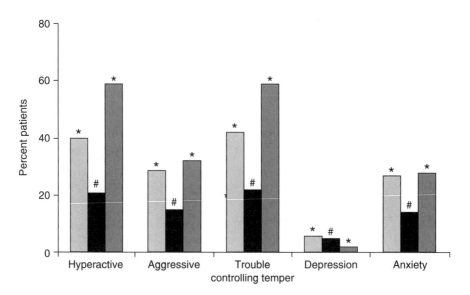

FIGURE 6   Psychopathology in children with PLMD. Percent patients with nocturnal complaints in the following groups: PLMD (light gray), SDB (black), and PLMD +SDB (medium gray), respectively. Bars marked with the same symbol are equivalent, while bars marked with different symbols are significantly different from each other for each variable in each panel (p < 0.05). The data presented are collected from either questionnaire data or chart review.

Prevalence of PLMD in Children

The true prevalence of PLMD based on the ICSD-2 criteria is unknown. Most studies defined PLMD as PLMS on PSG 5/hr (46–48). Based on this criterion, a prevalence of 1.2% (51) and 8.4% (48) have been reported from two different sleep medicine clinics and 11.9% identified from a community sample (48). A recent report of data retrospectively analyzed from a clinical practice of sleep medicine reported a much higher prevalence of 24 % increasing to 37% when children with comorbid

TABLE 4   PLMD Descriptors

Long history of poor sleep
  "Never been a good sleeper"
  "Gave up naps early"
Constant movement in sleep
  "Riding a bike"
  "Running a race"
  "Like a fish out of water"
  "No one wants to sleep with child"
  "Bed covers askew in the morning"
  "Had to sew sheets together"
  "Wore holes in the sheets"
  "Sheets constantly pushed to bottom of bed"
  "Legs always under me"

PLMD and SDB were considered (50). In this study, the diagnosis of PLMD was based on the ICSD-2 criteria (35); none of the children with PLMD had RLS.

Thus, it appears that PLMD has a higher prevalence in children than RLS, although both disorders clinically present with sleep disturbances; one (PLMD) without an urge to move the legs or unusual sensations, the other (RLS) associated with paresthesias/dysethesias, and an urge to move the affected limb. This raises interesting questions: are PLMD and RLS separate disorders? comorbid as they both share an underlying dopaminergic dysfunction (see Neuropathology)? Or are PLMD and RLS a spectrum of a single disorder with the motor component presenting earlier than the sensory component as suggested by recent data (52) (see also Current Controversies in Childhood RLS, PLMD)?

Diagnosis of PLMD in Children

PLMD is a polysomnographic and clinical diagnosis based on PLMS >5/hr on PSG and a clinical sleep complaint (35). However, there are some challenges in making a clinical diagnosis of PLMD that should be discussed.

Night-to-Night Variability in PLMS

This concept poses significant clinical challenges. The adult literature reports significant night-to-night variability of PLMS in adults with and without a diagnosis of RLS, although the variability was greater in the adults with RLS (53,54). In fact, the authors cautioned against using rigid cutoffs for the PLMI in making decisions about the clinical significance of PLMS in a specific individual. The concept of night-to-night variability is also relevant to children. Data from Home Limb Movement monitoring of children with RLS over five nights demonstrated considerable night-to-night variability in the PLMI (55) to the extent that on many nights the limb movements were < 5/hr. This fact should be taken into consideration when making a clinical diagnosis of PLMD especially in the context of a PSG with PLMS less than 5/hr, a clinical history suggestive of PLMD, and a parent report that the child had more restful sleep the night of the PSG. The parent should always be asked if the child's sleep the night of his/her PSG was typical of sleep at home; i.e., was the child's sleep comparable, less or more restful than sleep on most nights at home? If the PSG data is questionable and the clinical history suggestive of PLMD, it would be reasonable to confer a diagnosis of probable PLMD and initiate a treatment trial. Alternatively, Home Limb Movement monitoring over several nights would be extremely helpful. Currently there are no reliable Home Limb Movement monitors for children. Significant advancement in the diagnosis and treatment of PLMD would be the development of a home monitor that could reliably record limb movements during sleep over sequential nights.

Comorbidity

Children may have comorbid disorders such as SDB and PLMD, narcolepsy and PLMD, etc. The fact that PLMS are often associated with these other disorders does not negate the possibility of comorbidity. Children with PLMS and narcolepsy, for instance, may have symptomatic sleep disruption from the PLMS in addition to the daytime hypersomnolence of narcolepsy; PLMS may exacerbate daytime symptoms.

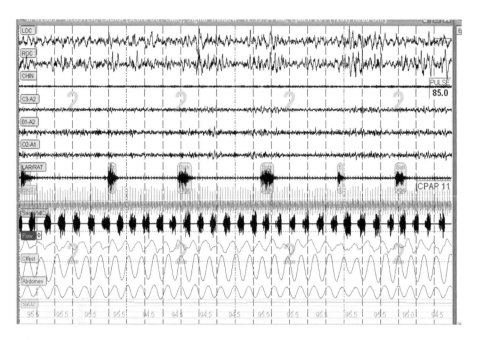

FIGURE 7   Co-occurence of PLMS and upper airway resistance.

In such a case, treatment of both disorders would be warranted. An example of comorbid disorders is seen in Figure 7 showing a polysomnogram from a child with both snoring/Upper Airway Resistance as well as rhythmic limb movements. A detailed clinical history is essential in assessing comorbidity.

One approach is to first address the chief presenting complaint; i.e., snoring/upper airway resistance/apnea. If the child continues to be symptomatic after treatment of the chief complaint (in this case, tonsillectomy and adenoidectomy) and had PLMS on PSG, he/she now meets the criteria for PLMD. At this time, treatment for PLMD is warranted. Similarly, children with narcolepsy who are unrefreshed in the morning after an adequate night's sleep and have PLMS on PSG may have comorbid disorders. Comorbidity is often seen in children with psychiatric diagnoses (56).

Differential Diagnosis of PLMS and PLMD

Care should be taken to identify known causes of PLMS such as Sleep-Disordered Breathing, Narcolepsy, and REM Sleep Behavior Disorder. Additionally, nocturnal epilepsy and nocturnal paroxysmal dystonia can manifest as rhythmic motor activity during sleep. Sleep starts occurring at sleep onset could be interpreted by the parent as limb movements in sleep, as could hypnagogic foot tremor and alternating leg muscle activation (24,35,57). Rhythmic movement disorder such as head banging, and/or body rocking should be easily differentiated from PLMS.

NEUROPHYSIOLOGY OF RLS AND PLMS

There have been excellent published reports on the proposed physiopathology of RLS and PLMD in the adult population (58,59). There is no evidence to suggest that these mechanisms are not applicable in children as well.

Significant data suggest a key role for the spinal cord in the neuropathology of RLS and PLMD. (The spinal cord is the site of primary sensory input and final motor output to the legs). The role of the spinal cord in the pathophysiology of RLS and PLMD has been supported by case reports of patients with complete spinal cord transections who demonstrated PLMS and PLMW on PSG similar to patients with RLS and PLMD. Transient RLS symptoms have also been reported during recovery from anaesthesia. Thus, the spinal cord, devoid of supraspinal input, is able to generate both the sensory symptoms of RLS and rhythmic limb movements. Incoming sensory afferents to the spinal cord and the final motor output are interconnected by the spinal interneuronal system that is modulated by both supraspinal, subcortical descending inhibitory and excitatory pathways and by peripheral input from the flexor reflex afferents (FRA). The role of the spinal cord has been eloquently reviewed by Paulus and Schomburg (58).

Supraspinal sites are also importantly involved in the physiopathogogy of RLS and PLMS although the exact neural structures involved have not definitely been defined. The hypothalamus has been implicated in the supraspinal modulation of the spinal cord neurons particularly the A11 neurons (60). These neurons are dopaminergic and project both to the dorsal (afferent site) and ventral horn (efferent site) in the spinal cord. Involvement of the hypothalamus could also explain the circadian component of RLS and PLMS. Earlier functional MRI studies revealed activation of other central nervous system (CNS) sites: thalamic and cerebellar regions associated with the sensory complaints of patients with RLS and activation of pontine sites and the red nucleus during PLMW (61).

Both the endogenous dopaminergic and opioidergic systems and iron metabolism have been implicated in the physiopathology of RLS and PLMD (58,59,62) based primarily on the therapeutic response of these disorders to pharmacologic treatment with dopaminergic and opiate medications (63,64) and to iron supplementation (65–68). Dopamine synthesis, for instance, demonstrates a circadian rhythm with dopamine levels being lowest at night when RLS symptoms are most severe. Iron also demonstrates a circadian rhythm. Also, iron is an essential cofactor in dopamine synthesis, and low iron stores, especially in the brain, have been implicated with increase RLS symptoms and with increase in PLMS.

Opiates have also shown therapeutic benefit especially in adult RLS patients with severe RLS or in patients who demonstrate augmentation (a phenomenon of worsening RLS symptoms when on dopaminergic agents) (59). Data suggest that the opiates may modulate RLS symptoms and PLMS, especially REM suppression, either via direct inhibition of spinal cord neurons (specifically FRA pathways) (58), or indirectly through dysinhibition of the dopaminergic neurons (59).

RLS, PLMD, AND ADHD

There is a well-established literature that suggests that children with ADHD have *some* type of sleep anomaly. Although sleepy adults may act groggily, most parents of young children know that sleepy children bounce off the wall. In a review of the literature, Owens (69) noted that there is overlap in the neural systems that regulate attention/arousal and sleep. Her review, based on over 50 articles, found that many children with ADHD have a co-occurring sleep disorder that may contribute to their symptoms of ADHD. Although parents of children with ADHD consistently complain of sleep problems in their children, objective measures of sleep often find no differences between children with ADHD and controls (69,70; however, see O'Brien et al. 71). This conjunction of sleep problems and ADHD is not universally accepted. A few studies find no connections between sleep and ADHD. Sangal et al. (72), for example, concluded that in the absence of indicators of a sleep disorder there is no reason to assume a connection between ADHD and sleep pathology.

There have been a number of studies that suggest inadequate and/or insufficient sleep may present as, cause, or co-exist with ADHD. For example, children whose parents or teachers have reported signs of inattention, hyperactivity, and impulsivity continue to show greater sleepiness than controls, even when they have experienced adequate sleep for the previous three nights (73). A study using a more objective measure of sleep than self- or parent-report (actigraphy) found that children with shorter sleep times showed more severe behavior problems than did children with more sleep (74). Despite having similar sleep latency, TST, and sleep efficiency, children with ADHD demonstrated greater daytime sleepiness, measured by a multiple sleep latency test, than controls (75).

Other work has examined whether ADHD can be associated with a specific sleep disorder. A substantial body of evidence associates symptoms of ADHD and SDB. Golan et al. (75) found that 50% of children with ADHD (vs. 22% of controls) had PSG documented signs of SDB. Chervin and colleagues (76,77) examined whether children with symptoms of ADHD (inattentiveness and hyperactivity) would show symptoms of sleep disorders. Using a validated, parent-completed sleep questionnaire, they found that habitual snoring was reported for children who had been diagnosed with ADHD (33% vs. 11% from the clinical sample and 9% from the community sample). A snoring score was associated with greater levels of inattention and hyperactivity. Complaints about restless legs (which may co-occur with PLMD) were associated with symptoms of ADHD, but less consistently so.

Evidence of a Link Between ADHD and RLS, PLMD

A number of studies report a co-occurrence of PLMs, PLMD, or RLS and ADHD or symptoms of ADHD, both in children (78) and adults. (79,80) As early as 1994 Walters et al. (17) were noting a connection between childhood RLS, ADHD, and growing pains. Picchietti et al. (46) found that 8 of 18 children with comorbid ADHD and PLMD had a personal history and a family history of symptoms of RLS. The authors concluded that daytime motor restlessness associated with RLS might contribute to inattention and hyperactivity.

Gaultney et al. (81) administered a validated sleep survey to 283 children from a community sample. Scales for SDB, PLMD, and bedtime resistance behaviors (BRB) were correlated with DSM-IV defined symptoms of ADHD. They found significantly stronger correlations between symptoms of PLMD and ADHD than between symptoms of SDB and PLMD. The connection between PLMD and ADHD remained even when controlling for age, SDB, sleepiness, and BRB.

Crabtree et al. (82) conducted a retrospective review of 97 children with ADHD. An overnight PSG of 69 of these children indicated that 35% of the children with ADHD had PLMD and 7% had SDB. They noted considerable variability in night-to-night sleep patterns. Crabtree et al. (48) examined children aged 5–7 with comorbid PLMD and ADHD (*N*=40), PLMD alone (*N*=50), and age-matched controls (*N*=52). Participants were selected from both clinical and community populations. The PLMD study group was identified as those with a PLMI >5. ADHD was indicated by parents' responses to the Conners Parent Rating Scale. The clinical group included 8.4% who had a PLMI >5, and 11.9% of the community group had a PLMI >5. Of the children with a PLMI >5, 44.4% also had a diagnosis of ADHD. The data indicated that children with PLMD had less REM sleep than controls. Children with comorbid ADHD and PLMD had more PLMs with arousals than did children with PLMD only. The authors concluded that although there did appear to be a connection between PLMD and ADHD, it was not a strong relation, and that it may be mediated by reduced REM sleep and sleep fragmentation.

Chervin et al. (83) surveyed parents of 866 children from two general pediatric clinics, using the PSQ, DSM-IV derived questions about symptoms of ADHD, and the hyperactivity index from the Conners Parent Rating Scale. Having a Hyperactivity Index score greater than 60 predicted symptoms of PLMD (OR=1.6), symptoms of restless legs (OR=1.9), and growing pains (OR=1.9). The fact that the association between symptoms of ADHD and symptoms of PLMD/RLS is similar to those found in a clinical population implies that comorbid sleep disorders and ADHD may be widespread.

Picchietti and Walters (47) conducted a retrospective chart review of 129 children and adolescents who had a PLMI >5/hr, and found that 91% also had ADHD. They then went on to examine the 16 children who had a PLMI >25/hr. Ninety-four percent of this more extreme group had ADHD. Of the 16 Ps with PLMS >25/hr, 15 had ADHD, 4 had RLS and 10/13 had a family history of RLS. Picchietti et al. (84) examined 14 children who had recently been diagnosed with ADHD, and 10 controls. All children received a PSG. Children with ADHD were more likely to have a family history of RLS than were control children. Children with ADHD produced more PLMs and PLMs with arousals than did controls. Over half of the children with ADHD (and none of the controls) had a PLMI >5/hr, and 21% had a PLMI >20/hr. The children with ADHD and PLMs >5/hr reported less sleep time, greater sleep onset latency, and more awakenings. Of the parents of children with ADHD, 32% had symptoms of RLS. The authors speculated that PLMs may contribute to symptoms of ADHD by means of sleep disruption or both conditions may share an underlying dopamine deficiency (also see 46).

One challenge in interpreting the studies of PLMD has been the way in which the study groups have been defined. Some studies (47,48,72,84) have operationalized PLMD by using a PLMI cutoff point of five. Others have defined study groups based on PLMI and the presence of sleep disruption. It is possible that these two different systems for establishing study groups introduce a confound into the literature. Preliminary analysis of data from our lab (49) of 251 children with either clinically diagnosed PLMD or SDB found that parent ratings of problems with daytime behavior and symptoms of internalizing and externalizing are significantly greater for children with PLMD. These group differences disappear or are diminished when (using scores from the same children) study groups are defined just by using a PLMI cutoff point of five.

Mechanisms

Lewin and Di Pinto (85) observed in an editorial that studies of ADHD and sleep can be divided into four categories (parenthetical statements added): those that offer evidence that children with ADHD have some type of sleep disorder that may, at least partially, explain some of the neurobehavioral deficits associated with ADHD (the "sleep problems cause ADHD" theory); those that cast ADHD as a disorder of hypoarousal (and, presumably, disordered inhibition), and suggest that the hypoarousal may interfere with sleep cycles (the "ADHD causes the sleep problem" theory); those that suggest that ADHD and sleep disorders share a common abnormality of brain structure or neurochemistry (the "ADHD and sleep disorder have a common cause" theory); and those that propose that the behavioral problems of ADHD and/or the medications used to treat ADHD disrupt sleep (another "ADHD and/or its treatment causes sleep problems" theory).

Picchietti et al. (46) proposed that the link may be due to sleep disruption. They screened 69 children diagnosed with ADHD for symptoms of PLMD. Twenty seven of these children underwent polysomnography. Sixty-seven percent of the 27 children had a PLMI >5/hr plus complaints of disrupted sleep. Eight of 18 children with comorbid ADHD and PLMD had a personal history and a family history of symptoms of RLS. The authors suggested that daytime motor restlessness associated with RLS might contribute to inattention and hyperactivity. In a review of the literature Cortese et al. (86) found strong connections between ADHD and RLS (up to 44% of patients with ADHD also had symptoms of RLS). These authors also suggested that sleep disruption due to RLS may produce daytime symptoms of ADHD. The effects of RLS (such as restlessness or inattention) may be manifest during the daytime, and interpreted as symptoms of ADHD. The authors also found evidence to suggest that ADHD and RLS may be comorbid disorders with a common underlying dopamine deficiency.

A number of studies have investigated the possibility of dopamine deficiency as the underpinning of both PLMD/RLS and ADHD. Dopaminergic therapy is often the treatment of choice for PLMD/RLS in children and adults (62,87). Nieoullon (88), in a review of the literature, noted several studies that suggest dopaminergic dysfunction underlies ADHD in children. Walters et al. (89) provided one of the few direct tests of mechanisms underlying a link between PLMD and ADHD. Working from the hypothesis that both conditions have an underlying dopamine deficiency, they treated seven children who had comorbid ADHD and PLMD/RLS with dopaminergic therapy. Treatment was associated with a significant decrease in symptoms of RLS, and a reduction in the PLMI and associated arousals. Successful treatment of the sleep disorder improved symptoms of ADHD (as measured by The Conners Parent Rating Scale and the Child Behavior Checklist) among all the children. Following treatment, three of the seven children no longer met the criteria for ADHD. In addition, they found that treatment was associated with oppositional-defiant disorder behavior, which frequently co-occurs with ADHD. The improvement could have been due to improved sleep or to increased levels of dopamine. The dopamine dysfunction theory has also been proposed for adults with ADHD (79).

Iron is an essential co-factor in the metabolism of dopamine. Both ADHD (90) and PLMD (87) have been associated with low levels of ferritin. Simakajornboon (87) notes that some children with PLMD have been successfully treated with iron. Some studies have examined the treatment of ADHD with iron supplements. Konofal et al. (91) presented a case study of a three-year-old child who was referred for hyperactivity, inattention, impulsivity, and sleep problems. The child had a low ferritin serum level. After treatment with ferrous sulfate his ferritin level increased and his symptoms of ADHD (as measured by both teachers and parents) improved.

Konofal et al. (90) compared ferritin levels in children with ADHD and in an age- and gender-matched control group. Serum ferritin levels were measured in 53 children with ADHD and 27 controls. The mean level was lower in children with ADHD, and 84% of this group had levels considered abnormal. Ferritin levels correlated with severity of ADHD symptoms. A review of the adult literature indicated self-reports of poor sleep quality and nighttime movement, although few objective measures of sleep corroborate these perceptions (79). The authors suggested that primary sleep disorders may be interpreted as ADHD or co-occur with ADHD. They noted a particular connection between ADHD and RLS and suggested a common underlying dopamine deficiency.

The iron/dopamine connection between PLMD and ADHD implies that the two disorders may be comorbid. Ongoing work from our lab is consistent with this interpretation (92). Symptoms of ADHD and several cognitive variables were measured in children with either SDB or PLMD, both before and after successful treatment for the sleep disorder. Preliminary analyses indicate that although children with either disorder show improvement in parent-ratings of symptoms of ADHD after treatment, the improvement is much more dramatic for children with SDB. After treatment, children with PLMD had significantly worse ADHD scores than children with SDB. Symptoms of ADHD among children with SDB appeared to be resolved after successful treatment, whereas the children with PLMD retained some symptoms. This supports the possibility that children with PLMD may have had comorbid ADHD that remained after the sleep disorder was resolved, whereas the symptoms among children with SDB were a "side effect" of their sleep disorder that disappeared once the sleep disorder was resolved. Support for the "common cause" theory was mixed; since symptoms of ADHD improved after successful treatment of PLMD, but scores remained significantly different from those of children who had been treated for SDB.

PLMD and Other Psychological Outcomes

There is a well-established, probably bidirectional, link between sleep and depression among children (56,93) as well as adults. In addition, depression and ADHD may co-occur (94). Most of the aspects of sleep that have been linked with depression are sleep loss and sleep fragmentation (not specific to a particular disorder). Work by Saletu et al. (95), however, found a connection between RLS and depression and a reduced quality of life, and between PLMD and generalized anxiety relative to controls in an adult sample. A review of the adult literature found that depression was frequently reported by individuals with RLS (24). Picchietti et al. (10) recently conducted a very large (N=10,523 families) online survey of a community sample of children aged 8–11 and 12–17, and found that children with RLS also reported comorbid ADHD (14.8% and 17.6%), depression (3.7% and 14.4%), and anxiety (4.9% and 8.0%). Rates of comorbid ADHD, depression, and anxiety were more likely to have been diagnosed among children in the United States than among children in the United Kingdom. Other work has found that parent reports of children with PLMD were more likely than those of children with SDB to display hyperactivity, aggression, temper, anxiety, and depression (50).

Very little work has been done examining links between PLMD and cognition. A study of adults by Saletu et al. (95) found that both RLS and PLMD patients had worse morning mental performance and fine motor scores compared to controls.

In addition, patients with RLS showed a slowed reaction time, while patients with PLMD exhibited deficits in numerical memory and variability of attention. Pearson et al. (96) looked for cognitive deficits among 16 adults with RLS and age- and gender-matched controls. They used tests that are known to be sensitive to prefrontal cortex functioning and sleep loss (two tests of verbal fluency and Trail Making), tests of executive function (Porteus Maze and Stroop) and general cognitive ability (Colored Progressive Matrices). Patients with RLS showed deficits in tests of prefrontal cortex functioning, but not in tests of executive cognition or general cognitive ability. This suggests deficits similar to those found after one night of sleep deprivation. It cannot be determined from these data whether the deficits were specific to RLS, or due to sleepiness associated with chronic sleep debt or disruption. A small study of children with RLS/PLMS and ADHD found that successful treatment produced improvements in visual but not verbal memory scores (89).

The connection between sleep and ADHD is likely complex and multifaceted. There is evidence to suggest that sleepiness, bedtime resistance, SDB, PLMD, RLS, as well as other sleep disorders, may play a role. Research is needed to isolate disorders, such as ADHD in the absence of any other pathology, or PLMD in the absence of any other sleep disorder, and then to examine connections between these "pure" groups. It may be that the picture varies with different subtypes of ADHD. Corkum et al. (97) addressed both these points. They found that psychopathology comorbid with ADHD may have explained more sleep features than did ADHD, and that the combined subtype (hyperactive/impulsive and inattentive) was associated with involuntary movements during sleep, but that the involuntary movements were better predicted by separation anxiety. Given the absence of a "litmus test" for ADHD, it will be difficult to distinguish between those who actually have ADHD, and those whose behavior presents as ADHD. It may be that some children with a sleep disorder appear to have ADHD but actually have ADHD-like symptoms secondary to the sleep disorder. Others will have ADHD comorbid with their sleep disorder. This distinction could be an important one in deciding courses of treatment for children. Although the relationship is not well understood yet, from a clinical standpoint, there seems to be sufficient evidence to warrant screening children for sleep disorders prior to beginning pharmaceutical treatment for ADHD (75,98).

TREATMENT OF RLS AND PLMD

Evidence-based practice parameters for treatment of RLS and PLMD for adults have been published. These were based on comprehensive reviews of the medical literature (62,63,64,100). Dopaminergic agents, specifically Levodopa with decarboxylase inhibitor, and the dopaminergic agonists specifically Premipexole and Ropinirole were considered effective treatments recommended as the first line therapy (63). Other agents such as opioids, benzodiazepine, anticonvulsant such as gabapentin and iron supplementation have demonstrated therapeutic effects, and treatment outcomes have been reviewed in the adult literature (64). There are no published evidence-based practice parameters for children with RLS and PLMD. To date also, there are no large-scale, cross over, blinded treatment studies in children and hence no specific recommendations regarding pharmacologic treatment of children with RLS and PLMD have been published.

There are, however, case reports on the potential efficacy of these agents in children. In 1999 (47), Picchietti and Walters reported on 16 children with moderate to severe PLMD. Seven of the 16 had daytime somnolence that resolved in all seven

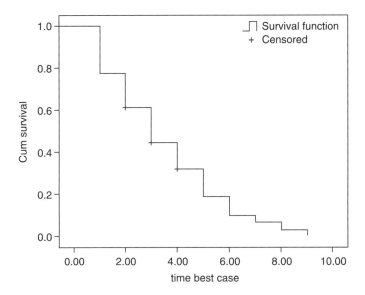

FIGURE 8 Survival analysis demonstrating successful treatment of PLMD: approximately 82% "cured," median time to cure was 3 visits (95% CI = 2–4 visits).

children with dopaminergic medication. Similarly, Walters et al. (89) reported a decrease in the number of PLMS in 7/7 children diagnosed with RLS and treated with dopaminergic agents, and Martinez and Guilleminault (99) reported benefit of pramipexol in decreasing the number of PLMS in 5/6 children with RLS. Simakajornboon (87) reviewed the potential benefit of dopaminergic agents, benzodiazepines, and iron supplementation in childhood PLMD. Konafel reported benefit of Ropinirole in a child with ADHD and RLS (101). Thus, case reports from the literature suggest potential benefit from pharmacologic treatment in children with RLS and PLMD.

A recent retrospective review of treatment outcome in children with diagnosed PLMD by the International Classification of Sleep Disorders (ICSD-2) criteria suggest excellent response to dopamine agonists (102). Figure 8 shows the survival analysis derived from treatment success of 44/54 children with PLMD and no other sleep disorder. Treatment success was defined as clinical resolution of the childrens' sleep disturbances; difficulty with sleep initiation, sleep maintenance, nonrestorative sleep, daytime sleepiness.

The survival analysis was derived from eight post diagnosis and treatment visits to a clinical practice of pediatric sleep medicine and demonstrates that treatment was successful in 82% of patients with a median time to response of three visits. The first line treatment choice in 89% of the children was a dopamine agonist (DA) and in 11% clonazepam; 82% of the children treated with DA versus 11% of children treated with clonazepam responded favorably to the initial medication. Of the 44 who were successfully treated, there was an average of two medication trials. Table 5 lists the agents used in patients successfully treated for PLMD. As in adults, dopamine agonists appear to be highly efficacious.

Other data report success of treatment when defined as improvement of daytime mood and behavioral difficulties (102). Twenty subjects diagnosed with

TABLE 5 Pharmacologic Agents Used for Successful Treatment of PLMD

	N	Percent
Dopamine agonists (DA) (ripinerole, pramepexole)	21	49%
Carbidopa/levidopa (DAminergic)	2	4%
Clonazepam	8	18%
DA + clonazepam	12	27%
DAminergic + clonazepam	1	2%

PLMD based on ICSD-2 criteria were enrolled into a behavioral study where cognition and daytime ADHD symptoms were assessed before and after treatment. Treatment consisted of a DA in 65%, benzodiazepam in 10%, dual treatment with DA and benzodiazepam in 15% and iron supplementation only in 10%. In children diagnosed with PLMD the parent-generated scores on the ADHD test showed significant improvement post-treatment in "hyperactivity" ($p < 0.003$), Impulsivity ($p < 0.05$), and "Inattention" ($p < 0.08$). There is also an anecdotal report of improvement in oppositional defiance symptoms in children with RLS and PLMD treated with dopaminergic agents (89). These data further support benefit from treatment and together underscore the need for large-scale, multi-center, double blind, cross-over pharmacolic studies in children. Table 6 summarizes statements from parents whose children had been successfully treated.

APPROACH TO TREATMENT OF CHILDREN WITH RLS OR PLMD

Healthcare professionals inclusive of family medicine physicians, pediatricians, psychiatrics, school psychologists, teachers, and other professionals who interact with children should be informed about these disorders. Screening questions should be asked during well-child evaluations and in children with sleep disturbances, daytime mood and behavioral difficulties and children with ADHD-like symptoms. Table 7 lists children who should be screened for these disorders and Table 8 lists suggested screening questions derived from validated sleep questionnaires (103).

TABLE 6 Parents' Report After Treatment

"I have a new family"
"I have a different child"
"Her smile is brighter"
"He is laughing more"
"No longer fighting with sibling"
"No longer grumpy"
"More pleasant"
"Teachers report improved behaviors"
"No more morning struggles"
"Feels better in the morning"
"Forgot to take Prozac"
"My legs don't hurt"
"More rested"
"Sleeping better"
"A pleasure to be with"

TABLE 7   Who to Screen

Daytime inattention, distractibility, inability to stay on task
ADHD-type symptoms
Whiny, mood swings
Excessive daytime sleepiness
Impulse control difficulties
Fidgetiness
Complaints of leg aches
Can't sit still
History of sleep disturbances
Report of growing pains
Other high risk groups
  Diabetes, renal failure, iron deficiency anemia, spinal cord problems
  Asperger's and William's Syndromes.

However, not all patients with RLS symptoms or PLMS on PSG need to be treated. Treatment is warranted for patients with sleep disturbances (sleep initiation or maintenance problems, nonrestorative sleep) and daytime consequences of nonrestorative sleep. For instance, if RLS symptoms occur infrequently without sleep disturbances or if a child with PLMS on PSG does not have a sleep disturbance (thus, by definition does not have PLMD), treatment is not indicated. This conundrum has been considered in a recent commentary about childhood RLS and is applicable, as well, to decision-making processes in children with PLMD (104).

RLS is a clinical diagnosis: a screening questionnaire has been proposed (22). Silber et al. published an algorithm for the management of restless legs syndrome in adults (105) that is applicable to children. There are no published algorithms for PLMD. Recently, an approach to the diagnosis of PLMD was developed by a panel of pediatric sleep specialists experienced in the diagnosis and treatment of RLS and PLMD (106). The approach was developed for a Clinical Workshop presented at the Sleep, 2007 meeting in Minneapolis, Minnesota and is summarized in Figure 9.

Firstly, the child should have a sleep complaint, typically sleep initiation or maintenance difficulties. Other clinical presentations include nonrestorative sleep, restless sleep, and daytime somnolence. A thorough clinical history should be obtained inquiring about other disorders that could be causal to the sleep disruption such as anxiety, depression, and others. If there is not another primary reason for the sleep complaint, a polysomnogram should be scheduled. An MSLT should be scheduled for those children with complaints of daytime hypersomnolence when

TABLE 8   Sleep screening questions

Does your child have difficulty falling or staying asleep?
Is your child unrefreshed in the morning after adequate sleep time?
Does your child have restless sleep?
Does your child kick excessively during sleep?
Is your child difficult to awaken in the morning?
Is your child tired, irritable, or grumpy in the morning?
Does your child report uncomfortable or funny feelings in his/her legs?
Does your child have growing pains?

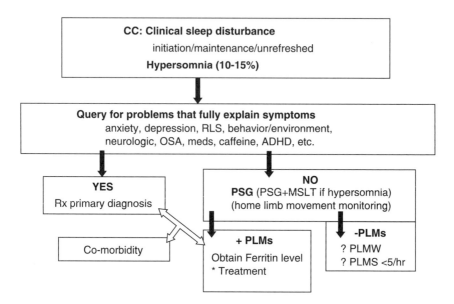

FIGURE 9 Diagnostic algorithm: PLMD in children.

a diagnosis of Narcolepsy is considered. A diagnosis of PLMD is conferred if PSG documents PLMS greater than 5/hr, limb movements are observed on video recording (important component of the pediatric PSG), and not accountable by another sleep disorder. The clinical challenge for diagnosis and treatment of PLMD is the child who presents with sleep complaints, PLMS on PSG < 5/hr, no RLS symptoms but a family history of RLS. Is this night-to-night variability and the PSG was performed "on a good night?" Or does the child have PLMD? What about PLMW on the PSG? Is this RLS with limb movements at rest? (see Current Controversies). The clinical decision to treat should consider all these factors.

If the child is clinically symptomatic, pharmacologic treatment should be considered. Once decision to treat is made, what treatment options are available? Figure 10 outlines an approach to treatment of PLMD proposed by a panel of pediatric sleep specialists and presented as part of a Clinical Workshop (105). This treatment approach is applicable to children with RLS as well.

Dopamine agonists such as ropinirole (Requip) and pramipexole (Mirapex) are considered first-line treatment medications. There are exceptions, especially in young children who cannot swallow a tablet. In this instance, treatment with gabapentin (liquid, 250 mg/5 cc) or clonazepam wafers (0.25 or 0.5 mg) may be considered as first-line treatment. Other agents with reported therapeutic benefits include clonidine and opioids, although the latter are seldom used in children.

In children with RLS or PLMD, a ferritin level should be obtained and iron supplementation initiated for ferritin < 50 ng/ml. A more conservative approach would be to use iron supplementation if ferritin is less than 35 ng/ml. In many instances, especially when the child is symptomatic, initial treatment will be with a pharmacologic agent and iron, assuming a low ferritin level. A reasonable approach

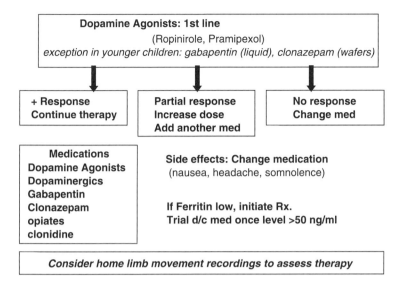

FIGURE 10   Treatment algorithm: RLS and PLMD in children.

would be to continue iron supplementation until the ferritn level is greater than 50 ng/ml at which time the child can be changed to a multivitamin with iron and treatment with a pharmacologic agent could be discontinued. If symptoms recur, then the child would be restarted on the pharmacologic agent.

Side effects should be discussed with the parents, and in certain patients the development of side effects would warrant a change in medication. The most common side effects to the DA are nausea that may be resolved by taking the medicine with crackers or a meal, headache, and a rare paradoxical alerting reaction. Also, DA can induce or aggravate tics. In children, clonazepam can have negative daytime mood and behavioral consequences such as depressed affect, aggression, and irrratibility. Clonazepam can also have a paradoxical alerting reaction at bedtime. Gabapentin has few adverse effects. The reader is directed to "A Clinical Guide to Pediatric Sleep: Diagnosis and Management of Sleep Problems" for a discussion of medication side effects (22).

SUMMARY
1. RLS and PLMD are more common than previously appreciated in the pediatric population.
2. RLS and PLMD are easily recognized by careful history (RLS and PLMD) and polysomnography (PLMD, supportive RLS)
3. RLS and PLMD have significant nocturnal and diurnal consequences that can negatively affect mood, behavior, academic and social success. A summary of the nocturnal and diurnal consequences is presented in Table 9.
4. RLS and PLMD are treatable childhood disorders.

TABLE 9 Nocturnal and Diurnal Clinical Complaints in Children with RLS and PLMD

Symptoms	RLS	PLMD
Bedtime complaints		
Difficulty falling asleep	+	++
"Want to, but cannot"		
Difficulty staying asleep	+	++
Bedtime Resistance Behaviors	+	++
Leg discomfort	+	–
Nocturnal symptoms		
Restless sleep	+	++
Awakenings after sleep onset	+	++
Leg movements in sleep	+	++
Daytime symptoms		
Difficult morning awakening	+	++
Fidgets, "can't sit still"	++	+
Leg discomfort	+	–
Daytime sleepiness	+	++
Daytime mood and behavioral difficulties		
ADHD	+	+
ADHD "symptoms complex"	+	+
Mood swings	+	++
Anxiety	?	+
Depression	+	+
ODD	+	+

CURRENT CONTROVERSIES IN CHILDHOOD RLS, PLMD
What Is Causal to the Insomnia Associated with RLS?

Currently, the diagnosis of RLS does not include a symptom frequency criterion. In cases of severe RLS, patients clearly state the insomnia is due to the unpleasant leg sensations and the need to move the limbs. However, in milder forms of RLS, the symptoms may occur rarely or infrequently yet the sleep disturbance is nightly. PSG may reveal significant PLMS. By current nosology, a diagnosis of RLS trumps PLMD. However, in this situation, the insomnia is nightly, RLS symptoms rare and PLMS on PSG are greater than 5/hr. Is this RLS with PLMS or PLMD with occasional RLS symptoms? Does it matter? Or, could this be a spectrum of a single disorder with the motor component preceding the sensory symptoms? As 80–90% of adults with RLS have associated periodic limb movements in sleep (PLMS) and 15% of patients with RLS will demonstrate PLMW; it is plausible that the sleep disruption associated with RLS is due to the PLMW (sleep initiation problems, insomnia and insufficient sleep) and/or the PLMS (cortical arousals, nonrestorative sleep or sleep maintenance problems). As PLMS are often associated with cortical arousals, the PLMS may have greater pathologic impact (36,107) than the RLS symptoms, especially if the RLS symptoms do not occur on a nightly basis yet the sleep disturbances occur nightly.

Can a Child Have Both RLS and PLMD Disorders?

Similar to the above discussion, patients with occasional RLS symptoms may have demonstrated PLMS on PSG. Is this RLS with PLMS or PLMD with RLS symptoms? Current nosology would say that any symptoms of RLS, regardless of frequency, would trump the diagnosis of PLMD. However, many children have nightly sleep disturbance, infrequent RLS symptoms, and PLMS on PSG, suggesting that the diagnosis should be PLMD with RLS symptoms. The concept of co-occurrence of RLS and PLMD has been proposed (18,87). It may well be that the disorders have overlap and that persons with RLS could also have PLMD although in current nosology, symptoms of RLS trump a diagnosis of PLMD. However, a sleep disturbance that occurs on a nightly basis, with rare RLS symptoms and PLMS on PSG: Is this RLS, PLMD or both?

Any Clinical Significance to Periodic Limb Movements in Quiet Wakefulness (PLMW)?

The significance of PLMS is controversial and has been recently debated (38,39). Less is known about the significance of PLMW. PLMW are often seen in persons with RLS and often used as a supportive diagnosis. Also, PLMW is the diagnostic feature in the immobilization test for RLS (29). Typically, PLMW are associated with RLS symptoms. In childhood, PLMW appear with greater frequency (28) although the functional sequelae are unknown. There have been recent case presentations of children with sleep initiation difficulties, no RLS symptoms, mild limb movements in sleep (less than 5/hr) and PLMW documented on PSG (108). Are PLMW causal to the insomnia or physiologic in childhood? Or are the PLMS demonstrating a night-to-night variability with the night of the PSG capturing mild movements in sleep? Does this matter for treatment considerations? Is a trial of RLS/PLMD treatment indicated? Should the clinician simply obtain a ferritin level? Treatment considerations should include the clinical history (what is the child's sleep history, restless, excessive kicking, was the night's PSG representative of a typical night's sleep?), PSG findings and daytime sequelae. A simple, first-line therapy could be to obtain a ferritin level and treat if less that 50 ng/ml. If the child is more symptomatic, then pharmacologic treatment would be indicated.

REFERENCES

1. Garcia-Borreguero d, Egatz R, Winkelmann J, et al. Epidemiology of "restless legs syndrome" The current status. Sleep Med Rev 2006, 10:153 67.
2. Walters AS, Hickey K, Maltzman J, et al. A questionnaire study of 138 patients with restless legs syndrome: The "night walkers" survey. Neurol 1996; 46:92–5.
3. Montplaisir J, Boucher Boucher S, Poirier G, et al. Clinical, polysomnographic, and genetic characteristics of restless legs syndrome: A study of 133 patients diagnosed with new standard criteria. Mov Disord 1997; 12:61–5.
4. Ekbom KA. Restless legs: A clinical study. Acta Med Scand 1945; 158(suppl):1–122.
5. Walters AS. Toward a better definition of the restless legs syndrome. Mov Disord 1995; 5:634–42.
6. Allen RP, Picchietti D, Hening WA, et al. Restless legs syndrome: Diagnostic criteria, special considerations, and epidemiology. A report from the restless legs syndrome diagnosis and epidemiology workshop at the National Institutes of Health. Sleep Med 2003; 4:101–19.

7. American Academy of Sleep Medicine. International classification of sleep disorders, 2nd edn Diagnostic and Coding Manual. Westchester, Illinois: American Academy of Sleep Medicine, 2005: pp. 178–81.

8. Hening WA. Restless legs syndrome: The most common and least diagnosed sleep disorder. Sleep Med 2004; 5:429–30.

9. Montplaisisir J, Michaud M, Petit D. New trends in restless legs syndrome research. Sleep Med Rev 2006; 10:147–51.

10. Picchietti D, Allen RP, Walters AS, et al. Restless legs syndrome: Prevalence and impact in children and adolescents. The Peds REST Study. Pediatr 2007; 120:253–66.

11. Winkelmann J, Ferini-Strambi L. Genetic of restless legs syndrome. Sleep Med Rev 2006; 10:179–83.

12. Merlino G, Fratticci L, Valente M, et al. Association of restless legs syndrome in Type 2 diabetes: A case-control study. Sleep 2007; 30(7):866–71.

13. Happe S, Treptau N, Ziegler R, et al. Restless legs syndrome and sleep problems in children and adolescents with insulin-dependent diabetes mellitus type 1. Neuropediatr 2005; 36:98–103.

14. Allen R, Earley C. Restless legs syndrome: A review of clinical and pathophysiologic features. J Clin Neurophysiol 2001; 18:128–47.

15. International Restless Legs Syndrome Study Group. Validation of the International Restless Legs Syndrome Study Group rating scale for restless legs syndrome. Sleep Med 2003; 4:121–32.

16. Kotagal S, Silber MH. Childhood-onset restless legs syndrome. Ann Neurol 2004; 56:803–7.

17. Walters AS, Picchietti DL, Ehrenberg BL, et al. Restless legs syndrome in childhood and adolescence. Pediatr Neurol 1994; 11:241–5.

18. Mindell JA, Owens JA. Resltess Legs Syndrome and Periodic Limb Movment Disorder. In: Mindell JA, Owens JA, eds A Clinical Guide to Pediatric Sleep: Diagnosis and Management of Sleep Problems. Philadelphia: Lippincott Williams & Wilkins, 2003: pp. 123–34.

19. Ekbom KA. Growing pains and restless legs. Acta Pediatr Scand 1975; 64:264–6.

20. Rajaram S, Walters AS, England S, et al. Some children with growing pains may actually have restless legs syndrome. Sleep 2004; 27:767–73.

21. Walters AS. Is there a subpopulation of children with growing pains who really have restless legs syndrome? A review of the literature. Sleep Med 2002; 3:93–8.

22. Mindell JA, Owens JA. AppendixD: Screening Questionnaire for Restless Legs Syndrome. In: Mindell JA, Owens JA, eds A Clinical Guide to Pediatric Sleep: Diagnosis and Management of Sleep Problems. Philadelphia: Lippincott Williams & Wilkins, 2003: pp. 230–321.

23. Michaud M, Paquet J, Lavigne G, et al. Sleep laboratory diagnosis of restless legs syndrome. Eur Neurol 2002; 48:108–13.

24. Picchietti D, Winkelman JW. Restless legs syndrome: Periodic limb movements in sleep and depression. Sleep 2005; 28(7):891–8.

25. Walters AS, Lavigne G, Hening W, et al. The scoring of movements in sleep. J Clin Sleep Med 2007; 3(2):155–67.

26. American Sleep Disorder Association (ASDA). Atlas task force of the American Sleep Disorders Association. Recording and scoring leg movements. Sleep 1993; 16:748–59.

27. Coleman RM, Pollak CP, Wertzman ED. Periodic movements in sleep (nocturnal myoclonus): Relation to sleep disorders. Ann Neurol 1980; 8:416–21.

28. Pennestri M-H, Whittom S, Adam B, et al. PLMS and PLMW in healthy subjects as a function of age: prevalence and interval distribution. Sleep 2006; 29 (9):1183–7.

29. Michaud M, Poirier GG, Lavigne, et al. Restless legs syndrome: Scoring criteria for leg movement recorded during the suggested immobilization test. Sleep Med 2001; 2:317–21.

30. Pollmacher T, Schulz H. Periodic leg movements (PLM): Their relationship to sleep stages. Sleep 1993; 16(6):572–7.

31. Symonds CP. Nocturnal myoclonus. J Neurol Neurosurg Psychiat 1953; 16:166–171.

32. Lugaresi E, Coccagna G, Mantovani M, et al. Some periodic phenomena arising during drowsiness and sleep in man. Electoencephalogr Clin Neurophysiol 1972; 32:701–5.
33. Coleman RM. Periodic movements in sleep (nocturnal myoclonus) and restless legs syndrome. In: Guilleminault C, ed. Sleep and waking disorders: Indications and techniques. Menlo Park, CA: Addison Wesley, 1982: pp. 265–95.
34. Zucconi M, Ferri R, Allen R, et al. The official world association of sleep medicine (WASM) standards for recording and scoring periodic leg movements in sleep (PLMS) and wakefulness (PLMW) developed in collaboration with a task force from the International restless legs syndrome study group (IRLSSG). Sleep Med 2006; 7(2):175–83.
35. American Academy of Sleep Medicine. International classification of sleep disorders, 2nd edn Diagnostic and Coding Manual. Westchester, Illinois: American Academy of Sleep Medicine, 2005: pp. 187–8.
36. Carrier J, Frenette S, Montplaisir J, et al. Effects of periodic leg movements during sleep in middle-aged subjects without sleep complaints. Mov Disord 2005; 20(9):1127–32.
37. Haba-Rubio J, Staner L, Krieger J, et al. What is the clinical significance of periodic limb movements during sleep? Neurophysiol Clin 2004; 34:293–300.
38. Hog B. Periodic limb movements are associated with disturbed sleep. J Clin Sleep Med 2007; 3(1):12–14.
39. Mahowald M. Periodic limb movements are not associated with disturbed sleep. J Clin Sleep Med 2007; 3(1):15–17.
40. Picchietti D. Periodic limb movements in sleep: irrelevant epiphenomenon, marker for a potential problem, or a disorder? J Clin Sleep Med 2006; 2(4):446–7.
41. Montgomery-Downs HE, O'Brien LM, Gulliver TE, et al. Polysomnographic characteristics in normal preschool and early school-aged children. Pediatr 2006; 117(3):741–53.
42. O'Brien LM, Holbrook CR, Jones VF, et al. Ethnic difference in periodic limb movements in children. Sleep Med 2007; 8:240–6.
43. Godbout R, Bergeron C, Limoges E, et al. A laboratory study of sleep in Asperger's syndrome. Neuroreport 2000; 11(1):127–30.
44. Arens R, Wright B, Elliott J, et al. Periodic limb movement in sleep in children with Williams syndrome. J Pediatr 1998; 133:670–4.
45. Tayag-Kier CE, Keenan GF, Scalzi LV, et al. Sleep and periodic limb movement in sleep in juvenile fibromyalgia. Pediatr 2000; 106(5):e70.
46. Picchietti DL, England SJ, Walters AS, et al. Periodic limb movement disorder and restless legs syndrome in children with attention-deficit hyperactivity disorder. J Child Neurol 1998; 13(12):588–94.
47. Picchietti DL, Walters AS. Moderate to severe periodic limb movement disorder in childhood and adolescence. Sleep 1999; 22(3):297–300.
48. Crabtree VM, Ivanenko A, O'Brien LM, et al. Periodic limb movement disorder of sleep in children. J Sleep Res 2003; 12(1):73–81.
49. Gaultney JF, Gingras JL, Merchant K. Does a periodic limb movement index (PLMI) > 5 uniquely define periodic limb movement disorder (PLMD) in children? Sleep 2006, 29 (abstract supplement), A89.
50. Gingras JL, Gaultney JK, Merchant K. Clinical Presentation, daytime sequelae among children with periodic limb movement disorder and sleep disrupted breathing: A comparative study. Sleep 2006; 29 (abstract supplement):A90.
51. VG Bohn S. Periodic limb movements in children: Prevalence in a referred population. Sleep 2004; 27(2):313–15.
52. Picchietti D, Stevens HE. Early manifestation of restless legs syndrome in childhood and adolescents. Sleep Med 2007; in press.
53. Hornyak M, Kopasz M, Feige B, et al. Variability of periodic leg movements in various sleep disorders: Implications of clinical and pathophysiologic studies. Sleep 2005; 28(3):331–5.
54. Mosko SS, Dickel MJ, Ashurst J. Night-to-night variability in sleep apnea and sleep in sleep-related periodic leg movements in the elderly. Sleep 1988; 11:340–8.

55. Durmer J. "Pathophysiology of RLS and PLMD " presented in a Clinical Discussion " RLS and PLMD in Childhood: Current Diagnostic and Treatment Considerations. Gingras J, Ivanenko A, Co-Chairs. Panelests: Durmer J, Walters A, Picchietti D, Chervin R. Sleep 2006, Salt Lake City, Utah.

56. Ivanenko A, Crabtree VM, Gozal D. Sleep in children with psychiatric disorders. Pediatr Clin N Am 2004; 51(1):51–68.

57. American Academy of Sleep Medicine. International classification of sleep disorders, 2nd edn Diagnostic and Coding Manual. Westchester, Illinois: American Academy of Sleep Medicine, 2005: pp. 213–15.

58. Paulus W, Schomburg E. Dopamine and the spinal cord in restless legs syndrome: Does spinal cord physiology reveal a basis for augmentation? Sleep Med Rev 2006; 10:185–96.

59. Walters AS. Review of receptor agonist and antagonist studies relevant to the opiate system in restless legs syndrome. Sleep Med 2002; 3:301–4.

60. Elrich J, Treede RD. Concergence of nociceptive and non-nociceptive inputs onto spinal reflex pathways to the tibialis anterior muscle in humans. Acta Physiol Scand 1998; 163(4):391–401.

61. Bucher SS, Seelos KC, Oertel WH, et al. Cerebral generators involved in the pathogenesis of the restless legs syndrome. Ann Neurol 1997; 41:639–45.

62. Chesson AL Jr, Wise M, Davila D, et al. Practice parameters for the treatment of restless legs syndrome and periodic limb movement disorder. An American Academy of Sleep Medicine Report. Standards of Practice Committee of the American Academy of Sleep Medicine. Sleep 1999; 22:961–8.

63. Littner MR, Kushida C, McDowell A, et al. Practice parameters for the dopaminergi treatment of restless legs syndrome and periodic limb movement disorder. Sleep 2004; 27(3):557–9.

64. Vignatelli L, Billiard M, Clarenbach P, et al. EFNS guidelines on management of restless legs syndrome and periodic limb movement disorder in sleep. Eur J Neurol 2006; 13:1049–65.

65. Earley C, Heckler D, Allen R. The treatment of RLS with intravenous iron dextran. Sleep Med 2004; 5(3):231–5.

66. Sun ER, Chen CA, Ho G, et al. Iron and the restless legs syndrome. Sleep 1998; 21:371–7.

67. Simakajomboon N, Gozal D, Blasic V, et al. Peirdic limb movment in sleep and iron status in children. Sleep 2003; 26:735–8.

68. Kryger MH, Otake K, Foerster J. Low body stores of iron on restless legs syndrome: A correctable cause of insomnia in adolescents and teenagers. Sleep Med 2002; 3:127–32.

69. Owens JA. The ADHD and sleep conundrum: A review. J Dev Behav Pediatr 2005; 26:312–22.

70. Wiggs L, Montgomery P, Stores G. Actigraphic and parent reports of sleep patterns and sleep disorders in children with subtypes of attention-deficit hyperactivity disorder. Sleep 2005; 28:1437–45.

71. O'Brien LM, Holbrook CR, Mervis, CB, et al. Sleep and neurobehavioral characteristics of 5- to 7-year-old children with parentally reported symptoms of attention-deficit/hyperactivity disorder. Pediatr; 2003; 111(3):554–63.

72. Sangal RB, Owens JA, Sangal J. Patients with attention-deficit/hyperactivity disorder without observed apneic episodes in sleep or daytime sleepiness have normal sleep on polysomnography. Sleep 2006; 28:1041–42.

73. Lecendreux M, Konofal E, Bouvard M, et al. Sleep and alertness in children with ADHD. J Child Psychol and Psychiat 2000; 41:803–12.

74. Aronen ET, Paavonen EJ, Fjallberg M, et al. Sleep and psychiatric symptoms in school-age children. J Am Acad Child Adolesc Psychiat 2000; 39:502–8.

75. Golan N, Shahar E, Ravid S, Pillar G. Sleep disorders and daytime sleepiness in children with attention-deficit/hyperactive disorder. Sleep 2004; 27:261–6.

76. Chervin RD, Dillon JE, Bassetti C, et al. Symptoms of sleep disorders, inattention, and hyperactivity in children. Sleep 1997; 20:1185–92.

77. Chervin RD, Dillon JE., Archbold, KH, Ruzicka DL. Conduct problems and symptoms of sleep disorders in children. J Am Acad Child Adolesc Psychiat 2003; 42:201–8.
78. Sadeh A, Pergamin L, Bar-Haim Y. Sleep in children with attention-deficit hyperactivity disorder: A meta-analysis of polysomnographic studies. Sleep Med Rev 2006; 10:381–98.
79. Philipsen A, Hornyak M, Riemann D. Sleep and sleep disorders in adults with attention deficit/hyperactivity disorder. Sleep Med Rev 2006; 10:399–405.
80. Wagner ML, Walters AS, Fisher BC. Symptoms of attention-deficit/hyperactivity disorder in adults with restless legs syndrome. Sleep 2004; 27:1499–504.
81. Gaultney JF, Terrell DF, Gingras JL. Parent-reported periodic limb movement, sleep disordered breathing, bedtime resistance behaviors, and ADHD. Behavi Sleep Med 2005; 3:32–43.
82. Crabtree VM, Ivanenko A, Gozal D. Clinical and parental assessment of sleep in children with attention-deficit/hyperactivity disorder referred to a pediatric sleep medicine center. Clin Pediatr 2003; 42:807–13.
83. Chervin RD, Archbold KH, Dillon JE, et al. Associations between symptoms of inattention, hyperactivity, restless legs, and periodic leg movements. Sleep 2002; 25:213–18.
84. Picchietti DL, Underwood DJ, Farris WA. et al. Further studies on periodic limb movement disorder and restless legs syndrome in children with attention-deficit hyperactivity disorder. Mov Disord 1999; 14:1000–7.
85. Lewin DS, Di Pinto M. Sleep disorders and ADHD: Shared and common phenotypes. Sleep 2004; 27:188–9.
86. Cortese S, Konofal E, Ledendreux M, et al. Restless legs syndrome and attention-deficit/hyperactivity disorder: A review of the literature. Sleep 2005; 28:1007–13.
87. Simakajornboon N. Periodic limb movement disorder in children. Paediatr Resp Rev 2006; 7:S55–S57.
88. Nieoullon, A. Dopamine and the regulation of cognition and attention. Prog Neurobiol 2002; 67:53–83.
89. Walters AS, Mandelbaum DE, Lewin DS, et al. Dopaminergic therapy in children with restless legs/periodic limb movements in sleep and ADHD. Dopaminergic Therapy Study Group. Pediatric Neurol 2000; 22:182–6.
90. Konofal E, Lecendreux M, Arnulf I, Mouren MC. Iron deficiency in children with attention-deficit/hyperactivity disorder. Arch Pediatr and Adolesc Med 2004; 158:1113–5.
91. Konofal E, Cortese S, Lecendreux M, et al. Effectiveness of iron supplementation in a young child with attention-deficit/hyperactivity disorder. Pediatr 2005; 116:732–4.
92. Gaultney JF, Gingras JL. Cognitive and behavioral outcomes associated with insufficient/disordered sleep among children. Talk presented at the American Association of SIDS Prevention Physicians meeting in Charlotte, NC, October 2006.
93. Ivanenko A, Crabtree VM., Gozal D. Sleep and depression in children and adolescents. Sleep Med Rev 2005; 9:115–29.
94. Ostrander R, Crystal DS, August G. Attention deficit-hyperactivity disorder, depression, and self- and other-assessments of social competence: A developmental study. J Abnorm Child Psychol 2006; 34:773–87.
95. Saletu M, Anderer P, Saletu M, et al. EEG mapping, psychometric, and polysomnographic studies in restless legs syndrome (RLS) and periodic limb movement disorder (PLMD) patients as compared with normal controls. Sleep Med 2002; 3:S35–S42.
96. Pearson VE, Allen RP, Dean, T, et al. Cognitive deficits associated with restless legs syndrome (RLS). Sleep Med 2006; 7:25–30.
97. Corkum P, Moldofsky H, Hogg-Johnson S, et al. Sleep problems in children with attention-deficit/hyperactivity disorder: Impact of subtype, comorbidity, and stimulant medication. Am Acad Child Adolesc Psychiat 1999; 38:1285–93.
98. Huang YS, Chen NH, Li HY, et al. Sleep disorders in Taiwanese children with attention deficit/hyperactivity disorder. J Sleep Res 2004; 13:269–77.

99. Martinez S, Guilleminault C. Periodic leg movements in prepubertal children with sleep disturbance. Dev Med Child Neurol 2004; 46:765–70.
100. Hornyak M, Feige B, Riemann D, et al. Periodic leg movements in sleep and periodic limb movement disorder: Prevalence, clinical significance and treatment. Sleep Med Rev 2006; 10:169–77.
101. Konofal E, Arnulf I, Lecendreux, et al. Ropinirole in a child with attention-deficit hyperactivity disorder and restless legs syndrome. Pediatr Neurol 2005; 32:350–1.
102. Gaultney JF, Gingras JL. "PLMD in Childhood: Does treatment alter outcome?" Talk presented in a Clinical Workshop entitled "Diagnostic and Clinical Challenges in Children with Periodic Limb Movement Disorder (PLMD): Toward a Rational Diagnosis and Treatment Approach. Chair: Gingras JL, Panelests: Durmer J, Gaultney J, Ivanenko A, Picchietti D, Walters A. The Association of Professional Sleep Societies, Sleep 2007. Minneapolis, MN.
103. Chervin RD, Hedger KR. Clinical prediction of periodic leg movements during sleep in children. Sleep Med 2001; 2:501–10.
104. Blum NJ, Mason T, II. Restless Legs Syndrome: What is a pediatrician to do? Pediatr 2007; 120:438–9.
105. Silber MH, Ehrenberg BL, Allen RP, et al. An algorithm for the management of restless legs syndrome. Mayo Clin Proc 20004; 79:916–22.
106. Gingras JL (Chair), Durmer J, Gaultney J, Ivanenko A, Picchietti D, Walters A. "Diagnostic and Clinical Challenges in Children with Periodic Limb Movement Disorder (PLMD): Toward a Rational Diagnosis and Treatment Approach." Clinical Discussion presented at the Association of Professional Sleep Societies, Sleep 2007, Minneapolis, MN.
107. Sforza E, Nicolas A, Lavigne G, et al. EEG and cardiac activation during periodic leg movements in sleep: Support for a hierarchy of arousal responses. Neurol 1999; 52:786–91.
108. Gingras JL. "Clinical significance of PLMW" case presentation in a Clinical Workshop entitled "Diagnostic and Clinical Challenges in Children with Periodic Limb Movement Disorder (PLMD): Toward a Rational Diagnosis and Treatment Approach." Chair: Gingras JL. Panelists: Durmer J, Gaultney J, Ivanenko A, Picchietti D, Walters A. Presented at the Association of Professional Sleep Societies, Sleep 2007, Minneapolis, MN.

Venkataramanujan Srinivasan,[a] Seithikurippu R. Pandi-Perumal,[b]
D. Warren Spence,[c] Marcel G. Smits,[d] Kristiaan B. van der Heijden,[e]
and Daniel P. Cardinali[f]

[a]Department of Physiology, School of Medical Sciences, University Sains
Malaysia, Kelantan, Malaysia
[b]Division of Clinical Pharmacology and Experimental Therapeutics, Department
of Medicine, College of Physicians and Surgeons of Columbia University, New
York, New York, U.S.A.
[c]Sleep and Alertness Clinic, University Health Network, Toronto, Ontario, Canada
[d]Centre for Sleep-Wake Disorders and Chronobiology, Hospital Gelderse Vallei,
Ede, The Netherlands
[e]Leiden University, Centre for the Study of Developmental Disorders, Leiden, The
Netherlands
[f]Department of Physiology, Faculty of Medicine, University of Buenos Aires,
Buenos Aires, Argentina

INTRODUCTION

Attention deficit hyperactivity disorder (ADHD) is a neurodevelopmental disability characterized by the occurrence of deficits in attention, hyperactivity or impulsivity or both. It co-occurs with many other developmental disorders such as mental retardation, cerebral palsy, autism, communication disorders, and learning disabilities (1).

A biological basis for the symptoms of ADHD was suspected ever since George Still described the salient features of ADHD (2). Study of neurobiology of ADHD is often based on anatomical, neurochemical and genetic bases (3). There is no single pathophysiological profile for ADHD. Dysfunction in fronto-subcortical pathways has been suggested as this pathway controls both attention and motor behavior (3,4).

Both dopamine (DA) and norepinephrine (NE) have been implicated in ADHD. Right sided frontal-striatal dysfunction due to impairment of mesocortical dopamine system has been proposed by Heilman and his co-workers (5). An altered role of DA systems in working memory and inhibitory processes may play a central role in ADHD (4).

ADHD is often associated with sleep problems, an initial insomnia characterized by long sleep onset latency (SOL). Of the 16 studies on subjective complaints by parents of children with ADHD, a majority indicate that sleep complaints are common in this disorder (6,7). Fragmented sleep and frequent nocturnal awakenings with disruption in circadian rhythms have been disturbing both to parents as well as to children. Children with ADHD and sleep onset insomnia have been found to have a delayed endogenous pacemaker as measured by delayed sleep onset and time of awakening (8–10). Chronic sleep onset insomnia in children with ADHD closely resembles the delayed sleep phase syndrome (DSPS), in that it is not only the sleep onset that is delayed but the onset of endogenous melatonin production (dim light melatonin onset [DLMO]) (11) is also delayed. It must be noted however that a tandem repeat polymorphism of the Per 3 gene, one of the major clock genes, has been found associated with DSPS but not with ADHD-related chronic sleep onset insomnia (12).

The close relationship between the nocturnal increase of endogenous melatonin and timing of sleep in humans suggests that melatonin is involved in the regulation of sleep/wake rhythm. Endogenous melatonin is considered as the best index of circadian timing in humans (13) and exogenous melatonin has been successfully used to treat a number of circadian rhythm sleep disorders (CRSD), such as DSPS, sleep disorders associated with shift-work, jet lag or mood disorders (14,15). Melatonin has been shown to be useful for the amelioration of sleep complaints in patients with various neurodevelopmental disabilities (16,17). Indeed, understanding the use of melatonin in a variety of pediatric patients will be helpful to evaluate the potential use of melatonin in pediatric sleep pharmacopeia (8,18).

MELATONIN

Melatonin is an ubiquitous biological signaling molecule that has been identified in all major taxa of organisms, different plants, invertebrates, and vertebrates (19,20). Melatonin has diverse physiological functions, signaling not only the time of day, or the season of the year, but also having immunomodulatory and cytoprotective roles. Because of its chronobiotic and sleep inducing properties, melatonin and its analogs are useful for the treatment of various CRSDs (14,15).

Though it is primarily synthesized in the pineal gland of all mammals, it also plays the role of autacoid, being locally synthesized in places like the retina, bone marrow cells, platelets, lymphocytes, skin, or the gastrointestinal tract (19,20). The enzymatic machinery for the biosynthesis of melatonin was first identified by Axelrod (21). Tryptophan is taken up from the blood and is converted into 5-hydroxytryptophan and then to 5-hydroxytryptamine (5-HT; serotonin).Subsequently, 5-HT is acetylated to form N-acetylserotonin by the enzyme arylakylamine N-acetyltransferase (AA-NAT). N-acetylserotonin is converted into melatonin through the action of hydroxyindole-O-methyl transferase (HIOMT). Once formed, melatonin is released from the pineal gland into the blood and also into the cerebrospinal fluid (CSF) (22).

Pineal melatonin production displays a very constant and remarkable circadian rhythm, with very low levels during daytime and high levels at night (23). This circadian rhythm persists in most animals as well as in humans under constant environmental conditions. The maximum plasma level occurs normally between 02.00 and 03.00 hrs (23) in adults, but earlier in children depending on age and, to a lesser extent, on behavioral and environmental factors. It is interesting to note that the melatonin rhythm is reproducible with great accuracy on successive nights in the same individual although considerable interindividual variations in the abundance of melatonin secretion occur. The genetic origin of these interindividual variations has been emphasised (24,25).

The half life of melatonin after intravenous infusion is about 30 minutes. Melatonin is metabolized mainly in the liver. It is first hydroxylated and then amalgamated with sulfate and glucuronide to form 6-sulfatoxymelatonin (aMT6s), which is the main metabolite found in the urine. Recent evidence shows that nearly 30% of overall melatonin is converted into pyrrole ring cleavage to form

N^1–acetyl-N^2–acetyl-5methoxykynuramine (AFMK). AFMK appears to be a major metabolite of melatonin oxidation in non-hepatic tissues (26). Since melatonin easily diffuses through biological membranes, it can exert actions on almost every cell in the body.

Environmental light/dark (LD) cycle acts as the pervasive and pre-eminent *Zeitgeber* that regulates melatonin synthesis by acting via the suprachiasmatic nucleus (SCN) of the hypothalamus. The circadian pattern of pineal AA-NAT and melatonin production and secretion is abolished by lesions of the SCN (27). The circadian activity of the SCN is synchronized to the LD cycle mainly by light that is perceived by the retina. The signal generated in the retina is then transmitted to the SCN through a monosynaptic retinohypothalamic tract that originates in the ganglion cell layer in the retina. These retinal ganglion cells contain a unique photopigment, melanopsin, and are involved in photic transmission of light signals to the SCN (28).

The neural pathway that connects SCN with the pineal gland starts by a GABAergic projection from the SCN to the subparaventricular zone and to the dorsomedial nucleus of the hypothalamus, which is crucial for producing circadian rhythms of sleep and waking (29). The neural pathway then follows to the spinal cord via the medial forebrain bundle and the reticular formation and makes synaptic connections with neurons in the intermediolateral columns of the cervical spinal cord, from where preganglionic sympathetic fibers to the superior cervical ganglion (SCG) emerge. The postganglionic sympathetic fibers from the SCG reach the pineal gland and release NE, which controls pineal melatonin synthesis (30). During the light phase, the SCN electrical activity is high and this inhibits discharge of NE from sympathetic fibers. During the scotophase, the electrical activity of SCN is inhibited and NE release from sympathetic nerve fibers is augmented (31). Melatonin is thus produced and released from the pineal gland during the time of electrical "quiescence" of the SCN occurring during the night.

Melatonin exerts its actions on various bodily systems in part through the membrane receptors MT_1 and MT_2 (32). Melatonin MT_1 and MT_2 receptors belong to the superfamily of G-protein coupled receptors displaying the typical seven transmembrane domains. The presence of MT_1 and MT_2 receptors in the SCN are responsible for the circadian pacemaker activity, MT_2 acting by inducing phase shifts and MT_1 acting by suppressing neuronal firing activity (32). Putative nuclear receptors have also been described. Additionally, direct effects of melatonin on intracellular proteins like calmodulin, tubulin or quinone reductase 2 (the "MT_3 receptor"), as well as actions on the mitochondria, underlie the complex effects of melatonin on the cells (19).

MELATONIN AND SLEEP

Among the various functions attributed to melatonin, its sleep/wake rhythm regulating function has received major attention. The close relationship between the nocturnal increase of endogenous melatonin and the timing of human sleep has prompted many investigators to implicate melatonin as a major regulator of sleep timing (33). The occurrence of human sleep is better if sleep is taken during the appropriate period of melatonin secretion. Measurement of melatonin or of urinary aMT6s rhythms has been found useful in diagnosing DSPS and non-24-hour sleep/wake disorders both in blind people as well as in sighted persons (23).

Melatonin regulates the quantity of sleep through its effects on MT_1 receptors in the SCN, inhibiting the firing of SCN neurons thus widening the differences between day and night. Melatonin also regulates the sleep timing mechanism, this phase shifting effect being attributed to its action on SCN MT_2 receptors (34). Altered melatonin secretion and sleep patterns have been documented in permanent night-shift workers (35).

Melatonin is now widely used to treat sleep disorders in children with central nervous system (CNS) disabilities. For example, melatonin has become a major therapeutic tool in many clinical neurophysiology departments of the UK (36). Melatonin has been found effective for inducing sleep during sleep electroencephalogram (EEG) recordings in uncooperative children (37). It is also used in pediatric neuroimaging studies, for inducing sleep in order to obtain successful brain magnetic resonance imaging in children with severe learning and behavioral difficulties (38). Melatonin use effectively replaces the need for employing sedation or general anesthetics and could be a safe effective method for analyzing not only normal sleep patterns but also for the treatment of pediatric sleep disorders (36).

So far, no significant adverse events of melatonin treatment have been found. However, the application of melatonin treatment in children remains a topic of considerable debate since its long-term effects have not been sufficiently investigated. Particularly, its effect on the gonadotropic system and onset of puberty (39), and on potential pro-convulsant properties requires closer scrutiny (40). One study systematically conducted a two-year follow-up in 24 children with ADHD and sleep onset insomnia (age 6–12 years). Two years after starting with melatonin treatment, 20 children (83%) still used melatonin. During the two-year treatment period no significant adverse events had occurred. More such systematic studies are needed to investigate long-term adverse effects of melatonin on younger children and on adolescents as well.

SLEEP DISTURBANCES IN ADHD
Sleep problems have frequently been encountered in children with learning difficulties. It is estimated that nearly 80% of children with neurodevelopmental disabilities have sleep problems. In a sample of 200 subjects examined, 51% of children had settling problems while 67% had waking problems (41). Sleep problems are associated with daytime behavioral problems, poor communication, irritability, or epilepsy, suggesting a neurological component of sleep disorder (42).

Studies undertaken in children with ADHD by employing objective sleep measures like polysomnography (PSG) or actigraphy, did not reveal major differences between ADHD and controls, in respect of sleep onset latency (SOL) or sleep duration (10). Concerning sleep architecture, there are studies indicating a significant decrease in rapid eye movement (REM) sleep in ADHD children while others did not find such a difference (for ref. see [10]). In a study employing the multiple sleep latency test (MSLT) in 32 boys with ADHD, there was a higher physiological tendency to fall asleep during the day as compared to 22 normal controls (43). The unstable sleep patterns seen in ADHD children have been attributed to arousal dysregulation (12).

The several parental observations studies in children with ADHD have shown abnormally high levels of activity during their sleep and this has been confirmed by objective methods using either actimetry or infrared camera recordings.

Motor restlessness during sleep can be a manifestation of periodic limb movement disorder (PLMD) (10). It can be concluded that despite methodological limitations, sleep disorder remains a major problem for many individuals with developmental disabilities (43). Indeed, the 16 studies that examined subjective complaints by parents of children with ADHD indicate clearly that sleep complaints are common among ADHD children (7). In a recent report, stimulant use, presence of depressive disorder, and bedtime resistance were the key risk factors of sleep onset insomnia in ADHD (44).

TREATMENT OF ADHD

Over the years, stimulant treatment remained as the first line of treatment for ADHD. In the United States 85% of children with ADHD receive stimulant medication (45). However, it has been noted by many investigators that use of stimulant medications actually increased SOL (46). Other medications include the a_2 agonist clonidine, bupropion, tricyclic antidepressants or guanfacine. A recent review and expert opinion on the use of atomoxetine (a highly selective NE reuptake inhibitor) in children with ADHD claim that this drug is safe and efficacious for treating ADHD in six to seven-year-old children, reducing the core symptoms of ADHD (47).

As there is some evidence that both ADHD and PLMD are genetically linked and are related to alteration of the DA system (48), dopaminergic agents have been used. Indeed, the use of dopaminergic therapy in children with PLMD and comorbid ADHD improved symptoms of PLMD as well as those of ADHD (49).

MELATONIN TREATMENT IN CHILDREN WITH ADHD AND RELATED DISORDERS

It has been found that children with ADHD and sleep onset insomnia have a delayed endogenous circadian pacemaker, as revealed by the findings of delayed sleep onset, dim light melatonin onset (DLMO) and time of awakening (8–10). Since melatonin plays a crucial role in regulating bodily rhythms it has been used as a drug to synchronize the internal bodily rhythms to the external LD cycles.

Jan and his co-workers were the first to propose the use of oral melatonin in the treatment of chronic sleep disorders in children with neural disabilities (6). Melatonin in doses ranging from 2.5 mg to 10 mg at bedtime was safe and effective to improve sleep in more than 80% of children suffering from chronic sleep–wake cycle disturbances (6). Some chronic sleep–wake cycle disorders in children with neurodevelopmental disabilities responded immediately to melatonin, whereas others waited 1–4 weeks for normalization of sleep pattern. Since oral administration appears to be safe, effective, and cost-efficient, it certainly has improved the management of sleep disorders in children and has helped to rescue the families from despair. The average number of hours asleep daily improved from a mean of 6.8 hours before melatonin to 7.9 hours after taking melatonin. In addition the average number of awakenings per night, average number of nights with delayed sleep onset, and average number of nights with early morning arousals were all remarkably decreased after initiation of melatonin therapy (16).

The efficacy of melatonin treatment in childhood sleep onset insomnia was evaluated by Smits et al. (8). In this double blind placebo controlled study, on 40 elementary school children, melatonin at a 5mg dose significantly advanced sleep onset time by 63 minutes (range 32–94); actigraphic sleep onset time by 75 minutes (range 36–114); DLMO by 57 minutes (range 24–89) and increased the total sleep time by 41 minutes (range 19–62). In the follow-up of this study, many parents reported that their child's behavior had considerably improved (8).

In an extended study on 79 children with idiopathic chronic sleep onset insomnia (some also having ADHD), sleep onset insomnia with a late melatonin onset was found (9). These children were obviously suffering from delayed sleep phase syndrome (DSPS). Melatonin treatment for four weeks was effective in improving health status and sleep in these children. It advanced both sleep onset and sleep offset time significantly. A lack of correlation between change in sleep onset and DLMO on one hand and changes in scores of health status scales RAND-GHRI and FS-II on the other suggested that melatonin can improve the health status of these children by properties other than its chronobiotic effects (9).

The Smith-Magenis syndrome is a genetic sleep disorder resulting from interstitial chromosomal deletion 17p11.2. A reduced sleep time has been documented in virtually all Smith-Magenis patients studied (50). Difficulty in falling asleep, staying asleep, or waking early have also been documented in children with Smith-Magenis syndrome. Nearly 50% of these individuals suffer from abnormalities of REM sleep (50). These patients are mentally retarded and hyperactive and exhibit behavioral abnormalities during the day, which correlate with insufficient sleep in the night (50–52). The study of the circadian pattern of melatonin secretion in these children has revealed an inverted pattern with elevated daytime levels and very low melatonin levels during the night. The inverted melatonin pattern seen in Smith-Magenis syndrome suggested that the sleep disturbance seen in this syndrome could be due to abnormalities in the production and secretion of melatonin (52,53).

It is interesting to note that Smith-Magenis patients display a major phase shift in their circadian rhythm of melatonin secretion. The time of onset of melatonin secretion is 06.00 hours ± 2 hours, whereas in normal children it is 21.00 hours ± 2 hours. Peak time of melatonin in Smith-Magenis patients is at 12.00 hours ± 1 hour versus 03.30 hours ± 1.30 hours in normal children. Melatonin is at 20.00 hours ± 1 hour in patients versus 06.00 hours ± 1 hour in normal children. In addition, an irregular pattern of melatonin secretion is also observed in Smith-Magenis patients during the day, sometimes with a second peak occurring between 18.00 hours and 20.00 hours (52). All children with Smith-Magenis display maladaptive behavior and sleep disturbances which are found to be extremely severe and difficult to manage. The abnormal behavior and sleep disturbances could not be controlled with medications like neuroleptics, antipsychotics, hypnotics or antiepileptic drugs (52). In contrast, the combination of morning β_1-adrenergic antagonist (to inhibit inappropriate melatonin synthesis) and evening melatonin administration not only restored a circadian pattern of plasma melatonin rhythmicity but also improved behavioral disturbances and sleep disturbances in these patients (53).

Hence for all practical reasons, melatonin appears to be a potentially useful and safe tool for treatment sleep disturbance seen in children with neurodevelopmental disabilities (36). The recommended dose of melatonin used to treat children with ADHD is not yet settled. In a systemic chart review conducted on 32 children and adolescents in the Kosair Children's Hospital Pediatric Sleep Medicine and Apnea Center, Louisville, KY, U.S.A., 27 (84%) of them had difficulties in falling asleep and 18 (56%) had frequent nocturnal awakenings. Melatonin was administered in doses (mean 2.0 ± 1.2 mg) ranging from 0.3 mg in the case of a two-year-old male with disturbed sleep cycle, to 6 mg in a 16-year-old patient with DSPS. The majority of these children had a comorbid diagnosis of ADHD. In this study melatonin was found to be an effective, safe and well-tolerated treatment of sleep initiation and maintenance (17). In another study, melatonin, in a dose of 3 mg, significantly reduced the time of falling asleep in 24 children with ADHD (54). Immediately after the start of melatonin treatment, the subjects fell asleep earlier than before, varying from 15 to 24 minutes.

The fact that regulation of the sleep/wake cycle has a beneficial impact on the health of children with ADHD has been demonstrated in almost all the studies in which melatonin was used. A melatonin dose of 5 mg/day in 33 children with ADHD (age range 6–4 years) was clinically and statistically superior to a placebo on SOL. Mean SOL on placebo was 62.1 minutes whereas after melatonin mean SOL was 46.4 minutes (46). A sleep hygiene approach on five patients was also shown to have a significant impact on mean SOL, thereby showing that behavioral aspects of ADHD also play a role in initial insomnia and regulation of the sleep/wake cycle (46).

In a four-week randomized, double blind, placebo-controlled study on 105 medication-free children with diagnosed ADHD aged 6–12 years and having chronic sleep onset insomnia, melatonin's efficacy on sleep (44), DLMO, behavior, cognitive performance, and quality of life were evaluated. Children received melatonin in a daily dose of 3 mg for body weight <40 kg or 6 mg for body weight > 40 kg. After melatonin treatment, 20 children showed an advance of sleep onset of more than 30 minutes. There was an increase in mean total time asleep of 19.8 ± 61.9 minutes with melatonin and a decrease of 13.6 ± 50.6 minutes with placebo (P=0.01). Sleep efficiency increased by $2.60 \pm 8.92\%$ with melatonin, whereas it decreased by $2.11 \pm 7.12\%$ with placebo (P=0.01). Melatonin-treated children showed a DLMO advance of 0.44 ± 1.07, whereas there was a delay of 0.13 ± 0.59 in placebo-treated children (P=0.0001) (44).

MELATONIN ON COGNITIVE AND BEHAVIORAL PROBLEMS IN CHILDREN WITH ADHD AND SLEEP ONSET INSOMNIA

In the study by van der Heijden et al. (44) the effect of melatonin treatment on measures of behavior, cognitive performance, and quality of life was evaluated. The most frequently observed problems were becoming easily angered (36.0%), sleep-onset problems (31.8%), and attention problems (23.3%). Melatonin alleviated these core problems, indicating that it reduced the burden on these children. However, no improvements on other behavioral or cognitive measures were found, not even in positive respondents in respect of sleep and who showed advances of sleep onset of more than 30 minutes. These findings indicate that in children with ADHD, melatonin can be used for the treatment of sleep onset insomia but not for behavioral or cognitive problems. Hence, melatonin treatment in children with ADHD may require supplementary psychostimulant treatment for ADHD-related dysfunction. One open-label study investigated the combined use of melatonin and stimulant treatment and showed robust effects of melatonin on sleep (54).

CONCLUSIONS

Sleep disorders in children with neurodevelopmental disabilities like ADHD and Smith–Magenis syndrome are very common and are often associated with many behavioral abnormalities during daytime. The analysis of published papers on the use of melatonin in children with ADHD and other neural developmental disabilities reveals that melatonin is safe and effective not only for the treatment of persistent and severe insomnia, but also in treating maladaptive behavior, especially in children with Smith–Magenis syndrome who have genetic abnormality, and have inverted melatonin with high daytime and low nocturnal melatonin secretion. Available evidence strongly indicates that melatonin can be beneficial in the treatment of pediatric sleep disorders.

ACKNOWLEDGMENTS
One of the authors (VS) wishes to acknowledge Mrs. Puan Rosnida Said, Department of Physiology, University Sains Malaysia, School of Medical Sciences, Kota Bharu, Malaysia, for her assistance in preparing a first version of this manuscript.

REFERENCES
1. Accardo PJ, Blondis TA. The Strauss syndrome, minimal brain dysfunction, and the hyperactive child: A historical introduction to attention deficit hyperactivity disorder. In: Accardo PJ, Blondis TA, Whitman BY, Stein MA, eds Attention Deficits and Hyperactivity in Children and Adults. New York: Marcel Decker, 2000: pp. 1–71.
2. Still GF. Some abnormal psychical conditions in children. Lancet 1902; i1008-1012:1163–68.
3. Levy F. The dopamine theory of attention deficit hyperactivity disorder (ADHD). Aus NZ J Psychiat 1991; 25:277–83.
4. Levy F, Swanson JM. Timing, space and ADHD: The dopamine theory revisited. Aus NZ J Psychiat 2001; 35:504–11.
5. Heilman KM, Voeller KK, Nadeau SE. A possible pathophysiologic substrate of attention deficit hyperactivity disorder. J Child Neurol 1991; 6(Suppl):S76–S81.
6. Jan JE, O'Donnell ME. Use of melatonin in the treatment of paediatric sleep disorders. J Pineal Res 1996; 21(4):193–9.
7. Cohen-Zion M, Ancoli-Israel S. Sleep in children with attention-deficit hyperactivity disorder (ADHD): A review of naturalistic and stimulant intervention studies. Sleep Med Rev 2004; 8:379–402.
8. Smits MG, Nagtegaal EE, van der HJ, et al. Melatonin for chronic sleep onset insomnia in children:A randomized placebo-controlled trial. J Child Neurol 2001; 16(2):86–92.
9. Smits MG, van Stel HF, van der HK, et al. Melatonin improves health status and sleep in children with idiopathic chronic sleep-onset insomnia: A randomized placebo-controlled trial. J Am Acad Child Adolesc Psychiatry 2003; 42(11):1286–93.
10. van der Heijden KB, Smits MG, Gunning WB. Sleep-related disorders in ADHD: A review. Clin Pediatr (Phila) 2005; 44 (3):201–10.
11. Pandi-Perumal SR, Smits M, Spence W et al. Dim light melatonin onset (DLMO): A tool for the analysis of circadian phase in human sleep and chronobiological disorders. Prog Neuropsychopharmacol Biol Psychiatry 2006.
12. van der Heijden KB, Blok MJ, Spee K, et al. No evidence to support an association of PER3 clock gene polymorphism with ADHD-related idiopathic chronic sleep onset insomnia. Biol Rhythm Res 2005; 36(5):381–8.
13. Klerman EB, Gershengorn HB, Duffy JF, et al. Comparisons of the variability of three markers of the human circadian pacemaker. J Biol Rhythms 2002; 17(2):181–93.
14. Zisapel N. Circadian rhythm sleep disorders: Pathophysiology and potential approaches to management. CNS Drugs 2001; 15(4):311–28.
15. Srinivasan V, Smits G, Kayumov L, et al. Melatonin in circadian rhythm sleep disorders. In: Cardinali DP, Pandi-Perumal SR, eds Neuroendocrine Correlates of Sleep/Wakefulness. New York: Springer, 2006: pp. 269–94.

16. Jan JE, Espezel H, Goulden KJ. Melatonin in sleep disorders in children with neurodevelopmental disabilities. In: Shafii M, Shafii SL, eds Melatonin in Psychiatric and Neoplastic Disorders. Washington DC: American Psychiatric Press, 1998: pp. 169–88.
17. Jan MM. Melatonin for the treatment of handicapped children with severe sleep disorders. Pediatr Neurol 2000; 23(3):229–32.
18. Ivanenko A, Crabtree VM, Tauman R, et al. Melatonin in children and adolescents with insomnia: A retrospective study. Clin Pediatr (Phila) 2003; 42(1):51–8.
19. Pandi-Perumal SR, Srinivasan V, Maestroni GJM, et al. Melatonin: Nature's most versatile biological signal? FEBS J 2006; 273:2813–38.
20. Reiter RJ, Tan DX, Pilar TM, et al. Melatonin and its metabolites: New findings regarding their production and their radical scavenging actions. Acta Biochim Pol 2007; 54:1–9.
21. Axelrod J. The pineal gland: Aneurochemical transducer. Science 1974; 184(144):1341–48.
22. Skinner DC, Malpaux B. High melatonin concentrations in third ventricular cerebrospinal fluid are not due to Galen vein blood recirculating through the choroid plexus. Endocrinology 1999; 140(10):4399–405.
23. Arendt J. Melatonin and human rhythms. Chronobiol Int 2006; 23(1–2):21–37.
24. Griefahn B, Brode P, Remer T, et al. Excretion of 6-hydroxymelatonin sulfate (6-OHMS) in siblings during childhood and adolescence. Neuroendocrinology 2003; 78(5):241–3.
25. Hallam KT, Olver JS, Chambers V, et al. The heritability of melatonin secretion and sensitivity to bright nocturnal light in twins. Psychoneuroendocrinology 2006; 31(7):867–75.
26. Tan DX, Manchester LC, Terron MP, et al. One molecule, many derivatives: A never-ending interaction of melatonin with reactive oxygen and nitrogen species? J Pineal Res 2007; 42(1):28–42.
27. Klein DC, Moore RY. Pineal N-acetyltransferase and hydroxyindole-O-methyltransferase: Control by the retinohypothalamic tract and the suprachiasmatic nucleus. Brain Res 1979; 174(2):245–62.
28. Berson DM, Dunn FA, Takao M. Phototransduction by retinal ganglion cells that set the circadian clock. Science 2002; 295(5557):1070–3.
29. Saper CB, Lu J, Chou TC, et al. The hypothalamic integrator for circadian rhythms. Trends Neurosci 2005; 28(3):152–7.
30. Cardinali DP, Pevet P. Basic aspects of melatonin action. Sleep Med Rev 1998; 2:175–90.
31. Gonzalez Burgos G, Rosenstein RE, Cardinali DP. Daily changes in presynaptic cholinergic activity of rat superior cervical ganglion. Brain Res 1994; 636:181–6.
32. Dubocovich ML, Markowska M. Functional MT1 and MT2 melatonin receptors in mammals. Endocrine 2005; 27(2):101–10.
33. Pandi-Perumal SR, Zisapel N, Srinivasan V, et al. Melatonin and sleep in aging population. Exp Gerontol 2005; 40:911–25.
34. Liu C, Weaver DR, Jin X, et al. Molecular dissection of two distinct actions of melatonin on the suprachiasmatic circadian clock. Neuron 1997; 19(1):91–102.
35. Burch JB, Yost MG, Johnson W, et al. Melatonin, sleep, and shift work adaptation. J Occup Environ Med 2005; 47(9):893–901.
36. Wassmer E, Whitehouse WP. Melatonin and sleep in children with neurodevelopmental disabilities and sleep disorders. Current Paediatrics 2006; 16(2):132–8.
37. Milstein V, Small JG, Spencer DW. Melatonin for sleep EEG. Clin Electroencephalogr 1998; 29(1):49–53.
38. Johnson K, Page A, Williams H, et al. The use of melatonin as an alternative to sedation in uncooperative children undergoing an MRI examination. Clin Radiol 2002; 57(6):502–6.
39. Luboshitzky R, Lavie P. Melatonin and sex hormone interrelationships: A review. J Pediatr Endocrinol Metab 1999; 12:355–62.
40. Sheldon SH. Pro-convulsant effects of oral melatonin in neurologically disabled children. Lancet 1998; 351:1254.
41. Quine L. Sleep problems in children with mental handicaps. J Mental Deficiency Res 1991; 35:286–90.

42. Turk J. Melatonin supplementation for severe and intractable sleep disturbance in young people with genetically determined developmental disabilities: Short review and commentary. J Med Genet 2003; 40(11):793–6.
43. Didden R, Sigafoos J. Review of the nature and treatment of sleep disorders in individuals with developmental disabilities. Res Develop Disabilities 2001; 22:255–72.
44. Van der Heijden KB, Smits MG, Van Someren EJ, et al. Effect of melatonin on sleep, behavior, and cognition in ADHD and chronic sleep-onset insomnia. J Am Acad Child Adolesc Psychiatry 2007; 46(2):233–41.
45. Olfson M, Gameroff MJ, Marcus SC, et al. National trends in hospitalization of youth with intentional self-inflicted injuries. Am J Psychiatry 2005; 162(7):1328–35.
46. Weiss MD, Wasdell MB, Bomben MM, et al. Sleep hygiene and melatonin treatment for children and adolescents with ADHD and initial insomnia. J Am Acad Child Adolesc Psychiatry 2006; 45(5):512–19.
47. Kratochvil CJ, Vaughan BS, Daughton JM, et al. Atomoxetine in the treatment of attention deficit hyperactivity disorder. Expert Rev Neurother 2004; 4(4):601–11.
48. Konofal E, Lecendreux M, Bouvard MP, et al. High levels of nocturnal activity in children with attention-deficit hyperactivity disorder: A video analysis. Psychiatry Clin Neurosci 2001; 55(2):97–103.
49. Walters AS, Mandelbaum DE, Lewin DS, et al. Dopaminergic therapy in children with restless legs/periodic limb movements in sleep and ADHD. Dopaminergic Therapy Study Group. Pediatr Neurol 2000; 22(3):182–6.
50. Potocki L, Glaze D, Tan DX, et al. Circadian rhythm abnormalities of melatonin in Smith-Magenis syndrome. J Med Genet 2000; 37(6):428–33.
51. Gropman AL, Duncan WC, Smith AC. Neurologic and developmental features of the Smith-Magenis syndrome (del 17p11.2). Pediatr Neurol 2006; 34(5):337–50.
52. De Leersnyder H. Inverted rhythm of melatonin secretion in Smith-Magenis syndrome: From symptoms to treatment. Trends Endocrinol Metab 2006; 17(7):291–8.
53. Smith AC, Dykens E, Greenberg F. Sleep disturbance in Smith-Magenis syndrome (del 17p,11.2). Am J Med Genet 1998; 81:186–91.
54. Tjon Pian Gi CV, Broeren JP, Starreveld JS, et al. Melatonin for treatment of sleeping disorders in children with attention deficit/hyperactivity disorder: A preliminary open label study. Eur J Pediatr 2003; 162(7–8):554–5.

17 Epidemiology of Insomnia

Cindy Phillips,[a] Lisa J. Meltzer,[b] and Jodi A. Mindell[c]

[a]Drexel University and Children's Hospital of Philadelphia, Philadelphia, Pennsylvania, U.S.A.
[b]Children's Hospital of Philadelphia and University of Pennsylvania School of Medicine, Philadelphia, Pennsylvania, U.S.A.
[c]Department of Psychology, Saint Joseph's University and Children's Hospital of Philadelphia, Philadelphia, Pennsylvania, U.S.A.

INTRODUCTION

Sleep problems are common in pediatric populations, with prevalence rates reported as high as 25–40% (1) in children and adolescents. Estimates are even higher in special populations, including children with medical and psychiatric disorders. Sleep problems for all children often result in decreased daytime functioning and poorer prognosis (1–2).

Insomnia in children and adolescents is not as well understood as in adult populations and it is difficult to extrapolate from adult studies to pediatric populations. Differences between adult and pediatric insomnia include the presentation, symptoms, and causes. Furthermore, treatments differ for children and adolescents compared to adults, which is complicated further by different presentations of sleep problems across the pediatric age span. For example, infants have more night wakings due to sleep-onset association disorder; preschoolers experience delayed sleep onset due to stalling and bedtime resistance, as well as nighttime fears and nightmares; school-aged children experience both difficulty falling and staying asleep; and adolescents are more likely to experience difficulties falling asleep related to a delayed sleep phase, which is compounded by early high school start times. All of these sleep disturbances may present as "insomnia," as described by the child or adolescent, or by parents/caregivers.

Defining Insomnia

Difficulty initiating or maintaining sleep is the hallmark feature of insomnia, although the name and diagnostic criteria vary slightly depending on the diagnostic manual used. The Diagnostic and Statistical Manual of Mental Disorders IV-TR (DSM-IV-TR) (3) calls this "Primary Insomnia," whereas the most common type of insomnia in the International Classification of Sleep Disorders (ICSD-2) (4) is "Psychophysiological Insomnia." The diagnostic criteria for each disorder can be found in Table 1.

Due to developmental issues and presentations, neither the ICSD-2 nor the DSM-IV-TR diagnostic criteria are always adequate in defining insomnia in children, although they may be more appropriate for adolescents (2). One of the main reasons why children fail to meet the diagnostic criteria for "insomnia" per se is that often they do not complain about their sleep, nor perceive it as problematic. Rather, it is usually the parents or caregivers who bring the issue to the attention of healthcare professionals. In addition, it is often difficult to ascertain the impact of

TABLE 1   Insomnia Definitions

DSM IV TR—Diagnostic Criteria: Primary Insomnia (307.42)
A. The predominant complaint is difficulty initiating or maintaining sleep, or nonrestorative sleep, for at least one month.
B. The sleep disturbance (or associated daytime fatigue) causes clinically significant distress or impairment in social, occupational, or other important areas of functioning.
C. The sleep disturbance does not occur exclusively during the course of Narcolepsy, Breathing-Related Sleep Disorder, Circadian Rhythm Sleep Disorder, or a Parasomnia.
D. The disturbance does not occur exclusively during the course of another mental disorder [e.g., major depressive disorder (MDD), generalized anxiety disorder (GAD), a delirium]
E. The disturbance is not due to the direct physiological effects of a substance (e.g., a drug of abuse, a medication) or a general medical condition.

ICSD II—Diagnostic Criteria: Psychophysiologic Insomnia (307.42-0)
A. A complaint of insomnia is present and is combined with a complaint of decreased functioning during wakefulness.
B. Indications of learned sleep-preventing associations are found and include the following:
   1. Trying to hard to sleep, suggested by an inability to fall asleep when desired, but ease of falling asleep during other relatively monotonous pursuits, such as watching television or reading.
   2. Conditioned arousal to bedroom or sleep-related activities, indicated by sleeping poorly at home but sleeping better away from the home or when not carrying out bedtime routines.
C. There is evidence that the patient has increased somatized tension (e.g., agritation, muscle tension, or increased vasoconstriction).
D. Polysomnographic monitoring demonstrates all of the following:
   1. An increased sleep latency
   2. Reduced sleep efficiency
   3. An increased number and duration of awakenings
E. No other medical or mental disorders accounts for the sleep disturbance.
F. Other sleep disorders can coexist with the insomnia, e.g., inadequate sleep hygiene, obstructive sleep apnea syndrome, etc.
Minimal Criteria: A plus B

ICSD II—Diagnostic Criteria: Behavioral Insomnia of Childhood—Limit-Setting Type (307.42-4)
A. The patient has difficulty in initiating sleep.
B. The patient stalls or refuses to go to bed at an appropriate time.
C. Once the sleep period is initiated, sleep is of normal quality and duration.
D. Polysomnographic monitoring demonstrates normal timing, quality, and duration of the sleep period.
E. No significant underlying mental or medical disorder accounts for the complaint.
F. The symptoms do not meet criteria for any other sleep disorder causing difficulties in initiating sleep (e.g., sleep-onset association type).
Minimal Criteria: B plus C

ICSD II—Diagnostic Criteria: Behavioral Insomnia of Childhood—Sleep-Onset Association Type (307.42-5)
A. The patient has a complaint of insomnia.
B. The complaint is temporally associated with absence of certain conditions (e.g., being held, rocked, or nursed at the breast; listening to the radio; or watching television).
C. The disorder has been present for at least three weeks.
D. With the particular association present, sleep is normal in onset, duration, and quality.
E. Polysomnographic monitoring demonstrates:
   1. Normal timing, duration, and quality of sleep period when the associations are present.
   2. Sleep latency and the duration or number of awakenings can be increased when the associations are absent.
F. No significant underlying mental or medical disorder accounts for the complaint.
G. The symptoms do not meet criteria for any other sleep disorder causing difficulties in initiating sleep (e.g., limit setting type).
Minimal Criteria: A plus B plus D plus F plus G

---

daytime functioning, especially for children and adolescents with special needs. In response to these concerns, a consensus definition was developed by experts in the field of pediatric insomnia (5). Based on the definition of insomnia according to the ICSD-2, pediatric insomnia is defined as "repeated difficulty with sleep initiation, duration, consolidation, or quality that occurs despite *age-appropriate* time and opportunity for sleep and results in daytime functional impairment for the *child and/or family*."

One major change in the ICSD-2 was the addition of the diagnosis Behavioral Insomnia of Childhood (BIC; see Table 1). The primary symptoms of BIC are difficulty falling asleep independently and/or frequent night wakings. The ICSD-2 defines three subtypes of BIC based on the behavioral etiology of the bedtime problem or night waking: sleep-onset association type, limit-setting type, and combined type. BIC sleep-onset association type is most often seen in infants and toddlers (ages six months to three years), although it can occur at any point during childhood or adolescence. Inappropriate sleep associations (e.g., rocking, nursing, watching TV, sleeping in the parents' bedroom) are needed for the child to fall asleep at bedtime, and then return to sleep following normal nighttime arousals. Thus, BIC sleep-onset association type typically presents with the complaint of frequent night wakings. Children with BIC limit-setting type are often described by their caregivers as refusing to go to bed or attempting to delay bedtime with repeated requests. BIC limit-setting type occurs most commonly in toddlers, preschoolers, and school-aged children. If bedtime routines and rules are not clear and consistent, and/or parents have difficulty enforcing limits, BIC limit-setting type can occur. Finally, there is combined type in which children display both subtypes. It typically occurs when a negative sleep association follows a prolonged bedtime that is caused by nonexistent or inconsistent limits (e.g., after two hours of bedtime struggles, the parent lies down with the child to help him/her fall asleep).

Unlike studies of insomnia in adults that adhere to strict diagnostic criteria for insomnia, pediatric studies have used a multitude of definitions to designate insomnia in children and adolescents. The majority of studies in the area of insomnia in children and adolescents have focused on "bedtime problems" and "night wakings." These studies have used definitions ranging from parental identification of their child experiencing a sleep problem to more empirically based definitions, such as a child waking three or more nights a week. No studies to date have used the designation of Behavioral Insomnia of Childhood. Studies on insomnia in adolescents have been more likely to use published diagnostic criteria (6).

Prevalence

Prevalence studies and national surveys have consistently found insomnia to be problematic for children and adolescents. In one survey (8), 69% of parents of children (ages 0 to 10 years) reported that their child experienced a sleep problem at least a few nights a week. Stalling and bedtime resistance (52% and 30% respectively) were the two most commonly experienced sleep problems, with preschoolers displaying them most frequently. Difficulties falling asleep were also common, with 13% to 16% of parents reporting this problem. In addition to difficulties getting to sleep, 30% of children were reported to wake at night at least once a week, requiring their parent's attention to fall back asleep. In a separate survey of adolescents (ages 11 to 17 years) (9), 51% of teens reported difficulty falling asleep at least once a week during the previous two weeks, while 31% reported having difficulty staying asleep at least once a week.

Empirical studies of bedtime problems and night wakings in infants and toddlers have consistently found prevalence rates of 20–30%, even when comparing studies across cultures (10–13). Multiple studies of school-aged children have also found prevalence rates in a similar range (14,15). In a clinical sample comprising two general pediatric clinics, Hedger Archibold et al. (16) found that 20% of children (ages 2 to 13.9 years) reported two or more insomnia symptoms. In addition, 25% of parents reported that their child resisted bedtime. A study by Blader et al. (17) found that one-third of school-aged children have difficulties sleeping and 27% of parents reported bedtime refusal at least three times per week. Finally, Sadeh and colleagues (18) report that 18% of school-aged children have poor sleep, as designated by low sleep efficiency or frequent night wakings on actigraphy.

Prevalance rates for insomnia in adolescents have ranged from 6% to 39%, depending on the definition used. Ohayon and colleagues (7) utilized DSM-IV criteria in a study of adolescents in the United Kingdom, France, Germany, and Spain. They found that 4% had insomnia in the past 30 days. Of these adolescents, approximately half were designated with primary insomnia, 27% had insomnia related to a psychiatric condition, 12% had insomnia associated with substance use, and 7% had insomnia related to a medical condition. In a more recent study of over 1000 adolescents (ages 13–16 years) in the United States utilizing DSM-IV-TR criteria, Johnson and colleagues (6) found a lifetime prevalence of primary insomnia of 10.7%, with the median age of onset 11 years. Of those who reported having a history of insomnia, 88% had current difficulties sleeping. In addition, 52.8% reported having a comorbid psychiatric condition. Insomnia is more prevalent in girls than in boys post-puberty, but few ethnic/racial differences have been found (6,7).

PSYCHIATRIC COMORBIDITY
Children and adolescents with sleep disturbances often have a comorbid psychiatric diagnosis (19). In a study conducted by Ivanenko and colleagues (19), 50% of children with insomnia had confirmed psychiatric comorbidity. For children without a psychiatric diagnosis, 40% scored in the clinical range on parent-report questionnaires for the presence of a co-occurring mental health illness.

Attention-Deficit/Hyperactivity Disorder (ADHD)
ADHD is one of the most common pediatric psychiatric disorders, affecting 8–10% of children and adolescents (3). Sleep problems, including insomnia, obstructive sleep apnea, and periodic leg movement disorder, have been reported in approximately 25% to 50% of children and adolescents with ADHD (20–24). It has been suggested that underlying sleep disruptions may be intrinsic to children with ADHD (22,25–27).

On a subjective basis, parents frequently complain of bedtime struggles and delayed sleep-onset, increased night wakings, restless sleep, and shortened sleep duration in children with ADHD. However, more objective measures, including actigraphy and polysomnography (PSG), do not support consistent differences between children with and without ADHD (20). One explanation for this discrepancy in findings may be due to the increased night-to-night variability in sleep found in children with ADHD (27). Furthermore, the discrepancy between parental reports and objective findings also may be related to comorbid psychiatric conditions and/or differences in the behaviors of children with ADHD at bedtime.

Developmental Disorders

Sleep problems are highly prevalent in children with developmental disorders, with estimates ranging from 30% to 84%. Similar to typically developing children, the most common sleep problems experienced by children with disabilities are difficulties with sleep-onset and sleep maintenance. The two areas that have been studied most within this range of disorders are Autism Spectrum Disorders (ASD) and Mental Retardation.

Autism Spectrum Disorders

Multiple studies have found increased rates of sleep disturbances in children and adolescents with ASDs (28–36), affecting approximately 44% to 83% of children with ASDs (28). The most commonly reported sleep problems include early morning wakings, shorter total sleep time, prolonged sleep-onset, and frequent and/or prolonged night wakings (28–32). Parents report children with ASDs have more sleep problems than typically developing children (28,33,34), as well as children with other developmental disabilities (30).

A study by Honomichl and colleagues (29) found that children with autism were more likely to take longer to fall asleep, have more night awakenings, have more time awake after sleep onset, and therefore have less total time asleep compared to controls. In addition, children with ASDs had greater bedtime refusal than controls by parent report.

Actigraphy, an objective measure of sleep patterns, has also been used to document differences in sleep onset latency, total sleep time, and early morning wakings in children with ASDs compared to typically developing children (28,31). For example, Allik and colleagues (35) studied 32 children with Asperger syndrome (AS) using actigraphy, reporting that children with AS had longer sleep-onset latencies compared to age and gender matched controls. Similar results (longer sleep latency and poorer sleep efficiency) were reported in a study of 21 children with ASD using PSG (36) compared to age-matched controls using PSG (36).

Mental Retardation (MR)

Difficulties falling asleep, maintaining sleep, and waking after sleep onset have been reported in up to 75% of children and adolescents with MR (37–40). A study by Stores and colleagues reported that children with Down syndrome and other intellectual disabilities had significantly poorer sleep than a control group of typically developing children (38). Another study of children with MR found the greatest cause of sleep difficulties to be bedtime resistance (39). Finally, the prevalence of sleep problems in a large group of children with developmental disorders was found to be four times higher compared to controls, with sleep maintenance the greatest problem for children with Down syndrome and familial intellectual disabilities (41).

Depression
Given that sleep disturbances are listed as one of the criteria for diagnosing depression according to the DSM-IV-TR (3), it is not surprising that between 66% and 90% of children and adolescents presenting with depression also report difficulties sleeping (42–48). The most common subjective complaints include difficulties initiating and/or maintaining sleep, hypersomnia (sleeping too much), and early morning awakening (44–48).

Considering the commonality of subjective sleep complaints in children and adolescents with depression, it is surprising that objective data do not provide complementary evidence. Although several studies report that the majority of children and adolescents (or their parents) complain of sleep difficulties (42–48), results from overnight sleep studies (PSG) find no significant differences between those with or without depression. In a sample of 51 children and adolescents (ages 8–17) with depression, and 42 age-matched controls, no differences in sleep were found on PSG (47). Conversely, those with depression displayed better sleep than the control group (although it was not significantly different), which they hypothesize was due to a first-night effect (sleeping better or worse because you are in new surroundings).

Other researchers believe that gender and developmental stage need to be accounted for when interpreting PSG findings (49). In one study of 173 participants, 97 children and adolescents with depression and 76 age-matched controls were evaluated with PSG. Adolescent boys with depression were found to have more sleep disruptions, including more arousals, than girls with depression. Sleep disruptions in girls with depression did not significantly differ from the control group.

Anxiety
Sleep disturbances are also a diagnostic criterion for anxiety and can perpetuate anxious behaviors (2). Children with anxiety often have difficulties falling asleep and are easily aroused once asleep (50–54). Similar to depression, sleep and anxiety are seen as having a bidirectional relationship. Fears and anxiety reduce the amount of sleep one gets, which then can increase the frequency and occurrence of anxiety symptoms.

There are, however, conflicting reports regarding the duration of sleep and its impact on anxiety. In a study by Iwawaki and colleagues (51), a negative relationship was found between anxiety level and actual sleep duration for adolescents (12–16 years), with a later bedtime and shorter sleep duration related to higher levels of anxiety. In contrast, Chattopadhyay and Dasgupta (52) found that children (ages 9–12) who were long sleepers reported higher levels of anxiety. The difference between these studies should be interpreted with caution however, due to the differences in developmental stage.

MEDICAL COMORBIDITY
Children with medical diagnoses are also highly likely to have comorbid insomnia. The underlying mechanisms of the varying diseases complicate the etiology of the accompanying sleep disorder. Furthermore, the reactions to medical issues can prolong and exacerbate the difficulties experienced with sleep. Three common medical problems (asthma, epilepsy, and pain) that are often accompanied by insomnia are presented here.

Asthma

The prevalence of asthma in children has increased over time, with current estimates of 5–15% (55–61). One study by Madge et al. (62) found that approximately 61% of children with symptoms of asthma report disturbed sleep. Other studies also have found that children with asthma report lower sleep quality compared to age-matched controls without asthma (63–65). As with other disorders discussed above, the results have not been consistent across studies, with some researchers failing to find a discrepancy in sleep problems between children with and without asthma (60).

Reduced pulmonary functioning seems to play a role in reduced sleep quality and quantity in asthma patients (55–65). Sadeh and colleagues (55) assessed 40 children with asthma and compared them to 34 controls using both subjective and objective measures. Based on actigraphy, they found that children with asthma displayed less quiet sleep and were more active during the night than the control subjects. In addition, they found that increased asthma severity and number of symptoms reported were associated with poorer sleep quality. However, no differences were found for insomnia symptoms or total sleep time.

In addition to reports of asthma-related sleep disruptions, Yeatts and colleagues (61) found that subclinical wheezing is also associated with increased sleep disturbance. In their study of 2059 8th graders from 25 middle schools, children who were diagnosed with asthma were 7.8 times more likely to report sleep disturbances, while those with wheezing were 4.7 times more likely to have sleep issues. It is, therefore, important to assess for sleep problems in children with both clinical and sub-clinical presentations for asthma.

Epilepsy

Epilepsy is a complex disease that has been described as analogous to an iceberg (66), in that epilepsy is merely a small part of the symptomology of a larger brain dysfunction. Another part of the picture is the sleep component (67), in that some children may only experience seizures during sleep. Lack of sleep also can precipitate the onset of seizure activity. Changes in sleep-related behaviors also occur with epilepsy. For example, with a new diagnosis of epilepsy, it has been reported that alterations to sleeping arrangements often occur due to increased parental anxiety and fears of reoccurrence of seizure activity. Williams and colleagues (68) found that 22% of families with a child with epilepsy moved to a less independent sleeping arrangement after diagnosis (such as co-sleeping or moving the child into the parental bedroom). Cottrell and Khan (69) also found that mothers were only sleeping an average of 4.5 hours and checking on their children approximately three times per night. These new patterns seem adaptive and protective in nature; however, they can cause increased anxiety in the child, as well as establish poor sleep hygiene and bedtime routines that may lead to behavioral insomnia of childhood.

Pain

Although sleep problems in children and adolescents who experience pain have received less attention in the literature, sleep disruptions are highly prevalent with pain disorders. Chambers, Icton, and Hayton (70) reported that more than half of children and adolescents with chronic pain have sleep issues, either difficulties initiating or maintaining sleep. In one study of children with sickle cell disease (SCD) (71), children who experienced pain had a shorter total sleep time compared to controls.

Migraines and headaches occur in approximately 10–13% of children (72,73), with sleep often disrupted in children who experience chronic headaches. One study (74) found that inadequate sleep, problems initiating sleep, restless sleep, and multiple night awakenings were reported more frequently in children with headaches than in controls. Miller and colleagues (75) studied 118 children diagnosed with migraines, finding that children with migraines, as compared to a normative population, reported more disturbances to their sleep, including reduced sleep latency, increased resistance at bedtime, decreased total sleep time, and multiple night wakings. In addition, they noted that the more intense the migraine, the shorter the total sleep time.

In a study of 26 adolescents with chronic musculoskeletal pain, adolescents with pain reported increased sleep-onset latency and later wake time on both weekdays and weekends compared to a normative population (76). In addition adolescents with pain also reported more daytime sleepiness, which was related to increased levels of depression and anxiety. The authors suggest that insufficient sleep appears to play a role in the maintenance of musculoskeletal pain.

It is unclear whether sleep affects pain or vice versa but many believe that there is a bidirectional relationship and that the two are interrelated (77–79). There have been several theories as to why pain may affect sleep, including the inability to manage a painful episode at bedtime, worrying about a possible pain episode, or not being able to find a position that will allow the child or adolescent to sleep (80). Children and adolescents with both pain and sleep disruptions are susceptible to daytime impairment, including changes to mood and functioning (81). When dealing with complex medical presentations, especially ones that include pain, it is difficult to tease apart the factors that affect both sleep and daytime functioning.

CONCLUSIONS

Insomnia is common in children and adolescents, with 20–30% of children of all ages experiencing some type of sleep disruption, including difficulties initiating and/or maintaining sleep. The clinical presentation of insomnia can vary greatly for children and adolescents compared to adults, as well as across developmental stages. Complicating the clinical presentation of insomnia in children and adolescents is that the complaint of sleep problems often comes from the parent and not the child. In addition, sleep disturbances can contribute to or be exacerbated by both psychiatric and medical comorbidities commonly found in children and adolescents.

There is still much work that needs to be done in the area of pediatric insomnia. Future research needs to further clarify appropriate diagnostic criteria for insomnia in children and adolescents, as well as conduct epidemiological studies on the prevalence and development of sleep difficulties across developmental stages.

REFERENCES

1. Meltzer LJ, Mindell JA. Sleep and sleep disorders in children and adolescents. Psychiatr Clin N Am 2006; 29:1059–76.

2. Mindell JA. Insomnia in children and adolescents. In: Szuba MP, Kloss JD, Dinges D, eds Insomnia: Principles and Management. United Kingdom: Cambridge University Press, 2003: pp. 125–35.

3. American Psychiatric Association Diagnostic and Statistical Manual of Mental Disorders–TR, 4th edn Washington, DC.

4. International Classification of Sleep Disorders 2nd edn American Society of Sleep Medicine, Westchester, IL, 2005.

5. Mindell JA, Emslie G, Blumer J, et al. Pharmacological management of insomnia in children and adolescents: Consensus statement. J Pediatr 2006; 117:1223–32.

6. Johnson EO, Roth T, Schultz L, et al. Epidemiology of DSM-IV insomnia in adolescence: Lifetime prevalence, chronicity, and an emergent gender difference. Pediatr 2006; 117:247–56.

7. Ohayon, MM; Roberts, RE; Zulley, J; Smirne, S; Priest, RG. Prevalence and patterns of problematic sleep among older adolescents. J Am Acad Child Psych 2000; 39(12):1549–56.

8. National Sleep Foundation. Children and sleep. Sleep in America Poll, 2004. http://www.sleepfoundation.org/polls/2004SleepPollFinalReport.pdf (accessed March 24, 2007).

9. National Sleep Foundation. Adolescents and sleep. Sleep in America Poll, 2006. http://www.sleepfoundation.org/site/c.huIXKjM0IxF/b.2419167/k.14D6/2006_Sleep_in_America_Poll.htm (accessed March 24, 2007).

10. Lozoff B, Wolf AW, Davis NS. Sleep problems seen in pediatric practice. Pediatr 1985; 75:477–83.

11. Armstrong, KL, Quinn, RA, Dadds, MR. The sleep patterns of normal children. Med J Australia 1994; 161:202–06.

12. Burnham MM, Goodlin-Jones BL, Gaylor EE, et al. Nighttime sleep-wake patterns and self-soothing from birth to one year of age: A longitudinal intervention study. J Child Psychol Psych 2002; 43:713–25.

13. Goodlin-Jones BL, Burnham MM, Gaylor EE, et al. Night waking, sleep-wake organization, and self-soothing in the first year of life. J Dev Behav Pediatr 2001; 22:226–33.

14. Owens JA. Epidemiology of sleep disorders during childhood. In: Sheldon SH, Ferber R, Kryger MH, eds Principles and Practices of Pediatric Sleep Medicine. Philadelphia: Elsevier Sanders, 2005: pp. 27–33.

15. Owens JA, Spirito A, McGinn M, et al. Sleep habits and sleep disturbance in elementary school-aged children. J Dev Behav Pediatr 2000; 21(1):27–36.

16. Hedger Archbold K, Pituch KJ, Panabi P, et al. Symptoms of sleep disturbances among children at two general pediatric clinics. J Pediatr 2002; 140:97–102.

17. Blader JC, Koplewicz HS, Abikoff H, et al. Sleep problems of elementary school children. Arch Pediatr Adolesc Med 1997; 151(5):473–80.

18. Sadeh A, Raviv A, Gruber R. Sleep patterns and sleep disruptions in school-aged children. Dev Psychol 2000; 36:291–301.

19. Ivanenko A, Barnes ME, Crabtree VM, et al. Psychiatric symptoms in children with insomnia referred to a pediatric sleep medicine center. Sleep Med Rev 2004; 5:253–9.

20. Chervin RD, Dillon JE, Bassetti C, et al. Symptoms of sleep disorders, inattention, and hyperactivity in children. Sleep 1997; 20(12):1185–92.

21. Bullock GL, Schall U. Dyssomnia in children diagnosed with attention deficit hyperactivity disorder: A critical review. Aust NZ J Psychiat 2005; 39:373–77.

22. Golan N, Shahar E, Ravid S, et al. Sleep disorders and daytime sleepiness in children with attention-deficit/hyperactivity disorder. Sleep 2004; 27(2):261–6.

23. Owens J. The ADHD and sleep conundrum: A review. J Dev Behav Pediatr 2005; 26(4):312–22.

24. McLaughlin Crabtree V, Ivanenko A, Gozal D. Clinical and parental assessment of sleep in children with attention-deficit/hyperactivity disorder referred to a pediatric sleep medicine center. Clin Pediatr 2003; 42:807–13.

25. Weiss MD, Wasdell MB, Bomben MM, et al. Sleep hygiene and melatonin treatment for children and adolescents with ADHD and initial insomnia. J Am Acad Child Adolesc Psychiatry 2006; 45(5):512–19.

26. Gruber R, Sadeh A. Sleep and neurobehavioral functioning in boys with attention-deficit/hyperactivity disorder and no reported breathing problems. Sleep 2004; 27(2):267–73.

27. Corkum P, Tannock, R, Moldofsky H, et al. Actigraphy and parental ratings of sleep in children with attention-deficit/hyperactivity disorder (ADHD). Sleep 2001; 24(3):303–12.

28. Hering E, Epstein R, Elroy S, Iancu DR, Zelnik N. Sleep patterns in autistic children. J Autism Dev Disord 1999; 29(2):143–7.

29. Honomichl RD, Goodlin-Jones BL, Burnham M, et al. Sleep patterns of children with pervasive developmental disorders. J Autism Dev Disord 2002; 32(6):553–61.

30. Patzold LM, Richdale AL, Tonge BJ. An investigation into sleep characteristics of children with autism and Asperger's Disorder. J Pediatr Child Hlth 1998; 34(6):528–33.

31. Wiggs L, Stores G. Sleep patterns and sleep disorders in children with autistic spectrum disorders: Insights using parent report and actigraphy. Dev Med Child Neurol 2004; 46(6):372–80.

32. Williams G, Sears L, Allard AM. Parent perceptions of efficacy for strategies used to facilitate sleep in children with autism. J Dev Phys Disabil 2006; 18(1):25–33.

33. Polimeni MA, Richdale AL, Francis AJP. A survey of sleep problems in autism, Asperger's disorder and typically developing children. J Intell Disabil Res 2005; 49(4):260–8.

34. Schreck KA, Mulick JA, Smith AF. Sleep problems as possible predictors of intensified symptoms of autism. Res Dev Disabil 2004; 25:57–66.

35. Allik H, Larsson J, Smedje H. Sleep patterns of school-aged children with Asperger syndrome or high-functioning autism. J Autism Dev Disord 2006; 36:585–95.

36. Maslow BA, Marzec ML, McGrew SG, et al. Characterizing sleep in children with autism spectrum disorder: A multidimensional approach. Sleep 2006; 29(12):1563–71.

37. Hayashi E, Katada A. Sleep in persons with intellectual disabilities: A survey. Jpn J Spec Edu 2002; 39(6):91–101.

38. Stores R, Stores G, Buckley S. The pattern of sleep problems in children with Down's syndrome and other intellectual disabilities. J App Res Intellect 1996; 9(2):145–59.

39. Gruber JC. Sleep and mental retardation: Towards a synthesis. Brain Dysfunct 1989; 2(2):73–83.

40. Bartlett LB, Rooney V, Spedding S. Nocturnal difficulties in a population of mentally handicapped children. J Ment Subnorm 1985; 31(60):54–9.

41. Cotton S, Richdale A. (2006). Brief report: Parental descriptions of sleep problems in children with autism, Down syndrome, and Prader-Willi syndrome. Res Dev Disabil 2006; 27(2):151–61.

42. Ryan N, Puig-Antich J, Ambrosini P, et al. The clinical picture of major depression in children and adolescents. Arch Gen Psychiat 1987; 44:54–861.

43. Armitage R. The effects of antidepressants on sleep in patients with depression. Can J Psychiat 2000; 45:803–09.

44. Tsuno N, Besset A, Ritchie K. Sleep and depression. J Clin Psychiat 2005; 66:1254–69.

45. Ivanenko A, Crabtree VM, Gozal D. Sleep and depression in children and adolescents. Sleep Med Rev 2005; 9:115–29.

46. Puig-Antich J, Goetz R, Hanlon C, et al. Sleep architecture and REM sleep measures in prepubertal children with major depression: A controlled study. Arch Gen Psychiat 1982; 39:932–9.

47. Bertocci MA, Dahl RE, Williamson DE, et al. Subjective sleep complaints in pediatric depression: A controlled study and comparison with EEG measures of sleep and waking. J Am Acad Child Psy 2005; 44(11):1158–66.

48. Lui X, Buysse DJ, Gentzler AL, et al. Insomnia and hypersomnia associated with depressive phenomenology and comorbidity in childhood depression. Sleep 2007; 30(1):83–90.

49. Roberts JJ, Hoffmann RF, Emslie GJ, et al. Sex and age differences in sleep macroarchitecture in childhood and adolescent depression. Sleep 2006; 29(3):351–8.
50. Gregory AM, Eley TC. Sleep problems, anxiety, and cognitive style in school-aged children. Infant Child Dev 2005; 14(5):435–44.
51. Iwawaki S, Sarmany Schuller I. Cross-cultural comparison of some aspects of sleeping patterns and anxiety. Stud Psychol 2001; 43(3):215–24.
52. Chattopadhyay PK, Dasgupta SK. Trait anxiety, neuroticism, and extraversion in long and short sleeper children. Bangladesh J Psych 1992; 13:1–5.
53. Liu X, Peng X, Guo C, et al. Insomnia in young students and associated factors. Chinese J Psychol 1995; 3(4):230–2.
54. Kellerman J. Rapid treatment of nocturnal anxiety in children. J Behav Ther Exp Psy 1980; 11:9–11.
55. Sadeh A, Horowitz I, Wollach-Benodis L, et al. Sleep and pulmonary function in children with well-controlled asthma. Sleep 1998; 21(4):379–84.
56. Crain EF, Weiss KB, Bijus PE, et al. An estimate of the prevalence of asthma and wheezing among inner-city children. Pediatrics 1994; 94:356–62.
57. Horowitz I, Wolach B, Eliakim A, et al. Children with asthma in the emergency department: Spectrum of disease, variation with ethnicity, and approach to treatment. Pediatr Emerg Care 1995; 11:240–4.
58. Smith JM. The prevalence of asthma and wheezing in children. Brit J Dev Disabil 1976; 70:73–7.
59. Strachan DP, Anderson HR, Limb ES, et al. A national survey of asthma prevalence, severity, and treatment in Great Britain. Arch Dis Child 1994; 70:174–8.
60. Tirosh E, Scher A, Sadeh A, et al. Sleep characteristics of asthmatics in the first four years of life: A comparative study. Arch Dis Child 1993; 68:481–3.
61. Yeatts KB, Shy CM. Prevalence and consequences of asthma and wheezing in African-American and white adolescents. J Adolescent Health 2001; 29:314–19.
62. Madge PJ, Nisbet L, McColl JH, et al. Home nebulizer use in children with asthma in two Scottish health board areas. Scott Med J 1995; 40:141–3.
63. Fitzpatrick MF, Engleman H, Whyte KF, et al. Morbidity in nocturnal asthma: Sleep quality and daytime cognitive performance. Thorax 1991; 46:569–73.
64. Janson C, Gislason T, Boman G, et al. Sleep disturbance in patients with asthma. Resp Med 1990; 84:37–42.
65. Kales A, Kales JD, Sly RM, et al. Sleep patterns of asthmatic children: All night EEG study. J Allergy 1970; 46:300–8.
66. Aicardi J. Epilepsy: The hidden part of the iceberg. Eur J Paediatr Neuro 1999; 3:197–200.
67. Dinner DS. Effect of sleep on epilepsy. J Clin Neurophysiol 2002; 19:504–13.
68. Williams J, Lange B, Sharp G, et al. Altered sleeping arrangements in pediatric patients with epilepsy. Clin Pediatr 2000; 39:635–42.
69. Cottrell L, Khan A. Impact of childhood epilepsy on maternal sleep and socioeconomical functioning. Clin Pediatr 2005; 44.613–16.
70. Chambers CT, Icton CD, Hayton K. The prevalence and nature of sleep disturbance among children with chronic pain: A review of the literature. Poster presented at the 4th International forum on Pediatric Pain, September 2002. White Point, NS, Canada.
71. Shapiro BS, Dinges DF, Carota Orne E, et al. Home management of sickle cell-related pain in children and adolescents: Natural history and impact on school attendance. Pain 1995; 61:139–44.
72. Abu-Arefeh I, Russell G. Prevalence of headache and migraine in schoolchildren. BMJ 1994; 309;765–9.
73. Lee L, Olness K. Clinical and demographic characteristics of migraine in urban children. Headache 1997; 37:269–76.
74. Bruni O, Fabrizi P, Ottaviano S, et al. Prevalence of sleep disorders in childhood and adolescence with headache: A case-control study. Cephalalgia 1997; 17:492–8.

75. Miller VA, Palermo TM, Powers SW, et al. Migraine headaches and sleep disturbances in children. Headache 2003; 43:362–368.
76. Meltzer LJ, Logan DE, Mindell JA. Sleep patterns in female adolescents with chronic musculoskeletal pain. Behav Sleep Med 2005; 3(4):193–208.
77. Pascualy R, Buchwald D. Chronic fatigue syndrome and fibromyalgia. In: Zorab R, Carroll C, eds Principles and Practice of Sleep Medicine. Philadelphia: Saunders, 2000, pp. 1040–9.
78. Moldofsky H, Scarisbrick P. Induction of neurasthenic musculoskeletal pain syndrome by selective sleep stage deprivation. Psychosom Med 1976; 38:35–44.
79. Affleck G, Urrows S, Tennen H, et al. Sequential daily relations of sleep, pain intensity, and attention to pain among women with fibromyalgia. Pain 1996; 68:363–8.
80. Lewin DS, Dahl RE. Importance of sleep in the management of pediatric pain. J Dev Behav Pediatr 1999; 20:244–51.
81. Dahl RE, Lewin DS. Pathways to adolescent health: Sleep regulation and behavior. J Adolescent Health 2002; 31:175–84.

18 Pharmacological Treatments of Pediatric Insomnia

Judith A. Owens

Division of Pediatric Ambulatory Medicine, Rhode Island Hospital, Providence, Rhode Island, U.SA.

INTRODUCTION

In a general sense, the operational definition of insomnia in children may be construed as similar to that in adults, i.e., significant difficulty initiating and/or maintaining sleep and/or non-restorative sleep (early morning awakening is an infrequent complaint in children). However, practically speaking, the most frequent clinical manifestations of childhood insomnia, particularly in younger children, are bedtime refusal or resistance, delayed sleep onset, and/or prolonged night wakings requiring parental intervention. It is estimated that overall 20% to 30% of children in cross-sectional studies are reported to have some significant bedtime problems and/or night wakings (1–7), and a recent study suggests that lifetime prevalence of insomnia in 13 to 16-year-old adolescents approaches 11% (8). These percentages are substantially higher in children with psychiatric comorbidities (9,10) and with a variety of neurodevelopmental disorders (11). Furthermore, there is clear evidence from both experimental laboratory-based studies and clinical observations that insufficient and poor quality sleep in children results in or exacerbates mood instability and behavioral dysregulation, impacts negatively on neurocognitive functions and academic performance (12–14), and affects caregivers, with significant repercussions on family functioning. Therefore, appropriate and effective management of insomnia in the pediatric population is an important therapeutic goal for mental healthcare providers.

Treatment of Pediatric Insomnia: General Considerations

There are several general principles regarding interventions for pediatric insomnia that should be considered before treatment is initiated. First, the treatment must be *diagnostically-driven*, as there are many potential etiologies for the same constellation of presenting complaints. "Insomnia" is a symptom and not a diagnosis. For example, sleep problems in children with attention-deficit/hyperactivity disorder (ADHD) are likely to be multi-factorial in nature, and potential etiologies range from psychostimulant-mediated sleep onset delay in some children to bedtime resistance related to a comorbid anxiety or oppositional defiant disorder in others (15). In some children, settling difficulties at bedtime may be related to deficits in sensory integration associated with ADHD, while in others, a primary sleep disorder such as circadian phase delay or restless legs syndrome may be the major etiologic factor in bedtime resistance. Furthermore, difficulty falling asleep related to psychostimulant use may respond to adjustments in the dosing schedule, as in some children the sleep onset delay is due to a "rebound" effect of the medication wearing off coincident with bedtime, rather than a direct stimulatory effect of the medication itself.

Second, it follows that all children and adolescents presenting with symptoms of insomnia must undergo a *thorough clinical evaluation*, in order to determine the etiology and guide treatment selection. In addition to the essential components of a medical and developmental history, the child's current level of functioning both in school and at home, and the impact of the child's sleep problem on the family should be assessed. A specific sleep history related to sleep habits, sleep hygiene practices, sleep schedules, and the sleeping environment, as well as the severity, frequency, and duration of the sleep complaint and any previous attempts at treatment, should be reviewed. Additional diagnostic tools such as polysomnography or multiple sleep latency testing are not indicated in the routine assessment of pediatric insomnia, but should be considered in those situations in which primary sleep disorders such as sleep disordered breathing or periodic limb movements are suspected on clinical grounds; sleep diaries are also often helpful in elucidating sleep patterns and behaviors. It should also be emphasized that more than one sleep disorder may be present in a given child; e.g., obstructive sleep apnea and behavioral insomnia. Referral to a sleep specialist for diagnosis and/or treatment should be considered for children in whom the diagnosis is unclear or complex.

Third, *behavioral interventions are the mainstay of treatment* in childhood insomnia. Consistent with the conclusions of two previous reviews (5,16), a recent review of 52 treatment studies indicates that behavioral therapies produce reliable and durable changes for both bedtime resistance and night wakings in young children (17). Ninety-four percent of the studies reported that behavioral interventions were efficacious, with over 80% of children treated demonstrating clinically significant improvement maintained for up to three to six months, and no study reported detrimental effects. A number of studies also found positive effects of sleep interventions on secondary child-related outcome variables, such as daytime behavior (18,19) as well as on the well-being of caregivers (20).

Fourth, whether or not pharmacological therapy is considered for pediatric insomnia, the importance of *sleep hygiene education* is critical in any discussion and should be viewed as paramount in treating children with sleep problems. Educating parents and children about normal sleep development and good sleep hygiene is key to successful treatment. The institution of appropriate sleep hygiene measures which revolve around the basic environmental (e.g., temperature, noise level, ambient light), scheduling (e.g., regular sleep–wake schedule), sleep practice (e.g., bedtime routine), and physiologic (e.g., exercise, timing of meals, caffeine use) factors promoting optimal sleep are a necessary component of every treatment package.

Medication Use in Clinical Practice

Although our knowledge base regarding the behavioral treatment of insomnia in the pediatric population has evolved significantly in the past two decades, very few empirical data regarding the efficacy, safety, and tolerability of pharmacologic interventions exist in the pediatric population, and there are currently no medications approved for use as hypnotics in children by the Food and Drug Administration (FDA). Despite this, medications are often used in clinical practice for pediatric sleep disorders (21–25). For example, a recent study (25) found that more than 75% of 671 community-based pediatric practitioners had recommended non-prescription medications and over 50% had prescribed a medication for "insomnia" (defined as significant difficulty falling or staying asleep) in the past six months; alpha-agonists were the most frequently prescribed sleep medications (31% of respondents). Another recent survey of 1271 practicing child and adolescent psychiatrists found that respondents prescribed a variety of medications to treat insomnia in a typical month, including alpha-agonist, sedating antidepressants, trazodone, atypical antipsychotics, and anticonvulsants (26). In a third study of nearly 10,000 pediatric inpatients at three centers, although only 3% of all medically hospitalized children were prescribed a sleeping medication, children with a psychiatric diagnosis were almost three times more likely to receive a sleep medication (27). In addition, it should be emphasized that herbal preparations and over-the-counter medication such as diphenhydramine and melatonin are frequently used by parents to treat sleep problems with or without the recommendation (or necessarily the knowledge) of the primary care or mental health provider.

General Guidelines for the use of Medications in Pediatric Insomnia

The following recommendations are adapted from the report of a 2003 consensus conference regarding use of hypnotics in children (28). The task force, supported by the American Academy of Sleep Medicine, included experts in pediatric sleep, child psychiatry, child neurology, general and developmental-behavioral pediatrics, and clinical pharmacology.

- Since the "ideal" pediatric hypnotic does not currently exist, rational treatment selection should be based on the clinician's judgment of the *best possible match* between the clinical circumstances (type of sleep problem, patient characteristics, etc.) and the individual properties of currently available drugs (onset and duration of action, safety, tolerability, etc.). This principle presumes some degree of familiarity on the part of the clinician with the pharmacologic profile of the available sedative/hypnotics currently available for use in the pediatric population (Tables 1 and 2). Prior to choosing a pharmacological agent for a targeted sleep symptom such as sleep onset, sleep duration, or night wakings, the risks and benefits should be weighed in the context of the clinical situation.
- In almost all cases, medication is *not* the first treatment choice or the sole treatment strategy. Medication use, except for very self-limited circumstances such as travel, should be viewed only within the context of a more comprehensive treatment plan.
- Medication should always be used *in combination* with non-pharmacologic strategies (behavioral interventions, parent education, etc.). This is analogous to a number of other conditions in children, such as (ADHD), in which a combination of pharmacologic and behavioral strategies is often superior to drug treatment alone.
- Treatment goals should be *realistic, clearly defined, discussed and agreed upon with the family* before treatment is initiated. In addition, there must be a clear plan for follow up and reassessment of therapeutic goals. In particular, the parental expectations regarding the degree of amelioration of the sleep problem by medication and the anticipated duration of drug treatment should be clearly established.
- Medication use should be for as *short a time as possible*; no prescription refills should be given without reassessment of the target symptoms and assessment of patient compliance with both pharmacologic and behavioral management.

TABLE 1 Pharmacology of Selected Medications Used for Pediatric Insomnia[1]

Drug	Class	Mechanism of action	Half-life (T 1/2) (hours)	Metabolism	Onset of action/peak level (min)	Drug-drug interactions	Sleep architecture effects
Clonazepam (Klonopin) Flurazepam (Dalmane) Quazepam (Doral) Temazepam (Restoril) Estazolam (ProSom) Triazolam (Halcion)	Benzodiazepines (BZD)[2]	Bind to central GABA (gama-aminobutyric acid) receptors	19–60 48–120 48–120 3–25 8–24 8–24	Hepatic	20–60 20–45 20–45 45–60 15–30 15–30 Rapid absorption; slowed by food	ETOH/ barbiturates increase CNS depression	Supress SWS; reduce frequency of nocturnal arousals
Chloral hydrate		Unknown; nonspecific CNS depression? interaction with GABA receptors	10 hr; decreases with increasing age in children; T1/2 infants 3–4x > adults	Hepatic/renal	Onset 30	Increases CNS & respiratory depressant effects; may alter effects of anticoagulants	Decreases SOL
Clonidine (Catapres)	Alpha agonists	Alpha adrenergic receptor agonists; (guanfacine more selective) decrease NE release	6–24	50–80% of dose excreted unchanged in urine	Rapid absorption; bioavailability 100%; onset action within 1 hr; peak effects 2–4 hrs	Reports of serious CVS effects with co-administration with psychostimulants[3]	Decreases SOL
Guanfacine (Tenex)			17				
Zolpidem (Ambien)	Pyrimidine derivatives	BZD-like	2–4	Hepatic	30–60	ETOH, CNS depressants may potentiate effects	Decrease SOL, little effects sleep archtecture
Zaleplon (Sonata)			1–2	No active metabolites			
Trazadone (Desyrel)	Atypical antidepressant	5HT, serotonin agonist	Biphasic; first T 1/2 3–6 hours; second T 1/2 5–9 hours 10–36 hours post ingestion	Hepatic	30–120	Potentiates effects ETOH, CNS depressants, digoxin, phenytoin, antihypertensives	Decreases SOL, improves sleep continuity, decreases REM, increases SWS

Drug	Class	Main effect	Metabolism			Interactions	Clinical effect
Melatonin[4]	Hormone analogue	circadian; weak hypnotic	Hepatic	30–50 min Returns to baseline levels in 4–8 hours biphasic elimination; 3 min and 45 min 90% excreted in 4 hours	30–60 (sustained release peak level 4 hours)	Largely unknown; NSAID's ETOH, Caffeine, BZD's may interfere with normal melatonin production	Decreases SOL; main effect on circadian rhythms
Diphenhydramine (Benadryl) Brompheniramine Chlorpheniramine Hydroxyzine (Atarax)	Antihistamines	H1 subtype receptor agonists; First generation drugs cross blood–brain barrier	Hepatic	Duration of action: 4–6 4–6 4–6 6–24	Rapid absorption and onset of action; Peak levels 2–4 hours	ETOH/CNS depressants (barbiturates, opiates)	Decreases SOL; may impair sleep quality

1. Reed MD, Findling RL. Overview of current management of sleep disturbances in children: I-Pharmacotherapy. *Current Therapeu Research*. 2002;63 (Supplement B):B18–B37.
2. Mendelson WB. Hypnotics: Basic mechanisms and pharmacology. In Principles and Practice of Sleep Medicine, 3rd edn, Philadelphia, PA: WB Saunders, 2000.
3. Popper CW. Combining methylphenidate and clonidine: Pharmacologic questions and news reports about sudden death. *J Child Adol Psychopharmacol*. 1995;5:157.
4. Czeisler CA, Cajochen C, Turek FW. Melatonin in the regulation of sleep and circadian rhythms. In Principles and Practice of Sleep Medicine, 3rd edn, Philadelphia, PA: WB Saunders, 2000.

Abbreviations: SWS = Slow Wave Sleep (Stage 3–4); SOL = Sleep Onset Latency; BZD = Benzodiazepine; NSAD = Non Steroidal Anti-inflammatory Drug; ETOH = Alcohol

TABLE 2 Clinical Properties of Selected Medications Used for Pediatric Insomnia

Drug	Adult dosing range (mg/d)	Formulation	Side effects	Development tolerance/ withdrawal effects	Safety profile/ (overdose)	Comments
Clonazepam	0.5–2.0	Tablets	Residual daytime sedation, rebound insomnia on discontinuation, psychomotor/ cognitive impairment, anterograde amnesia (dose dependent); impairment respiratory function	Yes, especially with shorter acting BZD; withdrawal effects include seizures	Marked abuse potential	Also used to control partial arousal parasomnias (night terrors, sleepwalking); use short half-life BZD for sleep onset; longer half-life for sleep maintenance
Flurazepam	15–30					
Quazepam	7.5–30					
Temazepam	15–30					
Estazolam	1–2					
Triazolam	0.125–0.25					
Chloral hydrate	50–75 mg/kg; max 1–2 gm per dose	Capsules, syrup, rectal suppository	Respiratory depression, GI (nausea, vomiting, especially if taken without food), drowsiness/dizziness	Yes, withdrawal after prolonged use may cause delerium, seizures	Poor tolerability safety profile; OD: CNS depression, cardiac arrythmias, hypothermia, hypotension	Reports of possible liver toxicity, respiratory depression limit use
Clonidine	0.025–0.3 (up to 0.8) Increase by 0.05 increments	Tablet, transdermal patch	Dry mouth, bradycardia, hypotension, rebound hypertension on discontinuation		Narrow therapeutic index; OD-bradycardia, decreased consciousness hypotension	Also used in daytime treatment of ADHD
Quanfacine	0.5–2					
Zolpidem	5–10		Headache, retrograde amnesia; few residual next-day effects	May develop tolerance/adaptation with extended use; May develop rebound insomnia on discontinuation	Well-tolerated in adults/OD: CNS depression; hypotension	Little clinical experience in children
Zaleplon	5–10					
Trazadone	20–50	Tablets	Dizziness, CNS overstimulation. Cardiac arrythmias, hypotension, priapism		OD: hypotension, cardiac effects	May be used with comorbid depression

Abbreviations: OD = overdose, BZD = benzodiazapine

- Medication selection, particularly in terms of duration of action, should be *appropriate for the presenting complaint*, i.e., for problems with sleep onset, a shorter acting medication is generally desirable. For problems with sleep maintenance, longer acting medications may be considered, but are more likely to result in "hang-over"effects the following morning.
- The use of medication is rarely, if ever, indicated when the insomnia is due to a *developmentally based normal sleep behavior*, or when there are inappropriate expectations regarding the child's sleep behaviors from the parent or practitioners. For example sleep problems in infants and very young children are almost always related to "developmental asynchrony" between the child's sleep development and parental expectations (e.g., development of nocturnal–diurnal sleep–wake rhythms, "sleeping through the night").

Safety Considerations

- Patients should also be screened for concurrent use of self-initiated non-prescription sleep medications (e.g., Tylenol PM, melatonin, herbals). Some of these medications have similar ingredients (e.g., diphenhydramine is the soporific ingredient in both Benadryl and Tylenol PM); while generally viewed by parents as "safe," the potential drug–drug interactions between most herbal preparations and sedative/hypnotics are largely unknown.
- Adolescents should be screened for alcohol and drug use and pregnancy prior to initiation of therapy. Many recreational substances may have synergistic clinical effects when combined with sedatives/hypnotics. In addition, hypnotics with high toxicity levels in overdose should be used with extreme caution in situations in which there is any risk of non-accidental overdose.
- All medications prescribed for sleep problems should be closely monitored for the emergence of side effects. Some medications may also precipitate or exacerbate additional problems such as sleepwalking, confusional arousals, and daytime sleepiness, or may further escalate behavioral problems (29,30). Furthermore, discontinuation of these agents may also result in increased sleep problems; for example, increased nightmares as a result of "rapid eye movement (REM) rebound" may occur if a REM-suppressing medication is withdrawn abruptly.
- Because the use of medication for one disorder could potentially exacerbate co-existing sleep problems (e.g., selective serotonin reuptake inhibitors (SSRIs) may increase symptoms in restless legs syndrome), the presence of both medically based and behaviorally based sleep disorders must be assessed and appropriately addressed.
- Medication should be avoided if the insomnia occurs in the presence of untreated sleep disordered breathing (e.g., obstructive sleep apnea). Not only is hypnotic medication often inappropriate for treating the underlying condition, but sedatives with respiratory depressant properties (e.g., chloral hydrate) may be dangerous in the situation of a comorbid sleep-related breathing disorder.
- Medication should also be used with caution in situations in which there may be potential drug interactions with concurrent medications (e.g., opiates) or unrecognized substance abuse or alcohol use, or if there is limited ability to follow-up with and monitor the patient; e.g., parent frequently misses scheduled appointments.

Special Considerations for Pharmacologic Treatment of Insomnia in Children with Comorbid Conditions

Not only do children with chronic physical and mental health problems have sleep problems similar to those occurring in normal children (31,32), unique factors related to the specific condition (hyperactivity, cognitive delays, pain, etc.) may result in sleep problems which are more severe, more chronic, and more difficult to treat. For example, children with severe neurodevelopmental deficits may be more challenging to actively engage in behavioral management or may have more difficulty complying with treatment.

A number of children with specific genetic, psychiatric and behavioral syndromes and conditions are susceptible to insomnia. For example, up to 70–80% of children with autism and pervasive developmental disorder (PDD) (33–35) have sleep problems, including irregular sleep–wake cycles, delayed sleep onset, prolonged night wakings, short sleep duration, and early morning wake times. Children with ADHD are often reported by parents to have sleep onset difficulties and restless sleep, and present one of the more common chronic conditions for which sedatives are recommended by pediatric practitioners (36–38). Psychiatric conditions (i.e., anxiety disorders or depression) can often present with either insomnia or hypersomnia; 75% of children and adolescents with major depressive disorder report insomnia—30% "severe"—and 25% of depressed adolescents report hypersomnia. Sleep problems may exacerbate the mood and anxiety symptoms; successful treatment of the sleep complaint may improve the psychiatric condition, and vice versa.

Children with other chronic medical conditions such as asthma (39) or atopy (40) and cystic fibrosis, can be prone to sleep disruption either from medication used to treat the underlying condition, or as a result of poor symptom control. In addition, other factors such as the psychological response to illness, family dynamics, hospitalization-related disruption of normal sleep routines, and related secondary symptoms, such as pain, can significantly impact sleep in these children. Medical conditions which may place children particularly at risk for sleep problems also include severe burns, sickle cell anemia, rheumatologic disorders, and chronic headaches.

The approach to insomnia in children with underlying medical or developmental conditions must be viewed in the context of the many challenges of the situation that involve the patient and family. Pharmacologic therapy should be considered for sleep problems as part of the overall management strategy, in conjunction with behavioral therapy and sleep hygiene. Sleep problems in these children often require aggressive management to avoid exacerbation of the underlying condition and to improve overall quality of life; longer duration of drug therapy is also often necessary in these children (21).

In addition, it should be kept in mind that many over-the-counter and prescription drugs used for a variety of medical and psychiatric conditions have potentially significant effects on sleep and alertness in children, including direct pharmacologic effects, disruption of sleep patterns (e.g., night wakings), exacerbation of a primary sleep disorder (e.g., obstructive sleep apnea or restless legs syndrome), withdrawal effects, and daytime sedation. Drugs commonly used in children which may have effects on sleep include: psychotropic drugs such as stimulants (amphetamines and methylphenidate may cause increased wakefulness and increased sleep onset latency) and antidepressants (tricyclic antidepressants suppress slow wave sleep and may cause daytime sedation; SSRIs are often activating and may result in sleep disruption;); antihistamines: (first generation drugs such as diphenhydramine, hydroxyzine, and chlorpheniramine cross the blood brain barrier and promote sleep; alternatively, they may also significantly reduce daytime alertness and impair performance); corticosteroids (may be associated with insomnia and subjective increases in wakefulness), opioids (associated with daytime sedation and disruption of sleep continuity, and may worsen obstructive sleep apnea; abrupt discontinuation may lead to insomnia and nightmares), and anticonvulsants (associated with excessive daytime sedation). It should also be noted that caffeine, the most widely used drug in the world, has potent effects on sleep resulting in difficulty initiating sleep and more frequent arousals.

PHARMACOLOGICAL AGENTS FOR PEDIATRIC INSOMNIA
A summary of pharmacologic and clinical properties of medications currently most commonly used in the treatment of pediatric insomnia are listed in Tables 1 and 2 and are discussed below. Although many different classes of medications have sedating properties, only those used in clinical practice for treatment of insomnia will be reviewed

Benzodiazepines
Benzodiazepines (BZD) activate gamma-aminobutyric acid (GABA) receptors and, as a result, shorten sleep onset latency and improve non-rapid eye movement (NREM) sleep maintenance; most disrupt slow wave sleep. They also have muscle relaxant, anxiolytic, and anticonvulsant properties. In pediatrics, these medications have been used primarily for sedation and as anticonvulsants, less often as hypnotics. The shorter onset of action of some benzodiazepines is useful for treating sleep onset insomnia, while agents with a longer half-life and duration of action are more useful in addressing maintenance of sleep. However, use of longer-acting BZDs may lead to morning "hangover," daytime sleepiness, and compromised daytime functioning. Anterograde amnesia may also occur. There is a risk of habituation or addiction with these medications, as well as withdrawal phenomena, making them of limited use in children and adolescents. In general, this class of medication should be used for short-term or transient insomnia, or in clinical situations in which their other properties (e.g., anxiolytic) are advantageous. Of note, benzodiazepines are occasionally used to treat intractable partial arousal parasomnias (e.g., sleep terrors) in children because of their slow wave sleep suppressant effects.

Pyrimidine Agents (Non-Benzodiazepines)
Zaleplon (Sonata) is a non-benzodiazepine medication that binds to the benzodiazepine receptor. It has a very short half-life, making it useful for sleep onset insomnia. Effects on sleep architecture appear minimal, although it may increase slow wave sleep. Side effects include dizziness, anterograde amnesia, confusion, and hallucinations; the most common adverse event reported in adults is headaches. Use of zaleplon has not been studied in children, except in one study where it was used for sedation purposes. Therefore, its potential role in the clinical treatment of pediatric insomnia is not known.

Zolpidem (Ambien) is also a hypnotic agent that acts at the $GABA_A$ receptor site by binding selective GABA receptors. It can be used for sleep maintenance insomnia or night awakenings because of its slightly longer half-life of two to three hours. Ambien-CR has a longer half-life which may make it more useful in sleep maintenance. No published efficacy studies in the pediatric population exist; a single case series which described 12 accidental ingestions in a group of children aged 20 months to five years and five intentional ingestions in 15–16-year-olds (41) reported onset of central nervous system symptoms but no fatalities. Recent reports of rare sleep-related events (sleep-eating, sleep-driving) in adults taking zolpidem have raised additional concerns about its use in children. Rebound insomnia may occur with either of these compounds.

Eszopiclone (Lunesta) is a newer GABA-ergic sleep medication which, because of its longer half-life, has been used in adults for both sleep initiation and sleep maintenance. Peak drug concentration occurs at 60 minutes; half-life and clinical effect are approximately six hours. Fatty foods tend to delay the absorption; side effects include unpleasant taste and headache. Abrupt withdrawl with prolonged use (>2 weeks) may be associated with rebound insomnia. Studies in adults have shown no development of tolerance effects at six months; this medication has been approved for longer-term use.

Tricyclic Antidepressants (TCAs)

Tricyclic antidepressants have been used to treat children with mood disorders, as well as with ADHD, for a number of years. Most TCAs are potent REM suppressants; thus, rapid withdrawal may lead to REM rebound and nightmares. TCAs also tend to suppress slow wave sleep. The choice of antidepressant for a mood disorder should take into consideration the presence of concurrent sleep problems, and whether insomnia or hypersomnia is part of the clinical picture. Treating the underlying mood disorder will often result in improved sleep, but the reverse is clearly true as well. Most TCAs are sedating, although they vary in the degree of sedating properties. Amitriptyline, doxepin, trimipramine are the most sedating TCAs. The most activating tricyclic is protriptyline; thus it should be avoided in the child with sleep onset or sleep maintenance difficulties. The most commonly reported side effects of tricyclics are anxiety and agitation as well as anticholinergic effects; because of their cardiotoxicity, TCAs should be used with extreme caution in clinical situations in which there is a risk of accidental or intentional overdose. TCAs may also exacerbate restless legs syndrome (RLS) symptoms.

Serotonin Antagonists/Reuptake Inhibitors (SSRIs)

These agents promote sleep by inhibiting uptake of serotonin. They vary widely in their propensity to cause sleep onset delay and sleep disruption (e.g., fluoxetine) and sedation (e.g., fluvoxamine, paroxetine, citralopram). They suppress REM sleep and often prolong REM onset while increasing the number of rapid eye movements; a characteristic polysomnographic finding in patients on SSRIs is so-called "Prozac eyes" due to this increased REM density. Most increase sleep onset latency and decrease sleep efficiency (time asleep/time in bed). SSRIs frequently are associated with motor restlessness, and may exacerbate pre-existing RLS and periodic limb movements (PLM).

Atypical Antidepressants

Trazadone, a 5HT agonist commonly used in child psychiatry clinical practice, is one of the most sedating antidepressants because it both inhibits binding of serotonin and blocks histamine receptors. Trazadone has suppressant effects on REM and may increase slow wave sleep. "Morning hangover" is a common side effect; it has rarely been associated with reports of priapism. Other classes of antidepressants also affect sleep; mirtazapine, for example, decreases sleep onset latency and increases sleep duration with relatively little effect on REM.

Clonidine

Clonidine, a central α_2 agonist, is one of the most widely used sedating medications in pediatric and child psychiatry practice, particularly in children with sleep onset delay and ADHD. Despite its widespread use, data regarding safety and efficacy in children with ADHD and sleep problems are limited (42,43). Pharmacokinetics show rapid absorption, with an onset action within one hour, peak effects at two to four hours and a half-life 6–24 hours. Effects on sleep architecture are fairly minimal but may include decreased REM, thus discontinuation can lead to REM rebound. Clonidine has a narrow therapeutic index and there has been a recent dramatic increase in reports of overdose with this medication (44). Potentially significant side effects include hypotension and bradycardia, and there have been reports in the literature of sudden death in combination with psychostimulant medication (45). Anti-cholinergic effects; irritability and dysphoria; and rebound hypertension may occur on abrupt discontinuation. Tolerance often develops, necessitating increases in dose.

Antihistamines

Both prescription and over-the-counter (OTC) antihistamines are the most commonly prescribed/recommended sedatives in pediatric practice. They bind to H_1 receptor central nervous system (CNS), with only the first generation medications crossing the blood–brain barrier. They are generally rapidly absorbed. Effects on sleep architecture are minimal, and side effects include daytime drowsiness, cholinergic effects, and paradoxical excitation. In general these drugs are rather weak soporifics; a recent study in 6–15-month-olds found that diphenhydramine was no better than a placebo in reducing night waking (46). However, parental and provider familiarity tend to make them a more acceptable choice for many families. It should also be noted that tolerance to antihistamines tends to develop, necessitating increasing doses. Parents should also be cautioned about inadvertently overdosing a child by giving multiple OTC medications with diphenhydramine as the active ingredient (e.g., Benadryl and Tylenol PM).

Melatonin

Melatonin is a hormone secreted by the pineal gland in response to decreased light, mediated through the suprachiasmatic nucleus. The mechanism of action of commercially available melatonin is to supplement the endogenous pineal hormone. Thus, clinical uses for melatonin are principally in acute or chronic circadian rhythm disturbances (e.g., delayed sleep phase syndrome, jet lag) in normal children and children with special needs (blindness, Rett's syndrome). A number of studies have demonstrated efficacy in reducing sleep onset latency in children with ADHD (46–50), based on the premise that at least some of these children have a circadian-medicated phase delay (i.e., delayed sleep onset and offset compared to developmental norms). In addition to effects on circadian regulation of sleep–wake cycles, melatonin has mild hypnotic properties. Thus it may be helpful in reducing sleep onset latency when taken at bedtime; sustained release preparations may assist in maintaining sleep. The plasma levels of exogenous melatonin peak within one hour of administration. Although generally regarded as safe, potential side effects of melatonin include lowering of seizure threshold in some individuals, and potential suppression of the hypothalamic-gonadal axis. Melatonin is not regulated by the FDA, therefore the commercially available formulations tend to vary in strength, and purity. Reported doses for melatonin include: 1 mg in infants, 2.5 to 3 mg in older children, and 5 mg in adolescents; use of melatonin in children with special needs have reported doses ranging from 0.5 mg to 10 mg, irrespective of age. It should be noted that studies of melatonin use in adults for advancing sleep phase have reported that smaller doses (e.g., 0.5 mg) five to seven hours before sleep onset may be more effective in circadian rhythm disorders.

Other classes of medications that may be used for pediatric insomnia include mood stablizers/anticonvulsants (carbamezapine, valproic acid, topiramate, gabapentin), atypical antipsychotics (risperidone, olanzapine), and chloral hydrate, as well as herbal preparations such as chamomile and valerian root. Many of the newer atypical antipsychotics have weight gain as a significant side effect, and thus can worsen obstructive sleep apnea; they also tend to suppress REM sleep and increase motor restlessness during sleep. Any of these medications should be used with caution for insomnia in children, as there are limited data on safety and tolerability for this indication. Chloral hydrate and barbiturates are rarely indicated in children because of significant side effects; the American Academy of Pediatrics (AAP) in 1993 recommended the use of chloral hydrate in children for short-term sedation only because of the risk of hepatotoxicity.

Most herbal preparations are generally considered safe. However, there have only been a handful of studies which have suggested that some herbal preparations may be useful for sleep in the pediatric population, and these products in general remain largely untested in children. Valerian root, St. John's Wort, and hops have been shown to have some evidence of efficacy in adult and/or pediatric studies; lemon balm, chamomile, and passionflower have limited to no evidence, and kava-kava and tryptophan have been associated with significant safety concerns (e.g., hepatotoxicity and eosinophilic myalgia syndrome, respectively) (51).

REFERENCES

1. Goodlin-Jones BL, Burnham MM, Gaylor EE, et al. Night waking, sleep-wake organization, and self-soothing in the first year of life. J Dev Behav Pediatr 2001; 22(4):226–33.
2. Burnham MM, Goodlin-Jones BL, Gaylor EE, et al. Nighttime sleep-wake patterns and self-soothing from birth to one year of age: A longitudinal intervention study. J Child Psychol Psychiatry 2002; 43(6):713–25.
3. Lozoff B, Wolf AW, Davis NS. Sleep problems seen in pediatric practice. Pediatrics 1985; 75(3):477–83.
4. Armstrong KL, Quinn RA, Dadds MR. The sleep patterns of normal children. Med J Aust 1994; 161(3):202–6.
5. Mindell JA. Empirically supported treatments in pediatric psychology: Bedtime refusal and night wakings in young children. J Ped Psychol 1999; 24(6):465–81.

6. Blader JC, Koplewicz HS, Abikoff H, et al. Sleep problems of elementary school children A community survey. Arch Pediatr Adolesc Med 1997; 151(5):473–80.
7. Owens JA, Spirito A, McGuinn M, et al. Sleep habits and sleep disturbance in elementary school-aged children. J Dev Behav Pediatr 2000; 21(1):27–36.
8. Johnson EO, Roth T, Schultz L, et al. Epidemiology of DSM-IV insomnia in adolescence: Lifetime prevalence, chronicity, and an emergent gender difference. Pediatrics 2006; 117(2):e247–56.
9. Dahl.RE, Ryan ND, Matty MK, et al. Sleep onset abnormalities in depressed adolescents. Biol Psychiatry 1996; 39(6):400–10.
10. Sadeh A, McGuire JP, Sachs H, et al. Sleep and psychological characteristics of children on a psychiatric inpatient unit. J Am Acad of Child Adolesc Psychiatry 1995; 34(6):813–19.
11. Wiggs L. Sleep problems in children with developmental disorders. J R Soc Med 2001; 94(4):177–9.
12. Fallone G, Owens J, Deane J. Sleepiness in children and adolescents: Cinical implications. Sleep Med Rev 2002; 6(2):287–306.
13. Valent F, Brusaferro S, Barbone F. A case-crossover study of sleep and childhood injury. Pediatrics 2001; 107(2):E23.
14. Spiegel K, Leprout R, Van Cauter E. Impact of sleep debt on metabolic function. Lancet 1999; 354(9188):1435–9.
15. Owens JA. The ADHD and sleep conundrum: A review. J Dev Behav Pediatr 2005; 26(4):312–22.
16. Kuhn BR, Elliott AJ. Treatment efficacy in behavioral pediatric sleep medicine. J Psychosom Res 2003; 54(6):587–97.
17. Mindell J, Kuhn B, Lewin D, et al. Behavioral treatment of bedtime problems and night wakings in infants and young children. An American Academy of Sleep Medicine Review. Sleep 2006; 29(10):1263–76.
18. Minde K, Faucon A, Falkner S. Sleep problems in toddlers: Effects of treatment on their daytime behavior. J Am Acad Child Adolesc Psychiat 1994; 33(8):1114–21.
19. Adams LA, Rickert VI. Reducing bedtime tantrums: Comparison between positive routines and graduated extinction. Pediatrics 1989; 84(5):756–61.
20. Hiscock H, Wake M. Randomised controlled trial of behavioural infant sleep intervention to improve infant sleep and maternal mood. BMJ 2002; 324(7345):1062.
21. Owens JA, Babcock D, Blumer J, et al. The use of pharmacotherapy in the treatment of pediatric insomnia in primary care: Rational approaches. A consensus meeting summary. J Clin Sleep Med 2005; 1(1):49–59.
22. Zito JM, Safer DJ, DosReis S, et al. Psychotropic practice patterns for youth: a 10-year perspective. Arch Pediatr Adolesc Med 2003; 157(1):17–25.
23. Rappley MD, Eneli IU, Mullan PB, et al. Patterns of psychotropic medication use in very young children with attention-deficit hyperactivity disorder. J Dev Behav Pediatr 2002; 23(1):23–30.
24. Ledoux S, Choquet M, Manfredi R. Self-reported use of drugs for sleep or distress among French adolescents. J Adolesc Health 1994; 15(6):495–502.
25. Owens J, Rosen C, Mindell J. Medication use in the treatment of pediatric insomnia: Results of a survey of community-based pediatricians. Pediatrics 2003; 111(5):e628–35.
26. Rosen C, Owens J, Mindell J. Pharmacotherapy for pediatric insomnia child psychiatrists. Sleep 2005, 8 (Abstract Supplement): A79.
27. Meltzer L, Mindell J, Owens J, et al. The use of sleep medications in pediatric inpatients. Pediatrics 2007; 119(6):1047–55.
28. Owens J, Babcock D, Blumer J, et al. The use of pharmacotherapy in the treatment of pediatric insomnia in primary care: Rational approaches. A consensus meeting summary. J Clin Sleep Med 2005; 1(1):49–59.
29. Sheldon S, Ferber R, Kryger M. Principles and Practice of Pediatric Sleep Medicine. United States: Elsevier Inc, 2005.

30. Kryger M, Roth T, Dement W. Principles and Practice of Sleep Medicine, 3rd edn Philadelphia, PA: WB Saunders Co, 2000.
31. Sachs H, McGuire J, Sadeh A, et al. Cognitive and behavioral correlates of mother reported sleep problems in psychiatrically hospitalized children. Sleep Res 1994; 23:207–13.
32. Johnson C. Sleep problems in children with mental retardation and autism. Child Adolesc Psychiatr Clin N Am 1996; 5(3):673–81.
33. Palermo TM, Koren G, Blumer JL. Rational pharmacotherapy for childhood sleep disturbances: Characteristics of an ideal hypnotic. Cur Ther Res 2002; 63 (Suppl B):B67–B79.
34. Johnson C. Sleep problems in children with mental retardation and autism. Child and Adolesc Psychiatr Clin of N Am 1996; 5(3):673–81.
35. Wiggs L. Sleep problems in children with developmental disorders. J R Soc Med 2001; 94(4):177–9.
36. Mick E, Biederman J, Jetton J, et al. Sleep disturbances associated with attention deficit hyperactivity disorder: The impact of psychiatric comorbidity and pharmacotherapy. J Child Adolesc Psychopharmacol 2000; 10(3):223–31.
37. Marcotte AC, Thacher PV, Butters M, et al. Parental report of sleep problems in children with attentional and learning disorders. J Dev Behav Pediatr 1998; 19(3):178–86.
38. Owens JA, Maxim R, Nobile C, et al. Parental and self-report of sleep in children with attention-deficit/hyperactivity disorder. Arch Pediatr Adolesc Med 2000; 154(6):549–55.
39. Sadeh A, Horowitz I, Wolach-Benodis L, et al. Sleep and pulmonary function in children with well-controlled stable asthma. Sleep 1998; 21(4):379–84.
40. Dahl R, Bernhisel-Broadbent J, Scanlon-Holdford S, et al. Sleep disturbances in children with atopic dermatitis. Arch Pediatr Adolesc Med 1995; 149(8):856–60.
41. Kurta DL, Myers LB, Krenzelok EP. Zolpidem (Ambien): A pediatric case series. J Toxicol Clin Toxicol 1997; 35(5):453–7.
42. Prince JB, Wilens TE, Biederman J, et al. Clonidine for sleep disturbances associated with attention-deficit hyperactivity disorder: A systematic chart review of 62 cases. J Am Acad Child Adolesc Psychiatry 1996; 35(5):599–605.
43. Hunt RD, Minderaa RB, Cohen DJ. Clonidine benefits children with attention deficit disorder and hyperactivity: Report of a double-blind placebo-crossover therapeutic trial. J Am Acad Child Psychiatry 1985; 24(5):617–29.
44. Kappagoda C, Schell DN, Hanson RM, et al. Clonidine overdose in childhood: implications of increased prescribing. J Paediatr Child Health 1998; 34(6):508–12.
45. Popper CW. Combining methylphenidate and clonidine: Pharmacologic questions and news reports about sudden death. J Child Adolesc Psychopharmacol 1995; 5:157–66.
46. Van der Heijden KB, Smits MG, Van Someren EJ, et al. Effect of melatonin on sleep, behavior, and cognition in ADHD and chronic sleep-onset insomnia. J Am Acad Child Adolesc Psychiatry 2007; 46(2):233–41.
47. Smits MG, Nagtegaal EE, Van der Heijden J, et al. Melatonin for chronic sleep onset insomnia in children: A randomized placebo-controlled trial. J Child Neurol 2001; 16(2):86–92.
48. Smits MG, van Stel HF, Van der Heijden K, et al. Melatonin improves health status and sleep in children with idiopathic chronic sleep-onset insomnia: A randomized placebo-controlled trial. J Am Acad Child Adolesc Psychiatry 2003; 42(11):1286–93.
49. Van der Heijden KB, Smits MG, Van Someren EJ, et al. Prediction of melatonin efficacy by pretreatment dim light melatonin onset in children with idiopathic chronic sleep onset insomnia. J Sleep Res 2005; 14(2):195–7.
50. Weiss MD, Wasdell MB, Bomben MM, et al. Sleep hygiene and melatonin treatment for children and adolescents with ADHD and initial insomnia. J Am Acad Child Adolesc Psychiatry 2006; 45(5):512–19.
51. Merenstein D, Diener-West M, Halbower AC, et al. The trial of infant response to diphenhydramine: The TIRED Study—A Randomized, Controlled, Patient-Oriented Trial. Arch Pediatr Adolesc Med 2006; 160(7):707–12.

19 Nonpharmacological Interventions for Sleep Disorders in Children

Brett R. Kuhn and Margaret T. Floress

Munroe-Meyer Institute, Department of Pediatric Psychology, University of Nebraska Medical Center, Omaha, Nebraska, U.S.A.

INTRODUCTION

An estimated 20–30% of children will experience sleep problems during the first three years of life (1–4). Although parents and professionals wish that sleep problems would simply "go away" as the child matures, research suggests they can be highly persistent, lasting even into adulthood (5–8). Although certain pediatric sleep disorders clearly demand medical attention (e.g., obstructive sleep apnea, narcolepsy), the majority call for clinical assessment and intervention skills that behavioral specialists are well-suited to provide. Principles of learning (e.g., reinforcement, extinction, shaping, fading, stimulus control) that have been shown successful in reducing daytime behavior problems can be highly effective in alleviating many forms of pediatric sleep disturbance (9). The purpose of this article is to review nonpharmacological interventions for pediatric sleep disturbance; namely, bedtime resistance and night waking, circadian rhythm disorders, and the parasomnias. We then review briefly a rapidly emerging literature on behavioral interventions to promote adherence with continuous positive airway pressure (CPAP) for sleep-related breathing disorders.

BEDTIME RESISTANCE AND FREQUENT NIGHT WAKING

Bedtime resistance and frequent night waking are considered a "clinical dyad" because they often co-exist, and treatments targeting one symptom appear to generalize to the other (10). The core skill that binds these two symptoms is independent sleep initiation, which is required at bedtime and again to re-initiate sleep following nighttime awakenings that are part of a child's normal sleep cycle (11).

Research has identified a long list of factors that adversely impact children's sleep. The obvious culprits include illness, pain, medical conditions, child temperament, and circadian preference. Among numerous bio-psychosocial factors studied, the strongest predictor of sleep disturbance among infants and young children is parental handling at bedtime and again in response to nighttime awakenings (12–17). Children miss important opportunities to develop adaptive sleep associations when their parents remain with them until they fall asleep, place them in bed already asleep, feed them to sleep, or take them into the parents' bed following nocturnal awakenings. Because parents play a key role in establishing and maintaining children's sleep problems, it is not surprising that the majority of effective interventions target parents as the primary agent of change (18,19).

Early Intervention/Prevention

Parent education programs typically take place during the prenatal period or first six months of life. They may also occur while working toward early intervention with an emerging sleep problem. Parent education focuses on promoting positive sleep habits. Caregivers are typically provided information on bedtime routines, sleep schedules, and how to instill appropriate sleep associations for infants and toddlers (20). A nearly universal recommendation is to place infants in bed "drowsy but still awake." This practice teaches infants to develop independent sleep initiation skills at bedtime which allows them to re-initiate sleep following naturally occurring nighttime arousals. The effects of early intervention/prevention on infant sleep have been examined across five studies involving over 1000 subjects (21). Results are not only statistically significant, but clinically impressive. A sixth, more recent, study randomized 268 families to either parent education or no-treatment control. The education component consisted of a single, 45-minute consultation that took place two to three weeks after the child's birth (22). Results indicated that infants whose parents received parent education slept 1.3 hours more per day, or nine hours more per week compared to control infants.

Dissassociating Feeding from Sleep–Wake Transitions

For infants and toddlers, it is important to examine the impact of feeding habits and feeding patterns on sleep continuity, as the two are closely linked (23). Infants who are fed until they fall asleep at bedtime and again to re-initiate sleep following night wakings will quickly begin to associate feeding with the process of sleep initiation. Once the link between feeding and sleep is established, infants may become dependent on fluid intake, or the act of feeding itself, to fall asleep. Most experts agree that healthy infants who are four to six months old no longer require nighttime nutritional intake (24), and therefore do not need to be fed in the middle of the night. Infants usually make up for reduced nocturnal caloric intake by increasing their consumption early in the morning (25).

Implementing this strategy involves feeding the child prior to bedtime, then placing infants in the crib drowsy, but still awake (26). Infants who fall asleep while feeding can be gently awakened just before placing them down to sleep. This strategy allows sleep initiation to occur in the crib or habitual sleep location, gently breaking the association between feeding or sucking and sleep onset.

Research indicates that disassociating feeding from sleep–wake patterns can be achieved with even very young infants. Success has been found when mothers are taught to gradually delay breast-feeding in response to nighttime awakenings by replacing feeding with other activities such as re-swaddling, diapering, or walking (25). Disassociating feeding is an early intervention strategy that may eliminate the need for more intense intervention later on. It should be noted, however, that some professionals have raised concerns about the safety of modifying the sleep and feeding schedules in newborn infants, even questioning contemporary parents' goal of getting the young infant to "sleep through the night" (27).

Unmodified Extinction

When extinction is used for pediatric sleep disturbance, the child is placed in bed while any sleep interfering behaviors (e.g., crying) are ignored until morning.

Ignoring is discontinued when children are ill, in danger of harming themselves, or become destructive. Extinction maintains the strongest empirical support for improving sleep disturbances (28) however, it is possibly the most difficult intervention for parents to administer (3).

Graduated Extinction

Douglas and Richman (29) first described a version of graduated extinction; then it was popularized by Ferber (30) in his self-help book entitled *Solve Your Child's Sleep Problems.* The extinction procedure is supplemented with a parent checking procedure that is faded over time. Two types of graduated extinction have been identified. In the first, parents wait for progressively longer periods of time prior to responding to their child (31). The second calls for the parent to immediately respond, but parents decrease the time they spend with the child over time (32). The quick check procedure (33) is similar to graduated extinction, except the waiting period between parental checks is maintained at a constant interval (e.g., every 10 minutes).

Advantages of graduated extinction include the convenience of keeping the child's regular bedtime and that positive results are usually evident within the first week of implementation. Disadvantages include possibly shaping the child's crying for longer periods of time or inadvertently increasing the "reinforcement value" across successive check-ins by intensifying or lengthening parent–child interactions (34).

Extinction with Parental Presence

During extinction with parental presence, the parent is instructed to sleep in the child's room but in a different bed, while ignoring the child's crying (35). This sleeping arrangement continues for one week until the child falls asleep consistently. The parent then returns to sleeping in a separate room. The underlying theory is that parental presence is reassuring, allowing children to fall asleep more quickly. Compared to unmodified extinction and extinction with checking, extinction with parental presence appears to reduce nighttime awakenings while limiting the post-extinction response burst (36). These findings have led some researchers to conclude that extinction with parental presence is the "treatment of choice" for infant sleep disturbance (36). Some parents, however, may be hesitant to change sleeping arrangements and find it more, not less, difficult to ignore their child while in close proximity. Another potential limitation is that the children may continue to depend on parental presence to initiate sleep. The literature has yet to describe how parents can make the transition back to an alternative bedroom without re-initiating the child's protests.

Scheduled Awakenings

The Scheduled Awakenings protocol involves having parents briefly awaken their child just prior to those times when the child would be expected to wake spontaneously. After completing a baseline diary of spontaneous nighttime wakings, a planned schedule of parent-initiated awakenings is implemented 15 to 30 minutes prior to each anticipated awakening. Once awake, the child is provided the usual parenting responses (e.g., rocking, patting, feeding) as if the child had awakened spontaneously (37). Gradually, the scheduled awakenings are delayed until the child sleeps for longer periods between awakenings, and finally sleeps through the night. Research supports scheduled awakenings as another treatment option for frequent nighttime awakenings (21). However, because Scheduled Awakenings is a more complicated protocol and takes longer to implement compared to extinction, parents may have more difficulty maintaining adherence. Another disadvantage is that this intervention does not address sleep initiation skills, thereby limiting its usefulness with children who present with both nighttime awakenings and bedtime resistance (28). Scheduled awakenings may be most beneficial for parents who are unwilling to use extinction-based interventions or for children who have become resistant to extinction-based procedures and exhibit gagging, vomiting, or self-injurious behaviors upon awakening at night (38).

Positive Bedtime Routines and Faded Bedtime

Positive bedtime routines and faded bedtime are similar strategies. Both rely heavily on sleep scheduling and stimulus control (28). Positive bedtime routines can be conceptualized as a differential reinforcement procedure designed to teach children appropriate and adaptive pre-bedtime behaviors and sleep onset skills. First, bedtime is temporarily moved later in the evening to correspond more closely with the child's natural sleep onset time. This increases homeostatic sleep drive which usually ensures more rapid sleep onset. Parents implement a positive and enjoyable pre-bedtime routine that teaches the child to engage in relaxing activities prior to bed. Parents attend to and praise the child after the completion of each step in the bedtime routine. Once the routine is well-established and the child is falling asleep quickly, bedtime is gradually faded earlier in the evening until the predetermined bedtime goal is reached.

The faded bedtime procedure is similar in that the child's bedtime is temporarily delayed approximately 30 minutes later than usual. A response cost component may be added by removing children from the bed and keeping them awake for 30–60 minutes if they do not fall to sleep quickly (e.g., 15–30 minutes) (39). Once a child begins to fall asleep more quickly, the bedtime is systematically faded 30 minutes earlier over successive nights until the bedtime goal is reached.

Positive bedtime routines and the faded bedtime protocol appear to decrease the duration of child crying episodes, bedtime struggles, and parental anxiety. Positive bedtime routines has been termed an "errorless" procedure (38), offering a decided advantage over extinction-based approaches. Specifically, children are provided attention when they demonstrate adaptive and appropriate bedtime behaviors. Potential disadvantages include interruptions (e.g., illness, family travel) to the systematic bedtime fading process, and occasional parental resistance to initially delaying a child's bedtime.

Bedtime Pass

The bedtime pass is a modified extinction protocol for children who exhibit bedtime resistance, including calling out or leaving the room after bedtime (40). The program involves providing the child a card or "free pass" exchangeable for one permitted trip out of their room to request one final good night hug or drink of water. The pass is then surrendered and parents are instructed to ignore additional requests or crying. Research indicates that children receiving the bedtime pass left their rooms less often and quieted more quickly than children in the control condition (41).

Advantages to the bedtime pass include increased likelihood of parent adherence compared to traditional extinction interventions. Reasons for this may include increased social acceptability as well as the absence of an extinction burst (40). The bedtime pass may be less effective with children younger than three years of age and children older than 10 years of age (42).

Reinforcement

Reinforcement refers to any event that follows the occurrence of a behavior, which increases the future probability or rate of that behavior (43). Tangible reinforcers such as candy, toys, or tickets can be used, however social reinforcers (hug, smile, praise) and activity reinforcers (reading, playing a game) should not be overlooked. Very little research has been conducted to evaluate positive reinforcement as the lone treatment component to target children's sleep. Rather, reinforcement is usually included as part of a multicomponent treatment package (21). Robinson and Sheridan used behavioral contracting in conjunction with a Mystery Motivator to effectively reduce bedtime noncompliance (44). Caregivers first identify a specific target behavior (e.g., in bed by 9 p.m. without getting up more than once before morning). Achieving the target allows a child to color in a pre-selected square using a "developer" pen with invisible ink that changes color to reveal the child's reward.

Preliminary research suggests that the sleep fairy, which combines the use of a social story with tangible rewards, may be another effective method in reducing children's disruptive bedtime behavior and frequent night waking (45). The social story consists of a bedtime story about the tale of a "Sleep Fairy," who leaves a small tangible reward under a child's pillow contingent upon age appropriate sleep compatible behaviors. Following introduction of the sleep fairy a rapid and consistent reduction in children's disruptive bedtime behaviors was observed (45).

Alternative Treatments

Although behavioral interventions are clearly effective in treating bedtime resistance and nighttime awakening, some parents have difficulty adhering to the principles. Alternative treatments such as massage and chiropractic manipulation have been explored, although this literature as a whole is immature, with less methodological rigor (46). Theoretically, massage could play a role by reducing stress hormones, by dampening physiological arousal prior to bedtime, or by entraining circadian rhythmicity (47,49). Preliminary research on massage therapy has been mixed, with some studies finding little to no effect on children's sleep (49–51) while others have reported improved circadian rhythms, reduced sleep latency, better bedtime behavior, and increased daytime alertness (47,48,52–56). Interestingly, Field et al. found that parent-delivered massage was more effective than rocking in getting young children to fall asleep quickly (54). It is possible that these discrepant findings can be accounted for by differences in study methodology. For example, massage has been delivered throughout the day in some studies while others provided it imme-diately before naptime or bedtime specifically to promote sleep. Although there are now a few methodologically sound studies, this literature could benefit from addi-tional randomized studies evaluating pure forms of the intervention (not con-founded by other treatments) targeting clinically referred children experiencing sleep problems. Future studies should also incorporate objective outcome measures of sleep and bedtime behavior. Nonetheless, an emerging literature indicates that massage therapy may represent an option for parents who do not mind intervening to help their child initiate sleep. Parents desiring solitary sleeping arrangements and independent child sleep initiation skills may be less enthused about massage, because it introduces non-adaptive sleep associations. Children may learn to require parental contact multiple times during the night when they awaken briefly at the completion of each sleep cycle.

The impact of chiropractic manipulation on pediatric sleep has also been explored, albeit to a much lesser degree (57–59). At this time no conclusions can be made regarding the efficacy of chiropractic manipulation on pediatric sleep because the literature consists entirely of uncontrolled case reports with no formal outcome measures.

CIRCADIAN RHYTHM DISORDERS

The circadian rhythm sleep disorders involve a misalignment between the timing of an individual's inherent 24-hour sleep pattern and environmental demands such as work, school, or social schedule. Children may be at increased risk for circadian-related sleep problems, because unlike adults, their bedtimes and wake times are usually imposed upon them (60).

Advanced Sleep Phase Syndrome

Advanced sleep phase syndrome (ASPS) describes a major sleep episode that occurs earlier than the desired clock time. Symptoms of ASPS include an inability to remain awake in the evening followed by waking earlier than the desired morning clock time (61). ASPS is thought to occur most commonly among infants, toddlers, and the elderly. Parents often don't mind when the infant falls asleep early, however they may complain about early awakening. The ASPS literature is devoid of treatment outcome studies with children. Anecdotally, clinicians gener-ally suggest systematically delaying the child's bedtime by 15-minute increments while also delaying naptimes and mealtimes. Introducing bright light in the evening and decreasing or eliminating light exposure in the morning are also recommended (62). Before settling prematurely on a diagnosis of ASPS, clinicians should consider other reasons for a child's early morning awakenings. Children with ASPS will fall asleep early then awaken early in the morning after obtaining a full night's sleep. Some early morning "risers," however, fall to sleep at a normal (later) clock hour yet awaken early regardless of the time they fell asleep. The reduced nocturnal sleep time may result in sleepiness later in the day. This pattern may be seen in children who choose to start their day rather than returning to sleep to complete their final sleep cycle, often to gain access to enjoyable activities (TV, movies, parent's bed) immediately upon leaving the bedroom.

Delayed Sleep Phase Syndrome

Delayed sleep phase syndrome (DSPS) is characterized by a later than normal sleep phase, creating difficulty falling asleep at the desired bedtime and inability to awaken at the desired morning wake time. DSPS is particularly prevalent among adolescents due to a biologically induced delay in their endogenous circadian rhythm, producing later sleep onset and awakening times (63,64). A history of school tardiness or absences is not uncommon due to extreme difficulty waking in the early morning. If they do make it to school on time, students with DSPS often have difficulty staying awake in class, particularly during morning classes that coincide with their preferred sleep phase. Individuals with DSPS typically exhibit normal sleep onset and sleep duration when they are allowed to follow their desired schedule (e.g., summer vacation). During the school year, however, they may carry a heavy sleep debt due to awakening early for school. They may attempt to "catch up" by sleeping significantly later on weekends, creating further delay in their circadian physiology (65).

A variety of nonpharmacological interventions have been used clinically for children and adolescents with DSPS; unfortunately they remain relatively untested with pediatric populations (28). Environmental accommodations can be made such as delaying the bedtime to more closely match the child's natural sleep initiation time, shortening the morning routine to allow for a later wake time, or, in some cases, making special allowances for later school attendance. On a larger scale, delaying the school start time is a proven countermeasure which affords students later wake times, more sleep, and a reduction in daytime sleepiness and school tardiness (66,67). Treatments targeting individuals with DSPS have relied primarily on bright light therapy and behavioral interventions to advance or delay the sleep schedule, then maintain that schedule once achieved. Timing of administration is important regardless of the chosen intervention, necessitating an assessment of the pre-treatment endogenous circadian rhythm (68). A reasonably accurate clinical estimate of a person's dim light melatonin onset (DLMO) can be obtained from sleep–wake diaries collected during self-selected sleep periods (69).

With appropriate timing, bright light therapy can be used to shift the circadian rhythm in either direction. The timing and duration of the light stimulus as well as the intensity and wavelength may be manipulated to induce phase shifts (68). Morning administration of white light at 2500 to 10000 lux successfully advances the endogenous circadian rhythm of people with DSPS, however, more recent studies are beginning to use shorter wavelengths (blue to green) (68). Comparatively, bright light therapy produces greater effects with a phase response curve about two to five times that of melatonin (70). Wyatt (71) aptly noted that most of the research on light therapy has been conducted under optimal laboratory conditions; further work is needed to adapt the technology for routine clinical use.

Behavioral therapy for DSPS has focused primarily on systematically advancing or delaying an individual's sleep phase until the desired sleep–wake schedule is achieved. Ferber has advocated phase advancing younger children with DSPS by gradually advancing the waking time to create a mild sleep debt, then slowly advancing the child's bedtime (72). Formal research has yet to evaluate this approach with children. For more severe cases of DSPS, the intervention of choice is phase delay chronotherapy (73). Chronotherapy involves placing the child on a

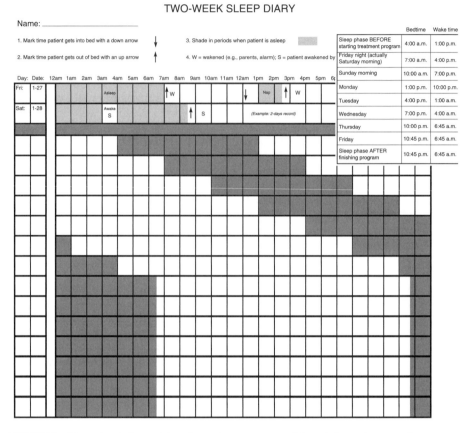

FIGURE 1   Example of phase delay chronotherapy to treat delayed sleep phase syndrome.

27-hour "day" by systematically moving the bedtime and wake times later until reaching the desired sleep–wake schedule (Fig. 1). Thorpy and colleagues devised an interesting alternative to daily chronotherapy that appears less disruptive to student's school attendance (74). Sleep deprivation with phase advance (SDPA) involves keeping a regular sleep schedule for six days, followed by one night of total sleep deprivation on the weekend. The following night, bedtime is advanced by 90 minutes and this new sleep schedule is maintained for six days. The process is repeated on successive weekends until the desired schedule is attained. SDPA was deemed "helpful," however the protocol still awaits scientific evaluation. Despite the widespread billing that chronotherapy has received as an effective treatment for DSPS, there has been surprisingly little formal research on the procedure. The pediatric literature consists of uncontrolled case studies and combination treatments (75–77).

Lack and Wright (68) noted that it can be a difficult decision whether to use phase advance (morning bright light, evening melatonin) or phase delay (chronotherapy) for individuals with DSPS. They recommend phase advancing for less extreme cases (e.g., <4 hr) and phase delay for more extreme delays (>6 hr), however, patient preference and convenience must also weigh into the decision (68).

Regardless of the choice to phase advance or phase delay, the challenge in treating most patients with DSPS is maintaining the desired schedule once it is achieved. Intervention is not complete unless clinicians address those factors that contributed to the delayed schedule in the first place. Maintaining a dark, quiet, sleep compatible bedroom environment can be a challenge for some. Regulating the timing of light exposure and managing caffeine intake become imperative. Bedtime management strategies such as stimulus control instructions for adolescents (78) or matching children's bedtime to coincide with their natural sleep onset time may be needed to extinguish conditioned insomnia. A reinforcement program or behavioral contracting can be useful in maintaining treatment effects over time. Finally, the evaluation and treatment of DSPS is never complete without considering motivational factors. Sleeping late may serve as an escape or avoidance function for children with learning problems, anxiety, social problems, or school refusal (79,80).

PARASOMNIAS

Parasomnias are undesirable events that occur during entry into sleep, during sleep, or during arousals from sleep (61). Common parasomnias in the pediatric population include sleepwalking, sleep terrors, nightmares, and sleep-related rhythmic movement disorder.

Sleep Terrors and Sleepwalking

Sleep terrors and sleepwalking are classified as non-rapid eye movement (NREM) parasomnias because they occur during incomplete arousal from sleep (81). Although appearing different, sleepwalking and sleep terrors share a number of characteristics including their genetics, typical age of onset, timing within the sleep cycle, behavioral manifestations, and pathophysiology (82). Young children who experience sleep terrors are likely to develop sleepwalking at an older age (83,84). Sleepwalking and sleep terrors occur most frequently during early to middle childhood when slow wave (deep) sleep is predominant, and the events are usually outgrown during puberty when slow wave sleep sharply declines. Event frequency appears to increase with factors that amplify a child's homeostatic sleep "pressure," such as insufficient sleep resulting from an irregular sleep schedule, staying up late, giving up a daily nap, or waking too early in the morning (85). Children with primary sleep disorders, such as obstructive sleep apnea (OSA) or periodic limb movement disorder (PLMD), are at increased risk for partial arousal parasomnias due to sleep fragmentation, as are children with behavioral sleep disturbances that compromise total sleep time (86–88).

Parents can be reassured that partial arousal parasomnias are rarely an indication of psychopathology in children. They can be encouraged to take safety precautions by removing items from stairways, securing doors and windows leading outside, and moving the child to the bottom bunk. Inexpensive motion-activated alarms can be installed to alert parents when a child leaves the bedroom.

Referral for an overnight sleep study is indicated whenever parasomnias are accompanied by symptoms suggestive of a primary sleep disorder such as OSA or

PLMD (89). Children with sleep terrors and sleepwalking respond well with identification and treatment of co-existing primary sleep disorders (87). When primary sleep disorders are not present, scheduled awakenings represent another treatment option. The protocol calls for the caregiver to awaken the child 15 to 30 minutes before an anticipated sleepwalking or sleep terror event (90–93). Finally, preliminary evidence suggests that treating behaviorally based sleep problems (e.g., bedtime resistance, night waking, circadian disorders, nap refusal) to restore a child's sleep duration can significantly decrease sleepwalking and sleep terrors (88).

Nightmares

Nightmares refer to vivid dreams marked by intense dread or terror that awaken the individual from sleep (94). Nightmares can be distinguished from sleep terrors because in the former case the child is more alert, coherent, interactive, and usually seeks parental reassurance and comfort. Nightmares typically occur during REM sleep which occurs during the latter part of the night (95). Frequent nightmares in children do not necessarily suggest underlying psychopathology; yet they may serve as a barometer of the child's overall level of adjustment (96). Stressful periods, especially traumatic events, are known to increase the frequency and severity of nightmares. Stress may be related to obvious family disruptions (e.g., death, marital conflict) however, it is thought that normal developmental transitions such as toilet training or starting school may also precipitate nightmares (97). Other common precipitants include certain illnesses, and psychological traumas such as physical or sexual abuse. Protective factors include good overall health, family/social support, and effective coping skills (96).

Families with children who experience an occasional nightmare usually require no more than reassurance that the events do not necessarily signify emotional disturbance. As with anything impacting a child's well-being (i.e., school performance, behavior); frequent or particularly distressing nightmares may require further attention. Unfortunately, there is no solid research base to guide professionals who treat children suffering from distressing nightmares. One cognitive–behavioral intervention, imagery rehearsal therapy (IRT), does appear to be promising, based on its utility with adult nightmare sufferers (98). The impact of IRT was tested on a population of adolescent females with chronic nightmares (99). Participants were taught to self-select a nightmare, change the nightmare any way they wish, and rehearse the new version for 5–20 minutes each day. By three months there was a significant decrease in nightmare frequency for those receiving IRT compared to the control group.

Sleep Related Rhythmic Movement Disorder

Sleep Related Rhythmic Movement Disorder (RMD) is a sleep–wake transition disorder that involves a group of stereotyped, repetitive movements of the large muscles, typically of the head and neck (61). Rhythmic movement is usually observed during the transition from wakefulness to sleep, but it clearly can occur in all stages of sleep (100,101). Episodes of muscle movement typically last from 5 to 30 minutes, but the topography of the movements varies greatly. The most common form involves head banging during which the head is repeatedly lifted and forcibly driven into the pillow, mattress, headboard, or wall. RMD typically emerges before two years of age and rapidly decreases by four years of age (102), however it has been documented in high-functioning adults (101). RMD likely represents a common end-point resulting from multiple etiologies. Interestingly, most children with RMD are typically developing and do not cry, even when banging becomes quite forceful or violent. Many children find the rhythmic movement to be a pleasant activity that develops into a self-soothing, over-learned habit that assists in sleep onset.

The treatment outcome literature for RMD in children suggests that carefully constructed behavioral interventions have the potential to produce rapid and substantial reductions in sleep-related rhythmic motor behavior, with durable and lasting effects (28). Several studies included some form of detection or increased awareness (i.e., verbal prompts, contingent light, auditory signals) (103–107). Other studies taught children to practice alternative sleep initiation behaviors, with rewards or mild punishers to maintain these new behaviors (103–105,108,109). The behavioral intervention components found in the RMD literature bear striking resemblance to a treatment package termed habit reversal, shown to be effective for other habit behaviors including motor tics, stuttering, thumb-sucking, and hair-pulling (110).

ADHERENCE TO CONTINUOUS POSITIVE AIRWAY PRESSURE

Adenotonsillar hypertrophy is the most common etiology of (OSA) in the pediatric population, and surgery (adenotonsillectomy) represents first line treatment. Continuous positive airway pressure (CPAP) affords a viable backup option for children who are not candidates for surgery (e.g., craniofacial abnormalities, neuromuscular problems, obesity) or who do not respond to surgery (111). The effectiveness of CPAP hinges greatly upon whether or not children accept and utilize the appliance in the manner it was intended. Contrary to verbal report, objectively monitored CPAP usage by adults is shockingly low (112). This pattern also holds true for children, as parents greatly overestimate actual nightly CPAP usage (7.6 hrs vs. 5.3 hrs) (113). Hopefully, a recent explosion in the literature will begin to provide professionals with effective tools to improve CPAP adherence.

The field of behavioral medicine has long made the distinction between "compliance" and "adherence" to medical intervention (114). Compliance derives from the traditional biomedical model, in which patients receive and carry out treatments or instructions prescribed by an all-knowing expert. The preferred term adherence refers simply to patient use and tends to be less judgmental in tone, accounting for today's increased access to technical information (115).

Increasing CPAP adherence involves patient education, continuous monitoring and feedback, and identifying barriers to regular usage. Fortunately, monitoring CPAP usage has become significantly easier since the introduction of sophisticated microchips and card counters (116).

Education is the first step in promoting CPAP adherence. Parents and children are provided information on sleep apnea and CPAP, delivered by nurses, videos, or printed material. Families can get additional information by attending patient support groups, through phone calls with medical staff, or by scheduling follow-up clinic appointments and home visits (115,117).

The most frequently cited reasons for poor CPAP tolerability involve problems related to the interface between man and machine (115). Proper fit becomes a challenge for some due to the lack of available pediatric masks and headgear for young children. Poorly fitted masks and improper air titration can result in air leakage, skin irritation, nasal stuffiness, and dryness of the eyes or throat. Technological improvements in the masks and headgear, titration methods (standard vs. auto), and delivery method (bilevel) have effectively addressed many of man–machine interface problems for adult CPAP users. Unfortunately, technological advances have not significantly impacted patient adherence rates (118). As a result, increased efforts have been made toward identifying cognitive–behavioral factors coupled with psychosocial treatment approaches (119). Effective treatment options have now been introduced and studied in pediatric populations.

Unfortunately, many parents introduce the CPAP machine to their child during the bedtime routine on the first night following the sleep study. They turn the air pressure to the maximum prescribed setting and tell the child to wear it all night long. If the child resists by head-turning, pushing the mask away, or removing the mask, parents respond by scolding, explaining the importance of CPAP, or threatening punishment.

There are numerous problems and inherent risks associated with the scenario described above. Fortunately, sleep professionals have turned their attention to the field of behavior analysis and are beginning to use principles of learning and child behavior to promote and maintain CPAP adherence (120). Graduated exposure, conditioning, shaping, and positive reinforcement have been heavily relied upon to increase children's adherence to CPAP. For example, a task analysis breaks complex behavioral chains into multiple steps or component skills. Prerequisite skills and behaviors can be further broken down to reduce the level of difficulty. Short-term, achievable goals can be set, and rewards can be used to reinforce successive approximations.

A number of variables can be skillfully manipulated to ensure initial child success and help gain behavioral momentum. Children can learn to tolerate wearing the CPAP equipment for increasing durations during the day, then during short naps, during part of the night, and finally through the entire night. Daytime practice sessions can be exceedingly short at first, gradually increasing in duration. Initially, children might participate in highly engaging activities (TV, movies, videogames) while they wear the mask, gradually reducing the "distraction value" over time. CPAP components can be introduced sequentially, starting by placing the mask to the child's face, then adding the headgear, the hose, and attaching the hose to the blower unit. Air pressure can be started at the lowest setting, increasing gradually until reaching the prescribed level. The use of positive reinforcement is critical, especially during early behavior-rehearsal sessions while CPAP-related stimuli are presented. Frequent delivery of high preference tangible or activity rewards can be used early, fading to less frequent delivery of social attention.

Preparation, practice, graduated exposure, shaping, and reinforcement are powerful tools for promoting adherence. However, it is only natural for children to attempt to escape or avoid uncomfortable situations or procedures (121). Preventing escape (escape extinction) may be necessary in some cases, such as ignoring the child's vocal protests, physically blocking the child's attempt to remove the mask, and directing the child's hands towards a different activity while encouraging the child, in a calm voice, "you can do it, you will be OK" (122).

A recent study demonstrated that escape extinction, in combination with other behavioral strategies, can successfully teach children to tolerate CPAP therapy (123).

REFERENCES

1. Adair R, Bauchner H, Philipp B, Levenson S, Zuckerman B. Night waking during infancy: Role of parental presence at bedtime. Pediatrics 1991; 87:500–4.
2. Armstrong KL, Quinn RA, Dadds MR. The sleep patterns of normal children. Med J Aust 1994; 161:202–6.
3. Johnson CM. Infant and toddler sleep: A telephone survey of parents in one community. J Dev Behav Pediatr 1991; 12:108–14.
4. Richman N. A community survey of characteristics of one- to two- year-olds with sleep disruptions. J Am Acad Child Psychiat 1981; 20:281–91.
5. Hauri P, Olmstead E. Childhood-onset insomnia. Sleep 1980; 3:59–65.
6. Kataria S, Swanson MS, Trevathan GE. Persistence of sleep disturbances in preschool children. J Pediatr 1987; 110:642–6.
7. Lam P, Hiscock H, Wake M. Outcomes of infant sleep problems: A longitudinal study of sleep, behavior, and maternal well-being. Pediatrics 2003; 111:e203–7.
8. Zuckerman B, Stevenson J, Bailey V. Sleep problems in early childhood: Continuities, predictive factors, and behavioral correlates. Pediatrics 1987; 80:664–71.
9. Kuhn BR, Elliott AJ. Efficacy of behavioral interventions for pediatric sleep disturbance. In: Perlis ML, Lichstein KL, eds. Treating Sleep Disorders: Principles and Practices of Behavioral Sleep Medicine. Hoboken, NJ: Wiley; 2003: pp. 415–51.
10. Mindell JA, Durand VM. Treatment of childhood sleep disorders: Generalization across disorders and effects on family members. Special issue: Interventions in pediatric psychology. J Ped Psychol 1993; 18:731–50.
11. Anders TF, Halpern LF, Hua J. Sleeping through the night: A developmental perspective. Pediatrics 1992; 90:554–60.
12. Atkinson E, Vetere A, Grayson K. Sleep disruption in young children: The influence of temperament on the sleep patterns of pre-school children. Child Care, Health Dev 1995; 21:233–46.
13. Fehlings D. Frequent night awakenings in infants and preschool children referred to a sleep disorders clinic: The role of non-adaptive sleep associations. Child Health Care 2001; 30:43–55.
14. Lozoff B, Wolf AW, Davis NS. Sleep problems seen in pediatric practice. Pediatrics 1985; 75:477–83.
15. Touchette E, Petit D, Paquet J, et al. Factors associated with fragmented sleep at night across early childhood. Arch Pediatr Adolesc Med 2005; 159:242–9.
16. Van Tassel EB. The relative influence of child and environmental characteristics on sleep disturbances in the first and second years of life. J Dev Behav Pediatr 1985; 6:81–5.
17. Wolke D, Meyer R, Ohrt B, Riegel K. The incidence of sleeping problems in preterm and fullterm infants discharged from neonatal special care units: An epidemiological longitudinal study. J Child Psychol Psychiatr 1995; 36:203–23.
18. Sadeh A. Cognitive-behavioral treatment for childhood sleep disorders. Clin Psychol Rev 2005; 25:612–28.
19. Owens JA. When child can't sleep, start by treating the parents. Curr Psychiatr 2006; 5:21–2, 7–30, 5–6.
20. Morgenthaler T, Alessi C, Friedman L, et al. Practice parameters for the use of actigraphy in the assessment of sleep and sleep disorders: An update for 2007. Sleep 2007; 30:519–29.
21. Mindell JA, Kuhn B, Lewin DS, Meltzer LJ, Sadeh A. Behavioral treatment of bedtime problems and night wakings in infants and young children. Sleep 2006; 29:1263–76.

22. Symon BG, Marley JE, Martin AJ, Norman ER. Effect of a consultation teaching behaviour modification on sleep performance in infants: a randomised controlled trial. Med J Aust 2005; 182:215–18.
23. Spasaro SA, Schaefer CE. Infant night waking. In: Schaefer CE, ed. Clinical Handbook of Sleep Disorders in Children. Northvale, NJ: Jason Aronson; 1995: pp. 49–68.
24. Schmitt BD. Your Child's Health: The Parents' One-Stop Reference Guide to: Symptoms, Emergencies, Common Illnesses, Behavior Problems, and Healthy Development. New York: Bantam Books; 2005.
25. Pinilla T, Birch LL. Help me make it through the night: Behavioral entrainment of breast-fed infants' sleep patterns. Pediatrics 1993; 91:436–44.
26. Adair R, Zuckerman B, Bauchner H, Philipp B, Levenson S. Reducing night waking in infancy: A primary care intervention. Pediatrics 1992; 89:585–8.
27. Walker M. Sleep, feeding, and opinions. Pediatrics 1993; 92:883–5.
28. Kuhn BR, Elliott AJ. Treatment efficacy in behavioral pediatric sleep medicine. J Psychosom Res 2003; 54:587–97.
29. Douglas J, Richman N. My Child Won't Sleep. Harmondsworth, England: Penguin Books; 1984.
30. Ferber R. Solve Your Child's Sleep Problems. New York: Simon & Schuster; 1985.
31. Durand VM, Mindell JA. Behavioral treatment of multiple childhood sleep disorders: Effects on child and family. Behav Mod 1990; 14:37–49.
32. Lawton C, France KG, Blampied NM. Treatment of infant sleep disturbance by graduated extinction. Child Fam Beh Ther 1991; 13:39–56.
33. Schaefer CE, Petronko MR. Teach Your Baby to Sleep Through the Night. New York: G.P. Putnam's Sons; 1987.
34. France KG. Fact, act, and tact: A three-stage approach to treating the sleep problems of infants and toddlers. Child Adolesc Psychiatr Clin N Am 1996; 5:581–99.
35. Sadeh A. Assessment of intervention for infant night waking: Parental reports and activity-based home monitoring. J Consult Clin Psychol 1994; 62:63–8.
36. France KG, Blampied NM. Modifications of systematic ignoring in the management of infant sleep disturbance: Efficacy and infant distress. Child Fam Beh Ther 2005; 27:1–16.
37. Kuhn BR, Weidinger D. Interventions for infant and toddler sleep disturbance: A review. Child Fam Beh Ther 2000; 22:33–50.
38. Durand VM. Sleep Better! A Guide to Improving the Sleep for Children with Special Needs. New York: Paul H. Brookes; 1998.
39. Piazza CC, Fisher WW. A faded bedtime with response cost protocol for treatment of multiple sleep problems in children. J Appl Behav Anal 1991; 24:129–40.
40. Freeman K. Treating bedtime resistance with the bedtime pass: A systematic replication and component analysis with 3-year-olds. J Appl Behav Anal 2006; 39:423–8.
41. Moore BA, Friman PC, Fruzzetti AE, MacAleese K. Brief report: Evaluating the bedtime pass program for child resistance to bedtime: A randomized, controlled trial. J Pediatr Psychol 2007; 32:283–7.
42. Friman PC, Hoff KE, Schnoes C, Freeman KA, Woods DW, Blum N. The bedtime pass: An approach to bedtime crying and leaving the room. Arch Pediatr Adolesc Med 1999; 153:1027–9.
43. Miltenberger RG. Behavior Modification: Principles and Procedures. Second edn. Pacific Grove, CA: Brooks/Cole; 2001.
44. Robinson KE, Sheridan SM. Using the Mystery Motivator to improve child bedtime compliance. Child Family Beh Ther 2000; 22:29–49.
45. Burke RV, Kuhn BR, Peterson JL. Brief Report: A "Storybook" ending to children's bedtime problems—The use of a rewarding social story to reduce bedtime resistance and frequent night waking. J Pediatr Psychol 2004; 29:389–96.
46. Forbes EA. Behavioral and massage treatments for infant sleep problems. Med Health R I 2006; 89:97–9.

47. Field T, Hernandez-Reif M. Sleep problems in infants decrease following massage therapy. Early Child Dev Care 2001; 168:95–104.

48. Ferber SG, Laudon M, Kuint J, Weller A, Zisapel N. Massage therapy by mothers enhances the adjustment of circadian rhythms to the nocturnal period in full-term infants. J Dev Behav Pediatr 2002; 23:410–15.

49. Scafidi FA, Field TM, Schanberg SM, Bauer CR, et al. Massage stimulates growth in preterm infants: A replication. Infant Behav Dev 1990; 13:167–88.

50. Scafidi FA, et al. Effects of tactile/kinesthetic stimulation on the clinical course and sleep/wake behavior of preterm neonates. Infant Behav Dev 1986; 9:91–105.

51. Williams TI. Evaluating effects of aromatherapy massage on sleep in children with autism: A pilot study. Evid-Based Compli Alt 2006; 3:373–7.

52. Agarwal KN, Gupta A, Pushkarna R, Bhargava SK, Faridi MM, Prabhu MK. Effects of massage and use of oil on growth, blood flow and sleep pattern in infants. Indian J Med Res 2000; 112:212–17.

53. Escalona A, Field T, Singer-Strunck R, Cullen C, Hartshorn K. Brief report: Improvements in the behavior of children with autism following massage therapy. J Autism Dev Disord 2001; 31:513–16.

54. Field T, Grizzle N, Scafidi F, Abrams S, et al. Massage therapy for infants of depressed mothers. Infant Behav Dev 1996; 19:107–12.

55. Field TM, Morrow CJ, Valdeon C, Larson S, et al. Massage reduces anxiety in child and adolescent psychiatric patients. J Am Acad Child Adolesc Psychiatry 1992; 31:125–31.

56. Dieter JNI, Field T, Hernandez-Reif M, Emory EK, Redzepi M. Stable preterm infants gain more weight and sleep less after five days of massage therapy. J Pediatr Psychol 2003; 28:403–11.

57. Jamison JR, Davies NJ. Chiropractic management of cows milk protein intolerance in infants with sleep dysfunction syndrome: A therapeutic trial. J Manipulative Physiol Ther 2006; 29:469–74.

58. Elster E. Upper cervical chiropractic care for a nine-year-old male with Tourette syndrome, attention deficit hyperactivity disorder, depression, asthma, insomnia, and headaches: a case report. J Vertebr Sublux Res 2003:11p.

59. Elster E. Treatment of bipolar seizure, and sleep disorders and migraine headaches utilizing a chiropractic technique. J Manipulative Physiol Ther 2004; 27:217.

60. Kuhn BR. Sleep disorders. In: Hersen M, Thomas JC, eds. Handbook of Clinical Interviewing with Children. New York: Sage Publications; 2007: pp. 420–7.

61. AASM. The International Classification of Sleep Disorders, Second Edn: Diagnostic and Coding Manual. Westchester, IL: American Academy of Sleep Medicine; 2005.

62. Ferber R. Circadian rhythm sleep disorders in childhood. In: Ferber R, Kryger M, eds. Principles and Practice of Sleep Medicine in the Child. Philadelphia: Saunders; 1995: pp. 91–8.

63. Carskadon MA, Vieira C, Acebo C. Association between puberty and delayed phase preference. Sleep 1993; 16:258–62.

64. Knutson KL. The association between pubertal status and sleep duration and quality among a nationally representative sample of US adolescents. Am J Hum Biol 2005; 17:418–24.

65. Burgess HJ, Eastman CI. A late wake time phase delays the human dim light melatonin rhythm. Neurosci Lett 2006; 395:191–5.

66. Wolfson AR, Spaulding NL, Dandrow C, Baroni EM. Middle school start times: The importance of a good night's sleep for young adolescents. Behav Sleep Med 2007; 5:194–209.

67. Wahlstrom K. Changing times: Findings from the first longitudinal study of later high school start times. NASSP Bulletin 2002; 86:3–21.

68. Lack LC, Wright HR. Clinical management of delayed sleep phase disorder. Behav Sleep Med 2007; 5:57–76.

69. Burgess HJ, Savic N, Sletten T, Roach G, Gilbert SS, Dawson D. The relationship between the dim light melatonin onset and sleep on a regular schedule in young healthy adults. Behav Sleep Med 2003; 1:102–14.

70. Revell VL, Eastman CI. How to trick mother nature into letting you fly around or stay up all night. J Biol Rhythms 2005; 20:353–65.

71. Wyatt JK. Delayed sleep phase syndrome: Pathophysiology and treatment options. Sleep 2004; 27:1195–203.

72. Ferber RA, Boyle MP. Phase shift dyssomnia in early childhood. Sleep Res 1983; 12:242.

73. Czeisler CA, Richardson GS, Coleman RM, et al. Chronotherapy: resetting the circadian clocks of patients with delayed sleep phase insomnia. Sleep 1981; 4:1–21.

74. Thorpy MJ, Korman E, Spielman AJ, Glovinsky PB. Delayed sleep phase syndrome in adolescents. J Adolesc Health Care 1988; 9:22–7.

75. Gruber R, Grizenko N, Joober R. Delayed sleep phase syndrome, ADHD, and bright light therapy. J Clin Psychiatry 2007; 68:337–8.

76. Dahl RE, Pelham WE, Wierson M. The role of sleep disturbances in attention deficit disorder symptoms: A case study. J Ped Psychol 1991; 16:229–39.

77. Okawa M, Uchiyama M, Ozaki S, Shibui K, Ichikawa H. Circadian rhythm sleep disorders in adolescents: clinical trials of combined treatments based on chronobiology. Psychiatry Clin Neurosci 1998; 52:483–90.

78. Bootzin RR, Epstein D, Wood JM. Stimulus control instructions. In: Hauri P, ed. Case Studies in Insomnia. New York: Plenum Press; 1991: pp. 19–28.

79. Kearney CA, Albano AM. The functional profiles of school refusal behavior: Diagnostic aspects. Behav Modif 2004; 28:147–61.

80. Ferber RA. Delayed sleep phase syndrome versus motivated sleep phase delay in adolescents. Sleep Res 1983; 12:239.

81. Rosen GM, Ferber R, Mahowald MW. Evaluation of parasomnias in children. Child Adolesc Psychiatr Clin N Am 1996; 5:601–16.

82. Broughton RJ. Sleep disorders: disorders of arousal? Science 1968; 159:1070-8.

83. Kales A, Soldatos CR, Bixler EO, et al. Hereditary factors in sleepwalking and night terrors. Br J Psychiatry 1980; 137:111–18.

84. Klackenberg G. Incidence of parasomnias in children in a general population. In: Guilleminault C, ed. Sleep and Its Disorders in Children. New York: Raven Press; 1987: pp. 99–113.

85. Rosen G, Mahowald MW, Ferber R. Sleepwalking, confusional arousals, and sleep terrors in the child. In: Ferber R, Kryger M, eds. Principles and Practice of Sleep Medicine in the Child. Philadelphia: Saunders; 1995: pp. 99–106.

86. Mehlenbeck R, Spirito A, Owens J, Boergers J. The clinical presentation of childhood partial arousal parasomnias. Sleep Med 2000; 1:307–12.

87. Guilleminault C, Palombini L, Pelayo R, Chervin RD. Sleepwalking and sleep terrors in prepubertal children: What triggers them? Pediatrics 2003; 111:e17–25.

88. Kuhn BR. Increasing sleep time effectively reduces sleepwalking and sleep terrors in children. Sleep 2001; 24:A220–A1.

89. Kushida CA, Littner MR, Morgenthaler T, et al. Practice parameters for the indications for polysomnography and related procedures: An update for 2005. Sleep 2005; 28:499–521.

90. Lask B. Novel and non-toxic treatment for night terrors. Br Med J 1988; 297:6648.

91. Durand VM, Mindell JA. Behavioral intervention for childhood sleep terrors. Beh Ther 1999; 30:705–15.

92. Frank NC, Spirito A, Stark L, Owens-Stively J. The use of scheduled awakenings to eliminate childhood sleepwalking. J Pediatr Psychol 1997; 22:345–53.

93. Tobin JD, Jr. Treatment of somnambulism with anticipatory awakening. J Pediatr 1993; 122:426–7.

94. Levin R, Fireman G. Nightmare prevalence, nightmare distress, and self-reported psychological disturbance. Sleep 2002; 25:205–12.

95. Spoormaker, Schredl, Bout. Nightmares: from anxiety symptom to sleep disorder. Sleep Med Rev 2006; 10:19–31.
96 Halliday G. Treating nightmares in children. In: Schaefer CE, ed. Clinical Handbook of Sleep Disorders in Children. Northvale, N.J.: Jason Aronson; 1995: pp. 149–76.
97. Blum NJ, Carey WB. Sleep problems among infants and young children. Pediatr Rev 1996; 17:87–92.
98. Krakow B, Zadra A. Clinical management of chronic nightmares: Imagery rehearsal therapy. Behav Sleep Med 2006; 4:45–70.
99. Krakow B, Sandoval D, Schrader R, et al. Treatment of chronic nightmares in adjudicated adolescent girls in a residential facility. J Adolesc Health 2001; 29:94–100.
100. Kohyama J, Matsukura F, Kimura K, Tachibana N. Rhythmic movement disorder: Polysomnographic study and summary of reported cases. Brain Dev 2002; 24:33–8.
101. Mayer G, Wilde-Frenz J, Kurella B. Sleep related rhythmic movement disorder revisited. J Sleep Res 2007; 16:110–16.
102. Klackenberg G. Rhythmic movements in infancy and early childhood. Acta Paediatr Scand 1971; 224:74–83.
103. Strauss CC, Rubinoff A, Atkeson BM. Elimination of nocturnal headbanging in a normal seven-year-old girl using overcorrection plus rewards. J Behav Ther Exp Psychiatry 1983; 14:269–73.
104. Balaschak BA, Mostofsky DI. Treatment of nocturnal headbanging by behavioral contractions. J Behav Ther Exp Psychiatry 1980; 11:117–20.
105. Lindsay SJ, Salkovskis PM, Stoll K. Rhythmical body movement in sleep: A brief review and treatment study. Beh Res Ther 1982; 20:523–6.
106. Martin RD, Conway JB. Aversive stimulation to eliminate infant nocturnal rocking. J Behav Ther Exp Psychiatry 1976; 7:200–1.
107. Linscheid TR, Copeland AP, Jacobstein DM, Smith JL. Overcorrection treatment for nighttime self-injurious behavior in two normal children. J Pediatr Psychol 1981; 6:29–35.
108. Bramble D. Two cases of severe head-banging parasomnias in peripubertal males resulting from otitis media in toddlerhood. Child Care, Health Dev 1995; 21:247–53.
109. Golding K. Nocturnal headbanging as a settling habit: The behavioural treatment of a 4-year old boy. Clin Child Psychol Psychiatr 1998; 3:25–30.
110. Miltenberger RG, Fuqua RW, Woods DW. Applying behavior analysis to clinical problems: Review and analysis of habit reversal. J Appl Behav Anal 1998; 31:447–69.
111. Marcus C, et al. Clinical practice guideline: Diagnosis and management of childhood obstructive sleep apnea syndrome. Pediatrics 2002; 109:704–12.
112. Kribbs NB, Pack AI, Kline LR, et al. Objective measurement of patterns of nasal CPAP use by patients with obstructive sleep apnea. Am Rev Respir Dis 1993; 147:887–95.
113. Marcus CL, Rosen G, Ward SLD, et al. Adherence to and effectiveness of positive airway pressure therapy in children with obstructive sleep apnea. Pediatrics 2006; 117:e442–51.
114. Lutfey KE, Wishner WJ. Beyond "compliance" is "adherence." Improving the prospect of diabetes care. Diabetes Care 1999; 22:635–9.
115. Engleman HM, Wild MR. Improving CPAP use by patients with the sleep apnoea/hypopnoea syndrome (SAHS). Sleep Med Rev 2003; 7:81–99.
116. Lin SK, Kuna ST, Bogen DK. A novel device for measuring long-term oxygen therapy adherence: a preliminary validation. Respir Care 2006; 51:266–71.
117. Richards D, Bartlett DJ, Wong K, Malouff J, Grunstein RR. Increased adherence to CPAP with a group cognitive behavioral treatment intervention: A randomized trial. Sleep 2007; 30:635–40.
118. Aloia MS, Arnedt JT, Riggs RL, Hecht J, Borrelli B. Clinical management of poor adherence to CPAP: Motivational enhancement. Behav Sleep Med 2004; 2:205–22.
119. Dinges DF, Weaver TE. Editorial: The critical role of behavioral research for improving adherence to continuous positive airway pressure therapies for sleep apnea. Behav Sleep Med 2007; 5:79–82.

120. Rains JC. Treatment of obstructive sleep apnea in pediatric patients: Behavioral intervention for compliance with nasal continuous positive airway pressure. 14th Annual Meeting of the Society of Behavioral Medicine (1993, San Francisco, California). Clin Pediatr (Phila) 1995; 34:535–41.
121. Kuhn BR, Allen KD. Expanding child behavior management technology in pediatric dentistry: A behavioral science perspective. Pediatr Dent 1994; 16:13–17.
122. Koontz KL, Slifer KJ, Cataldo MD, Marcus CL. Improving pediatric compliance with positive airway pressure therapy: The impact of behavioral intervention. Sleep 2003; 26:1010–15.
123. Slifer KJ, Kruglak D, Benore E, et al. Behavioral training for increasing preschool children's adherence with positive airway pressure: A preliminary study. Behav Sleep Med 2007; 5:147–75.

20 Sleep and Mood Disorders in Children and Adolescents

Anna Ivanenko

Department of Psychiatry and Behavioral Sciences, Feinberg School of Medicine, Northwestern University, Chicago, Division of Child and Adolescent Psychiatry, Children's Memorial Hospital, Chicago, Alexian Brothers Medical Center, Elk Grove Village, and Central DuPage Hospital, Winfield, Illinois, U.S.A.

INTRODUCTION

Sleep disturbance was identified as one of the main characteristics and biological markers of major depressive disorder (MDD) in adults. Sleep initiation, sleep maintenance and terminal insomnia with unrefreshed sleep and disturbing dreams have been consistently reported in the studies of adults with MDD. Hypersomnia has been reported in a subset of adult depressives. Although sleep disturbances may be present throughout all phases of a depressive disorder, they are most severe during an acute episode. Patients with depression who report sleep disturbances are more likely to attempt suicide than those who do not report difficulties with their sleep. Sleep disorders such as obstructive sleep apnea and periodic limb movement disorder can disrupt sleep to such a degree that patients may have vegetative symptoms of depression. Thus, it is important when assessing a depressed patient with sleep difficulties to consider a thorough sleep assessment to rule out a physiological cause of vegetative symptoms of depression and insomnia. Those with depression who also exhibit sleep disturbance can benefit from behavioral and relaxation training (1).

Numerous sleep electroencephalogram (EEG) studies demonstrated consistent changes in sleep characteristics that include prolonged sleep latency, reduced rapid eye movement (REM) sleep latency, increased amount of REM sleep, reduced slow wave-sleep (SWS) and delta-wave power, and increased sleep fragmentation.

Over the years, reduced REM latency has proved to be one of the most robust and specific features of sleep in depressed adult patients (1). However, not all groups of depressed patients have shown SWS abnormalities compared to controls. Further analysis has shown that SWS loss was most significant during the first non-rapid eye movement (NREM) period and that the number of delta waves was decreased in depressed patients (2,3).

The presence of sleep disturbances does not necessarily indicate that a patient is acutely ill at the time of study. Several studies have reported sleep parameters in patients in clinical remission as during episodes of acute illness. The results of these studies demonstrated that sleep abnormalities may be more severe in acute versus remitted states (4,5). Moreover, sleep abnormalities were shown to persist for prolonged periods of time in the asymptomatic recovered individuals (6).

Sleep disturbance and particularly reduced REM latency was proposed as a trait marker for some patients with depressive disorders. This hypothesis was further supported by family studies in which it was shown that first-degree relatives with major depression tend to show concordance in REM latency measures (7,8).

Regulation of the sleep–wake cycle is known to be closely associated with neurobehavioral and emotional development in children and adolescents. Bidirectional relationship between sleep and affective regulation has been proposed by Ronald Dahl (9) meaning that emotional problems can lead to sleep disruption, and sleep disturbances consistent of sleep loss and sleep fragmentation can cause dysregulation in mood and behavior creating a mutually interacting vicious cycle. From the clinical perspective, children presenting with affective problems should be thoroughly assessed for sleep disorders as they commonly accompany and complicate an array of psychiatric conditions.

Polysomnographic studies of early onset major depression, however failed to replicate findings described in adult patients with MDD. They are significantly fewer in number, with smaller sample sizes, greater variability in age, frequent lack of normal controls, and inconsistent use of standardized diagnostic criteria.

CLINICAL CHARACTERISTICS OF MAJOR DEPRESSION IN CHILDREN AND ADOLESCENTS

MDD is a common and frequently recurrent condition in children and adolescents with the estimated prevalence of approximately 2% in children and up to 8% in adolescents. In some community samples, incidence of major depression by age 18 is as high as 20% (10). The male to female ratio of MDD in children is 1:1 and reaches 1:2 during adolescence. According to the Diagnostic and Statistical Manual of Mental Disordsers (DSM-IV) criteria for MDD, an individual must demonstrate at least two weeks of either depressed mood or a loss of interest or pleasure. Other symptoms including change in appetite, weight, sleep pattern (insomnia or hypersomnia); impaired ability to focus or concentrate, diminished energy level, sense of guilt; poor self-esteem must be present and should not be attributable to other medical, psychiatric illness, or substance abuse (11).

The clinical presentation of childhood depression varies across different developmental stages, with younger children demonstrating more symptoms of anxiety with frequent phobias, separation anxiety, somatic complaints, irritability, temper tantrums, and behavioral problems. Changes in sleep and appetite, delusions, suicidal ideation, and attempts are more common among adolescents with MDD. Other psychiatric disorders are seen in as many as 40% to 90% of youths with MDD, with most common comorbid anxiety disorders, attention-deficit/hyperactive disorder (ADHD), disruptive disorders, and substance abuse (12). Major depression in children and adolescents significantly affects their social, emotional, and cognitive development. MDD, if untreated, increases risks of poor psychosocial functioning, substance abuse, early pregnancy, poor academic outcome, and suicide. (12–14).

SLEEP COMPLAINTS AND POLYSOMNOGRAPHIC CHARACTERISTICS IN CHILDREN WITH DEPRESSION

Few studies have assessed the prevalence and nature of subjective sleep complaints in children. In summary, between 13% and 27% of parents of 4- to 12-year-olds will indicate the presence of sleep difficulties in their children, including bedtime resistance, bedtime anxiety, delayed sleep onset, co-sleeping, snoring, enuresis, nighttime awakenings, nightmares, night terrors, sleepwalking, early morning awakening, and excessive daytime sleepiness (15–18). These sleep disturbances appear to be fairly stable across childhood, with no apparent effect of age on frequency of reported sleep problems (18,19). There have been some studies indicating association between sleep difficulties in children and maternal depression, as well as with general emotional distress and anxiety (15,18–20). A large community sample survey revealed that children with delayed sleep onset were significantly more likely to require the presence of an adult at bedtime, have nocturnal fears, bedtime resistance, and excessive daytime sleepiness. Those with sleep onset delay and sleep onset associated behavioral problems had a higher rate of psychiatric disorders (15).

Early studies of prepubertal children with major depression indicated that about two-thirds reported sleep onset and sleep maintenance insomnia, and almost 50% had terminal insomnia (21). Sleep difficulties in children with depression were found to be quite persistent over the course of a depressive episode with 10% of children continuing to exhibit insomnia following remission (6). In some cases, children will present with sleep initiation problems, nighttime wakening, and hypersomnia during the day (22). Comprehensive assessment of sleep related symptoms was recently conducted among 553 children diagnosed with a major disorder according to the DSM-IV criteria using the Interview Schedule for Children and Adolescents—Diagnostic Version. The study included children ages 7.3–14.9, recruited from 23 mental health centers (23). The results of the study revealed 72.7% of the sample had sleep disturbance, 53.5% had insomnia alone, 9% had hypersomnia alone, and 10.1% had both. Sleep disturbed children were found to have more severe depression with higher rates of comorbid anxiety. Those with insomnia and hypersomnia exhibited depressive episodes of longer duration with more profound symptoms of depression including anhedonia, psychomotor retardation, and weight loss. Interestingly enough, the finding of this most recent study corresponds with the earlier research by Ryan et al. (24) when sleep complaints were compared among children and adolescents across various age groups and subtypes of depression. Hypersomnia was more prevalent in adolescents than in pre-adolescents (34% vs. 16%), and more likely to be associated with symptoms of anhedonia, social withdrawal, fatigue, decreased appetite, and weight loss. However, children with comorbid anxiety symptoms like separation anxiety, excessive worrying, somatic complaints, and behavioral agitation had more pronounced insomnia.

Fewer polysomnographic studies were done in children with major depression compared to adolescents and yielded inconsistent results. Some studies demonstrated shortened REM sleep latency in children with MDD compared to normal controls (25–27) while others failed to reveal any significant differences (21,28,29). Severity of depression and inpatient status seemed to be associated with more changes in sleep architecture such as shortened REM sleep latency, increased duration of REM sleep, and a decreased amount of stage 4 sleep (27,29). Some prepubertal children were found to have shorter first REM period latency and an increased total number of REM sleep episodes both during an acute episode of major depression and after recovery (6).

In a recent study by Bertocci et al. (30) EEG sleep characteristics were compared to subjective sleep complaints in depressed children. There was no evidence of sleep disruption of depressed children versus healthy controls. Paradoxically children with depression and the highest ratings of insomnia demonstrated the best sleep quality according to the polysomnography (PSG) findings. The results of this study bring up an important issue of subjective perception of sleep versus EEG macroarchitectural sleep changes, as well as maturational factors that may unfold as children progress to adolescence.

To further support the hypothesis of maturational and gender influences on sleep in early onset MDD polysomnographic characteristics of 97 pediatric patients ages 8–18 years were compared to 76 healthy controls matched for sex and age (31). The depressed adolescent males had the greatest changes in PSG sleep measures with the shortest REM latency, highest amount of stage 1 sleep, fewer amounts of SWS during the first NREM period, and more frequent arousals compared to depressed females. There were no statistically significant changes found among pre-adolescent and adolescent girls with MDD and healthy female controls. The results of the study have also found that maturational age assessed by Tanner score correlated with sleep changes only in a subset of boys with MDD. Significant sex differences were previously found among adolescents and adults with major depression by the same group of authors where depressed females showed greater desynchronization of ultradian rhythms based on temporal coherence of the quantitative EEG measures (32,33).

Several actigraphic studies were conducted evaluating diurnal/nocturnal activity levels in children with major depression. Abnormal circadian rhythms were demonstrated in depressed children with decreased circadian amplitude and more blunted activity levels (34,35). Depressed pre-adolescents girls were shown to have damped circadian rhythms and lower light exposure compared to boys with MDD (35).

SLEEP COMPLAINTS AND POLYSOMNOGRAPHIC CHARACTERISTICS IN ADOLESCENTS WITH DEPRESSION

Compared to those in younger children, studies on sleep in adolescents with depression are far more represented in the literature. Symptoms of sleep disruption including delayed sleep onset, frequent nighttime awakenings, excessive daytime sleepiness, and unrefreshed sleep are common in the general population of adolescents. However, complaints of depressed mood, anxiety, internal tension, moodiness, excessive worry are more common among those with sleep difficulties. Nicotine, caffeine, and alcohol use are greater in adolescents who report sleep disturbances (36–41). Therefore sleep disturbances can be viewed as a potential marker for adolescents at high risk for psychopathology.

Longitudinal study of a large-scale community sample of adolescents revealed that sleep disturbance was one of the most prevalent major depressive symptoms; 89% of those who met criteria for major depression reported sleep disturbance (42). Approximately 76% of adolescents who had initially reported sleep disturbances during a 12-month period went on to develop symptoms that met criteria for a major depressive episode. Most adolescents with symptoms of a major depressive episode in this study reported significant sleep disturbance (42).

While only four well-controlled polysomnographic studies of prepubertal major depression were conducted, EEG sleep characteristics have been examined more extensively in adolescent depressives. Early studies revealed significantly shorter REM latency and increased REM density in depressed adolescents compared to non-depressed controls (43), with more drastic changes seen in female patients (44).

Additional studies of sleep in adolescent depression demonstrated heterogeneous EEG sleep findings (45–47). Changes in REM sleep similar to those in adults with major depression were observed in adolescents with endogenous type of MDD (48). Reduced REM latency, significantly longer sleep onset latency and greater REM density were associated with inpatient status and suicidality (49,50) as well as with psychotic depression (51) in adolescent patients.

Several studies examined the predictive value of EEG sleep changes in adolescent MDD. Prolonged sleep latency, decreased sleep efficiency, hypersomnia, and suicidality significantly predicted recurrence and lifetime depression (52,53). Spectral analysis of sleep EEG in a sample of depressed youth showed that temporal coherence of EEG rhythms was associated with recovery time and recurrence of depression (54).

Dahl et al. (55) integrated sleep findings across studies of childhood and adolescent depression and suggested that prolonged sleep latency may be the first and the most reliable macroarchitectural characteristic in early onset depression, with reduced REM latency occurring as a second level of sleep dysregulation, and delta sleep abnormalities becoming robust in adult depression (9,55).

TREATMENT APPROACH TO SLEEP PROBLEMS IN EARLY ONSET MAJOR DEPRESSION

There is virtually no research addressing treatment of insomnia in children and adolescents with major depression. It is also unclear whether antidepressants have a direct effect on sleep regulation in depressed individuals or their influence is mediated through the neuronal pathways involved in the modulations of emotions.

There are only a few studies examining sleep characteristics in children receiving antidepressants. REM sleep suppression, changes in sleep continuity, increases in stage 2 sleep, decreases in stage 4 sleep, were observed in children treated with imipramine (26,56). These findings are similar to those described in adults with depression, especially in respect of REM suppression. Interestingly, REM suppression was more pronounced in children who showed clinical improvement in depressive symptoms.

Serotonin reuptake inhibitors, like fluoxetine, have been demonstrated to significantly suppress REM sleep, increase NREM sleep, number of EEG arousals, frequency of periodic limb movements, and oculomotor abnormalities and bruxism in adult patients (57). A study of a small sample of children and adolescents treated with fluoxetine showed a significant increase in stage 1 sleep, number of arousals, and REM density with no signs of REM suppression (58).

Retrospective study was conducted in a group of adolescents with depressive disorder treated with a combination of fluoxetine and trazodone, and fluoxetine alone (59). The results of this study showed a significantly faster resolution of insomnia in subjects treated with combination therapy rather than fluoxetine. However, the analysis of the clinical course of illness revealed that the difference between the two groups, although statistically significant, was not clinically significant in the treatment of insomnia in depressed adolescents. This small study raised an important issue of the effectiveness of pharmacological treatment of insomnia in the context of major depression in children and adolescents.

From adult studies, it has become apparent that chronic insomnia commonly accompanies or complicates various psychiatric disorders, including depression. A two-year follow-up study of the emergence of insomnia in patients with medical and psychiatric conditions showed the odd ratio of patients with depression developing insomnia was 8.2 (60). A history of insomnia was also shown to be associated with a four times greater likelihood of developing MDD in a large cohort of young adults (61). A longer duration of insomnia is also known to be associated with higher incidence of psychiatric illness. Recognizing and addressing insomnia may prevent a new onset or relapse of mood disorders and other psychiatric conditions.

There are no large-scale, systematic studies examining treatment options of sleep disorders in children and adolescents with major depression. Simultaneous treatment of depression and insomnia in children with MDD appears to be the most rational approach to achieving a faster improvement in depressive symptomatology and entering remission state. Sleep hygiene, stimulus control and cognitive–behavioral therapies for insomnia should be considered first, prior to pharmacological intervention with sedative/hypnotics. Since there are no Food and Drug Administration (FDA) approved agents for the treatment of insomnia in the pediatric population, the choice of the hypnotic agent should be based on the best possible match between the type of sleep problem, patient characteristics, family circumstances, and the individual properties of currently available drugs (see chap. 12, this book, for the review of pharmacological treatments of insomnia). Short-term use of sedative/hypnotics should be encouraged to alleviate sleep disruption, while behavioral therapies should be applied to achieve and sustain healthy functional sleep habits.

Severe excessive daytime sleepiness is known to be associated with certain subtypes of depression and may require additional sleep laboratory assessment to objectively quantify the degree of hypersomnolence. In cases of documented clinically significant hypersomnia, use of alerting agents or antidepressants with alerting qualities may be warranted.

CLINICAL CHARACTERISTICS OF BIPOLAR DISORDER IN CHILDREN AND ADOLESCENTS

The exact prevalence of bipolar disorder in children is unknown, however, almost 20% of adult patients with bipolar disorder reported their first episode during adolescence (62), with the lifetime prevalence rate of bipolar disorder of approximately 1% (63). There are three distinct types of bipolar spectrum disorder: Bipolar I type, bipolar II type, and cyclothymic disorder. The same adult DSM-IV criteria are used to diagnose bipolar disorders in children and adolescents. However, the expression of the symptoms of bipolar illness is different in pediatric patients. For example, bipolar disorder in prepubertal children frequently has a course of long duration with rapid cycling (ultradian) or even continuous cycling and mixed state with simultaneous occurrence of both mania and depression (64). Children with mania commonly present with psychomotor agitation, irritability, belligerence, poor social boundaries, school failure, fighting and inappropriate sexualized behaviors. Retrospective review of clinical symptoms and response to treatment is very helpful in defining a course of illness and patterns of episodes in order to differentiate bipolar spectrum disorders from other affective conditions.

SLEEP CHARACTERISTICS IN EARLY ONSET BIPOLAR DISORDER

Sleep problems are commonly observed in children during manic episodes and are similar to those seen in children with ADHD. A decreased need for sleep along with symptoms of elated mood, grandiosity, racing thoughts/flights of ideas and hyper-sexuality are shown to be the best discriminators between ADHD, normal healthy controls, and prepubertal bipolar disorder (65,66). In the study by Geller et al. (65), about 40% of children diagnosed with mania presented with a substantially decreased need for sleep compared to only 6.2% among children with ADHD and 1.1% among normal healthy community controls.

Manic children, just like manic adults, continue to exhibit high energy during the day without complaints of fatigue or tiredness despite significantly reduced amounts of sleep. In contrast, children with ADHD or other types of behavioral or emotional disorders tend to exhibit symptoms of tiredness, fatigue, sleepiness, inat-tentiveness, increased irritability, impulsivity, and aggression in response to sleep loss. In certain cases a decreased need for sleep can be the first manifestation of emerging mania, and should be further explored in the clinical assessment of a child.

There have been only few studies examining sleep problems in children with early onset bipolar disorder. Meta-analysis of literature on the phenomenology of early onset bipolar disorder conducted by Kowatch et al. (67) revealed six studies, indicating a reduced need for sleep in children and adolescents with bipolar mania, and a high rate of sleep complaints in pediatric bipolar disorder. The highest preva-lence of a decreased need for sleep was reported in the study of 82 children with bipolar type 1, type 2, and cyclothymia (ages 3–17 years old) averaging 95.1%. A comparison of parent and child reports on sleep problems among children with bipolar disorder revealed a high discrepancy between parental and self-perception of sleep and a high prevalence of sleep complaints (96.2%) in children during depressed and manic phases of illness (68). Most sleep complaints were reported around most severe mood episodes, with more frequently reported sleep problems during the depressive phase (82%) versus manic (58%). Initial insomnia, middle, and terminal insomnia were among the most common sleep complaints in the sur-veyed sample of children.

Only two studies provided some polysomnographic data on children with bipolar disorder. Rao et al. (69) compared EEG sleep measures in 21 adolescents with unipolar depression, five adolescents with a later revised diagnosis of bipolar disorder, and 33 healthy controls. There were no statistically significant differences in REM sleep among the groups, with an increased percentage of stage 1 sleep and a reduced amount of stage 4 sleep in adolescents with bipolar disorder. Another study characterized sleep EEG and parental sleep questionnaires in 13 children ages six and seven years with a pediatric bipolar disorder profile based on the Child Behavior Checklist (70). Polysomnography revealed lower sleep efficiency, increased number of awakenings with reduced amount of REM sleep in children with bipolar profile versus controls. Children with bipolar profile had more parentally reported sleep problems including difficulties initiating sleep, more rest-less sleep, with more frequent nightmares and morning headaches.

TREATMENT APPROACH TO SLEEP PROBLEMS IN EARLY ONSET BIPOLAR DISORDER

Treatment approach to a child presenting with the complex clinical picture of affec-tive and sleep dysregulation should include the comprehensive psychiatric and sleep assessments to establish the diagnosis and formulate a treatment plan.

Stabilizing mood and behavioral symptoms in patients with bipolar disorders usually results in the substantial improvement of the sleep–wake pattern. However, in most patients presenting with sleep initiation and maintenance insomnia, nocturnal anxiety and bed refusal behavioral and pharmacological interventions for sleep can be initiated immediately to alleviate chronic severe sleep loss and to prevent further deterioration in daytime functioning.

Unfortunately there are no well-designed studies addressing treatment options in children and adolescents with early onset bipolar disorder and comorbid sleep dysfunction. Future research is needed to more successfully delineate types of sleep–wake dysfunction associated with different phases of bipolar illness and to develop treatment algorithms that would allow fast and successful resolution of mood and sleep problems in children and adolescents.

SEASONAL AFFECTIVE DISORDER IN CHILDREN AND ADOLESCENTS

Rosenthal et al. (71) described Seasonal Affective Disorder (SAD) as an affective disorder in which a depressive episode occurs during at least two consecutive autumns and/or winters with remittance during the spring or summer, with no other Axis I psychiatric disorder present and no obvious seasonal psychosocial influences on mood. This definition was established after having studied adult subjects with seasonal mood changes, and no children were included in the original description of the disorder.

To study seasonal mood changes in children, Carskadon and Acebo (72) surveyed parents regarding their children's seasonal moods. According to their survey, 4% of children, with a mean age of 10.6 years, in their sample met criteria for SAD. No gender disparity was present, which is different from reports of adult SAD, in which women are reported to have significantly greater incidence than men. It is interesting to note, however, that the older girls in the sample had significantly more symptoms of a mood disorder in the winter months than the younger girls, leaving one to wonder if puberty may be a factor in increasing winter depression. Although a smaller percentage of children met diagnostic criteria for SAD, nearly 25% of parents reported that their children ate more during the winter, and 23% reported that their children slept more and were more tired during the winter months. Older girls were reported to have significantly more symptoms of excessive sleep and withdrawal than were younger girls. Furthermore, significantly fewer symptoms were reported in the southern (below 36 latitude) than in the northern (above 42 latitude) United States.

Swedo et al. (73) assessed prevalence rates of SAD in adolescents through a survey of 1835 children in grades six through twelve and found an SAD rate of 3.3%. As with the children in the Carskadon and Acebo (72) study, there was no significant gender difference in the prevalence rate. SAD may be associated with puberty, as cases increased significantly between sixth and tenth grade but remained stable throughout the high school years. The most frequently reported symptoms included negative feelings, low energy, irritability, poor grades, and decreased social activity. There was no difference in the amount of sleep between those with SAD and those without, as all adolescents reported increased sleep in the summer, most likely as a result of the lack of school schedule. This similarity in sleep schedules is notably different than the pattern of symptoms present in adult cases of SAD.

To determine the nature and etiology of SAD, Glod et al. (74) studied 14 children between the ages of six and 17 with the disorder. Although children with SAD did not differ from controls in their nocturnal activity levels, they did have significantly lower diurnal activity levels and had less robust circadian rhythms with a reduction in the amplitude than control children. Therefore, Glod et al. asserted that the etiology of SAD in children is most likely related to an attenuation of the circadian amplitude. They further stated that this disturbance is more similar to the circadian rhythms of children with non-seasonal depression than it is to adults with SAD. They hypothesized that children's high levels of nocturnal melatonin may serve to signal their circadian rhythms differently than adults with lower levels of nocturnal melatonin.

In treating SAD in children, Swedo et al. (75) discovered that bright light therapy with two hours of dawn simulation plus one hour of bright light therapy in the early evening can be beneficial. Parents' ratings of their children's SAD symptoms on the Structured Interview Guide for the Hamilton Depression Rating Scale (SIGH-SAD), Seasonal Affective Disorders significantly decreased during active treatment of light therapy as compared with baseline, placebo, and washout periods. Side effects were only reported by "one or two" children and consisted of somatic complaints, fatigue, and insomnia.

CONCLUSION

Although the exact neurophysiological mechanisms of sleep disturbances in children with affective disorders remains unknown, it is apparent that children with mood disorders have a higher prevalence of sleep complaints with delayed sleep onset being the most consistent finding in youth with major depression. Polysomnographic studies in early onset depression revealed inconsistent results with more pronounced changes in adolescents compared to prepubertal children. There is an evidence of gender influences on sleep regulation with a greater degree of biological rhythm dysregulation seen in female adolescents with major depression. Very little is known about sleep and circadian organization in children and adolescents with bipolar disorder. Future studies of impaired sleep homeostasis may help to delineate various phenotypes of affective disorders and be potentially helpful in the identification of biological markers of early onset bipolar disorder and major depression.

Research on the management of sleep disturbances in children with mood disorders is currently unavailable. However, it is important to recognize and treat sleep problems in pediatric patients suffering from emotional disturbances that if left untreated may complicate the course of the mental illness and precipitate future relapse.

REFERENCES

1. Benca RM. Mood Disorders. In: Kryger MH, Roth T, Dement WC, eds Principles and Practice of Sleep Medicine, 3rd edn. Philadelphia: WB Saunders, 2000, pp. 1140–57.
2. Kupfer DJ, Reynolds CF 3rd, Ulrich RF, Grochocinski VJ. Comparison of automated REM and slow-wave sleep analysis in young and middle-aged depressed subjects. Biol Psychiatry 1986; 21:189–200.
3. Reynolds CF 3rd, Kupfer DJ, Taska LS, et al. Slow WAVE sleep in elderly depressed, demented, and healthy subjects. Sleep 1985; 8:55–9.

 4. Kerkhofs M, Hoffmann G, De Martelaere V, Linkowski P, Mendlewicz J. Sleep EEG recordings in depressive disorders. J Affect Disord 1985; 9:47–53.
 5. Knowles JB, Cairns J, MacLean AW, et al. The sleep of remitted bipolar depressives: Comparison with sex and age-matched controls. Can J Psychiatry 1986; 31:295–8.
 6. Puig-Antich J, Goetz R, Hanlon C, Tabrizi MA, et al. Sleep architecture and REM sleep measures in prepubertal major depressives studies during recovery from the depressive episode in a drug-free state. Arch Gen Psychiatry 1983; 40:187–92.
 7. Giles DE, Biggs MM, Rush AJ, Roffwarg HP. Risk factors in families of unipolar depression: I. Incidence of illness and reduced REM latency. J Affect Disord 1988; 14:51–9.
 8. Giles DE, Kupfer DJ, Roffward HP, et al. Polysomnographic parameters in first-degree relatives of unipolar probands. Psych Res 1989; 27:127–36.
 9. Dahl RE. The regulation of sleep and arousal: Development and psychopathology. Development and Psychopathology 1996; 8:3–27.
10. Lewinsohn PM, Hops H, Roberts RE, et al. Adolescent psychopathology, I: Prevalence and incidence of depression and other DSM-III-R disorders in high school students. J Abnorm Psychol 1993; 102:133–44.
11. Diagnostic and Statistical Manual of Mental Disorders, Fourth Edition-Text Revision (DSM-IV-TR), APA 1994
12. American Academy of Child and Adolescent Psychiatry, Practice parameters for the assessment and treatment of children and adolescents with depressive disorders, J Am Acad Child Adolesc Psychiatry 2007; 46:1503–26.
13. Birmaher B, Ryan ND, Williamson DE, et al. Childhood and adolescent depression: A review of the past 10 years. Part I. J Am Acad Child Adolesc Psychiatry 1996; 35:1427–39.
14. Practice parameters for the assessment and treatment of children and adolescents with depressive disorders. J Am Acad Child Adolesc Pscyhiatry 1998; 37(Suppl):63S–83S.
15. Blader JC, Koplewicz HS, Abikoff H, Foley C. Sleep problems of elementary school children: A community survey. Archives of Pediatrics & Adolescent Medicine 1997; 151:473–80.
16. Paavonen EJ, Aronen ET, Moilanen I, et al. Sleep problems of school-aged children: A complementary view. Acta Pædiatr 2000; 89:223–8.
17. Smedje H, Broman JE, and Hetta J. Parents' reports of disturbed sleep in 5–7-year-old Swedish children. Acta Pædiatr 1999; 88:858–65.
18. Stein MA, Mendelsohn J, Obermeyer WH, Amromin J, Benca R. Sleep and behavior problems in school-aged children. Pediatrics 2001; 107:e60, 766.
19. Zuckerman B, Stevenson J, Bailey V. Sleep problems in early childhood: Continuities, predictive factors, and behavioral correlates. Pediatrics 1987; 80:664–71.
20. Johnson EO, Chilcoat HD, Breslau N. Trouble sleeping and anxiety/depression in childhood. Psych Res 2000; 94:93–102.
21. Puig-Antich J, Goetz R, Hanlon C, et al. Sleep architecture and REM sleep measures in prepubertal children with major depression. A controlled study. Arch Gen Psychiatry 1982; 39:932–9.
22. Fava M. Daytime sleepiness and insomnia as correlates of depression. J Clin Psychiaty 2004; 65:27–32.
23. Liu X, Buysse DJ, Gentzler AL, et al. Insomnia and hypersomnia associated with depressive phenomenology and comorbidity in childhood depression. Sleep 2007; 30:83–90.
24. Ryan ND, Puig-Antich J, Ambrosini P, et al. The clinical picture of major depression in children and adolescents. Arch Gen Psychiatry 1987; 44:854–61.
25. Kane J, Coble P, Conners CK, Kupfer DJ. EEG sleep in a child with severe depression. Am J Psychiatry 1977; 134:813–14.
26. Kupfer DJ, Coble P, Kane J, et al. Imipramine and EEG sleep in children with depressive symptoms. Psychopharmacology 1979; 60:117–23.
27. Emslie GJ, Rush AJ, Weinberg WA, et al. Children with major depression show reduced rapid eye movement latencies. Arch Gen Psychiatry 1990; 47:119–24.

28. Young W, Knowles JB, MacLean AW, et al. The sleep of childhood depressives: Comparison with age-matched controls. Biol Psychiatry 1982; 17:1163–8.
29. Dahl RE, Ryan ND, Birmaher B, et al. Electroencephalographic sleep measures in prepubertal depression. Psych Res 1991; 38:201–14.
30. Bertocci MA, Dahl RE, Williamson DE, et al. Subjective sleep complaints in pediatric depression: A controlled study and comparison with EEG measures of sleep and waking. J Am Acad Child Adolesc Psychiatry 2005; 44:1158–66.
31. Robert JJT, Hoffmann RF, Emslie GJ, et al. Sex and age differences in sleep macroarchitecture in childhood and adolescent depression. Sleep 2006; 29:351–8.
32. Armitage R, Emslie GJ, Hoffman RF, et al. Ultradian rhythms and temporal coherence in sleep EEG in depressed children and adolescents. Biol Psychiatry 2000; 47:338–50.
33. Armitage R, Hoffmann R, Trivedi M, Rush AJ. Slow-wave activity in NREM sleep: Sex and age effects in depressed outpatients and healthy controls. Psychiatry Res 2000; 95:201–13.
34. Teicher MH, Glod CA, Harper D, et al. Locomotor activity in depressed children and adolescents: I. Circadian dysregulation. J Am Acad Child Adolesc Psychiatry 1993; 32:760–9.
35. Armitage R, Hoffman R, Emslie G, et al. Rest-sctivity cycles in childhood and adolescent depression. J Am Acad Child Adolesc Psychiatry 2004; 43:761–9.
36. Kirmil-Gray K, Eagleston JR, Gibson E, Thoresen CE. Sleep disturbance in adolescents: Sleep quality, sleep habits, beliefs about sleep, and daytime functioning. J Youth and Adolescence 1984; 13:375–84.
37. Manni R, Ratti MT, Marchioni E, et al. Poor sleep in adolescents: A study of 869 17-year–old Italian secondary school students. J Sleep Res 1997; 6:44–9.
38. Morrison DN, McGee R, Stanton WR. Sleep problems in adolescence. J Am Acad Child Adolesc Psychiatry 1992; 31:94–9.
39. Patten CA, Choi WS, Gillin JC, Pierce JP. Depressive symptoms and cigarette smoking predict development and persistence of sleep problems in US adolescents. Pediatrics 2000; 106:e23, 334.
40. Saarenpää-Heikkilä O, Laippala P, Koivikko M. Subjective daytime sleepiness and its predictors in Finnish adolescents in an interview study. Acta Pædiatr 2001; 90:552–7.
41. Price VA, Coates TJ, Thoresen CE, Grinstead OA. Prevalence and correlates of poor sleep among adolescents. American Journal of Diseases in Childhood 1978; 132:583–6.
42. Roberts RE, Lewinsohn PM, Seeley JR. Symptoms of DSM-III-R major depression in adolescence: Evidence from an Epidemiological Survey. J Am Acad Child Adolesc Psychiatry 1995; 34:1608–17.
43. Lahmeyer HW, Poznanski EO, Bellu SN. EEG sleep in depressed adolescents. Am J Psychiatry 1983; 40:1150–3.
44. Mendlewicz J, Hoffman G., Kerkhofs M, Linkowski P. Electroencephalogram and neuroendocrine parameters in pubertal and adolescent depressed children. A case report study. J Affect Disord 1984; 6:265–72.
45. Goetz RR, Puig-Antich J, Ryan N, et al. Electroencephalographic sleep of adolescents with major depression and normal controls. Arch Gen Psychiatry 1987; 44:61–8.
46. Appelboom-Fondu J, Kerkhofs M, Mendlewicz J. Depression in adolescents and young adults polysomnographic and neuroendocrine aspects. J Affect Disord 1988; 14:35–40.
47. Khan AU, Todd S. Polysomnographic findings in adolescents with major depression. Psychiatry Res 1990; 33:313–20.
48. Kutcher S, Williamson P, Marton P, Szalai J. REM latency in endogenously depressed adolescents. Br J Psychiatry 1992; 161:399–402.
49. Dahl RE, Puig-Antich J, Ryan ND, Nelson B, Dachille S, Cunningham SL, et al. EEG sleep in adolescents with major depression: The role of suicidality and inpatient status. J Affect Disord 1990; 19:63–75.

50. Goetz RR, Puig-Antich J, Dahl RE, Ryan ND, Ryan ND, Asnis GM, Rabinovich H, Nelson B. EEG sleep of young adults with major depression: A controlled study. J Affect Disord 1991; 22:91–100.

51. Naylor MW, Shain BN, Shipley JE. REM latency in psychotically depressed adolescents. Biol Psychiatry 1990; 28:161–4.

52. Goetz RR, Wolk SI, Coplan JD, et al. Premorbid polysomnographic signs in depressed adolescents: A reanalysis of EEG sleep after longitudinal follw-up in adulthood. Biol Psychiatry 2001; 49:930–42.

53. Emslie GJ, Armitage R, Weinberg WA, et al. Sleep polysomnography as a predictor of recurrence in children and adolescents with depressive disorder. Int J Neuropsychopharmacol 2001; 4:59–168.

54. Armitage R, Hoffman RF, Emslie GJ, et al. Sleep microarchitecture as a predictor of recurrence in children and adolescents with depression. Int J Neuropsychopharmacol 2002; 5:217–28.

55. Dahl RE, Ryan ND, Matty MK, et al. Sleep onset abnormalities in depressed adolescents. Biol Psychiatry 1996; 39:400–10.

56. Shain BN, Naylor M, Shipley JE, Alessi N. Imipramine effects on sleep in depressed adolescents: A preliminary report. Biol Psychiatry 1990; 28:459–62.

57. Dorsey CM, Lukas SE, Cunningham SL. Fluoxetine-induced sleep disturbance in depressed patients. Neuropsychopharmacol 1996; 14:437–42.

58. Armitage R, Emslie G, Rintelmann J. The effect of fluoxetine on sleep EEG in childhood depression: A preliminary report. Neuropharmacol 1997; 17:241–5.

59. Kallepalli BR, Bhatara VS, Fogas BS, et al. Trazodone is only slightly faster than fluoxetine in relieving insomnia in adolescents with depressive disorders. J Child Adolesc Psychopharmacol 1997; 7:97–107.

60. Katz DA, McHorney CA. Clinical correlates of insomnia in patients with chronic illness. Arch Intern Med 1998; 158:1099–107.

61. Breslau N, Roth T, Rosenthal L, Andreski P. Sleep disturbance and psychiatric disorders: A longituginal epidemiological study of young adults. Biol Psychiatry 1996; 39:411–8.

62. Practice Parameters for the Assessement and Treatment of Children and Adolescents with Bipolar Disorder. J Am Acad Child Adolesc Psychiatry 1997; 36(10 Suppl):157S–176S.

63. Lewinsohn PM, Klein D, Seeley JR. Bipolar disorders in a community sample of older adolescents: prevalence, phenomenology, comorbidity, and course. J Am Acad Child Adolesc Psychiatry 1995; 34:454–63.

64. National Institute of Mental Health Research Roundtable on Prepubertal Bipolar Disorder. J Am Acad Child Adolesc Psychiatry 2001; 40:871–8.

65. Geller B, Zimmerman B, Williams M, et al. DSM-IV mania symptoms in a prepubertal and early adolescent bipolar phenotype compared to attention-deficit hyperactive and normal controls. J Child Adolesc Psychopharmacol 2002; 12:11–25.

66. Geller B, Zimmerman B, Williams M, et al. Phenomenology of prepubertal and early adolescent bipolar disorder: Examples of elated mood, grandiose behaviors, decreased need for sleep, racing thoughts and hypersexuality. J Child Adolesc Psychopharmacol 2002; 12:3–9.

67. Kowatch RA, Youngstrom EA, Danielyan A, Findling RL. Review and meta-analysis of the phenomenology and clinical characteristics of mania in children and adolescents. Bipolar Disorders 2005; 7:483–96.

68. Lofthouse N, Fristad MA, Splaingard M, Kelleher K. Parent and child reports of sleep problems associated with early-onset bipolar spectrum disorders. J Fam Ther 2007; 21:114–23.

69. Rao U, Dahl RE, Ryan ND, et al. Heterogeneity in EEG sleep findings in adolescent depression: Unipolar versus bipolar clinical course. J Affect Dis 2002; 70:273–80.

70. Mehl RC, O'Brien LM, Jones JH, et al. Correlates of sleep and pediatric bipolar disorder. Sleep 2006; 29:193–7.
71. Rosenthal NE, Sack DA, Gillin JC, et al. Seasonal affective disorder: A description of the syndrome and preliminary findings with light therapy. Arch Gen Psychiatry 1984; 41:72–80.
72. Carskadon MA, Acebo C. Parental reports of seasonal mood and behavior changes in children. J Am Acad Child Adolesc Psychiatry 1993; 32:264–9.
73. Swedo SE, Pleeter JD, Richter DM, et al. Rates of seasonal affective disorder in children and adolescents. Am J Psychiatry 1995; 152:1016–19.
74. Glod GA, Teicher MH, Polcari A, et al. Circadian rest-activity disturbances in children with seasonal affective disorder. J Am Acad Child Adolesc Psychiatry 1997; 36:188–95.
75. Swedo SE, Allen AJ, Glod CA, et al. A controlled trial of light therapy for the treatment of pediatric seasonal affective disorder. J Am Acad Child Adolesc Psychiatry 1997; 36:816–21.

21 Quantitative EEG Studies of Attention Disorders and Mood Disorders in Children

Lukasz M. Konopka and Teresa J. Poprawski

Clinical Psychology Department, Chicago School of Professional Psychology and Department of Psychiatry and Behavioral Neuroscience, Loyola University Medical Center, Chicago, Illinois, U.S.A.

QUANTITATIVE EEG, A NEW USE FOR AN OLD CONCEPT

For many years, we have used classical electroencephalography (EEG) in clinical settings. Clinicians use classical EEG primarily to detect and classify seizure disorders. However, each EEG clearly contains additional significant information (1,2). A new approach to classical EEG, Quantitative EEG, views EEG data using acquisition systems and computers that store large quantities of data. To use these tools appropriately in electroencephalography, we need definitions of normality and abnormality (3–7). As a result, F. Duffy, E. John, and R. Thatcher developed several databases that are commercially available for clinical and research settings (8–10). Databases become important because one's EEG interpretation often depends on the choice of comparison groups. Only if we can replicate the results in other laboratories and test the results in the clinical realm does published data become of universal importance. Without common, universal, comparison groups, this is a very difficult task (11).

In these authors' opinion, several variables define qEEG's importance as a clinical instrument: One, the user must be trained, knowledgeable, and competent in the interpretation of classical EEGs. Interpretive skills begin when the reader can visually identify and describe classical EEG patterns in various montages to recognize potentially focal findings. After completing this task, the reader begins analyzing background activity. But, to do this, users must be familiar with EEG technology and be able to identify potential artifacts and shortcomings of this methodology. Second, the users must carefully select the control/comparison group. Third, when acquiring data from a study population, users must follow the same selection protocol they chose for the control group. Fourth, one must define the comparison subject or population that one wishes to investigate. Last, we have probably the most difficult variable; we must define the patient's disorder (12). In today's paradigm, when we look for discriminating factors or diagnoses, we rely solely on the patient's clinical presentation. For example, if we want to use qEEG for studying attention deficit disorder (ADD) patients, we need to decide what defines ADD. Thus, we should ask the question, "Is there a gold standard defining ADD?" The answer is "no."

"FROM THE BRAIN TO BEHAVIOR," A POTENTIAL PARADIGM SHIFT

Currently, we rely on behavioral measures for defining potential neuropathology; but in this respect, we do not do well. Generally, clinicians define the behavior and then look at the brain, but we propose shifting that diagnostic paradigm. We propose looking at brain physiology, first, and then identifying the behavior. For example, we know that there are many behavioral patterns that may co-exist with ADD, including bipolar illness, depression, conduct disorder, etc. Are these presentations on a continuum or are they distinct categories? We would argue that a continuum exists; however, each individual case has a significant, well-defined, neurobiological substrate related to the presentation. If we changed our approach by using qEEG, evoked potentials (EP), and imaging, and considered not only the behavior, but defined disorders using objective neurobiological substrates, we would find greater homogeneity in our diagnostic subgroups. We might also recharacterize clinical presentations and develop new diagnostic descriptors. Although not yet very popular, our "brain to behavior" concept deserves some attention.

QUANTITATIVE EEG, A FLEXIBLE AND NON-INVASIVE TOOL
Quantitative EEG offers significant advantages over other, perhaps, more trendy imaging techniques. Quantitative EEG is a non-invasive tool that provides true-time resolution of neuronal activity. Millisecond resolution is the standard. Quantitative EEG is available as an objective neurodiagnostic tool using large, normative databases. In addition, quantitative EEG provides information about potential pharmacological choices using the principles of pharmaco-EEG (13,14). Pharmaco-EEG defines EEG profiles generated by specific medication subtypes. Thus, when EEG patterns are well defined, we can select pharmaco-therapeutic interventions we anticipate will modify the patient's abnormal EEG pattern. Quantitative EEG may be used to objectively track treatment efficacy because Quantitative EEG helps us assess whether brain activity is improving in parallel with the clinical presentation. We can co-register Quantitative EEG results to other imaging modalities such as MRI, functional MRI (fMRI), positron emission tomography (PET), and single-photon emission-computed tomography (SPECT) in three-dimensional space. Also in three-dimensional MRI space, we can identify sources and/or abnormalities using low resolution electromagnetic tomography (LORETA) (15,16). Lastly, Quantitative EEG is portable and may be used in a strict laboratory environment or in a patient's home.

STANDARDIZED QUANTITATIVE EEG USE LEADS TO MEANINGFUL OUTCOMES
Standard patient evaluation procedures include traditional EEG with scalp electrodes placed according to the International 10/20 System. The potential use of database standards dictates the recording conditions. Usually, the protocol involves recordings with the eyes opened and eyes closed while closely monitoring the patient's arousal state and avoiding drowsy, transitional states. Quantitative pediatric EEG studies may be more challenging than adult studies, as the child's tolerance and cooperation often require us to adjust the protocol. Therefore, one should pay attention to issues, such as acute hypoglycemia, that may cause aberrant EEG patterns. A glucose-enriched drink, such as orange juice, easily remedies this state. In our laboratory, we also use basic activation procedures such as hyperventilation, photic stimulation, and sleep. Other laboratories have developed specific activation procedures using psychological tests or other cognitive tasks during the EEG. These laboratories have compiled in-house, normative databases; but to our knowledge,

these databases are not commercially available. Complicated activation procedures often cause considerable EEG artifact, and behavioral manipulations are critical to assure appropriate data quality. Therefore, the technologist must be skilled at recording EEGs free from artifact.

We describe basic data acquisition and processing in Figure 1. In Section A of Figure 1, we show a page of digitized EEG recorded from a child wearing an electrode cap. Section B shows FFT (Fast Fourier Transform) data with all the electrode traces superimposed and a well-defined peak at 9.5 Hz, representing the dominant frequency in the eyes-closed state. Next, Section C shows dominant frequency source localization displayed in LORETA. Then finally, Section D shows topographic maps comparing the patient to the normative database. The gray-scale defines the patient's findings within plus and minus three standard deviations of the norms. After acquisition, the data analysis is based on the study's purpose and the available database. In general, we first select artifact-free epochs during distinct states excluding drowsiness and then convert these epochs into their frequency domains using Fast Fourier Transform (Fig. 1-B). The spectral data are displayed in many ways. In addition to the most standard displays involving absolute power and relative power measures, we also use coherence, phase, symmetry, and power ratios (17); however, the discussion of these variables is outside the scope of this paper.

Using Fast Fourier Transform, quantitative EEG analysis relies on separating complex waveforms into individual frequencies, classically defined as Delta, Theta, Alpha, Beta, and Gamma (Fig. 2). The Delta frequencies, 0.5–4 Hz, are generally

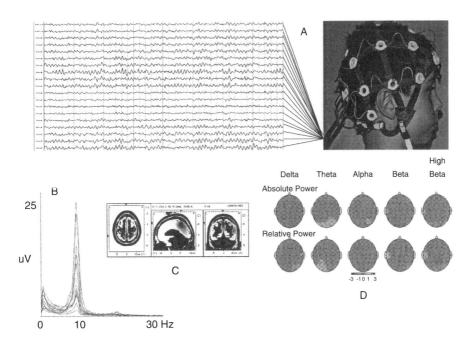

FIGURE 1 Diagram representing the steps in processing EEG data using classical acquisition and statistical comparisons.

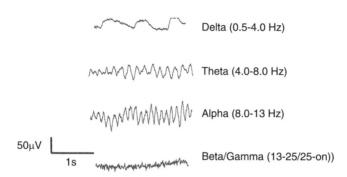

Delta (0.5-4.0 Hz)

Theta (4.0-8.0 Hz)

Alpha (8.0-13 Hz)

50μV

1s   Beta/Gamma (13-25/25-on))

FIGURE 2 Examples of classically divided frequencies observed in EEG recordings.

present in infants and during sleep, but when present in wake and focally distributed, they may reflect an underlying abnormality. Delta originates in cortical neurons and the thalamus. When the ascending reticular activating system is absent, it does not inhibit those brain structures and Delta occurs (18). Theta, 4–8 Hz, is often present in the transition from wake to drowsiness and may reflect normal memory acquisition patterns, however, large quantities of Theta in wake have been associated with abnormalities. Theta in the frontal and temporal regions is often associated with dysfunctions of these areas. The limbic system, specifically the hippocampus and anterior cingulate cortex, generate Theta (19,20). The Theta generator is inhibited by dopaminergic and serotoninergic innervations from the ventral tegmental area and the median raphe nucleus, respectively (Fig. 3). Originating in the septal nucleus and nucleus accumbens from neuronal connections, acetylcholine release positively influences the Theta generator (21). When eyes are closed, Alpha, 8–13 Hz, is often present as the dominant pattern in the occipital lobe. Frontal Alpha and asymmetric Alpha correlate with affective states. Presumably originating in the thalamus, a healthy, mature brain's dominant rhythm is an Alpha rhythm. The Alpha pacemaker's projections modulate cortical activity in an oscillatory and tonic fashion (22,23). Inhibitory GABA input from the striatum and excitatory cholinergic projections from the midbrain reticular formation influence the thalamus' activity. Beta frequencies, 13–25 Hz, often reflecting highly active brain states, may be contaminated by muscle activity, and are often observed in anxiety states. Beta frequencies originate in cortico-cortical and thalamo-cortical circuits and represent active information processing. Although we have not yet clearly defined the generators of Gamma frequencies, greater than 35 Hz, were recorded and interpreted as representing consciousness.

In the next step, we compare the frequency data to control groups composed of normal subjects or clinically defined populations, for example, traumatic brain injury patients (24,25) or patients with depression (27). First, we decide whether a patient belongs in the clinical population by comparing outcomes from the multivariate statistical analysis and, in some cases, we may also characterize the severity of the deficit (26). Prichep documented this process very well (28). Nevertheless, the multivariate approach has some potential drawbacks such as defining clinical comparison groups purely from the behavioral diagnosis.

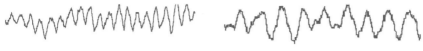

Alpha rhythm generator   Theta rhythm generator

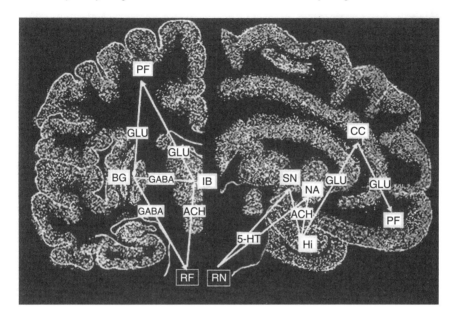

FIGURE 3 Potential neuroanatomical networks involved in generating Alpha and Theta frequencies observed in EEG.
Alpha Generator: Coronal cut, RF—midbrain reticular formation, Th—thalamus, PF—prefrontal cortex, BG—basal ganglia (dorsal striatum, globus pallidus, subthalamic nucleus, substantia nigra)
Theta Generator: Sagittal cut, RN—median raphe nucleus, SN—septal nucleus, NA—nucleus accumbens, Hi—hippocampus, CC—cingulate cortex, PF—prefrontal cortex
Neurotransmitters: 5-HT—serotonin, ACH—acetylcholine, GLU—glutamate, GABA—gamma-aminobutyric acid

EVOKED POTENTIALS

In addition to evaluating ongoing EEG activity, one can challenge the brain to perform tasks related to basic sensory functions by incorporating electrophysiological techniques called evoked potentials. As an adjunct to qEEG analysis, Frank Duffy developed evoked potentials by averaging a time-locked EEG signal to a presented stimulus. In his database, Dr. Duffy incorporated auditory, visual, and cognitive evoked potentials and then thoroughly described how these additional data were used for patient management (29).

PEDIATRIC QUANTITATIVE EEG

The following sections will summarize pediatric qEEG and address its potential diagnostic utility and subsequent therapeutic implications. With an eye for scientific design, we reviewed the literature from 1995 to 2007 using Medline and searched the key words: quantitative EEG, qEEG, pediatric, children, ADD, attention-deficit/hyperactive disorder (ADHD), depression, and bipolar disorder. Some recent studies focus on frontal lobe activities. Besides decreases or increases in frequencies, the authors evaluated amplitude relationships, defined as symmetry measures, and found that symmetry measures between hemispheres were associated with specific behaviors. In the literature, reports have focused primarily on Alpha asymmetry in the frontal lobes. The negative correlation between increased alpha power and cortical activation has been well documented. Studies by Davidson have shown that increased left frontal activity is associated with positive mood and active engagement, but also with anger and aggression. The presence of increased right frontal activity has been associated with negative mood and withdrawal behavior (30). Rybak et al. replicated these findings in the pediatric population (31). They analyzed frontal Alpha asymmetry in a group of sixty-five pediatric subjects, ranging in age from five to 17, diagnosed with affective disorders and disruptive behavior. They found a significant positive correlation between anger and aggression and left frontal activation, suggesting a fine balance in interhemispheric function. Its disruption may constitute a neurophysiologic process that leads to behavioral disinhibition and affective deregulation. Frontal EEG asymmetry may be clinically useful for identifying patients with hyperactivity of the approach motivational system, and may also function as a severity index. Some studies report a positive correlation between the intensity of frontal EEG abnormalities and the progressive severity of behavioral clinical presentation. We see a behavioral disruption continuum that seems to exist, beginning with impulsive and aggressive behavior, progressing to conduct disorder, and ending in psychopathic and criminal behavior (31).

Although qEEG is a valuable, non-invasive tool in psychiatric diagnosis, treatment selection, and monitoring of medication effectiveness, it has not been used enough in children. Most quantitative EEG literature focuses on adults, and pediatric EEG is limited mainly to children with ADHD.

QUANTITATIVE EEG IN ATTENTION DISORDERS

In the past three decades, peer-reviewed journals published more than 1000 research articles analyzing qEEG data in Attention Deficit Hyperactive Disorder, making it the most widely studied childhood behavioral disorder in children and adolescents; to study the brains of these children and adolescents, we have used electrophysiological measures. In their 2006, meta-analysis paper, Snyder and Hall cited nine articles (32) where they described highly variable research methodology. Yet, several issues concern us: First, the articles in the meta-analysis paper used two, variable, diagnostic classifications, the Diagnostic and Statistical Manual of Mental Disorders (DSM) III and the DSM IV. Second, the acquisition parameters used in the articles ranged from single electrodes to full electrode sets. Third, some studies recorded in the eyes-closed state, while others recorded with eyes open. Fourth, only one article mentioned recording state, which may indicate potential problems with drowsiness. Despite these shortcomings, when compared to normal children, these findings show that most children with ADHD display fairly consistent EEG abnormalities in brain electrical activity. The most common qEEG findings were increased absolute and relative Theta power in the frontal and central regions, which indicate decreased frontal cortical activity (33–37). In addition, studies have reported increased frontal Theta/Beta and Theta/Alpha ratios that may reflect the cortical arousal level, defined by increased frontal Theta/Beta, and maturational delay defined by Theta/Alpha ratios (38,39,35).

In a recent paper, Loo and Barkley (40) reviewed qEEG studies related to ADHD and demonstrated inconsistencies in patient selection, diagnostic criteria, acquisition, and the processing of EEG data. In frequencies other than Theta, we see variable observations. For example, in children with ADHD, Delta increased, decreased or was seen at normal levels. Also, Alpha findings were variable and age- and gender-dependent (33,35,36,38). Beta findings were mixed and both Alpha and Beta decreased. Moreover, the findings showed no changes in Beta in the fronto-central regions (33,34,37,41).

The DSM IV defines three subtypes of ADHD: combined, predominantly inattentive, and hyperactive–impulsive. Within the DSM IV subdivisions, Clark and his collaborators identified different qEEG patterns, reporting that inattentive ADHD could be subdivided into two EEG subtypes (42): Subtype One showed increased Theta, with Delta and Beta deficiencies, and Subtype Two showed increased slow wave and fast wave deficiencies. Among ADHD combined type pediatric populations, Clarke et al. have reported three different EEG subtypes (43). In these populations, consistent with other electrophysiological studies, they showed increased frontal Theta and decreased Beta and used the amount of Theta and Beta as a differentiating factor. Using the Theta/Beta ratio for defining ADHD pediatric subpopulations was not independently replicated (39). This discrepancy may be due to methodological issues. When compared to normal controls, the third pediatric ADHD EEG group, the combined type, demonstrated distinct increased frontal Beta activity. In the combined type, but not the inattentive type, developmental studies suggest that electrophysiologic abnormalities appear to normalize with age (44). In children with ADHD, clinicians also observe this phenomenon. When children mature, hyperactivity often decreases, but inattention often persists into adulthood (45).

When using behavioral definitions, classifying pediatric disorders is highly non-specific. So, it is not surprising that objective measures, such as EEG, may readily detect subtle differences in neuropathophysiology. For different ADHD groups, the EEG classifies subgroups better than behavioral assessments. The "brain to behavior" approach appears more logical than classifying psychiatric disorders based solely on subjective measures. Recently, Chabot and his colleagues attempted the former approach by using qEEG abnormalities to classify 344 children with ADHD or ADD and 245 children with learning disabilities (LD) (46). For the analysis, he used 35 qEEG variables, showing the greatest variance across the entire pediatric population. Based on the analysis, he detected five different EEG patterns. Table 1 summarizes these findings. He made no attempt to correlate specific EEG patterns with potential behavior variance and/or diagnosis, including potential comorbidities, family history, and other psychosocial factors. We also see evidence for ADHD population heterogeneity in medication response studies where approximately 75% of ADHD patients show a positive response to stimulants. Several studies analyzed EEG differences between unmedicated and medicated patients, and also between stimulant responders and non-responders (47,48). After therapeutic intervention begins, the studies showed that stimulants generally normalized EEG patterns in individuals who responded to medication. In general, normalization leads to decreased frontal and central Theta and Alpha absolute power, and frontal Beta increase, but non-responders exhibit the reverse pattern. EEG normalization also parallels the performance on tasks requiring sustained attention (49,50).

TABLE 1 EEG Patterns Observed in Subpopulations of Patients Diagnosed with Deficits of Attention

	Delta rhythm	Theta rhythm	Alpha rhythm	Beta rhythm	Coherence
Cluster 1	deficit (absolute and relative power)	excess in the frontal region	generalized excess	no findings	increased frontal theta and alpha
Cluster 2	no findings	generalized excess(absolute and relative power)	decreased mean frequency	no findings	increased frontal theta
Cluster 3	generalized excess	generalized deficit	generalized deficit	generalized deficit	decreased frontal alpha
Cluster 4	excess in fronto-central region	excess in fronto-central region	generalized deficit and decreased mean frequency		decreased fronto-central alpha
Cluster 5	no findings	no findings	no findings	no findings	no findings

Source: Adapted From Ref. (46).

ACUTE CHALLENGE STUDIES

Using a one-day session, we propose to provide information on medication effectiveness. For example, when we consider methylphenidate pharmacokinetics, with its action onset within 20–60 minutes and short half-life of 2–3 hours, we can assess instantaneously both qEEG and behavioral responses to this medication by performing a methylphenidate challenge. In 1999, Loo et al. published this approach (49). In our laboratory, we also utilize this paradigm (51). The protocol considers qEEG and behavioral studies before and after the medication administration, providing clinicians with a useful tool that allows medication evaluation without lengthy therapeutic trials. When new therapeutic agents become available, we should apply these approaches to medication evaluation. For example, clinicians are considering a new use for modafinil in ADD treatment. In 2006, Saletu et al. showed that modafinil decreased frontal Delta and increased Theta, Alpha, and Beta powers (52). So, by applying their pharmaco-EEG principles of lock and key, we may predict responses in defined patient subpopulations. Therefore, using response-matching patterns, we suggest that medication only benefits patients with reverse EEG findings, e.g., patients with narcolepsy or ADHD (Cluster 3, Table 1).

QUANTITATIVE EEG IN CHILDHOOD DEPRESSION

Although we have much data defining qEEG findings in depressed adults, we have very limited qEEG data reported in pediatric depression. Davidson (30) has shown that increased left frontal activity is associated with positive mood and active engagement, but also with anger and aggression. Conversely, the presence of increased right frontal activity has been associated with negative mood and withdrawal behavior. As discussed above, Rybak et al. replicated these findings in the pediatric population (31). Graae et al. studied Alpha asymmetry in depressed adolescents who attempted suicide (53). The study analyzed EEG data from 16 adolescent Hispanic girls who attempted suicide and compared them to a group of normal adolescent girls of the same ethnicity. They found that the degree of Alpha asymmetry differed between the normal controls and the study group, with the normal controls showing statistically significant asymmetric Alpha activity and greater Alpha power over the right hemisphere. The depressed, suicidal patients did not show this pattern of interhemispheric asymmetry in this patient population. These findings demonstrate frontal lobe involvement and potentially reduced interhemispheric activity in this patient population. As with the other studies presented in this paper, Rybak et al. and Graae et al. utilized the DSM IV diagnoses as their primary grouping criteria. If Rybak and Graae had selected groupings using EEG features, they may have reported different outcomes.

QUANTITATIVE EEG IN CHILDHOOD BIPOLAR ILLNESS

Treating bipolar illness differs significantly from the treatment of major depression or ADD, and the precise diagnosis of bipolar illness is critical. Unfortunately, the scientific community does not currently use qEEG in studies of pediatric bipolar illness. Existing research on the neurobiology of pediatric mood disorders mainly utilizes MRI, fMRI, and magnetic resonance spectroscopy (MRS) (see review article by DelBello et al.) (54). The results of these studies suggest the involvement of two main brain circuits in the neuropathophysiology of bipolar disorder. The first includes a network potentially engaged in mood regulation involving the ventro-medial prefrontal cortex, orbitalfrontal cortex, and amygdala. The second circuit involves cognition and includes the dorsolateral prefrontal cortex, thalamus, and basal ganglia. Based on the proposed circuits, we would expect to observe qEEG defined electrophysiological patterns reflecting alterations in these circuits.

CONCLUSION

Because children experience highly unstable, physiological stages driven by developmental variability, we find it difficult to evaluate pediatric studies. A child's chronological age does not necessarily correlate with the development of their brains. For example two 7-year-old children may present with very different, basic, dominant frequencies, potentially implying a difference in brain maturation. So, should we consider these individuals in the same group? Often, this question is not addressed. Another issue is the use of medications. We should not consider the quantitative EEG of children treated with psychotropic agents as reflecting a specific neurobiological marker. One might argue that if we see focal findings in a medicated child's EEG, we have eliminated the confounding factors of pharmacological treatment. This may be particularly true when one uses current density mapping. Yet in the absence of other converging data, we must exercise significant care in interpreting such findings. Although focal findings may give us a guide to subsequent diagnostic evaluations, they cannot stand alone. When combined with the "brain to behavior model," the pediatric qEEG is valuable for objectively defining potential abnormalities that lead to more precise therapeutic decisions. Therefore, in treating and studying children, we need to establish uniform protocols and use standardized databases so that scientists can easily replicate published results and clinicians can employ them in practice.

REFERENCES

1. Gordon E. Brain imaging technologies: How, what, when, and why? Aust NZ J Psychiatry 1999; 33:187–96.
2. Kaiser DA. QEEG: State of the art, or state of confusion. J Neurother 2001; 4:57–75.
3. Gordon E, Cooper N, Rennie C, et al. Integrative neuroscience: The role of a standardized database. Clin EEG Neurosci 2005; 36(2):64–75.
4. Prichep LS. Use of normative databases and statistical methods in demonstrating clinical utility of QEEG: Importance and cautions. Clin Electroencephalogr Neurosci 2005; 36:82–7.
5. Johnstone J, Gunkelman J. Use of databases in QEEG evaluation. J Neurother 2003; 7:31–52.
6. Lorensen TD, Dickson P. Quantitative EEG databases: A comparative investigation. J Neurother 2004; 8:53–68.
7. Johnstone J, Gunkelman J, Lunt J. Clinical database development: Characterization of EEG phenotypes. Clin Electroencephalogr Neurosci 2005; 36:99–107.
8. John ER, Karmel BZ, Corning WC, et al. Neurometrics: Numerical taxonomy identifies different profiles of brain functions within groups of behaviorally similar people. Science 1977; 196:1383–410.
9. John E, Prichep L, Friedman J, et al. Neurometrics: Computer assisted differential diagnosis of brain dysfunctions. Science 1988; 293:162–9.

10. John ER, Prichep LS. Principles of neurometric analysis of EEG and evoked potentials, in EEG: Basic Principles, Clinical Applications, and Related Fields. Edited by Niedermeyer E, Lopes da Silva F, Baltimore, Williams and Wilkins, 1993, pp. 989–1003.
11. Gordon E, Konopka LM. EEG databases in research and clinical practice: Current status and future directions. Clin Electroencephalogr Neurosci 2005; 36:53–4.
12. Coburn KL, Lauterbach EC, Boutros NN, et al. The value of quantitative electroencephalography in clinical psychiatry: A report by the Committee on Research of the American Neuropsychiatric Association. J Neuropsychiatry Clin Neurosci 2006; 18:460–500.
13. Saletu B, Anderer P, Kinsperger K, et al. Topographic brain mapping of EEG in neuro-psychopharmacology-Part II. Clinical applications (pharmaco EEG imaging). Methods & Findings in Experimental & Clinical Pharmacology 1987; 9(6):385–408.
14. Saletu B, Anderer P, Saletu-Zyhlarz GM. EEG topography and tomography (LORETA) in the classification and evaluation of the pharmacodynamics of psychotropic drugs. Clin EEG Neurosci 2006; 37 (2):66–80.
15. Pascual-Marqui RD, Michel CM Lehmann D. Low resolution electromagnetic tomography: A new method for localizing electrical activity in the brain. International Journal of Psychophysiology 1994; 18:49–65.
16. Thatcher W, North D, Biver C. Parametric vs. non-parametric statistics of low resolution electromagnetic tomography (LORETA). Clin EEG Neurosci 2005; 36:1.
17. Hughes JR, John ER. Conventional and quantitative electroencephalography in psychiatry. J Neuropsychiatry Clin Neurosci 1999; 11:190–208.
18. John ER, Prichep LS. The relevance of QEEG to the evaluation of behavioral disorders and pharmacological interventions. Clin EEG Neurosci 2006; 37(2):135–43.
19. Buzaki G. Theta oscillations in the hippocampus. Neuron 2002; 33:325–40.
20. Pizzagalli DA, Oakes TR, Davidson RJ. Coupling of theta activity and glucose metabolism in the human rostral anterior cingulate cortex: An EEG/PET study of normal and depressed subjects. Psychophysiology 2003; 40(6):939–49.
21. John ER. Consciousness: From synchronous neural discharge to subjective awareness? Prog Brain Res 2005; 150:143–72.
22. Thatcher R, John ER. The genesis of alpha rhythm and EEG synchronizing mechanisms. Foundation of Cognitive Process. LEA, Hillsdale 1977, pp. 53–82.
23. Michele F, Prichep L, John ER, et al. The neurophysiology of attention-deficit/hyperactivity disorder. Int J Psychophysiol 2005; 58:81–93.
24. Thatcher RW, Cantor DS, McAlaster R, et al. Comprehensive predictions of outcome in closed head-injured patients: the development of prognostic equations. Ann N Y Acad Sci 1983; 432:82–101.
25. Thatcher RW, Walker RA, Gerson I, et al. EEG discriminant analyses of mild head trauma. Electroencephalogr Clin Neurophysiol 1989; 73:94–106.
26. Thatcher RW, North DM, Curtin RT, et al. An EEG severity index of traumatic brain injury. J Neuropsychiatry Clin Neurosci 2001; 13:77–87.
27. Prichep LS, John ER, Essig-Peppard T, et al. Neurometric subtyping of depressive disorders, in Plasticity and Morphology of the Central Nervous System. Edited by Cazzullo CL, Sacchetti E, Conte G, et al. London, Kluwer Academic Publishers 1990, pp. 95–107.
28. Prichep LS. Use of normative databases and statistical methods in demonstrating clinical utility of QEEG: Importance and cautions. Clin EEG Neurosci 2005; 36(2):82–7.
29. Duffy FH. Long latency evoked potential database for clinical applications: justification and examples. Clin EEG Neurosci 2005; 36(2):88–98.
30. Davidson RJ. Anterior electrophysiological asymmetries, emotions, and depression: Conceptual and methodological conundrums. Psychophysiology 1998; 35:607–14.
31. Rybak M, Crayton JW, Young IJ, et al. Frontal alpha power asymmetry in aggressive children and adolescents with mood and disruptive behavior disorders. Clin EEG Neurosci 2006; 37(1):16–24.

32. Snyder SM, Hall JR. A meta-analysis of quantitative EEG power associated with attention-deficit hyperactivity disorder. J Clin Neurophysiol 2006; 23(5):440–55.
33. Chabot RJ, Serfontein G. Quantitative electroencephalographic profiles of children with attention deficit disorder. Biol Psychiatry 1996; 40:951–63.
34. Clarke AR, Barry RJ, McCarthy R, et al. EEG analysis in attention-deficit/hyperactivity disorder: A comparative study of two subtypes. Psychiatric Research 1998; 81:19–29.
35. Clarke AR, Barry RJ, McCarthy R, et al. Age and sex effects in the EEG: Differences in two subtypes of attention-deficit/hyperactivity disorder. Clin Neurophysiol 2001; 112:815–26.
36. El-Sayed E, Larson JO, Persson HE, et al. Altered cortical activity in children with attention–deficit/hyperactivity disorder during attentional load task. J Am Acad Child Adolesc Psychiatry 2002; 41:811–19.
37. Lazzaro I, Gordon E, Whitmont S, et al. Quantified EEG activity in adolescent attention deficit hyperactivity disorder. Clin Electroencephalogr 1998; 34:123–34.
38. Bresnahan SM, Anderson JW, Barry RJ. Age-related changes in quantitative EEG in attention-deficit/hyperactivity disorder. Biol Psychiatry 1999; 46:1690–7.
39. Monastra VJ, Lubar JF, Linden M. The development of a quantitative electroencephalographic scanning process of attention-hyperactivity disorder: Reliability and validity studies. Neuropsychology 2001; 15:136–44.
40. Loo SK, Barkley RA. Clinical utility of EEG in attention deficit hyperactivity disorder. Applied Neuropsychology 2005; 12(2):64–76.
41. Kuperman S, Johnson B, Arndt S, et al. Quantitative EEG differences in a nonclinical sample of children with ADHD and undifferentiated ADD. J Am Acad Child Adolesc Psychiatry 1996; 35:1009–17.
42. Clarke AR, Barry RJ, McCarthy, et al. EEG evidence for a new conceptualization of attention deficit hyperactivity disorder. Clin Neurophysiol 2002; 113:1036–44.
43. Clarke AR, Barry RJ, McCarthy, et al. EEG-defined subtypes of children with attention-deficit/hyperactivity disorder. Clin Neurophysiol 2001; 112:2098–105.
44. Barry RJ, Clarke AR, Johnstone SJ. A review of electrophysiology in attention-deficit/hyperactivity disorder: I Qualitative and quantitative electroencephalography. Clin Neurophysiol 2003; 114:171–83.
45. Hart EL, Lahey BB, Loeber R, et al. Developmental change in attention-deficit hyperactivity disorder in boys: A four-year longitudinal study. J Abnorm Child Psychol 1995; 23:729–49.
46. Chabot RJ, di Michele F, Prichep L. The role of quantitative electroencephalography in child and adolescent psychiatric disorders. Child Adolesc Psychiatr Clin N Am 2005; 14(1):21–53.
47. Clarke AR, Barry RJ, Bond D, et al. Effect of stimulant medications on the EEG of children with attention-deficit/hyperactivity disorder. Psychopharmacology (Berl) 2002; 164:277–84.
48. Clarke AR, Barry RJ, McCarthy R, et al. EEG differences between good and poor responders to methylphenidate and dexamphetamine in children with attention-deficit/hyperactivity disorder. Clin Neurophysiol 2002; 113(2):194–205.
49. Loo SK, Teale PD, Reite ML. EEG correlates of methylphenidate response among children with ADHD: A preliminary report. Biol Psychiatry 1999; 45:1657–60.
50. Winsberg BG, Javitt DC, Silipo GS. Electrophysiological indices of information processing in methylphenidate responders. Biol Psychiatry 1997; 42:434–45.
51. Goforth HW, Konopka L, Primeau M, et al. Quantitative electroencephalography in frontotemporal dementia with methylphenidate response: A case study. Clin EEG Neurosci 2004; 35(2):108–11.
52. Saletu B, Anderer P, Saletu-Zyhlarz GM. EEG topography and tomography (LORETA) in the classification and evaluation of the pharmacodynamics of psychotropic drugs. Clin EEG Neurosci 2006; 37(2):66–80.
53. Graae F, Tenke C., Bruder G, et al. Abnormality of EEG alpha asymmetry in female adolescent suicide attempters. Biol Psychiatry 1996; 40:706–13.
54. DelBello MP, Adler CM, Strakowski SM. The neurophysiology of childhood and adolescent bipolar disorder. CNS Spectrums 2006; 11(4):298–311.

22 | Parasomnias in Childhood

Rupali Bansal[a] and Stephen H. Sheldon[b]

[a]*Division of Pediatric Pulmonology, Phoenix Children's Hospital, Phoenix, Arizona, U.S.A.*
[b]*Northwestern University, Feinberg School of Medicine and Division of Pulmonary Medicine, Children's Memorial Hospital, Chicago, Illinois, U.S.A.*

BACKGROUND

Parasomnias are unpleasant or undesirable behavioral, experiential, or motor phenomena that occur predominantly or exclusively during the sleep period (1). They may be classified as dysfunctions associated with transitions into sleep, partial arousals during sleep, or following arousals from sleep (2,3). Parasomnias can be categorized either as primary or secondary. Transitional parasomnias typically occur during wake-to-sleep transitions and can persist into N1 (Stage 1) sleep. Primary parasomnias can be subdivided by the sleep from which they appear, e.g., rapid eye movement (REM) sleep, non-REM (NREM) sleep, or both. Secondary parasomnias are more commonly associated with other organ system dysfunction and manifest symptoms during the sleep period.

Transitional parasomnias are quite common and rhythmic movements prior to sleep onset occur in older infants and some toddlers. Spells are infrequent and typically cease as the child matures. Rarely do rhythmic movements prior to sleep onset persist into later childhood. When this occurs symptoms may range from simple head rolling to violent head banging and body rocking.

Primary parasomnias are more common in children than adults (4). Common childhood parasomnias include sleepwalking, sleep terrors, nightmares, and confusional arousals. Few pathological abnormalities or objective diagnostic criteria can be identified, despite the presence of intense and often striking symptoms. No obvious clinical abnormalities are present during wakefulness. Although symptoms can be significant, spontaneous remission is typical (3). Frequency can vary from a single isolated episode to multi-nightly events and that may persist for a protracted period of time. Parasomnias based on the International Classification of Sleep Disorders (2nd edition) are listed in Table 1.

ETIOLOGY

Etiology of most parasomnias is unknown. A maturational cause is likely due to the decremental nature of symptoms and spontaneous resolution. It is thought that many of these undesirable motor spells during sleep are due to state dissociation and the intensity of the arousal threshold in children when compared to adults. Nonetheless, many different hypotheses have been proposed. Often a familial pattern can be seen in some parasomnias. Familial occurrence is every so often seen in sleepwalking and night terrors (5,6,7). Developmental factors and psychological factors may account for some parasomnias such as sleep terrors (8). Environmental factors that contribute to parasomnias in children include excitement, stress, and/or anxiety (4).

TABLE 1 Classification of Parasomnias

Sleep-wake transition disorders	Arousal disorders	Parasomnias usually associated with REM sleep	Other parasomnias
1) Rhythmic Movement Disorder 2) Sleep starts 3) Sleep talking 4) Nocturnal leg cramps	1) Confusional arousals 2) Sleepwalking 3) Sleep terrors	1) Nightmares 2) Sleep paralysis 3) Impaired sleep-related penile erections 4) Sleep-related painful erections 5) REM sleep related sinus arrest 6) REM sleep behavior disorder	1) Sleep bruxism 2) Sleep enuresis 3) Sleep related abnormal swallowing syndrome 4) Nocturnal paroxysmal dystonia 5) Sudden unexplained nocturnal death 6) Primary snoring 7) Infant sleep apnea 8) Congenital central hypoventilation syndrome 9) Sudden infant death

Source: *ICSD—International classification of sleep disorders: Diagnostic and coding manual.* Diagnostic Classification Steering Committee, Thorpy MJ, Chairman. Rochester, Minnesota: American Sleep Disorders Association, 1990.

EVALUATION

Evaluation begins with a comprehensive medical history and physical examination. These are essential and can likely result in an accurate diagnosis without elaborate testing. Attention should be placed on a detailed description of the characteristics, timing, frequency, and duration of the spells. Additionally, the history should include, but not be limited to: whether the child is easily soothed or symptoms become worse after caretaker's intervention; presence or absence of agitation; symptoms following awakening; amnesia for the events; and presence or absence of stereotypic activity. Morning wake time, evening bedtime, number of nighttime arousals and naptime rituals require description. Sleep diaries are frequently very helpful in assessment. Although not always possible, videotaping of the events may often reveal identifiable characteristics. A review of symptoms including presence of daytime sleepiness, sleep attacks, snoring, restlessness, or limb movement during sleep, may help in determining precipitating factors. Family history is also important since some parasomnias have a familial predisposition. Physical examination is essential but is usually normal. Emphasis should be placed on neurological function and developmental assessment. Medical or surgical history may suggest an organic cause for sleep disorders. Social history may reveal psychosocial stressors that may be contributing to a disrupted sleep state.

DIAGNOSIS/TREATMENT

Imaging studies are of little utility in diagnosing a parasomnia, unless it is to detect the primary medical illness that may be causing the parasomnia. A drug screen might be helpful if there is concern that the symptoms may be a side effect or adverse reaction to a medication. It may also be helpful in the adolescent patient with persistent symptoms. Polysomnography with video recordings may be helpful for some of the parasomnias. An expanded electroencephalogram (EEG) electrode array can assist in differentiating partial arousals or transitional sleep disorders from sleep-related seizures. Concurrent video recording of the patient while sleeping may demonstrate symptoms and document movements. Reassurance, psychotherapy, and good sleep hygiene are all that are needed to treat most parasomnias. They usually resolve spontaneously without significant intervention. In severe cases, medical management may be necessary. In REM sleep motor disorder, clonazepam is used to control symptoms. In severe nocturnal leg cramps, quinine sulfate is usually recommended.

SLEEP/WAKE TRANSITION DISORDERS

These disorders usually occur while falling asleep, during the wake-to-sleep transition. Most commonly they appear at the beginning of the major nocturnal sleep period, but they may occur following arousals, while waking up from sleep, or during naps.

Rhythmic Movement Disorder

Rhythmic movement disorder is defined as a group of stereotyped repetitive movements involving large muscles, usually of the head and neck, that typically occur prior to sleep onset and are sustained into light sleep (2). This includes but is not limited to body rocking, head rolling, or head banging. Rhythmic movements surrounding sleep are very common and have been reported in about two-thirds of normal children (9). Rhythmic movements typically resolve spontaneously by four years of age (10). The pathophysiologic mechanisms of rhythmic movements remain obscure. Polysomnography is generally not indicated since diagnosis can be made on history and physical examination alone. It may, however, be helpful to rule out a seizure disorder particularly when stereotypic behaviors are noted. Movements are usually seen in NREM sleep, and are rare in REM sleep (11). Focal, paroxysmal, or epileptiform activity is notably absent. Sleep architecture, progression of states and state percentages as proportions of the total sleep time are normal for age. Treatment other than parental reassurance is rarely necessary (12).

Somniloquy

Somniloquy refers to talking in one's sleep. Talking during sleep is extremely common, and of little concern to parents or child healthcare practitioners. Exact incidence is unknown, but recent epidemiology literature suggests that the overall prevalence for children ages three to 13 years is about 55.5% (13). Somniloquy itself is not associated with pathology but may be associated with sleep terrors, confusional arousals, or sleepwalking. It usually occurs in the lighter stages (1 and 2) of NREM sleep. Diagnosis is clinical, and based on typical manifestations of coherent speech or incoherent mumbling. The individual usually has no recollection of the event. Somniloquy is most often self-limited. Polysomnography is rarely indicated, and treatment is unnecessary.

Nocturnal Leg Cramps

These cramps are sudden, painful, involuntary contractions of the calf muscles that occur at night or while resting. They can last for a few seconds and up to 10 minutes. Usually, nocturnal leg cramps occur in middle age to older individuals, but they can occur at any age. Previous studies have shown an incidence of 7.3% in children; the incidence increases at 12 years and peaks at 16–18 years of age (14). Causes of leg cramps include overexertion, structural (flat feet), endocrine disorders, dehydration, and some medications. It can be treated by leg movement and/or local massage (15). Persistent or severe leg cramps often are treated with Quinine sulfate but this has many side effects and should be used with caution (16).

Nocturnal leg cramps should not be confused with restless leg syndrome (RLS). RLS causes unpleasant sensations in the legs and an uncontrollable urge to move while at rest in order to relieve these feelings. People have described these sensations as burning, creeping, tugging, or like insects crawling inside the legs. It is not, however, associated with severe pain like nocturnal leg cramps. Additionally, in younger children, complaints of growing pains may indicate either nocturnal leg cramps or periodic limb movements of sleep (Sheldon and Davis 2007, unpublished data).

PARASOMNIAS ASSOCIATED WITH NREM SLEEP/AROUSAL DISORDERS

Parasomnias during NREM sleep (typically N3/slow wave sleep) are considered to be part of a continuum of undesirable manifestations of arousal or partial arousal that occur during sleep. Symptoms typically begin in childhood and resolve spontaneously.

Confusional Arousals

Confusional arousals are often seen in children and are characterized by movements in bed and include thrashing about, or inconsolable crying (17). Confusion and disorientation are prominent, and with toddlers, may resemble a temper tantrum. It usually occurs in the first half of the night, but may occur at any time. Attempts to awaken the child are futile, and may exacerbate the symptoms; the episode just needs to run its course. The episodes can last anywhere from five to 45 minutes, but usually subside after five to 10 minutes. Organic pathology is rarely present, but it does occur more commonly in the setting of other sleep disorders such as obstructive sleep apnea syndrome (OSAS), hypnagogic or hypnopompic hallucinations, insomnia, and hypersomnia (18). Diagnosis is based on identification of classical symptoms of confusion, disorientation, agitation, and/or combativeness upon arousal typically occurring in the first half of the sleep period. Polysomnography is rarely indicated but might reveal sudden arousal from N3/slow wave sleep, brief episodes of hypersynchronous delta activity, theta delta sleep, recurrent micro-sleep episodes, or a poorly reactive alpha activity. Epileptiform activity is absent from the EEG. There is no treatment for confusional arousals, and children usually outgrow the episodes after middle childhood. Ensuring adequate rest and regular sleep habits can help to reduce the chances of an attack.

Somnambulism

Sleepwalking, formally known as somnambulism, is a primary sleep parasomnia that originates during deep sleep (N3/SWS) and can range from simply sitting up in bed, quiet walking about the home, to performing complex behaviors while asleep. Sleepwalking occurs most commonly in middle childhood and pre-adolescence, with a peak incidence in children aged 11–12 years (19). Between 10% and 15% of children 5–12 years of age have at least one episode of somnambulism (19). Most children do not actually walk, but sit up in bed, and make repetitive movements such as rub their eyes or fumble with their clothes (20). Some children may get up and walk around their bedroom, or even around the house. Eyes are typically open and the youngster may appear awake. Motor activity can quickly cease and the child may lay down on the floor or return to sleep at unusual places around the home. Enuresis and voiding at unusual places around the house often occur. Upon awakening from sleepwalking, children usually have no memory or only a vague awareness of what has happened. There are substantial genetic effects in sleepwalking in both childhood and adulthood. One study showed, for sleep-walking in childhood, the probandwise concordance rate to be 0.55 for mono-zygotic and 0.35 for dizygotic pairs (21). Precipitating factors associated with sleepwalking include fever, sleep deprivation, OSA, environmental noise, and certain medications. Evaluation of a patient should include a thorough medical, psychiatric, and sleep history. Sleep laboratory evaluation is not generally required. Treatment is usually reassurance, and supportive treatment including safety measures. A psychotherapeutic approach may be used to identify and relieve stressors that may be exacerbating the sleepwalking episodes. Children eventually outgrow sleepwalking.

Sleep Terrors

A sleep terror, also known as pavor nocturnes, is a sleep disorder characterized by extreme terror and a temporary inability to regain full consciousness(22). The prevalence of sleep terrors is greater in childhood than adulthood, with a peak between five and seven years and resolution typically before adolescence (13). Sleep terrors have been reported to affect approximately 3% of children, with no preference for age or race (13). Risk factors for night terrors include stress, fever, sleep deprivation, certain medications, intrinsic sleep disorders such as OSA, periodic limb movement disorder (PLMD), and genetic predisposition (23). A typi-cal history includes the child sitting up in bed and screaming approximately 90 minutes after falling asleep. Prominent autonomic activity (e.g., tachycardia, tachypnea, diaphoresis, flushing) may occur. The child appears awake but may be confused, disoriented, and unresponsive to stimuli. Most episodes last 1–2 minutes, but the child may remain inconsolable for 5–30 minutes before relaxing and returning back to quiet sleep. If the child wakes up during the episode, he may recall fragmented pieces of the "bad dream." In the morning, the child typically has no memory of the experience. Management is targeted towards parental reassur-ance and guidance. Sleep hygiene should be reviewed and implemented as needed. For children who continue to have frequent night terrors, polysomnogram should be done to evaluate for intrinsic sleep disorders. Medication should be reserved for extreme cases when the child has sustained an injury secondary to the spell, is at significant risk for injury, and/or when the spells are quality of life threatening. Common medications recommended have included benzodiazepines or gabapentin.

PARASOMNIAS ASSOCIATED WITH REM SLEEP
Nightmares
Nightmares are vivid and terrifying nocturnal episodes in which the dreamer is suddenly awakened. In general, the child wakes up from REM sleep, and can describe in full detail the events of the dream. Nightmares occur in 35–45% of children aged 2–18 years (24). In older children and adults, causes of nightmares include emotional stressors, post-traumatic stress disorders, certain drugs, neurocognitive deficits, and/or genetic predisposition (25). The differences between night terrors and nightmares are outlined in Table 2. The evaluation of nightmares includes extensive history taking and the physical examination which usually show no specific findings. The family of a child who has nightmares needs to be reassured that this is a common finding in childhood and that it is a normal part of development. Parents should be encouraged to spend time reading, relaxing, and talking with the child after the event. Behavioral approaches such as insight oriented psychotherapy can be used in extreme cases. Medical management is usually not indicated.

Isolated Sleep Paralysis
Isolated sleep paralysis (ISP) consists of a period of inability to perform voluntary movements either at sleep onset or upon awakening. Patients are able to breathe spontaneously and are fully aware of what is happening. An episode can last for seconds or minutes, and resolves spontaneously. Episodes can be associated with hypnagogic hallucinations (26). Sleep paralysis is most often associated with narcolepsy, however, there are many people who experience sleep paralysis without having signs of narcolepsy (27). Diagnosis can be made by clinical history. Therapeutic intervention involves reassurance. Although it may be frightening to the patients, it is not harmful. Episodes can be reduced by good sleep hygiene. Patients should be encouraged to get enough sleep, reduce stress, and maintain a regular sleep schedule.

REM Sleep Motor Disorder
In REM sleep motor disorder (RMD) (also referred to as REM-sleep behavior disorder in adults) the brainstem mechanisms generating the muscle atonia normally

TABLE 2 Clinical Characteristics of Night Terrors Versus Nightmares

Sleep terrors	Nightmares
Occur in the 1st two hours of sleep (usually in NREM sleep)	Occur in later stages of sleep (usually REM sleep)
Usually end in confusion/daze, with no recollection of the dream	Events can be recalled in extensive detail
During the event, do not restrain or hold him, since this will exacerbate the episode. Let him go through the screaming episode till he returns to peaceful sleep	With nightmares, immediate reassurance is helpful. Hold and comfort the child and reassure him that he is safe
Kicking, tossing/turning, and vocalizations are not uncommon	Child is still usually until the point of awakening with fear. No association with vocalizations

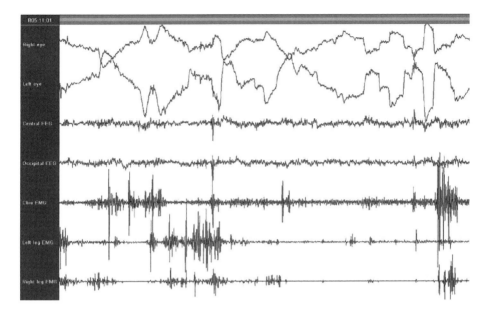

FIGURE 1 Eye leads show rapid movements and central and occipital leads show desynchronized electroencephalographic activity; both are features of REM sleep. Chin and leg electromyographic leads represent the excessive muscle activity that characterizes REM sleep motor disorder. From Ref. (30).

seen in REM sleep are lost. Therefore, you see the appearance of elaborate motor activity associated with dream mentation. Dramatic and often violent motor behaviors occur during sleep and associated vivid and striking dreams are the most common presenting complaints of RMD (28). It can often cause self-injury or injury to the bed partner. The dream-enacting behaviors are usually nondirected and may include punching, kicking, leaping, or running from bed while still in REM sleep. RMD occurs predominantly in elderly males, although the disease may occur at all ages, including childhood (29). RMD may be idiopathic, or may occur in association with various neurological conditions, such as brainstem neoplasm, Alzheimer dementia, Shy–Drager syndrome, and Parkinson's disease (30). Polysomnogram is the most important diagnostic test in RMD, and will show some tonic or phasic abnormalities of muscle tone during REM (Fig. 1). The treatment of RMD typically involves small doses of clonazepam (31). The prognosis of RMD depends on etiology. In idiopathic cases, the symptoms are controlled with medications. In secondary cases, the prognosis depends on the primary disease.

OTHER PARASOMNIAS
Bruxism
Bruxism is characterized by grinding or clenching of the teeth during sleep. Symptoms associated with bruxism include abnormal wear of the teeth, and jaw muscle discomfort. Usual treatment involves wearing a rubber mouthguard over the teeth at night to prevent dental complications.

Enuresis

Nocturnal enuresis is the involuntary loss of urine that occurs only at night. It is a common problem, affecting an estimated five to seven million children in the United States and occurring three times more often in boys than in girls (32). At five years of age, 15% to 25% of children wet the bed (33). With each year of maturity, the percentage of bed-wetters declines by 15%. Enuresis may be primary or secondary. There are many causes, including diabetes, urinary tract infections, low bladder capacity, psychological factors, and sleep disordered breathing. Treatment is geared towards behavioral therapy such as positive reinforcement, alarms, and medical management such as desmopressin.

REFERENCES

1. Mahowald M, Bornemann MC, Schenck C. Parsomnias. Semin Neurol 2004; (3):283–92
2. American Academy of Sleep medicine. International classification of sleep disorders, 2nd edn: Diagnostic and Coding Manual. Westchester, Illinois: American Academy of Sleep Medicine, 2005, p. 137.
3. Sheldon SH. The parasomnias. In Sheldon SH, Ferber R, Kryger MH, eds. Principles and Practice of Pediatric Sleep Medicine. Philadelphia: Elsevier/Saunders, 2005, pp. 305–15
4. Parkes JD. The parasomnias. Lancet 1986; 2(8514):1021–5.
5. Lecendreux M, Bassetti C, Dauvilliers Y, et al. HLA and genetic susceptibility to sleepwalking. Mol Psychiatry 2003; 8(1):114–7.
6. Hublin C, Kaprio Jaakko. Genetic aspects and genetic epidemiology of parasomnias. Sleep Med Rev 2003; 7(5):413–21.
7. Guilleminault C, Palombini L, Pelayo R, Chervin RD. Sleepwalking and sleep terrors in prepubertal children: What triggers them? Pediatrics 2003; 111(1):17–25.
8. Kales JD, Kales A, Soldatos CR, et al. Night terrors. Clinical characteristics and personality patterns. Arch Gen Psychiatry 1980; 37(12):413–17.
9. Sallustro F, Atwell CW. Body rocking, head banging and head rolling in normal children. J Pediatr 1978; (93):704–8.
10. Parkes JD. Sleep and its Disorders. London: WB Saunders, 1985, p. 195
11. Stepanova I, Nevsimalova S, Hanusova J. Rhythmic movement disorder in sleep persisting into childhood and adulthood. Sleep 2005; 28(7):851–7.
12. Manni R, Terzaghi. Rhythmic movements during sleep: a physiological and pathological profile. Neurol Sci 2005; (26):s181-s185.
13. Laberge L, Tremblay RE, Vitaro F, et al. Development of parasomnias from childhood to early adolescence. Pediatrics 2000; 106(1):67–74.
14. Leung AK, Wong BE, Chan PY, et al. Nocturnal leg cramps in children: Incidence and clinical characteristics. J Natl Med Assoc 1999; 91(6):329–32.
15. Giglio P, Undevia N, Spire JP. The primary parasomnias. A review for neurologists. Neurologist 2005; 11(2):90–7.
16. Man-Son-Hing M, Wells G, Lau A. Quinine for nocturnal leg cramps: A meta-analysis including unpublished data. J Gen Intern Med 1998; 13(9):600–6.
17. Rosen G, Mahowald MW, Ferber R. Sleepwalking, confusional arousals, and sleep terrors in the child. In Ferber R, Kryger M, eds Principles and Practice of Sleep Medicine in the Child. Philadelphia: WB Saunders, 1995, pp. 99–106.
18. Ohayon MM, Priest RG, Zulley J, et al. The place of confusional arousals in sleep and mental disorders: Findings in a general population sample of 13,057 subjects. J Nerv Ment Dis 2000; 188(6):340–8.
19. Simonds F, Parraga H. Prevalence of sleep disorders and sleep behaviors in children and adolescents. J Am Acad Child Psychiatry 1982; (21):383–8
20. Masand P, Popli AP, Weilburg JB. Sleepwalking. Am Fam Phys 1995, 51(3):649–54.

21. Hublin C, Kaprio J, Partinen M, et al. Prevalence and genetics of sleepwalking: A population-based twin study. Neurology 1997; 48(1):177–81.
22. Robinson A, Guilleminault C. Disorders of arousal. In Chokraverty S, Hening WA, Walters AS, eds Sleep and Movement Disorders. Philadelphia: Butterworth Heinemann, 2003, pp. 265–72.
23. Kales A, Soldatos CR, Bixler EO, et al. Hereditary factors in sleepwalking and night terrors. Br J Psychiatr 1980, (137):111–18.
24. http://www.emedicine.com/ped/topic1609.htm (accessed January, 2007)
25. Hublin Christer, Kaprio Jaakko, Partinen Markku, et al. Nightmares: Familial Aggregation and Association with Psychiatric Disorders in a Nationwide Twin Cohort. Am J Med Genet 1999; (88):329–36.
26. Stores G. Sleep paralysis and hallucinosis. Behav Neurol 1998; 11(2):109–12.
27. Sturzenegger C, Bassetti CL. The clinical spectrum of narcolepsy with cataplexy: A reappraisal. J Sleep Res 2004; 13(4):395–406.
28. Mahowald NW, Schenck CH. REM sleep behavior disorder. In Kryger, MH, Roth T, Dement WC eds Principles and practice of sleep medicine. 2nd edn Philadelphia: WB Saunders, 1994, pp. 574–88.
29. Schenck CH, Hurwitz TD, Mahowald MW. REM sleep behaviour disorder: An update on a series of 96 patients and a review of the world literature. J Sleep Res 1993; 2(4):224–31.
30. Gagnon JF, Postuma RB, Mazza S, et al. Rapid-eye-movement sleep behaviour disorder and neurodegenerative diseases. Lancet Neurol 2006; 5(5):424–32.
31. Chokroverty S. Diagnosis and treatment of sleep-disorders caused by co morbid disease. Neurology 2000; 54(suppl. 1):S8–S15.
32. Miller K. Concomitant nonpharmacologic therapy in the treatment of primary nocturnal enuresis. Clin Pediatr (Phila) 1993; 32–7.
33. Wan J, Greenfield S. Enuresis and common voiding abnormalities. Pediatr Clin North Am 1997; (44):1117–31.

23   Sleep in Children with Anxiety Disorders

Candice A. Alfano[a] and Daniel S. Lewin[b]

[a]Department of Psychiatry, Children's National Medical Center, The George Washington University School of Medicine, Washington, D.C., U.S.A.
[b]Pediatric Behavioral Sleep Medicine and Department of Pediatrics and Psychiatry, Children's National Medical Center, The George Washington University School of Medicine, Washington, D.C., U.S.A.

INTRODUCTION

As is evident from the current volume, a growing body of research indicates that emotional and behavioral problems and sleep disturbance commonly co-occur in children with different forms of psychopathology (1–7). As a result, there is now compelling evidence for linkages between the regulation of sleep, emotion, attention, and behavior in children. To date however, research examining sleep in youth with psychiatric disorders has primarily focused on children and adolescents with depression (e.g., 8–11), and more recently, attention deficit hyperactivity disorder (ADHD) (12). Meanwhile, a recent series of studies demonstrate robust associations between early and chronic sleep disruption and anxiety. The current chapter is aimed at providing an overview of the existing research on sleep and anxiety during childhood including the potential role of specific mechanisms and developmental factors implicated in the etiology of these problems. Suggestions for clinical practice and research also are provided. When relevant, findings from the adult literature also will be discussed.

FEATURES AND PREVALENCE OF CHILDHOOD ANXIETY DISORDERS

As the most common childhood psychiatric disorders, anxiety disorders occur in 12% to 20% of children (13,14). They are associated with significant impairments in functioning across multiple domains including academics, family relationships, and social interactions (15,16). Anxiety and associated impairments often persist into adulthood and predict adult anxiety and depressive disorders, suicide attempts, substance abuse, chronic illness, and psychiatric hospitalization (17–22). Although anxiety disorders may occur alone, they are most commonly comorbid with other anxiety disorders and phobias (23).

Anxiety symptoms may be viewed on a continuum ranging from transient, developmentally appropriate periods of worry, avoidance, and fear to chronic symptoms that cause interference in daily functioning. State anxiety refers to temporary symptoms of arousal that occur in a specific situation or in response to a unique stressor. These symptoms are generally transient and do not necessarily generalize to other situations or cause impaired functioning. However, an acute or severe stressor or repeated stressors may result in an anxiety disorder such as post-traumatic stress disorder (PTSD) or acute stress disorder (ASD) requiring clinical intervention. By comparison, trait anxiety (i.e., a temperamentally anxious child) is characterized by an innate propensity toward hypervigilance and hyperarousal across a number of settings and situations. Children with elevated levels of trait anxiety are at an increased risk of developing anxiety disorders based on both biological and environmental (e.g., anxious children often have parents with anxiety disorders who model anxious responses) risk factors.

The Diagnostic and Statistical Manual of Mental Disorders (DSM-IV) (24) includes several anxiety disorder categories that are frequently diagnosed in children including separation anxiety disorder (SAD), generalized anxiety disorder (GAD), social phobia (SOC), specific phobias, obsessive compulsive disorder (OCD), PTSD, panic disorder with or without agoraphobia, and ASD. Despite diagnostic differences, all anxiety disorders are represented by a tripartite model that includes the interaction of physiological (rapid heart beat, sweating, and somatic complaints), cognitive (excessive worry and catastrophizing thoughts), and behavioral symptoms (avoidance) (93). Criteria for SAD, GAD and PTSD specifically include sleep-related symptoms that are commonly present, such as recurrent nightmares, refusal to sleep alone, and non-specific sleep disturbance. However, given the polythetic nature of the DSM, sleep problems are not required for any anxiety diagnosis.

SLEEP IN CHILDREN WITH ANXIETY DISORDERS

Research examining the associations and unique mechanisms of early sleep problems and anxiety disorders in children is quite limited. Preliminary data are nonetheless suggestive of a bidirectional relationship involving the role of physiologic, cognitive, and environmental and familial factors. Children with anxious temperaments commonly manifest chronic sleep disturbances early in life which may persist for years in the absence of clinical attention (26). Similarly, up to 85% of children and adolescents with anxiety disorders experience some form of sleep disruption (1); a rate that is similar to that found among anxiety-disordered adults (27,28). Historically, the frequent overlap of sleep and anxiety symptoms has been assumed to reflect an inherent incompatibility between hyperarousal and hypervigilance-defining features of anxiety disorders—and sleep onset and maintenance (29). Although anxious arousal may indeed result in either acute or chronic sleep disruption, disturbed sleep also has been shown to produce increases in anxiety and fear in both humans and animals (30–34). For example, among adults with anxiety disorders, acute sleep restriction results in significant increases in anxiety and panic the following day (35). Even in children and adolescents with no history of anxiety, increases in negative affective responses (including fear) following mild to moderate amounts of sleep restriction have been reported (31,36), and greater emotional intensity and lower levels of vagal suppression (a physiologic index of emotion regulation) have been shown to independently predict sleep problems (37). Collectively, these data reveal a complex relationship between regulatory systems governing sleep and arousal that is best understood as reciprocal.

In general, children's fears and anxiety are frequently associated with the presence of sleep disruption. Transient nighttime fears (e.g., monsters under the bed, the dark, burglars) are considered to be developmentally appropriate and occur in approximately 70% of young children (38,39). Normal fears and worry are frequently associated with delayed sleep onset, multiple calls to parents and less frequently, repeated middle of the night awakenings. Although most will overcome or outgrow these fears, a proportion of children experience persistent fears that interfere with sleep and family functioning on an ongoing basis. Such persistent nighttime fears may be indicative of an underlying anxiety disorder. For example, Muris et al. (39) found severe nighttime fears to be related to one or more DSM anxiety disorders in 11% of a community sample of children ages 4–12 years. SAD, GAD, and specific phobias were the most common diagnoses, respectively.

The common presentation of bedtime anxiety for many children is closely associated with separation from caregivers, darkness, strange noises, disinhibition of imagination, and poorer cognitive control related to tiredness. However, parental response to bedtime fears also may play a crucial role in the course of both sleep problems and anxiety. Parents may inadvertently reinforce children's nighttime fears by responding to bedtime avoidance and reassurance-seeking behaviors with a spectrum of responses typified by either loving support or increased frustration; each of which may be equally reinforcing. Parents who are anxious themselves or ambivalent about separating from their children at night may further reinforce a child's bedtime resistance by sending subtle or overt messages communicating their discomfort and increasing the child's own anxiety. These patterns may in turn lead to increased tiredness, more chronic sleep problems and greater difficulty regulating anxiety both during the day and night (39,40). For this reason, effective treatment is often focused on setting firm parental limits surrounding sleep and providing reinforcement for "brave" nighttime behaviors (41,42). Among older children and adolescents who are more advanced cognitively, self-control techniques including relaxation, emotive imagery, and correcting maladaptive sleep onset associations and thoughts may be more effective.

Among youth with DSM-IV anxiety disorders, approximately 85% experience intermittent sleep disturbances, while one half experience a persistent sleep problem (1,44). The most prevalent sleep-related problems found among youth with anxiety disorders include difficulty initiating and/or maintaining sleep, nightmares, and refusal to sleep alone. However, individual types of sleep problems vary based on children's level of cognitive and physical development and specific anxiety disorder. For example, young children with SAD commonly have difficulty sleeping alone and experience nightmares, children with GAD have problems initiating sleep, and children with PTSD frequently exhibit parasomnias (e.g., enuresis and night terrors) (43–45). Evidence for sleep disruption in children with other anxiety disorders including OCD and SOC also is available, though more limited (1,46).

Sleep disruption is well documented among adults with anxiety disorders (27,28,47), yet data based on the use of objective methods of assessment have only begun to emerge in children. One early study by Rapoport and colleagues (46) reported reduced sleep efficiency and increased sleep latency among nine adolescents (ages 13–17) with OCD compared to matched healthy controls based on the use of polysomnography (PSG). Adolescents with OCD required twice as long as control adolescents to initiate sleep. In addition, two studies have examined sleep patterns among children with PTSD based on the use of wrist actigraphy. Both Glod et al. (48) and Sadeh et al. (49) found poorer sleep efficiency among children with PTSD who were exposed to physical abuse compared to those exposed to sexual abuse. However, both groups had poorer sleep compared to control children. Glod and colleagues also reported that children with PTSD exhibited more nocturnal activity, longer sleep onset latencies, and reduced sleep efficiency compared to children with both PTSD and depression. Most recently, Forbes et al. (50) compared

24 youths (ages 7–17) with anxiety disorders to both depressed and control youth based on two consecutive nights of PSG. Anxious youth exhibited a significantly greater number of arousals compared to depressed youth, and significantly less slow wave sleep and greater sleep onset latency compared to both depressed and control groups. Interestingly, despite objective findings, youth with anxiety disorders were most likely to underreport sleep problems on subjective measures of sleep. Collectively, findings indicate that data based on objective assessment of sleep are necessary in order to understand the severity and specific mechanism of sleep disturbance among anxiety-disordered youth.

MECHANISMS OF SLEEP AND ANXIETY DISORDERS

From a clinical standpoint, a bidirectional relationship between sleep disruption and anxiety suggests not only that problems in one domain may result in problems in the other, but also the possibility of a progressive worsening of both disorders and associated impairments over time. There is increasing evidence to support this contention. Persistent early sleep problems have been shown to predict the later development of anxiety and anxiety disorders during childhood, adolescence, and adulthood even after controlling for childhood anxiety symptoms (26,51,52). Additionally, anxiety disorders pose specific risk for the later development of insomnia, with approximately 40% of adults reporting symptoms of insomnia following the onset of an anxiety disorder (53). This bidirectional relationship implies shared pathophysiology that may be influenced by biological, cognitive, environmental, and familial factors.

Environmental and familial factors appear to account for a significant portion of the variance in childhood sleep problems and anxiety (26,54). In a large twin study, longitudinal associations between sleep problems at ages 3–4 and anxiety at age seven were largely mediated by familial factors (26). In a separate study, both parental psychopathology and family disorganization (i.e., lack of structure and routine within the home) were highly correlated with sleep disturbance and anxiety; each accounted for 30% of the variance in the association between these childhood problems (26). However, the specific nature of these associations is less clear. One possibility includes the prospect that parents with psychiatric symptoms have greater difficulty imposing structure within the home, both in relation to daytime and nighttime routines. Lack of structure may result both in increases in child anxiety and inadequate sleep (55–57).

Parental over-control also has been linked with both childhood sleep problems and anxiety. Over-control (i.e., overly-involved, intrusive behavior that grants little autonomy) has consistently been identified among parents of anxiety-disordered children, who are less promoting of independence than parents of non-anxious children (58–60). Although less often examined in relation to sleep, Warren and colleagues (61) reported parents of infants and young children at-risk for the development of anxiety (based on having an anxiety-disordered parent) to be overly involved in bedtime routines (e.g., co-sleeping). Such parenting behaviors were associated with significantly higher rates of child sleep problems. For anxious children, providing excessive reassurance at night, delaying bedtimes, or permitting co-sleeping with parents or siblings may serve to reinforce children's fears and worries and may ultimately interfere with the development of necessary self-regulatory skills (62).

In terms of neurophysiological aspects of these childhood problems, hypothalamic pituitary adrenal (HPA) axis dysregulation is an important and burgeoning area of investigation. Although data are limited, available studies provide evidence of a link between higher levels of cortisol secretion and risk for childhood anxiety disorders (63–64). Two recent studies have examined cortisol secretion among anxiety-disordered children during the sleep period found altered patterns of nocturnal cortisol. Specifically, anxiety-disordered children, but not adolescents, evidenced increased levels of cortisol during the pre-sleep period compared to both depressed and non-psychiatric control adolescents (66). The authors hypothesized that increases in pre-sleep cortisol among anxious children may be associated with elevated levels of stress and arousal at bedtime, whereas chronic anxiety may result in adjustments in the HPA axis by adolescence. A second study reported decreases in cortisol secretion during the early morning hours among anxious youth compared to the same two groups of children (67). These data suggest that, in addition to having implication for the development of anxiety disorders, HPA dysregulation may impact the timing and patterns of children's sleep. Results from animal studies indicating a bidirectional association between alterations in sleep and regulation of the HPA axis are consistent with this hypothesis (68). Although more data are ultimately needed, collectively, neurohormonal factors appear to be an important feature of co-occurring sleep and anxiety disorders in youth.

A well-recognized feature of anxiety disorders, cognitive factors represent an important dimension of sleep disturbance as well (69–71). Difficulty with excessive mentation or worry prior to sleep onset independent of physiological activity is common among adults with both anxiety disorders and insomnia (71–73). Although nocturnal worry has not been examined among children with anxiety disorders, clinical and preliminary empirical evidence suggest important associations between sleep problems and daytime cognition among school-aged children (26). Among normally developing children, general increases in cognition and worry around the age of seven are evident and highlight the parallel maturation of cognitive and affective systems throughout development (74,75). In addition to daytime worry, this increase in metacognitive ability also may be associated with an increase in pre-sleep cognitive arousal among anxious children. In clinical settings, anxiety-disordered children as young as seven report excessive fears and worries at bedtime that interfere with sleep onset and maintenance. Concern regarding the potential impact of sleep loss on daytime performance is also common and may result in increased arousal at bedtime. The presence, persistently, of nocturnal cognitive activity may also interact with physiological systems, leading to a state of both cognitive and physiologic inflexibility that may predispose anxious children for the development of insomnia.

ASSESSMENT AND TREATMENT

Because earlier research indicated inadequate reliability in diagnosing anxiety disorders in children (e.g., 76) several structured and semi-structured interview schedules have been developed for this purpose. The Anxiety Disorders Interview Schedule for Children (ADIS-C) (77), which assesses a broad range of anxiety, mood, and externalizing disorders in youth (ages 7–17), possesses the best psychometric profile of available interviews and has been described as the premier instrument for assessing childhood anxiety disorders (78). In addition, several child and parent report questionnaires have been developed to screen for potential anxiety disorders including the Screen for Child Anxiety-Related Emotional Disorders (SCARED) (79) and the Multidimensional Anxiety Scale for Children (MASC) (80). Both the SCARED and the MASC include several items that assess common sleep difficulties in anxious children.

There are several highly efficacious treatment modalities for childhood anxiety disorders that include cognitive behavioral and psychosocial techniques, and pharmacological management. In terms of pharmacological interventions, selective serotonin reuptake inhibitors (SSRIs) are often the treatment of choice and have been shown to produce significant improvement in a majority of children (81,82). Cognitive behavioral therapy (CBT) also has been shown to be highly effective (83,84) and includes psychoeducation (corrective information about anxiety), exposure methods (graduated, systematic, and controlled exposure to feared situations/stimuli), management of somatic complaints (relaxation training), cognitive techniques (identifying and replacing maladaptive, fearful thoughts), and social modeling. Treatment gains are often maintained several years after the completion of CBT (85).

Although sleep disruption is a common feature of childhood anxiety disorders, few studies have specifically examined the impact of treatment on co-occurring sleep problems. Alfano and colleagues (1) reported that compared to placebo, fluvoxamine produced significantly greater reductions in sleep problems among youth treated for an anxiety disorders after eight weeks of treatment. However, more than 30% of youth continued to report at least mild levels of insomnia at post-treatment, suggesting the role of potentially unique mechanisms and a need for better intervention. Because other studies have reported sleep disturbance (most commonly insomnia) as a common side effect of treatment with SSRIs (82), more research is ultimately needed to determine the impact of pharmacologic interventions for childhood anxiety on sleep problems.

Both case reports and controlled studies have reported significant reductions in nighttime fears and associated sleep difficulties following the use of behavioral treatments (41,86). However, studies examining the impact of behavioral or cognitive behavioral treatments for heterogeneous anxiety disorders on co-occurring sleep problems have not been conducted. In many cases, use of these interventions may be most appropriate based on their attention to behavioral, somatic, cognitive, and familial factors that may serve to maintain both anxiety and sleep problems. For example, identifying and eliminating parental reinforcement of children's avoidant nighttime behaviors and fears that delay sleep onset and maintenance are often important foci of treatment for behavioral sleep problems (87,88). However, controlled studies among anxiety-disordered children are lacking and at present it is unknown whether sleep disruption may remit or persist following intervention that does not specifically target co-occurring sleep problems. Because sleep efficiency and sleep onset latency, in particular, appear to be unique predictors for relapse within 12 months of successful treatment among depressed adolescents (89) and because a substantial proportion of anxious youngsters remain symptomatic following completion of anxiety treatment, this is a critical area for future research.

It also is noteworthy that unaddressed, co-occurring sleep problems may negatively impact anxiety-related treatment outcomes. Because sleep loss in children commonly manifests as hyperactivity and an inability to maintain attention during the daytime, key components of CBT that require anxious children to stay focused and engage in behavioral tasks may be undermined when persistent sleep disturbance is present. Along these lines, it also has been demonstrated that deprivation of REM sleep following a learning task directly interferes with the extinction of both cued (90) and contextually conditioned fears (91) in animals. These data have important clinical significance in suggesting that the effects of comorbid sleep disturbance may extend beyond impairments in behavioral and emotional regulation to interfere with the implementation and long-term effectiveness of psychosocial treatments for anxiety.

CASE EXAMPLE

Harry is a nine-year-old male with a history of difficulty initiating and maintaining sleep independently and daytime tiredness. Harry's bedtime is 9:00 p.m. On a nightly basis, Harry requests that one (or both) of his parents sit on his bed with him until he falls asleep. If his parents refuse this request, he becomes inconsolable, waking up his five-year-old brother with his crying and screaming. Harry explains that he is afraid of something happening to him or his parents while he is sleeping, robbers breaking into the house and strange images he sees in the dark in his room. When a parent is present, Harry requires approximately 20 minutes to initiate sleep. On the few occasions he has attempted to initiate sleep on his own, Harry lies awake in his bed for up to 120 minutes listening for unusual noises in the house. Harry is a good student but is commonly tired during the day. He worries about his sleep and feels "different" because the other kids "don't have these sleep problems." Harry is able to sleepover at friends' houses but only if he sleeps in close proximity to his friend. Other fears and worry are present during much of the day and include being alone on one level of the house if family members are on another level, talking to strangers, burglars, and academic performance.

Assessment procedures within a sleep specialty clinic included: (1) a clinical interview with Harry and his parents including assessment of sleep behaviors, current stressors and overall functioning, psychiatric symptoms, medical history, development, and academic history; (2) completion of several child- and parent-report questionnaires; and (3) completion of a daily sleep log during a one-week period prior to the clinical assessment. Evaluation procedures led to a diagnosis of Psychophysiological Insomnia and Limit Setting Sleep Disorder.

A behavioral intervention protocol was implemented targeting Harry's sleep problems. First, general parent management skills were discussed and reviewed with Harry's parents including inadvertent reinforcement of his fearful behaviors and rumination. Next, progressive muscle relaxation training (PMR) (92) and "worry journaling" were reviewed and practiced with Harry. PMR was demonstrated and practiced over the course of several sessions to help Harry focus on relaxing his body instead of focusing on his fears at bedtime. Harry was also instructed to set aside 15–20 minutes each afternoon for writing down his specific fears and worries in a journal, including "examining the evidence" that such things will occur. Finally, graduated extinction procedures were implemented both at night and during the daytime. At night, Harry's parents were directed to sit in a chair next to his bed at bedtime and to gradually move the chair away from the bed over successive nights. After one week, the chair was to be outside the bedroom.

Over a second week, Harry's parents checked on him at regular intervals and the duration of the intervals increased over the course of the week. If Harry did not remain calm and in his bed, his parents were instructed to leave the room until Harry stopped crying or calling out to them, then returned as soon as he calmed to provide verbal praise. During the daytime, Harry was required to stay in his room alone while family members were downstairs for successively longer periods of time. A table-top timer was used to show Harry how long he should stay in his room before going to find a parent. A sticker chart was used to track Harry's progress and reward his brave behavior.

Treatment progress was tracked with daily sleep logs and child and parent report of daytime and nighttime behavior. Harry's sleep problems were significantly reduced within two weeks of beginning treatment (including less bedtime resistance and a reduction in sleep onset latency). Based on the extent of Harry's anxiety and fears, he was also referred to a clinical psychologist for further evaluation and treatment of anxiety. The psychologist diagnosed Harry with SAD and GAD and used a cognitive-behavioral intervention to help him face and cope with his general fears and worries. Initially, both clinics worked together to coordinate treatment and ensure consistency, i.e., in the use of daytime and nighttime interventions.

CONCLUSIONS

There is now compelling evidence of important links and reciprocal effects of anxiety and sleep problems in adults as well as children. Early sleep problems appear to presage the later emergence of anxiety disorders, and anxiety disorders often lead to the development of chronic sleep problems. The underlying pathophysiology of these problems likely involves shared and common mechanisms including hypervigilance and hyperarousal, environmental contingencies, inability to inhibit negative cognition, and specific neurophysiological changes. Collectively, data suggest that assessment and effective treatment requires attention to these unique and shared factors. Given the shared developmental course of these disorders, early screening and intervention is of particular importance, as there is the potential for intervention to prevent the emergence of chronic psychopathology. Further research at the level of specific mechanisms is particularly important as it may not only lead to prevention and positive outcomes, but to the elucidation of underlying causes of two chronic and common problems that can persist throughout the lifespan and cause significant impairment.

REFERENCES

1. Alfano CA, Ginsburg GS, Kingery JN. Sleep-related problems among children and adolescents with anxiety disorders. J Am Acad Child Adolesc Psychiatry 2007; 46(2):224–32.
2. Steenari MR, Vuontela V, Paavonen EJ, Carlson S, Fjallberg M, Aronen E. Working memory and sleep in 6- to 13-year-old schoolchildren. J Am Acad Child Adolesc Psychiatry 2003; 42(1):85–92.
3. Corkum P, Moldofsky H, Hogg-Johnson S, Humphries T, Tannock R. Sleep problems in children with attention-deficit/hyperactivity disorder: Impact of subtype, comorbidity, and stimulant medication. J Am Acad Child Adolesc Psychiatry 1999; 38(10):1285–93,

4. Gaultney JF, Terrell DF, Gingras JL. Parent-reported periodic limb movement, sleep disordered breathing, bedtime resistance behaviors, and ADHD. Behav Sleep Med 2005; 3(1):32–43.
5. Johnson EO, Chilcoat HD, Breslau N. Trouble sleeping and anxiety/depression in childhood. Psychiatry Res 2000; 94(2):93–102.
6. Roberts RE, Lewinsohn PM, Seeley JR. Symptoms of DSM-III-R major depression in adolescence: Evidence from an epidemiological survey. J Am Acad Child Adolesc Psychiatry 1995; 34(12):1608–17.
7. Morrison DN, McGee R, Stanton WR. Sleep problems in adolescence. J Am Acad Child Adolesc Psychiatry 1992; 31(1):94–9.
8. Dahl R. The regulation of sleep and arousal: Development and psychopathology. Dev Psychopathol 1996; 8:3–27.
9. Emslie GJ, Rush AJ, Weinberg WA, Rintelmann JW, Roffwarg HP. Sleep EEG features of adolescents with major depression. Biol Psychiatry 1994; 36(9):573–81.
10. Puig-Antich J, Goetz R, Hanlon C, Tabrizi MA, Davies M, Weitzman ED. Sleep architecture and REM sleep measures in prepubertal major depressives. Studies during recovery from the depressive episode in a drug-free state. Arch Gen Psychiatry 1983; 40(2):187–92.
11. Puig-Antich J. Sleep and neuroendocrine correlates of affective illness in childhood and adolescence. J Adolesc Health Care 1987; 8(6):505–29.
12. Owens JA. The ADHD and sleep conundrum: A review. J Dev Behav Pediatr 2005; 26(4):312–22.
13. Costello EJ, Egger H, Angold A. 10-year research update review: The epidemiology of child and adolescent psychiatric disorders: I. Methods and public health burden. J Am Acad Child Adolesc Psychiatry 2005; 44(10):972–86.
14. Shaffer D, Fisher P, Dulcan MK, Davies M, Piancentini J, Schwab-Stone ME, Lahey BB, Bourdon K, Jensen PS, Bird HR, Canino G, Regier DA. The NIMH diagnositc inteview schedule for children version 2.3 (DISC-2.3). Description, acceptability, prevalence rates, and performance in the MECA Study. Methods for the epidemiology of child and adolescent mental disorders study. J Am Acad Child Adolesc Psychiatry 1996; 35:865–77.
15. Ialongo, N, Edelsohn, G, Werthamer-Larsson, L, Crockett, L, Kellam, S. The significance of self-reported anxious symptoms in first-grade children. J Abnorm Child Psychol 1994; 22(4):441–55.
16. Ialongo N, Edelsohn G, Werthamer-Larsson L, Crockett L, Kellam S. The significance of self-reported anxious symptoms in first grade children: Prediction to anxious symptoms and adaptive functioning in fifth grade. J Child Psychol Psychiatry 1995; 36(3):427–37.
17. Bovasso G. The long-term treatment outcomes of depression and anxiety comorbid with substance abuse. J Behav Health Serv Res 2001; 28(1):42–57.
18. Ferdinand RF, Verhulst FC. Psychopathology from adolescence into young adulthood: An 8-year follow-up study. Am J Psychiatry 1995; 152(11):1586–94.
19. Pine DS, Cohen P, Gurley D, Brook J, Ma Y. The risk for early-adulthood anxiety and depressive disorders in adolescents with anxiety and depressive disorders. Arch Gen Psychiatry 1998, 55(1):56–64.
20. Strauss CC, Last CG, Hersen M, Kazdin AE. Association between anxiety and depression in children and adolescents with anxiety disorders. J Abnorm Child Psychol 1988; 16(1):57–68.
21. Wittchen HU, Fehm L. Epidemiology and natural course of social fears and social phobia. Acta Psychiatr Scand Suppl 2003; (417):4–18.
22. Woodward LJ, Fergusson DM. Life course outcomes of young people with anxiety disorders in adolescence. J Am Acad Child Adolesc Psychiatry 2001; 40(9):1086–93.
23. Brady EU, Kendall PC. Comorbidity of anxiety and depression in children and adolescents. Psychol Bull 1992; 111(2):244–55.
24. Diagnostic and Statistical Manual of Mental Disorders. Washington, D.C: American Psychiatric Association, 1994.

25. Barlow D. Chapter 8: The Process of Fear and Anxiety Reduction: Affective Therapy. The Process and Origins of Anxiety. New York: Routledge, 2004.
26. Gregory AM, Eley TC, O'Connor TG, Plomin R. Etiologies of associations between childhood sleep and behavioral problems in a large twin sample. J Am Acad Child Adolesc Psychiatry 2004, pp. 744–51, 2004 Jun.
27. Ohayon MM, Caulet M, Priest RG, Guilleminault C. DSM-IV and ICSD-90 insomnia symptoms and sleep dissatisfaction. Br J Psychiatry 1997; 171:382–8.
28. Uhde TW. Genetics and brain function: Implications for the treatment of anxiety. Biol Psychiatry 2000; 48(12):1142–3.
29. Dahl RE, Lewin DS. Pathways to adolescent health sleep regulation and behavior. J Adolesc Health 2002; (6 Suppl):175–84.
30. Dinges DF, Pack F, Williams K, Gillen KA, Powell JW, Ott GE, Aptowicz C, Paci AI. Cumulative sleepiness, mood disturbance, and psychomotor vigilance performance decrements during a week of sleep restricted to 4-5 hours per night. Sleep 1997; (4):267–77.
31. Leotta C, Carskadon MA. Effects of acute sleep restriction on affective response in adolescents: Preliminary results. Sleep Research 1997; 26:201.
32. Cole DA, Peeke LG, Martin JM, Truglio R, Seroczynski AD. A longitudinal look at the relation between depression and anxiety in children and adolescents. J Consult Clin Psychol 1998; 66(3):451–60.
33. Philip P, Sagaspe P, Moore N, Taillard J, Charles A, Guilleminault C, Bioulac B. Fatigue sleep restriction and driving performance. Accid Anal Prev 2005; 37(3):473–8.
34. Carvalho LB, Prado LB, Silva L, Almeida MM, Silva TA, Vieira CM, Atallah AN. & Prado GF. Cognitive dysfunction in children with sleep disorders. Arq Neuropsiquiatr 2004; 62:212–16.
35. Roy-Byrne PP, Uhde TW, Post RM. Effects of one night's sleep deprivation on mood and behavior in panic disorder. Patients with panic disorder compared with depressed patients and normal controls. Arch Gen Psychiatry 1986; 43(9):895–9.
36. Wolfson AR. Sleeping patterns of children and adolescents: developmental trends, disruptions, and adaptations. Child Adolesc Psychiatric Clini N Am 1996; pp. 549–68.
37. El-Sheikh M, Buckhalt JA. Vagal regulation and emotional intensity predict children's sleep problems. Dev Psychobiol 2005; 46(4):307–17.
38. Coplan JD, Rosenblum LA, Friedman S, Bassoff TB, et al.. Behavioral effects of oral yohimbine in differentially reared nonhuman primates. Neuropsychopharmacology 1992; 6(1):31–7.
39. Muris P, Merckelbach H, Ollendick TH, King NJ, Bogie N. Children's nighttime fears: Parent-child ratings of frequency, content, origins, coping behaviors and severity. Behav Res Ther 2001; 39(1):13–28.
40. Steen RG, Ogg RJ, Reddick WE, Kingsley PB. Age-related changes in the pediatric brain: Quantitative MR evidence of maturational changes during adolescence. Am J Neuroradiol 1997; 18(5):819–28.
41. Graziano AM, Mooney KC. Family self-control instruction for children's nighttime fear reduction. J Consult Clin Psychol 1980; 48(2):206–13.
42. King N, Cranstoun F, Josephs A. Emotive imagery and children's night-time fears: A multiple baseline design evaluation. J Behav Ther Exp Psychiatry 1989; 20(2):125–35.
43. Alfano CA, Beidel DC, Turner SM, Lewin DS. Preliminary evidence for sleep complaints among children referred for anxiety. Sleep Medicine 2006; 7(6):467–73.
44. Connell HM, Persley GV, Sturgess JL. Sleep phobia in middle childhood – a review of six cases. J Am Acad Child Adolesc Psychiatry 1987; 26(3):449–52.
45. Goenjian AK, Yehuda R, Pynoos RS, Steinberg AM, Tashjian M, Yang RK, Najarian LM, Fairbanks LA. Basal cortisol, dexamethasone suppression of cortisol, and MHPG in adolescents after the 1988 earthquake in Armenia. Am J Psychiatry 1996; 153(7):929–34.
46. Rapoport J, Elkins R, Langer DH, Sceery W, Buchsbaum MS, Gillin JC, Murphy DL, Zahn TP, Lake R, Ludlow C, Mendelson W. Childhood obsessive-compulsive disorder. Am J Psychiatry 1981; 138(12):1545–54.

47. Anderson DR. Stability of behavioral and emotional disturbance in a sample of disadvantaged preschool-aged children. Child Psychiatry Hum Dev 1984; 14(4):249–60.
48. Glod CA, Teicher MH, Hartman CR, Harakal T. Increased nocturnal activity and impaired sleep maintenance in abused children. J Am Acad Child Adolesc Psychiatry 1997; 821:1236–43.
49. Sadeh A, Hauri PJ, Kripke DF, Lavie P. The role of actigraphy in the evaluation of sleep disorders. Sleep 1995; 18(4):288–302.
50. Forbes EE, Bertocci MA, Gregory AM, Ryan ND, Axelson DA, Birmaher B, Dahl RE. Objective sleep in pediatric anxiety disorders and major depressive disorder. J Am Acad Child Adolesc Psychiatry 2008; 47(2) 148–55.
51. Ford DE, Kamerow DB. Epidemiologic study of sleep disturbances and psychiatric disorders. An opportunity for prevention? [see comments]. JAMA 1989; 262(11): 1479–84.
52. Ong HS, Wickramaratne P, Min T, Weissman MM. Early childhood sleep and eating problems as predictors of adolescent and adult mood and anxiety disorders. 2006; J Affect Disord 2006; 96(1–2):1–8.
53. Ohayon MM, Roth T. Place of chronic insomnia in the course of depressive and anxiety disorders. J Psychiatr Res 2003; 37(1):9–15.
54. Van den Oord EJC, Boomsma DI, Verhulst F.C. A study of genetic and environmental effects on the co-occurrence of problem behaviors in three-year-old-twins. J Abnorm Child Psychol 2000; 109:360–72.
55. Klackenberg G. Sleep behaviour studied longitudinally. Data from 4–16 years on duration, night-awakening and bed-sharing. Acta Paediatr Scand 1982; 71(3):501–6.
56. Meijer AM, Habekothe RT, van den Wittenboer GL. Mental health, parental rules and sleep in pre-adolescents. J Sleep Res 2001; 10(4):297–302.
57. Owens-Stively J, Frank N, Smith A, Hagino O, Spirito A, Arrigan M, Alario AJ. Child temperament, parenting discipline style, and daytime behavior in childhood sleep disorders. J Dev Behav Pediatr 1997; 18(5):314–21.
58. Dumas JE, LaFreniere PJ, Serketich WJ. "Balance of power": A transactional analysis of control in mother-child dyads involving socially competent, aggressive, and anxious children. J Abnorm Psychol 1995; 104(1):104–13.
59. Hudson JL, Rapee RM. Parent-child interactions and anxiety disorders: An observational study. Behav Res Ther 2001; 39(12):1411–27.
60. Siqueland L, Kendall PK, Steinberg L. Anxiety in children: Perceived family environments and observed family interaction J Child Clinical Psychology 1996; 25:225–37.
61. Warren SL, Gunnar MR, Kagan J, Anders TF, Simmens SJ, Rones M, Wease S, Aron E, Dahl RE, Sroufe LA. Maternal panic disorder: infant temperament, neurophysiology, and parenting behaviors. J Am Acad Child Adolesc Psychiatry 2003; 42:814–25.
62. Dahl RE. The regulation of sleep and arousal: Development and psychopathology. Dev Psychopathol 1996; 8:3–27.
63. Goldsmith HH, Lemery KS. Linking temperamental fearfulness and anxiety symptoms: A behavior-genetic perspective. Biol Psychiatry 2000; 48(12).1199–209.
64. Kagan J, Reznick JS, Snidman N. Biological bases of childhood shyness. Science 1988; 240(4849):167–71.
65. Schmidt LA, Fox NA, Rubin KH, Sternberg EM, Gold PW, Smith CC, Schulkin J. Behavioral and neuroendocrine responses in shy children. Dev Psychobiol 1997; 30(2):127–40.
66. Forbes EE, Williamson DE, Ryan ND, Birmaher B, Axelson DA, Dahl RE. Peri-sleep-onset cortisol levels in children and adolescents with affective disorders. Biol Psychiatry 2006; 59(1):24–30.
67. Feder A, Coplan JD, Goetz RR, Mathew SJ, Pine DS, Dahl RE, Ryan ND, Greenwald S, Weissman MM. Twenty-four-hour cortisol secretion patterns in prepubertal children with anxiety or depressive disorders. Biol Psychiatry 2004; 56(3):198–204.

68. Meerlo P, Koehl M, van der Borght K, Turek FW. Sleep restriction alters the hypothalamic-pituitary-adrenal response to stress. J Neuroendocrinol 2002; 14(5):397–402.

69. Gross RT, Borkovec TD. Effects of a cognitive intrusion manipulation on the sleep-onset latency of good sleepers. Behavior Therapy 1982; 13:112–6.

70. Harvey AG. A cognitive model of insomnia. Behav Res Ther 2002; 40(8):869–93.

71. Wicklow A, Espie CA. Intrusive thoughts and their relationship to actigraphic measurement of sleep: towards a cognitive model of insomnia. Behav Res Ther 2000; 38(7):679–93.

72. Leckman JF, Sholomskas D, Thompson WD, Belanger A, Weissman MM. Best estimate of lifetime psychiatric diagnosis: A methodological study. Arch. Gen. Psychiatry 1982; 39(8):879–83.

73. Harvey KJ, Espie CA. Development and preliminary validation of the Glasgow Content of Thoughts Inventory (GCTI): A new measure for the assessment of pre-sleep cognitive activity. Br J Clin Psychol 2004; 43(Pt 4):409–20.

74. Cicchetti D, Ackerman B, Izard C. Emotions and emotion regulation in developmental psychopathology. Developmental and Psychopathology 1995; 7:1–10.

75. Vasey, MW. Development and Cognition in Childhood Anxiety: The Example of Worry. New York: Plenum, 1993.

76. Costello AJ, Edelbrock CS, Dulcan MK, Kalas R, Klaric SH. Report to NIMH on the NIMH diagnostic interview schedule for children (DISC). Washington, DC: National Institute of Mental Health, 1984.

77. Silverman WK, Albano AM. The Anxiety Disorders Interview Schedule for Children for DSM-IV: (Child and Parent Versions). San Antonio, TX: Psychological Corporation, 1996.

78. Stallings P, March JS. Assessment In March, JS. ed. Anxiety Disorders in Children and Adolescents. New York: Guilford Press, 1995, pp. 125-47.

79. Birmaher B, Khetarpal S, Brent D, Cully M, Balach L, Kaufman J, Neer SM. The Screen for Child Anxiety Related Emotional Disorders (SCARED): Scale construction and psychometric characteristics. J Am Acad Child Adolesc Psychiatry 1997; 36(4):545–53.

80. Lamarche CH, Ogilvie RD. Electrophysiological changes during the sleep onset period of psychophysiological insomniacs, psychiatric insomniacs, and normal sleepers. Sleep 1997; 20(9):724–33.

81. Research Units in Pediatric Psychopharmacology Anxiety Study Group. Fluvoxamine for the treatment of anxiety disorders in children and adolescents. New Eng J Med 2001; 344:1279–85.

82. Wagner U, Gais S, Born J. Emotional memory formation is enhanced across sleep intervals with high amounts of rapid eye movement sleep. Learn Mem 2001; 8(2):112–19.

83. Kendall PC. Treating anxiety disorders in children: Results of a randomized clinical trial. J Consult Clin Psychol 1994; 62(1):100–10.

84. Silverman WK, Kurtines WM, Ginsburg GS, Weems CF, Lumpkin PW, Carmichael DH. Treating anxiety disorders in children with group cognitive-behaviorial therapy: A randomized clinical trial. J Consult Clin Psychol 1999; 67(6):995–1003.

85. Kendall PC, Southam-Gerow MA. Long-term follow-up of a cognitive-behavioral therapy for anxiety-disordered youth. J Consult Clin Psychol 1996; 64(4):724–30.

86. Ollendick TH, Hagopian LP, Huntzinger RM. Cognitive-behavior therapy with nighttime fearful children. J Behav Ther Exp Psychiatry 1991; 22(2):113–21.

87. Kuhn BR, Elliott AJ. Treatment efficacy in behavioral pediatric sleep medicine. J Psychosom Res 2003, 54:587–97.

88. Mindell JA, Owens JA, Carskadon MA. Developmental features of sleep. Child Adolesc Psychiatr Clin N Am 1999; 8(4):695–725.

89. Emslie GJ, Armitage R, Weinberg WA, Rush AJ, Mayes TL, Hoffmann RF. Sleep polysomnography as a predictor of recurrence in children and adolescents with major depressive disorder. Int J Neuropsychopharmacol 2001; 4(2):159–68.

90. Silvestri AJ. REM sleep deprivation affects extinction of cued but not contextual fear conditioning. Physiol Behav 2005; 84(3):343–9.
91. Graves LA, Heller EA, Pack AI, Abel T. Sleep deprivation selectively impairs memory consolidation for contextual fear conditioning. Learn Mem 2003; 10(3):168–76.
92. Rosen RC, Lewin DS, Woolfolk R, Goldberg L. Psychophysiological insomnia: Combined effects of pharmacotherapy and relaxation-based treatments. Sleep Med 2000; 1(4):279–88.

24 Autism Spectrum Disorders and Sleep

Kyle P. Johnson[a] and Darryn M. Sikora[b]

[a]Department of Psychiatry, [a,b]Oregon Health & Science University, Portland, Oregon, U.S.A.

INTRODUCTION

Without enough sleep, we all become tall 2-year-olds. JoJo Jensen, *Dirt Farmer Wisdom*, 2002

As discussed in previous chapters, sleep disorders occur across many different psychiatric disorders. The focus of the present chapter will be on sleep disorders in children and adolescents with autism spectrum disorders (ASD). We begin with a description of ASD and how the prevalence of ASD has changed over the past 10 to15 years. We then focus on how sleep problems in this population may be different than other groups of children and adolescents with psychiatric disorders, and why recognizing and treating sleep problems in individuals with ASD are important. We follow with information about the frequency and possible etiology of sleep problems in children and adolescents with ASD, and end with an explanation of different assessment instruments and strategies.

DESCRIPTION OF ASD

Diagnosis

ASD are a group of developmental disorders defined by impairments in the areas of communication and socialization, as well as patterns of restricted or repetitive behaviors (1). Historically referred to as Pervasive Developmental Disorders (PDD), a term still used in the Diagnostic and Statistical Manual of Mental Disorders (DSM-IV-TR) (1), most professional and parent/community groups prefer the term ASD. Therefore, ASD will be used throughout this chapter to include all five of the PDDs outlined in the DSM-IV-TR (1). Although symptoms of ASD were first described by Dr. Leo Kanner in 1943, the diagnostic description first appeared in the Diagnostic and Statistical Manual of Mental Disorders, 3rd edition (DSM-III) (2), under the label of "infantile autism". Subsequent editions have included a broader spectrum of symptom presentation and diagnoses. The DSM-IV (3) was the first revision to include criteria for five diagnoses on the autism spectrum: Autistic Disorder, Rett's Disorder, Childhood Disintegrative Disorder (CDD), Asperger's Disorder, and Pervasive Developmental Disorder—Not Otherwise Specified (PDD—NOS). However, two of these diagnoses are rarely, if ever, included in studies on ASD: Rett's Disorder and Childhood Disintegrative Disorder. Rett's Disorder is the only ASD to have a known genetic etiology. Therefore, genetic testing, rather than clinical presentation, most often secures the diagnosis. Mental health professionals rarely diagnose Childhood Disintegrative Disorder, making the number of children and adolescents with the diagnosis very small.

The ASD diagnostic criteria will be described briefly. In order to diagnose Autistic Disorder, as defined in the DSM-IV-TR (1), a specified number of criteria must be met in each of three areas; more specifically, two in the area of social impairment, one in the area of communication impairment, and one in the area of restricted or repetitive behaviors, with an overall total of six out of 12 (see Table 1). In addition, symptoms in the areas of communication, socialization, or play must have been present before the age of three years. Diagnosing Rett's Disorder or CDD precludes a diagnosis of Autistic Disorder. A diagnosis of Asperger's Disorder requires normal cognitive and early language development, no delays in functional daily living skills, and clinically significant impairment (see Table 2). In addition, out of the 12 criteria used to diagnose Autistic Disorder, two in the area of social impairment and one in the area of restricted or repetitive behaviors must be met. Finally, a diagnosis of PDD-NOS is given when there is a significant delay in social interaction, communication, or when stereotyped behaviors are present (1), but not to the degree that warrants a more specific diagnosis. It is also referred to as "atypical autism" in the International Classification of Diseases, 10th edition. The diagnosis of PDD-NOS is generally used in four different situations: (a) if the individual displays some, but not enough, criteria for another ASD, (b) if some unusual behaviors are present but not enough to warrant another psychiatric disorder due to the age of the individual, (c) when the onset criterion for Autistic Disorder is not met, or (d) when the individual does not have enough symptoms for Autistic Disorder but has cognitive or language delays precluding a diagnosis of Asperger's Disorder.

Epidemiology

Over the past few decades, the reported number of children identified as having ASD has increased exponentially, from approximately 5/10,000 in the 1980s to 50–70/10,000 presently (4). Several different possible reasons for the increase in ASD diagnosis have been postulated. These include: (a) increased awareness of ASD through the media, autism advocacy groups such as the Cure Autism Now Foundation and Autism Speaks, and physician training, (b) the broadening of the definition of ASD to include milder forms, such as Asperger's Disorder, (c) the process of diagnostic substitution, whereby a child that previously would have been given a different diagnosis is now given an ASD diagnosis, and (d) genetic and/or environmental factors. While none of these potential reasons alone explains the increase in ASD, in combination they provide a logical explanation for the phenomenon.

Neurobiology

A growing number of known genetic disorders are associated with ASD, including Fragile X syndrome, Smith-Lemli-Opitz syndrome, tuberous sclerosis, Angelman syndrome, duplication of 15q11-q13, Rett syndrome, Down syndrome, and Cohen syndrome (5). In addition, upwards of 15–20 genes have been associated with idiopathic ASD, and the risk of recurrence of autism within the same nuclear family now stands at 10–16%. These findings suggest a very strong genetic component to ASD. In addition, ASD is considered a neurological disorder of brain development (6), which appears to affect neuronal organization events occurring both pre- and post-natally. Imaging studies demonstrate an increase in total brain volume,

TABLE 1 DSM-IV-TR Diagnostic Criteria for Autistic Disorder

A. A total of six (or more) items from (1), (2), and (3), with at least two from (1), and one each from (2) and (3):
   (1) qualitative impairment in social interaction, as manifested by at least two of the following:
      (a) marked impairment in the use of multiple nonverbal behaviors such as eye-to-eye gaze, facial expression, body postures, and gesture to regulate social interaction
      (b) failure to develop peer relationships appropriate to developmental level
      (c) a lack of spontaneous seeking to share enjoyment, interests, or achievements with other people (e.g., by a lack of showing, bringing, or pointing out objects of interest)
      (d) lack of social or emotional reciprocity
   (2) qualitative impairments in communication as manifested by at least one of the following:
      (a) delay in, or total lack of, the development of spoken language (not accompanied by an attempt to compensate through alternative modes of communication such as gesture or mime)
      (b) in individuals with adequate speech, marked impairment in the ability to initiate or sustain a conversation with others
      (c) stereotyped and repetitive use of language or idiosyncratic language
      (d) lack of varied, spontaneous make-believe play or social imitative play appropriate to developmental level
   (3) restricted repetitive and stereotyped patterns of behavior, interests, and activities, as manifested by at least one of the following:
      (a) encompassing preoccupation with one or more stereotyped and restricted patterns of interest that is abnormal either in intensity or focus
      (b) apparently inflexible adherence to specific, nonfunctional routines or rituals
      (c) stereotyped and repetitive motor mannerism (e.g., hand or ginger flapping or twisting, or complex whole-body movements)
      (d) persistent preoccupation with parts of objects
B. Delays or abnormal functioning in at least one of the following areas, with onset prior to age three years: (1) social interaction, (2) language as used in social communication, or (3) symbolic or imaginative play.
C. The disturbance is not better accounted for by Rett's Disorder or Childhood Disintegrative Disorder.

Source: From Ref. (1) with permission.

coinciding with the onset of symptoms during the first and second years of life. It has been suggested that increased white matter, related to intrahemispheric and corticocortical connectivity, may explain why young children with ASD (under the age of five) on average have a greater head circumference when compared to their peers (7). The measurement of specific brain structures has yielded inconsistent results, most often due to small sample sizes and heterogeneous samples; however, the range of clinical presentations in ASD suggests widespread brain pathology, particularly in areas that allow for information integration.

IMPACT OF SLEEP PROBLEMS

While sleep problems are considered part of the diagnostic criteria for several psychiatric disorders, including mood disorders, they are not part of the diagnostic criteria for ASD. However, research suggests that sleep problems in individuals

TABLE 2   DSM-IV-TR Diagnostic Criteria for Asperger's Disorder

---

A. Qualitative impairment in social interaction, as manifested by at least two of the following:

    (1) marked impairment in the use of multiple nonverbal behaviors such as eye-to-eye gaze, facial expression, body postures, and gestures to regulate social interaction

    (2) failure to develop peer relationships appropriate to developmental level

    (3) a lack of spontaneous seeking to share enjoyment, interests, or achievements with other people (e.g., by a lack of showing, bringing, or pointing out objects of interest to other people)

    (4) lack of social or emotional reciprocity

B. Restricted repetitive and stereotyped patterns of behavior, interest, and activities, as manifested by at least one of the following:

    (1) encompassing preoccupation with one or more stereotyped and restricted patterns of interest that is abnormal either in intensity or focus

    (2) apparently inflexible adherence to specific, nonfunctional routines or rituals

    (3) stereotyped and repetitive motor mannerisms (e.g., hand or finger flapping or twisting, or complex whole-body movements)

    (4) persistent preoccupation with parts of objects

C. The disturbance causes clinically significant impairment in social, occupational, or other important areas of functioning.

D. There is no clinically significant general delay in language (e.g., single words used by age two years, communicative phrases used by age three years).

E. There is no clinically significant delay in cognitive development or in the development of age-appropriate self-help skills, adaptive behavior (other than in social interaction), and curiosity about the environment in childhood.

F. Criteria are not met for another specific Pervasive Development Disorder or Schizophrenia.

Source: From Ref. (1) with permission.

with ASD do affect daytime behavior and overall functioning. As mentioned in previous chapters, even typically developing children with sleep problems evidence a wide range of consequences during the day including behavior difficulties, depressed mood, mood swings, and cognitive dysfunction such as impairments in cognitive flexibility, memory and attention (8–12). Decreased sleep in children with developmental disabilities has been related to negative mood and irritability, self-injury, and aggression (13). Several studies have emphasized the negative impact of childhood sleep disorders on the daytime cognition and behavior of these children with developmental disabilities and on the quality of life for the child and the family (14,15). Robinson and Richdale also indicate that improvement in sleep is associated with improvement in these domains (15). Few studies evaluating the effect of sleep disorders on daytime behavior have focused exclusively on children with ASD. However, in a recent study completed as part of the Autism Treatment Network (unpublished), children with ASD were divided into two groups based on their scores on the Children's Sleep Habits Questionnaire (CSHQ) (16), a well-validated, parent report measure of pediatric sleep behaviors. Children with ASD and sleep problems were found to have higher scores on the Aberrant Behavior Checklist (17,18), several factors from the Child Behavior Checklist (19), and a higher Pervasive Developmental Behavior Inventory (20) Repetitive, Ritualistic, and Pragmatic Problems composite score.

In addition, several associations were observed between sleep problems and scores from the Behavior Inventory of Executive Functioning (21). Children in the Sleep Problems group had higher T-scores on the factor of Emotional Control (p = 0.034) than children without sleep problems. Additionally, children with sleep problems showed a trend toward difficulties in planning and organizing (p = 0.054). Taken together, these preliminary results suggest that children with ASD who demonstrate sleep problems also evidence greater impairment in a number of daytime activities and behaviors when compared to children with ASD who do not have sleep problems.

PREVALENCE OF SLEEP PROBLEMS

It has been estimated that between 44% and 83% of children with ASD have sleep problems, particularly sleep initiation and maintenance difficulties (22–24). Additionally, children with ASD suffer from irregular sleep–wake patterns, early morning awakenings, and poor sleep routines (25–29). Because the majority of this research has examined children with classic autism, most of which also have intellectual deficits (ID), these prevalence rates need to be evaluated in the context of the prevalence of sleep problems in patients with ID. Attempts have been made to control for the confounding variable of ID, and it appears that ASD is an independent risk factor for sleep problems (24,30). A recent study examined parental perception of sleep problems of children with ASD and normal intelligence compared with age-matched controls. Sleep problems in the ASD group occurred at a significantly higher rate than the comparison group and the sleep problems were more severe (31). Further evidence that sleep-related problems are associated with ASD independent of intellectual deficits was demonstrated in a study of children and adults of normal intelligence with Asperger's Disorder. When compared to a control group matched for age, gender, and IQ, the participants with Asperger's Disorder evidenced more severe sleep onset and maintenance insomnia (23).

Since by definition patients with Asperger's Disorder do not have intellectual deficits, a number of studies have looked at the prevalence of sleep problems in this population to help determine if ASD is an independent risk factor for sleep problems. One study compared the sleep of 50 children with Asperger's Disorder and 43 controls using a sleep questionnaire. Average sleep duration was significantly less in the Asperger's Disorder group and sleep latency was significantly longer, while sleep-related breathing problems, parasomnias, and excessive daytime sleepiness were not more common (32). These findings were replicated in a recent study comparing the quality of sleep as measured by parental surveys of children with autism, children with Asperger's Disorder, and typically developing controls (33). Approximately 73% of children with autism and Asperger's Disorder had sleep problems compared with 50% of typically developing children. The children with Asperger's Disorder had sleep problems more resistant to behavioral interventions, more disoriented waking, and more symptoms of sleep disturbance compared to children with autism and typically developing children. These findings, however, may have been confounded by the fact that the subjects with Asperger's Disorder were statistically significantly older than the other two subject groups.

Adults with Asperger's Disorder frequently experience insomnia, and according to sleep diaries, greater night-to-night variability of sleep parameters (34,35). A recent study compared 8–12-year-old children with Asperger's Disorder or high functioning autism with age and gender matched controls (36). Difficulties initiating sleep and daytime sleepiness were more commonly reported by parents of children with ASD than parents of typically developing children. Of the children with ASD, 31% met criteria for the definition of pediatric insomnia while none of the controls did. The insomnia reported by parents corresponded to objective findings obtained with actigraphy. The results of these studies suggest that the primary sleep problem in ASD is insomnia.

As with children who are developing typically, children with ASD are prone to have behavioral insomnia of childhood, either sleep onset association type, limit-setting type, or a combination of both. In some cases, these behavioral issues may be the underlying cause of insomnia, but in many cases behavioral issues may be compounded by neurobiologically determined insomnia. Inadequate sleep hygiene is often the result of parents struggling with insomnia in their special needs child. Inadvertently, inappropriate sleep onset associations may be established such as putting a television in the child's room and having it on as the child falls asleep. Addressing these sleep hygiene issues is an important part of any treatment plan.

PROPOSED ETIOLOGIES OF SLEEP PROBLEMS IN ASD

Studies to date all indicate high rates of sleep disorders among children and adolescents with ASD. More specifically, studies suggest the primary sleep problem in ASD is insomnia, which by recent consensus has been defined as "repeated difficulty with sleep initiation, duration, consolidation, or quality that occurs despite age-appropriate time and opportunity for sleep and results in daytime functional impairment for the child and/or family" (37). Problematic insomnia reported by parents has been substantiated by a recent study using polysomnography. Malow and colleagues evaluated the sleep of children with ASD and age-matched controls, dividing the ASD group into "good sleepers" and "poor sleepers" based on parental responses on the CSHQ (38). "Poor sleepers" as rated by parents showed prolonged sleep latency and decreased sleep efficiency on overnight polysomnography compared with ASD "good sleepers" and the typically developing controls. Research to date has not demonstrated an increased risk in this population for obstructive sleep apnea outside of other known risk factors (31,34,38).

Circadian rhythm dysfunction may contribute to the insomnia observed in patients with ASD (39,40,41). The circadian master clock, housed in the suprachiasmatic nucleus of the hypothalamus, determines the timing of melatonin production. Melatonin secretion from the pineal gland is suppressed by bright light; therefore, measuring dim light melatonin onset (DLMO) is a means of determining circadian timing (42–47). Several studies have demonstrated abnormal melatonin regulation in individuals with ASD compared with controls, including elevated daytime melatonin and significantly lower nocturnal melatonin (39–41). A recent study shows significantly lower excretion rates of urinary 6-sulphatoxymelatonin, the major metabolite of melatonin, in children and adolescents with autism compared to age-and-gender matched controls, with more marked differences in pre-pubertal subjects (48). While these studies support abnormalities in circadian rhythm physiology in subjects with ASD, they have several limitations. Most importantly, these studies have focused on the amplitude, or amount of melatonin production, and not on the phase of melatonin production relative to sleep. Moreover, the numbers of subjects in these studies are small, the sleep problems are not well defined, and ASD phenotypes are not well characterized. The methodology across studies is not consistent, making comparison of results less reliable.

Outside of circadian rhythm abnormalities, only a few case series reports suggest other sleep pathology in patients with ASD. One case series demonstrated an increased prevalence of rapid eye movement (REM) sleep without atonia on overnight polysomnograms (49). This finding is seen in patients with REM sleep behavior disorder. In this case series, patients with REM sleep without atonia were treated with clonazepam, a benzodiazepine, leading to an improvement in their sleep and daytime behavior. Another study reported that three of eight subjects (including a seven-year-old child with Asperger's Disorder) had an increased number of periodic limb movements noted on overnight polysomnogram (50).

ASSESSMENT OF SLEEP PROBLEMS IN CHILDREN AND ADOLESCENTS WITH ASD

Given the high prevalence rate of sleep disturbances in this population, all children with ASD should be screened for sleep problems. There are a number of published sleep questionnaires designed for use with children. One particular questionnaire is included in the text "The Clinical Guide to Pediatric Sleep" by Mindell and Owens in PDF on the accompanying CD-Rom (51). If sleep disturbances are discovered in the screening process, they should be made part of the problem list and addressed in the treatment plan. Treatment for some children and adolescents may only require changes in the sleep environment or improved sleep hygiene. Other children and adolescents may require more detailed behavioral interventions such as stimulus control, relaxation techniques, or sleep restriction. If symptoms or signs of sleep-disordered breathing are discovered, the individual should be referred to a sleep program for further assessment, which would likely include overnight polysomnography. Although ASD in and of itself does not appear to be an independent risk factor of obstructive sleep apnea, there will be children with ASD who have other risk factors including adenotonsillar hypertrophy and craniofacial abnormalities such as micrognathia. If restless legs syndrome or excessive movements while asleep are suspected, a referral to a sleep specialist is warranted. The most common sleep problem in this population will be insomnia. Behavioral interventions should be offered to all children with ASD and insomnia but they may not be adequate to address the problem in some children. In those children, pharmacotherapy may be indicated. If the clinician assessing the child with ASD and severe insomnia is not comfortable prescribing medications for insomnia, a referral to a sleep specialist should be made. Detailed information on the treatment of sleep problems in children and adolescents with ASD is presented in the Chapter 25.

REFERENCES

1. American Psychiatric Association: Diagnostic and Statistical Manual of Mental Disorders, Fourth Edition Text Revision. Washington, DC, American Psychiatric Association, 2000.
2. American Psychiatric Association: Diagnostic and Statistical Manual of Mental Disorders, Fourth Edition. Washington, DC, American Psychiatric Association, 1980.

3. American Psychiatric Association: Diagnostic and Statistical Manual of Mental Disorders, Fourth Edition. Washington, DC, American Psychiatric Association, 1994.
4. Center for Disease Control and Prevention. Prevalence of Autism Spectrum Disorders — Autism and Developmental Disabilities Monitoring Network, Six Sites, United States. Morbidity and Mortality Weekly Report 2007, 56, 1–11.
5. Cohen D, Pichard N, Tordjman S, et al. Specific genetic disorders and autism: clinical contribution towards their identification. J Autism Dev Disord 2005; 35:103–16.
6. Minshew NJ, Sweeney JA, Bauman ML, et al. Neurological aspects of autism. In: Volkmar FR, Paul R, Klin A, Cohen D, eds Handbook of Autism and Pervasive Developmental Disorders, 3rd edn Vol. 1. Hoboken, NJ: John Wiley & Sons, 2005: pp. 473–514.
7. Herbert MR, Ziegler DA, Makris N, et al. Localization of white matter volume increase in Autism and Developmental Language Disorder. Ann Neurol 2004; 55:530–40.
8. Zuckerman B, Stevenson J, Bailey V. Sleep problems in early childhood: Continuities, predictive factors, and behavioral correlates. Pediatrics 1987, 80(5):664–71.
9. Hansen DE, Vandenberg B. Neuropsychological features and differential diagnosis of sleep apnea syndrome in children. J Clin Child Psychol 1997; 26(3):304–10.
10. Owens J, Opipari L, Nobile C, et al. Sleep and daytime behavior in children with obstructive sleep apnea and behavioral sleep disorders. Pediatrics 1998; 102(5):1178–84.
11. Smedje H, Broman JE, Hetta J. Associations between disturbed sleep and behavioral difficulties in 635 children aged six to eight years: A study based on parents perceptions. Eur Child Adolesc Psychiatry 2001; 10:1–9.
12. Halbower AC, Mahone EM. Neuropsychological morbidity linked to childhood sleep-disordered breathing. Sleep Med Review 2006; 10(2):97–107.
13. Didden R, Sigafoos J. A review of the nature and treatment of sleep disorders in individuals with developmental disabilities. Res Dev Disabil 2001; 22(4):255–72.
14. Didden R, Korzilius H, van Aperlo B, et al. Sleep problems and daytime problem behaviours in children with intellectual disability. J Intellect Disabil Res 2002; 46(7):537–47.
15. Robinson AM, Richdale AL. Sleep problems in children with an intellectual disability: Parental perceptions of sleep problems, and views of treatment effectiveness. Child Care, Health & Development 2004; 30(2):139–50.
16. Owens J, Spirito A, McGuinn M. The Children's Sleep Habits Questionnaire (CSHQ): Psychometric properties of a survey instrument for school-aged children. Sleep 2000; 23:1043–51.
17. Aman MG, Singh NN. Aberrant Behavior Checklist: Manual. East Aurora, NY: Slosson Educational Publications, 1986.
18. Aman M. Aberrant Behavior Checklist—Community. In: Supplementary Manual. East Aurora, NY: Slosson Educational Publications, 1994.
19. Achenbach T, Rescorla L. Child Behavior Checklist. Burlington VT: ASEBA, 2000.
20. Cohen IL, Sudhalter V. The PDD Behavior Inventory. Psychological Assessment Resources 2005.
21. Gioia GA, Isquith PK, Guy SC, Kenworthy L. The Behavior Rating Inventory of Executive Function. Psychological Assessment Resources. 2000, Odessa, FL.
22. Wiggs L, Stores G. Severe sleep disturbance and daytime challenging behavior in children with severe learning disabilities. J Intellect Disabil Res 1996; 40(6): 518–28.
23. Patzold LM, Richdale AL, Tonge BJ. An investigation into sleep characteristics of children with autism and Asperger's Disorder. J Paediatrics Child Health 1998; 34:528–33.
24. Richdale AL, Prior MR, The sleep/wake rhythm in children with autism. Eur Child Adolesc Psychiatry 1995; 4(3):175–86.
25. Quine L, Sleep problems in children with mental handicap. J Ment Deficiency Res 1991; 35(4):269–90.

26. Clements J, Wing L, Dunn G. Sleep problems in handicapped children: A preliminary study. J Child Psychol Psychiatry 1986; 27(3):399–407.
27. Honomichl RD, Goodlin-Jones BL, Burnham M, et al. Sleep patterns of children with pervasive developmental disorders. J Autism Dev Disord 2002; 32(6):553–61.
28. Hoshino Y, Watanabe H, Yashima Y, et al. An investigation on sleep disturbance of autistic children. Folia Psychiatrica et Neurologica Japonica 1984; 38(1):45–51.
29. Schreck KA, Mulick JA. Parental report of sleep problems in children with autism. J Autism Dev Disord 2000; 30(2):127–35.
30. Bradley EA, Summers JA, Wood HL, et al. Comparing rates of psychiatric and behavior disorders in adolescents and young adults with severe intellectual disability with and without autism. J Autism Dev Disord 2004; 34(2):151–61.
31. Couturier JL, Speechley KN, Steele M, et al. Parental perception of sleep problems in children of normal intelligence with pervasive developmental disorders: Prevalence, severity, and pattern. J Am Acad Child Adolesc Psychiatry 2005; 44(8):815–22.
32. Paavonen EJ, Nieminen-von Wendt T, Vanhala R, et al. Effectiveness of melatonin in the treatment of sleep disturbances in children with Asperger disorder. J Child Adolesc Psychopharmacol 2003; 13(1):83–95.
33. Polimeni MA, Richdale AL, Francis AJP. A survey of sleep problems in autism, Asperger's disorder and typically developing children. J Intellect Disab Res 2005; 49(4):260–8.
34. Limoges E, Mottron L, Bolduc C, et al. Atypical sleep architecture and the autism phenotype. Brain Dev 2005; 128(5):1049–61.
35. Tani P, Lindberg N, Nieminen-von Wendt T, et al. Insomnia is a frequent finding in adults with Asperger syndrome. BMC Psychiatry [electronic resource] 2003; 3(1):12.
36. Allik H, Larsson JO, Smedje H. Insomnia in school-age children with Asperger syndrome or high-functioning autism. BMC Psychiatry 2006; 6:18.
37. Mindell JA, Emslie G, Blumer J, et al. Pharmacologic management of insomnia in children and adolescents: Consensus statement. Pediatrics 2006; 117;e1223–32.
38. Malow BA, Marzec ML, McGrew SG, et al. Characterizing sleep in children with autism spectrum disorders: A multidimensional approach. Sleep 2006; 29(12):1563–71.
39. Ritvo ER, Ritvo R, Yuwiler A, et al. Elevated daytime melatonin concentrations in autism: a pilot study. Eur Child Adolesc Psychiatry 1993; 2(2):75–8.
40. Nir I, Meir D, Zilber N, et al. Brief report: Circadian melatonin, thyroid-stimulating hormone, prolactin, and cortisol levels in serum of young adults with autism. J Autism Dev Disord 1995; 25:641–54
41. Kulman G, Lissoni P, Rovelli F, et al. Evidence of pineal endocrine hypofunction in autistic children. Neuroendocrin Letters 2000; 20:31–4.
42. Leibenluft E, Feldman-Naim S, Turner EH, et al. Salivary and plasma measures of dim light melatonin onset (DLMO) in patients with rapid cycling bipolar disorder. Biol Psychiatry 1996; 40:731–5.
43. Lewy AJ, Sack RL, Boney RS, et al. Assays for measuring the dim light melatonin onset (DLMO) in human plasma. Sleep Res 1997; 26:733.
44. Lewy AJ, Cutler NL, Sack RL. The endogenous melatonin profile as a marker for circadian phase position. J Biol Rhythms 1999; 14:227–36.
45. Lewy AJ, Bauer VK, Hasler BP, et al. Capturing the circadian rhythms of free-running blind people with 0.5 mg melatonin. Brain Res 2001; 918:96–100.
46. Lewy AJ, Emens J, Sack RL, et al. Low, but not high, doses of melatonin entrained a free-running blind person with a long circadian period. Chronobiol Int 2002; 19:649–58.
47. Lewy AJ, Emens J, Sack RL, Hasler, et al. Zeitgeber hierarchy in humans: Resetting the circadian phase positions of blind people using melatonin. Chronobiol Int 2003; 20:837–52.
48. Tordjman S, Anderson GM, Pichard N, et al. Nocturnal excretion of 6-sulphatoxy-melatonin in children and adolescents with autistic disorder. Biol Psychiatry 2005; 57:134–8.

49. Thirumalai SS, Shubin RA, Robinson R. Rapid eye movement sleep behavior disorder in children with autism. J Child Neurol 2002; 17(3):173–8.
50. Godbout R, Bergeron C, Limoges E, et al. A laboratory study of sleep in Asperger's syndrome. Neuroreport 2000; 11(1):127–30.
51. Mindell JA, Owens J. A Clinical Guide to Pediatric Sleep: Diagnosis and Management of Sleep Problems. Philadelphia: Lippincott Williams & Wilkins, 2003.

25 Sleep Interventions in Children with Autism Spectrum Disorders

Beth A. Malow[a] and Susan G. McGrew[b]

[a]Department of Neurology and Kennedy Center, Vanderbilt University, Nashville, Tennessee, U.S.A.
[b]Department of Pediatrics and Kennedy Center, Vanderbilt University and Monroe Carell Jr. Children's Hospital, Nashville, Tennessee, U.S.A.

INTRODUCTION

Disordered sleep affects daytime health and behavioral functioning in a variety of neurologic and psychiatric conditions, and autism spectrum disorders (ASD) are no exception. Treatment of sleep disorders in this population may not only improve sleep, but daytime behavior and autism symptoms as well. Furthermore, treatment of sleep problems in children with developmental disabilities and challenging daytime behavior may reduce parental stress and heighten their sense of control and ability to cope with their child's sleep. The causes of disrupted sleep in ASD are discussed in a separate chapter (chap. 24); this chapter will emphasize non-pharmacologic and pharmacologic treatment options to promote sleep. Two points should be emphasized. First, defining the cause of the sleep disturbance is critical to appropriate intervention. For example insomnia due to poor sleep hygiene may be responsive to behavioral interventions, insomnia due to impaired circadian control of sleep may be responsive to treatment with supplemental melatonin or light, daytime sleepiness due to obstructive sleep apnea should respond to treatment with adenotonsillectomy or continuous positive airway pressure (CPAP), and nocturnal events due to epileptic seizures should be treated with antiepileptic drugs. Second, pharmacologic and non-pharmacologic treatments often go hand-in-hand in the treatment of sleep disturbances in ASD. Whenever possible, behavioral treatments, which provide the foundation for proper sleep, should precede pharmacologic treatments to minimize adverse effects and maximize benefits achieved from pharmacologic treatments (Table 1).

TREATMENT OF INSOMNIA
Identify and Treat Underlying Causes

Symptoms of insomnia, defined as difficulty initiating or maintaining sleep, are the major sleep concerns reported by parents of children with ASD (1) and will be emphasized in this chapter. The cause of insomnia in a given child with ASD is often multifactorial, requiring a variety of treatment modalities. An important first step in formulating a treatment plan is to identify specific sleep disorders, as well as medical, neurological, and psychiatric conditions and medications that may be causing or contributing to insomnia.

This work was supported by a grant from the Autism Speaks Foundation/National Alliance for Autism Research.

TABLE 1   Treatment Guidelines for Children with ASD and Insomnia

Step 1: Identify and treat underlying causes of insomnia
- Neurological conditions (e.g., seizures)
- Psychiatric conditions (e.g., anxiety)
- Medical conditions (e.g., gastroesophageal reflux disease [GERD])
- Medications.

Step 2: Have parents initiate behavioral treatments for insomnia
- Promote healthy daytime habits (e.g., exercise)
- Promote healthy evening habits (e.g., limit stimulating activities)
- Selection of an appropriate bedtime (e.g., avoid the forbidden zone)
- Establishment of a bedtime routine
- Teach child to fall asleep on his or her own
- Minimize sleep aids (e.g., television)
- Promote effective interactions during night wakings (e.g., comfort, but keep interactions brief and boring).

Step 3: Recommend supplemental melatonin to parents
- Choose a reputable brand that does not contain other active ingredients (e.g., diphenhydramine).
- Start at 1 mg 30 minutes before bedtime.
- Increase by 1 mg every two weeks, following sleep diaries and parental report. Doses up to 10 mg have been documented in the literature without adverse effects.
- Consider giving melatonin earlier in children with delayed bedtimes to entrain the circadian cycle.
- Consider sustained release melatonin in children with night wakings.
- Continue behavioral treatments for insomnia during melatonin therapy.

Step 4: Consider trial of other sleep-promoting medications
- Prescribe a medication that also treats a coexisting condition (e.g., sedating antiepileptic medication given at night).
- Use lowest possible doses and monitor carefully for adverse effects.
- Continue behavioral treatments for insomnia during melatonin therapy.

Step 5: Consider light therapy
- Have parents purchase a commercially available light box if bright light not available.
- Administer light in early morning to promote an earlier bedtime.
- Light given in the late afternoon and evening delays sleep onset.
- Light of 2500 lux administered for one to two hours in the morning is recommended and is safe.
- Dosage may be increased by 1000 lux every three days to a maximum of 10000 lux.
- Monitor child for adverse effects: photosensitivity and mania.

Examples of sleep disorders that contribute to difficulty falling asleep or to night wakings include circadian rhythm disorders, restless legs syndrome, obstructive sleep apnea, or non-rapid eye movement (NREM) arousal disorders (eg. sleepwalking, sleep terrors). Psychiatric disorders or symptoms coexisting in children with ASD, such as anxiety or hyperactivity may interfere with sleep initiation, and depression may contribute to early morning awakening. A common or presenting symptom of bipolar phenotype is a decreased need for sleep. Medical conditions such as gastrointestinal reflux can contribute to night wakings, and neurological conditions such as epilepsy may impact on sleep (2). Insomnia may result from a variety of medications used to treat co-existing conditions. Examples include corticosteroids and asthma medications, stimulants for attention-deficit hyperactivity disorder, activating serotonin uptake inhibitors for depression, and stimulating antiepileptic drugs for epilepsy or mood stabilization.

Diagnosis and treatment of an underlying sleep, medical, neurological, or psychiatric disorder often is done in conjunction with consultants (e.g., sleep specialists, gastrointestinal specialists) with confirmatory ancillary tests (e.g., polysomnography) as needed. In the case of co-existing epilepsy, ensure that the child's seizures are being appropriately treated, as even daytime seizures can affect sleep the following night (3). Whenever possible, a medication that will help promote sleep as well as treat a co-existing medical, neurological, or psychiatric disorder should be utilized. For example, use an antiepileptic drug (AED) that promotes sleep onset, consolidates non-rapid eye movement (NREM) sleep, and minimizes arousals and awakenings, such as one of the newer AEDs (e.g., pregabalin for complex partial seizures). In the case of depression, use of an antidepressant that is either sleep neutral (e.g., citalapram) or sleep-promoting (e.g., mirtazapine) may be more effective with co-existing insomnia. Bupropion, venlafaxine, fluoxetine, and sertraline are relatively stimulating (4) and should be avoided if possible in those with insomnia and reserved for those with daytime sleepiness without insomnia. To help promote sleep, adjust the dose, timing, or specific medications that the child is already taking. For example, move the dosing of stimulating medications to the morning.

Initiate Behavioral Sleep Therapies

Once other causes of insomnia in ASD are excluded (or treated), first-line treatment involves behavioral therapy to promote sleep. Behavioral therapy for sleep has been beneficial for typically developing children (5) and small studies of children with developmental disorders, including ASD; for suggestions regarding its utility in this population, see (6,7).

A cornerstone to the behavioral treatment of insomnia in ASD is identifying sleep hygiene (habit) problems and educating parents to pay attention to the basic principles of sleep hygiene. These include daytime habits, evening habits, selection of an appropriate bedtime, establishment of a bedtime routine, minimizing sleep aids such as the television, which may promote sleep but result in night wakings once turned off, and promoting non-reinforcing interactions with the child during night wakings.

Daytime habits include attention to the quantity and timing of exercise (e.g., daytime exercise promotes sleep but evening exercise may be stimulating), light (e.g., helpful in the morning but best avoided in the evening when it can promote alertness), dietary choices (e.g., limiting caffeine in late afternoon and evening), naps (e.g., limit in afternoon and evening as may interfere with sleep drive), and bedroom use (avoid timeouts and engaging in schoolwork in bed and bedroom whenever possible to avoid conditioning the child to associate negative or stimulating activities with the bedroom).

Evening habits include promotion of calming "wind down" activities and avoidance of stimulating activities such as video games, minimizing light exposure, and engaging in a bedtime routine to condition the child to sleep. The bedtime should be selected based on the child's optimal time window to fall asleep. The interval before the optimal sleep window, also called the "forbidden zone" is a time of maximum alertness when children are too awake to easily fall asleep. The choice of a bedtime ideally also needs to take into account the family schedule, including the need to put other children to bed and the parent(s) need for wind down time in the evenings. Equally important to the choice of a bedtime is paying attention to the consistency of the bedtime, which promotes a regular sleep–wake cycle.

Difficulty initiating sleep may also result from hypersensitivity to environmental stimuli, including noises in the bedroom or elsewhere in the home, or tactile hypersensitivity to bedclothes or blankets. Weighted blankets may sometimes be helpful in children with tactile sensitivities. The sleep environment should take into account temperature, texture of the pajamas and bed sheets (in children with tactile sensitivities), and optimal noise and light. Some children will benefit from having their bedroom doors left open so that they can be comforted by the sounds coming from other areas of the home. A dim nightlight (15 watts) may reduce anxiety, without inhibiting the secretion of endogenous melatonin (necessary to maintain sleep).

Effective parental interactions to promote sleep at bedtime and with night wakings are critical to the success of any behavioral sleep intervention. Parents can be instructed to teach their children to fall asleep on their own by helping the child settle into a relaxed state and by providing no stimulation or reinforcement for resisting sleep. Educational techniques using first/then approaches, a timer with gradually lengthening quiet time, and a reinforcer for cooperation may be necessary for the child who does not understand how to lie quietly in the bed. Visual supports showing what is expected of the child are a critical part of this approach in ASD. A visual schedule for the bedtime routine and visual "back to bed" reminders on the door will communicate to the child the parental expectations (Figure 1). The child should be trained to follow the visual schedule after a cue from parents. This may be accomplished using physical prompts. Morning reinforcers

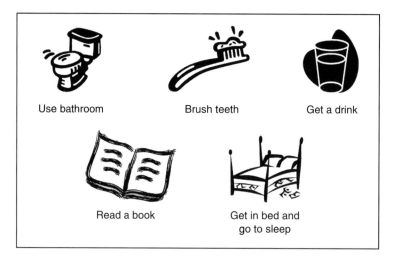

Use bathroom	Brush teeth	Get a drink
Read a book	Get in bed and go to sleep	

FIGURE 1 Example of a bedtime routine visual support designed for a child with ASD. The pictures convey to the child expectations for the bedtime routine as well as the order in which the steps of the bedtime routine will occur.

(e.g., wrapped presents) for successfully meeting expectations may be incorporated into the routine. If the child has anxiety about falling asleep alone, parents may temporarily set up a bed or rocking chair next to the child's bed. No physical contact or eye contact should be made during this phase of treatment. The rocking chair can be gradually moved closer to the door on successive nights until it is through the door. Limiting naps may also be effective in promoting more consolidated sleep at night. For more detailed information on behavioral treatment of sleep disturbances in children with ASD, the reader is referred to a comprehensive text (8).

If behavioral treatment of insomnia is not fully effective, pharmacological treatments should be initiated in conjunction with (rather than in place of) behavioral treatment, since one of the keys to successful maintenance of sleep involves being able to fall asleep on one's own. Medications to promote sleep given in the absence of behavioral therapy can actually interfere with sleep maintenance once the pharmacological agent has dissipated. Pharmacological treatment should be reserved for children who fail to have complete responsiveness to behavioral therapy because of possible adverse effects, in a population sensitive to medications and less able to communicate adverse effects.

Consider Trial of Supplemental Melatonin

Melatonin, a neurohormone which promotes sleep, is produced in the pineal gland from serotonin (9). Supplemental melatonin has shown promise in promoting sleep, although controlled studies of its efficacy and tolerability are limited. Its relative availability (does not require a prescription), its low expense, and its favorable safety profile make it an attractive choice for promoting sleep in children with ASD. Although melatonin is a dietary supplement, is not approved by the Food and Drug Administration (FDA), and has not been rigorously tested for safety, efficacy, or purity of preparation, no serious long term adverse effects have been seen in this widely used supplement.

The mechanisms whereby melatonin may promote sleep in ASD are not known. Melatonin may be acting to entrain the circadian clock. Alternatively, supplemental melatonin may be treating a deficiency state. Melatonin may act non-specifically as a hypnotic to promote sleep, or may promote sleep by decreasing core body temperature or through anxiolytic mechanisms (10). Two studies of repeated venous blood sampling of melatonin in young adults (11) and children (12) with ASD showed blunting of the nocturnal physiological increase in melatonin. Decreased nocturnal excretion of 6-sulphatoxymelatonin, the major metabolite of melatonin, has been observed in children and adolescents with ASD compared to controls matched on age, gender, and Tanner stage (13).

Several small studies of melatonin in neurodevelopmental disabilities and ASD have been conducted, with favorable results, although large controlled trials are needed to definitely establish its efficacy in ASD. Reductions in sleep latency (time to fall asleep) and improvements in total sleep time and sleep efficiency (time asleep/time in bed), with no or minimal adverse effects, have been observed in studies of children with neurodevelopmental disorders given supplemental melatonin (14–17). Epileptic seizures did not occur in children who had been seizure-free, and seizures did not increase in those with epilepsy in these studies. Only one study of five children with refractory seizures reported increased epileptic seizures during melatonin treatment (18). A large retrospective study of over 100 children with ASD treated with melatonin documented minimal adverse effects, with improved sleep in 85% of children treated (19).

Two trials of supplemental melatonin have been performed exclusively in children with ASD. One open-label trial administered 3 mg of immediate-release melatonin 30 minutes prior to bedtime for two weeks in 15 children with Asperger's syndrome (ages 6–17 years) (20). All children had severe sleep problems and none were taking psychotropic medications. Sleep latency, as measured by actigraphy, significantly decreased from 40 to 21 minutes during treatment. Improvement in behavior also occurred, as measured by several domains on the Child Behavior Checklist (CBCL) (21). Two children experienced mild tiredness and difficulty awakening, and one also had headaches. Another child dropped out due to extensive tiredness, difficulty staying awake, dizziness, and diarrhea, with symptoms resolving immediately after melatonin discontinuation. No other adverse effects were reported. A second open-label study of combined fast- and controlled-release melatonin (3–6 mg) in autism showed improvement in sleep diaries and questionnaires in all children (22). One month after melatonin was discontinued, 16 children returned to pre-treatment sleep scores.

Because melatonin's half life is less than an hour, it is recommended that melatonin initially be given 30 minutes prior to the desired bedtime. In addition to its sedating effects, melatonin also has a chronobiotic (phase-shifting) effect and therefore may be more effective in individuals with delayed sleep phase when given several hours before bedtime. Doses as low as 300 mcgs are physiologic and may be effective at promoting sleep, although doses of 1–3 mg are more sedating and more commonly used. Dosage is usually started at 1 mg and titrated up to 3 mg if needed, by 1 mg every two weeks. Occasionally, doses of 6 mg or higher are needed. When using melatonin, it is important to continue to use the same formulation, as the bioavailability of melatonin may vary widely among manufacturers. Because it is available over the counter, and not regulated by the FDA, it is important to instruct parents to read the label carefully and avoid choosing a brand with other active ingredients (e.g., diphenhydramine). Oral melatonin is rapidly metabolized, and extended release melatonin, also available over the counter, may be helpful for the child with sleep maintenance difficulties, although studies have been limited (23). Once a sleep cycle is established for six weeks or more, the melatonin may be discontinued, although long term use appears safe and may be necessary to maintain the sleep cycle.

Consider Other Pharmacological Treatments for Insomnia

Apart from melatonin, there is a wide range of options for pharmacologic treatment, best used in conjunction with behavioral techniques, and tailored to the cause of the individual child's sleep problem. As with all medications, it is important to start with low doses and increase gradually, monitoring carefully for adverse effects, as children with autism may be sensitive to certain classes of medications and unable to communicate side effects.

A helpful principle for prescribing sleep medications in children with ASD is to consider the overlapping neurological and psychiatric systems that are affected. Wherever possible, prescribe a medication that also assists with the co-existing condition. In children with co-existing epilepsy or bipolar disorder, mood stabilizing antiepileptics with sedating properties can be used. The antiepileptic regimen can be adjusted to administer a bedtime dose of medication that provides sedation and promotes sleep. Options include carbamazepine, gabapentin, or topiramate, which are usually dosed two or three times a day but can be adjusted to give the higher dose at bedtime. Valproic acid comes in an extended release form which can be given once a day, at bedtime. Lamotrigine tends to be more stimulating and may interfere with sleep, but may be an excellent choice in children with daytime sleepiness.

Children with comorbid bipolar disorder, extreme mood irritability, aggression, or self injurious behavior may benefit from treatment with the sedating atypical neuroleptics such as risperidone, olanzapine, or quetiapine. The dosages of these medications can be adjusted to give the higher dose at bedtime.

In the anxious or depressed child, specific antidepressants that promote sleep may be considered. These include the highly sedating drugs mirtazapine, trazadone (should be avoided in males who cannot communicate reliably because of the risk of priapism), the mildly sedating serotonin reuptake inhibitor (SRI) fluvoxamine, and the tricyclic antidepressants (such as clomipramine, imipramine, and nortryptilline). The selective SRIs (SSRI) or tricyclic antidepressants may also be useful for children with obsessional thoughts that interfere with sleep onset. Clonidine is also useful for sleep initiation problems in the child who is mildly anxious or overaroused at night. Diphenhydramine and benzodiazepines are other options.

Consider Light Therapy

Light therapy may be useful for children with circadian rhythm abnormalities in combination with chronotherapy, where the sleep–wake cycle is delayed over the course of several days until the desired bedtime is reached. Bright light administered in the morning "resets" the circadian clock and facilitates an earlier bedtime (24). There are several commercial light boxes which emit UV free light. An alternative to purchasing a commercial light box is for the patient to get exposed to bright light each morning. Although no definitive studies have been performed in autism, light of 2500 lux administered for 30 minutes to two hours in the morning is recommended and is safe, based on experience from the pediatric seasonal affective disorder literature (25). Dosage may be increased by 1000 lux every three days to a maximum of 10,000 lux. Lower dosages may require the longer treatment times. Cautions include the small risk of precipitating a manic episode in co-existing or unrecognized bipolar disorder (26) or the risk of a photosensitivity reaction (usually precipitated by UV light exposure) (27). If a child has a photosensitizing condition or is taking photosensitizing medications (such as tetracyclines, sulfonamides, nonsteroidal anti-inflammatory agents, and phenothiazines), the risk–benefit should be carefully weighed and a non-UV emitting light source should be used. Adherence to sleep hygiene measures including a strict bedtime and wake time routine is necessary to prevent the return of a delayed bedtime. Close follow up is recommended in children receiving light therapy to prevent relapse.

TREATMENT OF OTHER SLEEP DISORDERS IN CHILDREN WITH ASD

The International Classification of Sleep Disorders lists a variety of sleep disorders that may present in childhood. This section will focus on two categories of sleep disorder—parasomnias and obstructive sleep apnea—because they are common disorders that have unique relevance for children with ASD. Parasomnias can be confused with other conditions prevalent in ASD, such as epileptic seizures or repetitive / stereotyped behaviors. Obstructive sleep apnea may be under-recognized in children with ASD.

Parasomnias

Parasomnias need to be distinguished from epileptic seizures in this population, given the increased prevalence of epilepsy in autism (28). Such events include the non-REM (NREM) arousal disorders, rhythmic movement disorder, and REM sleep behavior disorder. Nocturnal events can usually be distinguished by history, although video-electroencephalography (EEG)-polysomnography in a sleep center is occasionally warranted. One of the cardinal distinguishing features of epileptic seizures is their stereotyped appearance, as well as the presence of tonic or dystonic limb posturing.

The non-REM arousal disorders consist of a spectrum of events of aberrant arousal arising from non-REM sleep stages 3 and 4 (deep) sleep, ranging from confusional arousals to sleepwalking to night terrors. There is often a family history of similar spells in parents or siblings, supporting a genetic predisposition. Precipitants include sleep deprivation, emotional stress, medical illness, and other conditions that contribute to disruption of normal sleeping patterns (29). Clonazapam is often effective for treatment; the tricyclic antidepressants given at night can also be useful.

In rhythmic movement disorder, children exhibit repetitive, stereotyped, and rhythmic motor behaviors that occur predominantly during drowsiness or sleep. These behaviors can include bodyrolling, bodyrocking, headrolling, and headbanging, and injury can occur. Episodes usually occur at sleep onset but can occur at any time during the night. While common in infants (59%) and small children (prevalence 5% at five years), when rhythmic movement disorder persists to older childhood, ASD, mental retardation, or related disorders are usually present and these children may have similar behaviors during the day (30). Treatment should be initiated when the potential for injury is present—clonazapam is the recommended choice, although not universally effective.

In REM sleep behavior disorder, individuals "act out their dreams" due to an interruption of physiological muscle atonia during REM sleep. This disorder has been reported in one case series of children with ASD and disrupted sleep who were studied with polysomnography (31). REM sleep behavior disorder is usually associated with older age and has been related to degeneration of dopaminergic neurons in the substantia nigra, a subcortical region involved in motor control. REM sleep behavior disorder can also occur in association with psychotropic medications that affect REM sleep, such as the selective SRIs (32). Related abnormalities, such as increased phasic muscle activity in REM sleep in mentally retarded individuals with autism (33), raise the possibility that neurostructural or neurochemical abnormalities involving the brainstem or subcortical regions may be associated with autism. REM sleep behavior disorder often responds to clonazapam, although dopaminergic agents and melatonin have also been tried.

In all of these parasomnias, attention to safety issues is also important, especially if injury can occur when a child may wander. Bedside monitors, as well as alarms or bells placed on a door that indicate to parents when a child has left the room, may be necessary.

Obstructive Sleep Apnea

This common sleep disorder may affect up to 3% of children in the general population, and is characterized by loud snoring or noisy breathing (usually worse in the supine position) in association with restless sleep, frequent awakenings, and sweating in sleep. Pauses in respiration are not always evident. Diagnosis can be made by overnight polysomnography, with monitoring of respiratory airflow and effort, as well as oxygenation, during sleep. While the prevalence of obstructive sleep apnea in children with ASD is unknown, identifying the presence of this sleep disorder can be very rewarding in caring for a child with ASD in that improvements in sleep as well as in daytime behavior may occur. While daytime sleepiness is common in adults with obstructive sleep apnea, due to disrupted sleep at night, children may not appear sleepy but instead exhibit symptoms of hyperactivity and other problematic behaviors. These behaviors may improve with treatment (see next section).

In children who continue to exhibit symptoms of obstructive sleep apnea after adenotonsillectomy, a repeat polysomnogram is warranted. Children with obesity or craniofacial abnormalities may not respond fully to adenotonsillectomy, but may be candidates for treatment with continuous positive airway pressure (CPAP). In CPAP therapy, a steady stream of air pressure administered through the nasal passages into the back of the throat keeps the airway open. Although it may appear that children with ASD would have great difficulty adjusting to a CPAP mask due to tactile sensitivities, success can be achieved. At our institution, we have set up a dedicated CPAP clinic, staffed by a physician or nurse practitioner in partnership with a sleep technologist (34). This team provides a combination of parent education and CPAP desensitization. A variety of CPAP interfaces, including nasal interfaces that do not involve a "mask," are available for children.

IMPACT OF TREATING SLEEP DISORDERS IN ASD ON DAYTIME BEHAVIOR

Treatment of a sleep disorder may improve daytime behavior in children with ASD, although definitive studies have not been carried out. In typically developing children, associations between sleep apnea and hyperactivity and aggressiveness are documented in typically developing children (35,36), with improvement in problem behaviors after adenotonsillectomy (37). In ASD, short sleep duration has been associated with stereotypic behavior, as well as higher overall autism scores and social skills deficits (38). There appears to be a relation between sleep problems and repetitive behaviors (stereotyped, self-injurious, compulsive, ritualistic, restricted) and craving for sameness in children with autism (39), although this relation may be moderated by their level of cognitive ability. In one case report of a girl with ASD and obstructive sleep apnea, an improvement in daytime behavior was documented after treatment with adenotonsillectomy (40). Although she still retained her autism diagnosis on the Autism Diagnostic Observation Schedule (ADOS) (41), her performance on this test and the Child Behavior Checklist (21) as well as parental report, documented improvement in a variety of domains, including social interaction and the ability to focus.

CONCLUSIONS

Sleep concerns are common in children with autism, with a variety of behavioral, pharmacological, and other options for therapy. The cornerstone of treatment is to establish the etiology of the sleep concern, which is often multifactorial. Identifying and treating sleep disorders may result not only in improved sleep, but also impact favorably on daytime behavior and functioning within the family.

REFERENCES

1. Richdale AL. Sleep problems in autism: Prevalence, cause, and intervention. Dev Med Child Neurol 1999; 41(1): 60–6.
2. Malow BA. Sleep disorders, epilepsy, and autism. Ment Retard Dev Disabil Res Rev 2004; 10(2): 122–5.
3. Bazil CW, Castro LH, Walczak TS. Reduction of rapid eye movement sleep by diurnal and nocturnal seizures in temporal lobe epilepsy. Arch Neurol 2000; 57:363–8.
4. Schwietzer PK. Drugs that disturb sleep and wakefulness. In: Kryger MH, Roth T, Dement WC, eds Principles and Practice of Sleep Medicine, 4th edn Philadelphia: Elsevier/Saunders, 2005: pp. 499–518.
5. Mindell JA, Kuhn B, Lewin DS, et al. Behavioral treatment of bedtime problems and night wakings in infants and young children. Sleep 2006; 29(10):1263–76.
6. Christodulu KV, Durand VM. Reducing bedtime disturbance and night waking using positive bedtime routines and sleep restriction. Focus Autism Other Dev Disab 2004; 19(3):130–9.
7. Weiskop S, Richdale A, Matthews J. Behavioural treatment to reduce sleep problems in children with autism or fragile X syndrome. Dev Med Child Neurol 2005; 47:94–104.
8. Durand VM. Sleep Better: A Guide to Improving Sleep for Children with Special Needs. Baltimore: Paul H. Brookes, 1998.
9. Claustrat B, Brun J, Chazot G. The basic physiology and pathophysiology of melatonin. Sleep Med Rev 2005; 9:11–24.
10. Heuvel CJvd, Ferguson SA, Macchi MM, et al. Melatonin as a hypnotic: Con. Sleep Med Rev 2005; 9:71–80.
11. Nir I, Meir D, Zilber N, Knobler H, Hadjez J, Lerner Y. Brief report: Circadian melatonin, thyroid-stimulating hormone, prolactin, and cortisol levels in serum of young adults with autism. J Autism Dev Disord 1995; 25(6):641–54.
12. Kulman G, Lissoni P, Rovelli F, Roselli MG, Brivio F, Sequeri P. Evidence of pineal endocrine hypofunction in autistic children. Neuroendocrinol Lett 2000; 21(1):31–4.
13. Tordjman S, Anderson GM, Pichard N, Charbuy H, Touitou Y. Nocturnal excretion of 6-sulphatoxymelatonin in children and adolescents with autistic disorder. Biol Psychiatry 2005; 57:134–8.
14. Jan JE, Esperzedl H, Appleton RE. The treatment of sleep disorders with melatonin. Dev Med Child Neurol 1994; 36:97–107.
15. Ross C, Davies P, Whitehouse W. Melatonin treatment for sleep disorders in children with neurodevelopmental disorders: An observational study. Dev Med Child Neurol 2002; 44:339–44.
16. Phillips L, Appleton R. Systematic review of melatonin treatment in children with neurodevelopmental disabilities and sleep impairment. Dev Med Child Neurol 2004; 46:771–5.
17. Dodge NN, Wilson GA. Melatonin for treatment of sleep disorders in children with developmental disabilities. J Child Neurol 2001; 16:581–4.
18. Sheldon S. Pro-convulsant effects of oral melatonin in neurologically disabled children. Lancet 1998; 351:1254.
19. Andersen I, Kaczmarska J, McGrew SG, Malow, BA. Melatonin for insomnia in children with autism spectrum disorders. J Child Neurol, prepublished 8 January 2008.
20. Paavonen E, von Wendt T, Vanhala N, et al. Effectiveness of melatonin in the treatment of sleep disturbances in children with Asperger disorder. J Child Adolesc Psychopharmacol 2003; 13:83–95.

21. Achenbach TM, Rescorla LA. Manual for the ASEBA Preschool Forms and Profiles. Burlington: University of Vermont, Research Center for Children, Youth, and Families, 2001.

22. Giannotti F, Cortesi F, Cerquiglini A, et al. An open-label study of controlled-release melatonin in treatment of sleep disorders in children with autism. J Autism Dev Disord 2006; 36(6):741–52.

23. Jan JE, Hamilton D, Seward N, et al. Clinical trials of controlled-release melatonin in children with sleep-wake cycle disorders. J Pineal Res 2000; 29(1):34–9.

24. Chesson AL, Littner M, Davila D, et al. Practice parameters for the use of light therapy in the treatment of sleep disorders. Sleep 1999; 22(5):1999.

25. Swedo SE, Allen AJ, Glod CA, et al. A controlled trial of light therapy for the treatment of pediatric seasonal affective disorder. J Am Acad Child Adolesc Psychiatry 1997; 36(6):816–21.

26. Schwitzer J, Neudorfer C, Blecha H-G, et al. Mania as a side effect of phototherapy. Biol Psychiatry 1990; 28:532–4.

27. Bickers DR. Photosensitivity and Other Reactions to Light. In: Kasper DL, Braunwald E, Fauci AS, et al., eds Harrison's Principles of Internal Medicine. New York: McGraw-Hill, 2004.

28. Tuchman R, Rapin I. Epilepsy in autism. Lancet Neurology 2002; 1:352–8.

29. Mahowald MW, Bornemann MAC. NREM Sleep-Arousal Parasomnias. In: Kryger M, Roth T, Dement W, eds Principles and Practice of Sleep Medicine. Philadelphia: Elsevier/Saunders, 2005: pp. 889–96.

30. Mayer G, Wilde-Frenz J, Kurella B. Sleep related rhythmic movement disorder revisited. J Sleep Res 2007; 16:110–6.

31. Thirumalai SS, Shubin RA, Robinson R. Rapid eye movement sleep behavior disorder in children with autism. J Child Neurol 2002; 17:173–8.

32. Mahowald M, Schenck C. REM Sleep Parasomnias. In: Kryger M, Roth T, Dement W, eds Principles and Practice of Sleep Medicine. 3rd edn. Philadelphia: Elsevier/Saunders, 2005: pp. 897–916.

33. Diomedi M, Curatolo P, Scalise A, et al. Sleep abnormalities in mentally retarded autistic subjects: Down's syndrome with mental retardation and normal subjects. Brain Dev 1999; 21(8):548–53.

34. Zimmerman M, Goldman S, Sumpter T, et al. CPAP clinic: A novel strategy designed to improve CPAP compliance. Sleep 2007; 30:A161.

35. Chervin RD, Ruzicka DL, Giordani BJ, et al. Sleep-disordered breathing, behavior, and cognition in children before and after adenotonsillectomy. Pediatrics 2006; 117(4):769–78.

36. Gottlieb DJ, Vezina RM, Chase C. Symptoms of sleep-disordered breathing in 5-year-old children are associated with sleepiness and problem behaviors. Pediatrics 2003; 112(4):870–7.

37. Goldstein NA, Fatima M, Campbell TF, et al. Child behavior and quality of life before and after tonsillectomy and adenoidectomy. Arch Otolaryngol Head Neck Surg 2002; 128(7):770–5.

38. Schreck KA, Mulick JA, Smith AF. Sleep problems as possible predictors of intensified symptoms of autism. Res Dev Disabil 2004; 24:57–66.

39. Gabriels RL, Cuccaro ML, Hill DE, Ivers BJ, et al. Repetitive behaviors in autism: Relationships with associated clinical features. Res Dev Disabil 2005; 26:169–81.

40. Malow BA, McGrew SG, Harvey M, et al. Impact of treating sleep apnea in a child with autism spectrum disorder. Pediatric Neurol 2006; 34:325–8.

41. Lord C, Risi S, Lambrecht L, et al. The autism diagnostic observation schedule-generic: A standard measure of social and communication deficits associated with the spectrum of autism. J Autism Dev Disord 2000; 30(3):205–23.

26 | Sleep and Substance Abuse in Adolescents

Irina Gromov[a] and Dmitriy Gromov[b]

[a]Matrix Alliance, Inc., Dallas, Texas, U.S.A.
[b]Center for Addiction Medicine, Massachusetts General Hospital, Boston, Massachusetts, U.S.A.

INTRODUCTION

Sleep disorders and substance use disorders remain among the most prevalent psychiatric disorders in children and adolescents. According to recent data, approximately 5.7% of children and adolescents suffer from clinically diagnosable insomnia, and 9.9% of youth between ages 12 and 17 reported the use of substances during the past month. Six in ten 9th–12th graders have less than eight hours of sleep on school nights and only 9% of students get the recommended nine hours of sleep. Among students who drive to school, 15% report fighting sleepiness while driving. Untreated insomnia in children and adolescents can lead to serious social and psychological consequences (1–3). Ivanenko et al. suggested that disruptions in the sleep–wake cycle during its maturation period in childhood and adolescence may indicate early development of psychopathology and should be identified and addressed appropriately (4). Indeed, rates of irritability, impulsivity, depression, anxiety, hyperactivity, substance abuse, and risk for suicide are higher in children and adolescents with sleep disturbances. Adolescents with frequent sleep difficulties were more likely to report use of inhalants, alcohol, marijuana, and cigarettes in comparison to those with no sleep problems (4,5).

Sleep disorders and substance use have strong reciprocal relationships. Both acute and chronic patterns of substance use contribute to significant changes in sleep architecture and can have long-term consequences. On the other hand, unrecognized and untreated sleep disorders increase the likelihood of initiating substance abuse with subsequent development of disorders of abuse and dependence.

Bidirectional relationships between sleep disorders and substance use disorders were examined by several researchers. In the review of substance abuse and sleep disturbances in adolescents, Bootzin et al. indicated that sleep problems in adolescence can present a pathway for substance abuse and also create obstacles for treatment of addictions by increasing rates of relapse. Sleep problems were found to be universal in their study of treatment of 55 adolescents with sleep disturbances and substance abuse. All study participants had increased sleep latency, increased awakenings, and diminished sleep efficiency. In addition to genetic factors, a self-medication mechanism for use of drugs to deal with consequences of sleep problems (stimulants for day time sleepiness and use of alcohol and marijuana for depression and insomnia, for example) was mentioned as one of the potential mechanisms of these interrelationships (6). Reciprocity between sleep disturbances and substances of abuse was also reported by Tynjala et al. where the authors studied 4,000 Finnish adolescents aged 11, 13, and 15. Structural equation models were used for the analysis. Strong interrelationships between irregular sleep schedules, substance use (alcohol, tobacco, and caffeine), and perceived tiredness among 15-year-olds were found. Irregular sleep and perceived tiredness explained 26% of the variance for substance abuse in boys and 12% in girls. On the other hand, substance use and irregular sleep explained 24% of the variance of perceived tiredness in boys and 20% in girls (7).

A strong relationship between sleep problems early in life and early initiation of alcohol and other drugs use was found in the longitudinal study of 257 boys from high-risk families by Wong et al. In the study, 33.5% of children had difficulty sleeping or complained of being overtired. Children with sleep problems, in comparison to those with no sleep problems, were 2.3 times more likely to have used alcohol by age 12–14, 2.3 times more likely to have smoked, 2.6 times more likely to have used marijuana, and 2.2 times more likely to have tried illicit substances. Due to significant consistency of sleep difficulties in the early onset of substance abuse, authors proposed that childhood sleep problems can be considered an early risk identifier for substance abuse in adolescents (8).

Both substance use and sleep problems are often associated with comorbid psychiatric conditions. Johnson et al. explored the possibility that the presence of co-existing psychiatric problems can lead to an association between substance use and sleep problems in adolescents. Data from the survey of adolescents ages 12–17 were used and adjusted for the "internalizing (depression and anxiety)" and "externalizing (deviance and aggression)" factors. Illicit drug use, either in combination with alcohol and cigarettes or by itself, was associated with sleep problems independently of psychiatric problems. In comparison to nonsmoking, daily smoking was associated with 57% greater probability of having sleep problems. The authors pointed to the complexity of associations between sleep and substance use in adolescents and proposed that sleep problems, substance use, and psychiatric problems may "cluster within individuals" (5).

The notion that there exists a connection between sleep, substance abuse, and emotional dysregulation was further explored by Haynes et al. In their study, 23 adolescents ages 13–19, who recently completed outpatient substance abuse treatment, were enrolled in a sleep-treatment protocol. Measures of sleep, substance use, and psychological status were taken at baseline, both during treatment and post treatment. The authors found that inadequate sleep led to later aggression in adolescents with recently treated substance abuse. It was proposed that sleep problems can contribute to affective and behavioral instability and subsequent substance abuse in adolescents (9).

Each drug of abuse has a unique influence on the health and development of adolescents. A description of use and effects of individual substances follows.

SUBSTANCES OF ABUSE
Alcohol
Alcohol remains the main substance of abuse among adolescents. Epidemiologic surveys demonstrated high and stable prevalence of underage drinking. In 2006, 66.5% of 12th graders reported alcohol use during the previous year, and 45.3% of 12th graders reported alcohol use in the previous month. There were about 10.8 million underage drinkers (age 12–20) in 2005. Among them, 7.2 million were binge drinkers (defined as consuming five or more alcoholic drinks on one occasion on at least one day during the past month), and 2.3 million were heavy drinkers (defined as five or more alcoholic drinks on one occasion on each of five or more

days in the past month). Of those college students still legally under age, 57.8% used alcohol in the past month. A first alcoholic drink was tried by 88.9% when they were younger than 21. Heavy drinking was engaged in by 16.6% of full-time college students. Alcohol was involved in 42% of drug-related Emergency Department (ED) visits in adolescents ages 12–20, 10% of which resulted in admission for inpatient care. Youth, who were in need of treatment but did not receive it, were not likely to recognize the need for treatment (1,10).

Early alcohol use increases the probability of developing alcohol dependence later in life. According to the analysis of data from the National Epidemiologic survey in 2001–2002, 47 % of individuals with onset of drinking before age 14 eventually became alcohol dependent, as compared to 9% of those who started drinking at age 21 and after. Initiation of alcohol use at an early age increases the likelihood of developing dependence within 10 years of drinking onset and before age 25. Of all alcohol-dependent responders, 46% started their drinking at 16 years or younger (11).

Alcohol dependence developed earlier in life may also lead to a smaller probability of treatment. In a comparative study of age at the time of diagnosis of alcohol dependence in relation to pursuit of treatment in 4778 persons with alcohol dependence, researchers found that people who became alcohol dependent at age 25 or younger were less likely to seek treatment than those diagnosed at age 30 or older. In addition, early alcohol dependence correlated with a significantly greater probability of relapse, long lasting dependence episodes, and additional symptoms of addiction. Study results also showed that approximately half of the analyzed patients developed alcohol dependence disorder before age 21, and about two-thirds developed the disorder before age 25 (12). As the human brain continues to develop into middle 20s, early alcohol consumption negatively affects its maturation. There are reports of diminished memory, visuospatial relations, executive functioning, and decreased hippocampal development in alcohol-dependent adolescents in comparison to non-dependent controls (13,14). Adolescents who start drinking before age 13 are more likely to drink to intoxication level and undertake high risk behaviors such as not wearing safety belts, drinking and driving, getting involved in fights, having unprotected sex, and experimenting with illicit drugs. Heavy adolescent drinkers tend to underachieve academically more frequently than other students (11,15). In addition to the above-mentioned effects, alcohol also influences sleep patterns.

Sleep depends on complex interrelationships between various neurotransmitters and sleep factors. Since alcohol influences the majority of these neurotransmitters, its influence on sleep is profound and has been studied extensively in adults. K.J.Brower described acute, chronic, and withdrawal effects of alcohol on sleep in the review of the topic. In general, changes in sleep during drinking include suppressed rapid eye movement (REM) sleep, increased time spent (%) in stages 3 and 4 of the non-REM (NREM) sleep, prolonged sleep latency, and decreased total sleep time. Both NREM and REM sleep returned to baseline during withdrawal, but sleep latency and total sleep remained disrupted. Most persistent sleep changes during recent abstinence (2–8 weeks) included decreased total sleep time, sleep efficiency, and various degrees of REM sleep disruptions. These sleep changes tend to normalize with maintained abstinence (more than three months) but can persist for years after alcohol cessation. Sleep problems during abstinence can contribute to a relapse to chronic drinking. Changes in both objective (increased proportion of REM sleep during total sleep time, decreased REM latency, increased REM density, decreased stage 4 of NREM sleep, and prolonged sleep latency) and subjective (difficulty falling asleep) sleep measures have been shown to predict relapse (16). Results of several studies found higher prevalence of alcohol abuse in adults with persistent insomnia, suggesting that self-medication of insomnia by alcohol in some people can contribute to the development of alcoholism. Alcohol-dependent patients are more likely to have sleep-disordered breathing and periodic leg movements during sleep than healthy controls (16,17,18).

Sleep problems were shown to correlate with alcohol drinking in adolescents. Reports of subjective day sleepiness were evaluated in 20 adolescents ages 12–19 three years after the initial interview. Frequent alcohol drinking was identified as one of the predictors of chronic day sleepiness in addition to the delayed sleep rhythm, presence of sleep disorders, and frequent medication intake (19).

Effects of alcohol on sleep and wakefulness in infants were studied by D'Angiullu et al. Generalized electroencephalographic (EEG) hypersynchrony was found in all three stages of sleep, with the most significant increases occurring during REM sleep. Both REM and NREM were affected differently depending on the pattern and the timing of alcohol use (occasional, moderate, binge, or chronic). Alcohol exposure during the first trimester caused a decrease in "irregular active sleep" in infants, and alcohol exposure during first and second trimester was associated with increase in arousals (20). Evidence exists that deficits in sleep EEG in infants with prenatal alcohol exposure correlate with impairment in neurocognitive development. Increased EEG power during REM sleep had an inverse relationship with motor development during the first 10 months of life. Increased EEG power during quiet sleep was associated with lower scores on verbal, quantitative, cognitive, and memory measures at ages 4–7 (21). Alcohol remains the main substance of abuse and affects development, behavior, sleep, and overall health in infants, adolescents, and adults.

Tobacco Smoking

Following alcohol, tobacco smoking is the second drug of choice after alcohol for adolescents. In 2006, 21% of 12th graders reported cigarette use during the past month (10). Mathers et al. examined long-term consequences of adolescent tobacco use in the review of 16 published behavioral studies. It was demonstrated that tobacco use in adolescence predicted subsequent social and health problems. There was a strong relationship between tobacco use in adolescence and early adult smoking. Youth smoking also strongly correlated with alcohol initiation and development of alcohol-related problems in adulthood. Authors proposed that tobacco use may contribute to modification of developing brain reward pathways and thus elevate the risk of alcohol use disorders. Social interactions between smoking peers may create opportunities for underage drinking by increasing availability of alcohol in the peer group (22).

It is known that tobacco causes more preventable deaths than any other drug. Increased morbidity among smoking teenagers has been documented. According to the study of health problems in 8040 daily smoking and nonsmoking teenagers ages 13–18, daily smoking among both sexes and all age groups correlated with use of more medications and health services. Smokers reported significantly poorer health and complained of respiratory symptoms, sleep problems, nausea, nervousness, and restlessness. Both boys and girls who smoked daily were 2.6–3.0 times more likely to experience difficulty falling asleep or waking up earlier than nonsmokers (23).

Strong relationships between cigarette smoking and sleep disturbances have been established. Nicotine as a stimulant decreases total sleep time and REM sleep and increases sleep latency. Phillips et al. reported results of a survey completed by 484 smokers, 99 of whom were high school students. Smokers had significant increase in initial and middle insomnia, daytime sleepiness, and minor accidents during the preceding year. Also, smokers were more likely to feel depressed and reported drinking more caffeine than nonsmokers. Authors proposed that poor sleep reported by smoking adolescents may have reflected a tendency to engage in unhealthy behavior in general. Suggestions have been made into inquiring about smoking habits in individuals complaining of sleep difficulties (24). Obstructive sleep apnea (OSA) can be a significant risk for youth who use nicotine, according to J.R. Schrand. Nicotine has a tendency to stimulate breathing and also to reduce somnolence and prevent weight gain due to sleep apnea. It might appeal to youth to smoke to reduce the symptoms of sleep apnea, but the habit of smoking can eventually lead to the development of nicotine dependence. The author proposed that treatment of sleep apnea should be a necessary step for a successful tobacco cessation program in youth (25). Both active and passive smoking can lead to snoring due to initial inflammation and subsequent narrowing of the pharyngeal airway. Habitual snoring can be one of the manifestations of OSA. In the study of 3871 11th graders in Korea, prevalence and correlates of habitual snoring were investigated. Of those who smoked, 13.2% were male students and 9.2% were female students. In addition to increased body mass index (BMI>23) and witnessed apneic events, cigarette smoking was one of the independent risk factors for habitual snoring. Habitual snoring in students contributed to significant decline in school performance in the studied population (26). Patten et al. reported that cigarette smoking and depressed mood were predictors of sleep problems in adolescents. Experimental and frequent smokers with no sleep problems at baseline (age 15) were found to have either occasional or frequent sleep problems at age 18.5. Teenagers who reported sleep problems at baseline had more frequent sleep problems by age 18.5 (27). In addition to adversely affecting general health and sleep patterns, tobacco smoking may also contribute to other sleep-related disorders.

Caffeine

Caffeine is a well known and most widely consumed psychoactive drug readily available to almost anyone. Of the U.S. adult and adolescent population, 75% uses it at least daily, and 98% of 5–18-year-olds consume it at least weekly (28). Many people do not believe caffeine is a drug and are unaware that caffeine dependence may be established with frequent use. In fact, according to The Utah Poison Control Center, caffeine was among the most frequently abused substances from 1991 to 1999 and was the number one abused substance in 1995. During the same time span, 23.4% of 6–19-year-olds, who intentionally abused a substance, abused caffeine (29). Caffeine has been reported to have negative effects on behavior and mood, and has been linked to headaches and increased blood pressure (30,31).

A familiar negative effect of caffeine is disruption of sleep. Caffeine causes cortical arousal by competing with adenosine receptors (32). Karacan et al. showed that caffeine-induced increased sleep latency and awakenings during the night were dose-related (33). In adults, ingestion of 300 mg of caffeine may decrease total sleep time by two hours and increase periods of wakefulness during the night (34).

Caffeine also has effects on "temporal organization" of both REM and NREM sleep (35). Orbeta et al. have shown that higher levels of caffeine intake among adolescents were positively correlated with sleep problems. 15,396 students from grades 6–10 were asked about their caffeine consumption and the number of times they had difficulty sleeping and felt tired in the morning. Students with high caffeine intake were 1.9 times more likely to have difficulty sleeping and were 1.8 times more likely to feel tired in the morning than those students who reported low caffeine intake (36). Pollack et al. asked 191 seventh, eighth, and ninth grade students to keep a two-week diary of their sleep times and caffeine-containing drinks and food. The authors found that higher caffeine intake resulted in shorter nighttime sleep and longer daytime sleep. They also found that those with high caffeine intake had more disturbed sleep and that sleep was more interrupted following a day of high caffeine intake, such as a weekend (35). Caffeine withdrawal after habitual use caused increased feelings of tiredness and being less alert in healthy volunteers, as was shown by James et al. (28).

In addition, taking caffeine in combination with other substances can have more profound effects on sleep. Pronounced insomnia has been observed when caffeine and alcohol were taken together due to the substances' separate half lives and opposite pharmacological actions. Alcohol is metabolized at roughly one unit (one glass of wine) per hour, and caffeine has a half life of five hours. Caffeine's arousal effect may be reversed by alcohol's immediate sedative properties. When the alcohol is completely metabolized, cortical arousal increases, adding to the stimulating effects of caffeine, which may only be half metabolized (32). Keeping in mind that caffeine is easily obtainable through soft drinks that fill the numerous vending machines in our schools, it maybe worthwhile to take a closer look at caffeine's effects on the adolescent population.

Marijuana

Marijuana is the most widely used illicit drug. In 2006, 31.5% of 12th graders reported marijuana use during the previous year and 18.3% of 12th graders reported marijuana use in the past month. The average age of onset is 17.4 years. Of 12th grades, 5% used marijuana daily, and 42% had tried it at least once (1,10). Marijuana use is so common among adolescents that it is perceived by many of them as a normal part of behavior (37). There is a growing body of evidence that marijuana use has significant adverse consequences. Marijuana intoxication causes cognitive impairment, which can extend beyond the acute stage and cause persistent deficits in specific cognitive functioning, especially when marijuana use commences before ages 16 or 17. Early onset cannabis users were shown to have changes in function (impaired attention, verbal learning, working memory, and response inhibition) and structure (smaller brain volume, lower percentage of cortical grey matter, and higher percentage of white matter) of the brain (38). Cognitive deficits were more likely to persist beyond 28 days if cannabis use was initiated before age 17 (39). Solowij et al. proposed that cannabis use can potentially trigger psychotic symptoms in vulnerable individuals and exacerbate schizophrenia symptoms. The authors based this proposal on similarities between cannabis-induced cognitive dysfunction and "cognitive endophenotypes of schizophrenia" (38). In addition to the consequences already mentioned, marijuana affects sleep.

The effects of cannabis extracts on nocturnal sleep, early-morning performance, memory, and sleepiness were evaluated in eight healthy young adults by Nicholson et al. Treatment with 15 mg Delta-9-tetrahydrocannabinol (THC), 5 mg THC in combination with 5 mg cannabidiol (CBD), and 15 mg THC in combination with 15 mg CBD were compared to placebo. Concomitant administration of THC and CBD in both dose ranges caused a decrease in stage 3 sleep with an increase in wakefulness with the higher concentration. While THC alone did not show change in nocturnal sleep, it caused decreased sleep latency, impaired memory, increased sleepiness, and changes in mood the next day (40).

Prenatal marijuana exposure caused significant sleep disruptions in three-year-olds, as was shown by Dahl et al. Eighteen children with prenatal marijuana exposure had significantly more frequent nocturnal arousals, increased awake time after sleep onset, and lower sleep efficiency in comparison to 20 control children (41). Marijuana abstinence symptoms, described by Budney et al. in 12 daily heavy marijuana smokers, included difficulty sleeping and strange dreams during both smoking and abstinence phases (42). Symptoms of cannabis withdrawal were assessed in 72 adolescents ages 14–19 in outpatient treatment by Vandrey et al. In this study, cannabis was the primary drug of abuse with a mean use of 18.1 out of 30 days prior to intake assessment. Of study subjects, 61% were current tobacco smokers, and 49% reported using alcohol at least once during the month prior to treatment. Cravings for marijuana, depressed mood, irritability, and sleep difficulty were among the most frequent symptoms of withdrawal and were of moderate or greater severity in 30% of patients (43).

Despite the widespread notion that marijuana is harmless, it in fact may cause severe cognitive impairments and sleep disruptions.

Narcotics/Prescription Pain Relievers

Recent literature indicates dramatic increase in the non-medical use of pain relievers by adolescents and young adults. In 2006, 4.3% of 12th graders reported the use of Oxycontin. In senior high school, 1 in 10 students (9.7%) used Vicodin. Abuse of over-the-counter cough and cold medicines containing dextromethorphan was experienced by 7% of 12th graders. Heroin use in adolescents has been reported by 0.8% of 12th graders (1,10). Serious concern exists about the use of opioids by teenagers. Exposure to opioids during rapid brain development may lead to yet unknown neurobiological and behavioral consequences, which may significantly differ from those in adults (44). Wu et al. pointed to a new developing pattern of drug use among adolescents. In the study of prevalence of drug use in adolescents ages 12–17, the authors demonstrated that a significant proportion of adolescents used pain relievers non-medically without having used marijuana and/or inhalants first (45). Dependence on alcohol, cocaine, benzodiazepines, and other substances is very common in opioid-dependent patients and contributes to morbidity and social malfunctioning (46).

Opioids have a profound influence on sleep architecture and are suggested to be involved in both sleep initiation and sleep maintenance. Opioid use causes reduction in REM and NREM sleep stages during induction and maintenance of opioid use. Rebound in REM sleep persisted longer than 13 weeks following opioid use (47). Withdrawal from opioids causes insomnia. Central sleep apnea (CSA) has been reported in chronic opioid users. An estimated 30% of patients on methadone maintenance are diagnosed with CSA (48). Occurrence of new patterns of addiction involving prescription pain relievers and significance of opioid use effects on general health and sleep warrant further studies in the adolescent population.

Amphetamines

Stimulant medications such as amphetamine-dextroamphetamine and methylphenidate are well established as effective treatments for Attention Deficit Hyperactivity Disorder (ADHD). Appropriate pharmacotherapy may reduce the risk of future substance use disorders by 85% in ADHD youth (49). However, stimulant medications are known to be diverted and abused. In 2006, 8.1% of 12th graders abused amphetamine and 4.4% of 12th graders abused methylphenidate during the previous year (10). A Drug Abuse Warning Network (DAWN) survey reported 7873 drug-related ED visits that involved methylphenidate or amphetamine-dextroamphetamine in 2004. The rate of visits for patients ages 12–17 was higher than the rate for patients ages 18 or older for both medical and non-medical use. These patients used a higher than prescribed dose or a drug prescribed for another person and evidence of misuse or abuse was present in their medical records. About 68% of ED visits for non-medical use of stimulant medications involved use of other substances (illicit drugs—26%, alcohol—20%, other pharmaceuticals—57%) (50). In the retrospective file review of 450 adolescents treated at the Addiction Centre in Calgary, Alberta, Canada, 23% of adolescents reported non-medical use of methylphenidate or dextroamphetamine at some point in their lives. Of adolescents prescribed stimulant medications, 44% reported non-medical use. Abuse of other substances, school absences, and concurring eating disorders were related to the significantly increased risks for abuse of stimulant medications. The authors suggested the use of non-stimulant medications to treat these higher-risk groups of adolescents (51). Despite their widespread use as therapeutic agents for treatment of ADHD, amphetamines are yet to be studied extensively for their effects on sleep. Nonetheless, EEG sleep changes after administration of a single dose of amphetamine were described by Valverde et al. A single dose of 15 mg of amphetamine was administered in eight obese but otherwise healthy volunteers for seven days. The authors showed that amphetamine increased sleep stage 2 and significantly reduced stages 3 and 4 and REM sleep. Amphetamine withdrawal caused a rebound in REM sleep and prolonged stage 3 of NREM sleep after 24 hours (52). Use of amphetamines is common in treatment of children and adolescents. Because of significant complications of amphetamine misuse and its effects on general well-being, there is need to conduct more studies on long-term consequences of amphetamine use in adolescents.

Inhalants

Inhalants include aerosols containing butane and propane, solvents, and chemicals found in gasoline, spray paints, shoe polish, and glues. They can be easily abused due to their wide availability. In 2006, 9.1% of 8th graders reported using inhalants during the previous year. The average age of first-time users is approximately 15 years (30% of 12–13 year-olds, 39% of 14–15 year-olds, 31% of 16–17 year-olds). Of inhalant users, 35.9% have previously used cigarettes, alcohol, and marijuana (1,10). Neurobiological complications of inhalant use can be serious and include convulsions, encephalopathy, organ failure, blindness, and sudden death. Deaths due to inhalant use are often underreported due to social stigma and a lack of awareness of use. Sleep disturbances have been described during inhalant withdrawal. Shah et al. presented a case report of nine children and adolescents with gasoline abuse by inhalation (mean age was 13.6 years). In addition to sleep problems, withdrawal symptoms included irritability, psychomotor retardation, anhedonia, dry mouth, cravings, and increased lacrimation (53). Due to the potential dangers of inhalant use and the rising numbers of inhalant users, awareness and knowledge about inhalant use in adolescents is very important.

Tranquilizers

Medications from this class include benzodiazepines (BDZ), which are also known as minor tranquilizers. Most commonly abused BDZ are diazepam, alprazolam, and lorazepam. Misuse of minor tranquilizers by adolescents has recently decreased but still remains at significantly high levels. In 2006, 6.6% of senior high school students reported use of tranquilizers during the previous year (10). BDZ use is common in opioid and cocaine abusers and correlates with a history of more severe drug abuse and higher levels of psychological distress. Concomitant use of BDZ, alcohol, and barbiturates is common and can be particularly dangerous in overdose (46) due to the additive sedative properties of these drugs.

BDZ's sedative effect is caused by the inhibitory impact on the brain stem and reticular formation of the brain. Changes in EEG sleep architecture due to BDZ administration consist of depression of REM sleep and stage 4 of NREM sleep. The latter effect of BDZ has significant clinical implications because sleepwalking and night terrors occur during this sleep stage. It has been shown that treatment of night terrors with 15 mg of midazolam in children ages 6–15 leads to increase in total sleep time, decrease in REM latency and nocturnal awakenings, and elimination of night terrors in the majority of cases (54,55). Due to the fact that BDZs have therapeutic value in certain cases and also possess addictive potential, clinical use of these substances should be considered with caution.

Cocaine

Use of cocaine in adolescents remains at high level. In 2006, 5.7% of 12th graders reported cocaine use during the previous year, and 2.1% reported crack cocaine use, which is the most addictive form of cocaine and can be smoked (10). A study of 28 adolescents with cocaine addiction demonstrated a strong connection between heavy cocaine use and youth delinquent behaviors like vandalism and stealing. School dropout and runaway rates were also high. Twenty-one percent of adolescents initiated their cocaine use at age 14, and 54% of study subjects reported weekly cocaine use. Eight weeks after onset, the rate of cocaine use progressed to at least weekly (56). In 479 adolescents ages 14–19, 84% of heavy users reported use of crack cocaine, and 23% used cocaine intravenously. Of heavy cocaine users, 65% progressed to weekly use in less than three months. Rapid progression in frequency of cocaine use in adolescents may indicate its greater addictive potential in adolescents than in adults. Sleep disturbances in cocaine users included sleeplessness and fatigue.

Psychiatric symptoms of dysphoria, suspiciousness, aggressiveness, and suicide attempts progressed as cocaine use increased. More than two thirds of heavy cocaine users reported using cannabis and sedative hypnotics to achieve a calming effect (57).

Sleep disturbances following cocaine administration in adults were described by Johanson et al. The authors evaluated the influence of cocaine on mood and sleep in three volunteers in a controlled environment. Insomnia-like patterns of EEG were seen immediately following cocaine use. The effects included increased sleep latency, decreased sleep efficiency, increased REM latency, and decreased % (time spent) in REM sleep. During the initial abstinence phase, day sleepiness was high and REM latency decreased. Decreased REM latency was not related to depression and remained diminished even after two weeks of abstinence (58). In addition to serious psychosocial and health consequences of cocaine use, it has profound influence on sleep architecture and can lead to permanent sleep alteration.

Club Drugs

Drugs from this class include methamphetamine, MDMA, and others. These drugs are used by teenagers and young adults to maintain energy and to achieve an altered state of consciousness at clubs, parties, and concerts. The term "club drugs" was introduced by The National Institute on Drug Abuse (NIDA) in 2005. It symbolizes the circumstances under which the drugs are used and not their psychotropic effects. Use of club drugs by adolescents is increasing and causes particular concern. Studies have shown that club drug users consume multiple drugs, engage in criminal behaviors, develop substance dependence, and engage in risky sexual behaviors, which include heightened risk of acquiring and transmitting HIV (59,60). In a recent study, Wu et al. investigated trends of club drug use in19,084 youth aged 16–23. Twnety percent of youth reported using at least one club drug in their lifetime. Nearly all club drug users (99%) reported other drug use. Of these, 97–100% used alcohol and marijuana, 63–87% used pain relievers, 45–84% used inhalants, and 35–79% used cocaine (60).

Methamphetamine

This is also known as "speed" or "ice," is inexpensive and can be easily made in clandestine laboratories. In 2006, methamphetamine use was reported by 2.5% of 12th graders (10). McGregor et al. investigated the effect of methamphetamine withdrawal on sleep. In a study of 21 methamphetamine-dependent inpatient adults, the authors described increased total sleep during the acute phase of withdrawal ("crash") and decreased quality of sleep during the sub-acute phase of withdrawal, which was accompanied by increased sleep latency and frequent awakenings during the night. No insomnia was observed following the "crash" period (61).

MDMA (3,4-methylenedioxymethamphetamine)

This also known as ecstasy, is a hallucinogenic stimulant, which in 2006 had been taken by 4.1% of 12th graders (10). Ecstasy targets serotonergic neurons in the brain and acts to release large amounts of serotonin from the neurons very quickly.

Damage to these neurons and depletion of serotonin by MDMA can cause vulnerability to a wide range of long-term neuropsychiatric sequelae, such as sleep disturbance (insomnia), affective dysregulation (depression, anxiety), and cognitive deficits (confusion, impaired memory), especially in adolescents (62). In a study of 12 heavy ecstasy users by Parrott et al., researchers reported significantly elevated scores for paranoid ideation, anxiety, altered appetite, and restless sleep. Authors suggested that these psychobiological problems were caused by reduced serotonin activity due to regular ecstasy use (63). Sleeplessness and bruxism (grinding of teeth) were associated with recreational ecstasy use (64). Recent findings confirmed that even a small amount of ecstasy can be harmful to the brain. According to de Win, low doses of ecstasy in first-time users caused prolonged vasoconstriction in the frontal cortex and increased impulsivity scores when compared to nonusers (65). Use of club drugs in adolescents is becoming a new area of child and adolescent medicine. Extensive research needs to be done to evaluate the effects of club drug use on the physical and emotional health of adolescents.

Anabolic Steroids
Prevalence of anabolic steroid use remains high in adolescents. Of senior high school students, 2.7% reported use of steroids at least once in their lives, and 1.8% of seniors used steroids in 2006 (1,10). Improvement of athletic performance and physical appearance were the main reasons for use (47.1% and 26.7% respectively) (66). Psychiatric consequences of steroid use are numerous and consist of depression, hypomania, rage, anger, unexpected violence, and dependent pattern of use. Unfortunately, there is no clear understanding of underlying biological mechanisms of psychological disturbances due to anabolic steroid use. In an attempt to shed some light on the issue, Daly et al. described the correlation between behavioral symptoms and increased levels of 5-hydroxyindoleacetic acid (5-HIAA) in the cerebrospinal fluid (CSF) of 17 healthy men six days after administration of methyltestosterone. "Activation" symptoms were observed and included increased energy, increased sexual feelings, and diminished sleep. These symptoms positively correlated with increased levels of 5-HIAA in CSF. These preliminary findings identified change in serotonergic function as a potential mechanism of some of the effects of steroid use on behavior and sleep (67). Anabolic steroid use remains a significant health problem in adolescents. Further studies need to be conducted to explore the mechanisms and consequences of steroid-induced psychiatric symptoms.

CONCLUSION
Prevalence of sleep and substance use disorders is high in adolescents. Consequences of unrecognized and untreated disorders of sleep and substance abuse lead to significant health, behavioral, and psychosocial complications not only during adolescence but also later in life. There exists a considerable rate of under-diagnosis of these disorders; also, a lack of understanding of their bidirectional relationships hinders the best treatment options and methods. This is why exploration and counseling about sleep patterns and substance use in youth is very important in medical care. Early screening, assessment, and treatment of both of these disorders during adolescence are essential.

REFERENCES

1. Substance Abuse and Mental Health Services Administration. Results from the 2005 National Survey on Drug Use and Health: National Findings. Office of Applied Studies, NSDUH Series H-30, DHHS Publication No. SMA 06–4194). Rockville, MD, 2006.
2. Mindell JA, Emslie G, Blumer J, et al. Pharmacological management of insomnia in children and adolescents: Consensus statement. Pediatrics 2006; 117(6):1223–32.
3. National Sleep Foundation. 2006 Sleep in America poll. Available at: www. sleepfoundation.org. Accessed 03/10/07.
4. Ivanenko A, Crabtree VM, Gozal D. Sleep in children with psychiatric disorders. Pediatr Clin N Am 2004; 51:51–68.
5. Johnson EO, Breslau N. Sleep problems and substance use in adolescence. Drug and Alcohol Dependence 2001; 64:1–7.
6. Bootzin RR, Stevens SJ. Adolescents, substance abuse, and the treatment of insomnia and daytime sleepiness. Clinical Psychology Review 2005; 25:629–44.
7. Tynjala J, Kannas L, Levalahti E. Perceived tiredness among adolescents and its association with sleep habits and use of psychoactive substances. J Sleep Res 1997; 6(30):189–98.
8. Wong MM, Brower KJ, Fitzgerald HE, et al. Sleep problems in early childhood and early onset of alcohol and other drug use in adolescence. Alcohol Clin Exp Res 2004; 28(4):578–87.
9. Haynes PL, Bootzin RR, Smith L, et al. Sleep and aggression in substance-abusing adolescents: Results from an integrative behavioral sleep-treatment pilot program. Sleep 2006; 29(4):512–20.
10. Johnston LD, O'Malley PM, Bachman JG, et al. Monitoring the future national results on adolescent drug use: Overview of key findings, 2006 (NIH publication No. 07–6202). Bethesda, MD: National Institute on Drug Abuse, 2007.
11. Hingson RW, Heeren T, Winter MR. Age at drinking onset and alcohol dependence. Arch Pediatrics Adolesc Med 2006; 160(7):39–746.
12. Hingson RW, Heeren T, Winter MR. Age of alcohol-dependence onset: Associations with severity of dependence and seeking treatment. Pediatrics 2006; 118(3):e755–63.
13. Brown SA, Tapert SF, Grandholm E, et al. Neurocognitive functioning of adolescents: Effects of protracted alcohol use. Alcohol Clinical Exp Res 2000; 24:164–71.
14. De Bellis MD, Clark D, Beers S, et al. Hippocampal volume in adolescent-onset alcohol use disorders. Am J Psychiatry 2000; 157:737–44.
15. Grunbaum J, Kaun L, Kinchen S, et al. Youth Risk Behavior Surveillance- United States, 2003. MMWR Surveill Summ 2004; 53:1–96.
16. Brower KJ. Alcohol's effects on sleep in alcoholics. Alcohol Res Health 2001; 25(2):110–25.
17. Gillin JC, Smith TL, Irwin M, et al. Increased pressure for rapid eye movement sleep at time of hospital admission predicts relapse in non-depressed patients with primary alcoholism at 3-month followup. Arch General Psychiatry 1994; 51:189–97.
18. Brower KJ, Aldrich MS, Robinson EAR, et al. Insomnia, self-medication, and relapse to alcoholism. Am J Psychiatry 2001; 158:399–404.
19. Saarenpaa-Heikkila O, Laippala P, Koivikko M. Subjective daytime sleepiness and its predictors in Finish adolescents in an interview study. Acta Paediatr 2001; 90(5):552–7.
20. D'Anguinni A, Grunau P., Maggi S, et al. Electroencephalographic correlates of prenatal exposure to alcohol in infants and children: A review of findings and implications for neurocognitive development. Alcohol 2006; 40:127–33.
21. Ioffe S., Chernik V. Prediction of subsequent motor and mental retardation in newborn infants exposed to alcohol in utero by computerized EEG analysis. Neuropediatrics. 1990; 21:11–17.
22. Mathers M., Toumbourou JW, Catalano RF, et al. Consequences of youth tobacco use: A review of prospective behavioral studies. Addiction 2006; 101(7):948–58.
23. Holmen TL, Barrett-Connor E, Holmen J, et al. Health problems in teenage daily smokers versus nonsmokers, Norway, 1995–197: The Nord-Trondelag Health Study. Am J Epidemiol 2000; 15, 51(2):148–55.

24. Phillips BA, Danner FJ. Cigarette smoking and sleep disturbance. Arch Intern Med 1995; 10, 155(7):734–7.
25. Schrand JR. Is sleep apnea a predisposing factor for tobacco use? Med Hypotheses 1996; 47(6):443–8.
26. Shin C, Joo S, Kim J, et al. Prevalence and correlates of habitual snoring in high school students. Chest 2003; 124(5):1709–15.
27. Patten CA, Choi WS, Gillin C, et al. Depressive symptoms and cigarette smoking predict development and persistence of sleep problems in US adolescents. Pediatrics 2000; 106(2):1–9.
28. James JE. Acute and chronic effects of caffeine on performance, mood, headache, and sleep. Neuropsychobiology 1998; 38(1):32–41.
29. Crouch BI, Caravati EM, Booth J. Trends in child and teen nonprescription drug abuse reported to a regional poison control center. Am J Health Syst Pharm 2004; 15, 61(12):1252–7.
30. Millichap JG, Yee MM. The diet factor in pediatric and adolescent migraine. Pediatr Neurol 2003; 28(1):9–15.
31. Savoca MR, MacKey ML, Evans CD, et al. Association of ambulatory blood pressure and dietary caffeine in adolescents. Am J Hypertens 2005; 18(1):116–20.
32. Strading JR. ABC of sleep disorders. Recreational drugs and sleep. BMJ 1993; 27, 306(6877):573–5.
33. Karacan I, Thornby JI, Anch M, et al. Dose-related sleep disturbances induced by coffee and caffeine. Clin Pharmacol Ther 1976; 20(6):682–9.
34. Morgan KJ, Stults VJ, Zabik ME. Amount and dietary sources of caffeine and saccharin intake by individuals ages 5 to 18 years. Regul Toxicol Pharmacol 1982; 2(4):296–307.
35. Pollak CP, Bright D. Caffeine consumption and weekly sleep patterns in US seventh-, eighth- and ninth-graders. Pediatrics 2003; 111(1):42–6.
36. 9.Orbeta RL, Overpeck MD, Ramcharran D, et al. High caffeine intake in adolescents: Associations with difficulty sleeping and feeling tired in the morning. J Adolesc Health 2006; 38(4):451–3.
37. Kandel DB. Marijuana users in young adulthood. Arch Gen Psychiatry, 1984; 41:200–9.
38. Solowij N, Michie P. Cannabis and cognitive dysfunction: Parallels with endopheno-types of schizophrenia? J Psychiatry Neurisci 2007; 32(1):30–52.
39. Pope HG, Gruber AJ, Hudson JI, et al. Early-onset cannabis use and cognitive deficits: What is the nature of the association? Drug Alcohol Dependence 2003; 69(3):303–10.
40. Nicholson AN, Turner C, Stone BM, et al. Effect of Delta-9-tetrahydrocannabinol and cannabidiol on nocturnal sleep and early-morning behavior in young adults. J Clin Psychopharmacology 2004; 4(3):305–13.
41. Dahl RE, Scher MS, Williamson DE, et al. A longitudinal study of prenatal marijuana use. Effects on sleep and arousal at age 3 years. Arch Pediatr Adolesc Med 1995;149(2):145–50.
42. Budney AJ, Hughes JR, Moore BA, et al. Marijuana abstinence syndrome effects in marijuana smokers maintained in their home environment. Arch Gen Psychiatry 2001; 58(10):917–24.
43. Vandrey R, Budney AJ, Kamon JL, et al. Cannabis withdrawal in adolescent treatment seekers. Drug and Alcohol Dependence 2005; 78(2):205–10.
44. Compton WM, Volkow ND. Major increases in opioid analgesic abuse in the United States: Concerns and Strategies. Drug and Alcohol Dependence 2006; 81(2):103–7.
45. Wu LT, Pilowsky WE, Schlenger WE. High prevalence of substance use disorders among adolescents who use marijuana and inhalants. Drug and Alcohol Dependence 2005; 78, 23–32.
46. Backmund M, Meyer K, Henkel C, et al. Co-consumption of benzodiazepins in heroin users, methadone-substituted and codeine-substituted patients. J Addictive Dis 2005; 24 (4):17–29.
47. Kay DC, Eisenstein RB, Jasinski DR. Morphine effects on human REM state, waking state and NREM sleep. Psychopharmacologia 1969; 14, 404–16.

48. Wang D, Teichtahl H. Opioids, sleep architecture and sleep-disordered breathing. Sleep Medicine Review 2007; 11(1):35–46.
49. Biederman J, Wilens T, Mick E, et al. Pharmacotherapy of attention-deficit/hyperactivity disorder reduces risk for substance use disorder. Pediatrics 1999; 104:e20.
50. Substance Abuse and Mental Health Administration, Office of Applied Studies. Drug Abuse Warning Network. The New DAWN Report: Emergency Department Visits Involving ADHD-Stimulant Medications. September, 2006. Available at http://DAWNinfo. samhsa.gov. Accessed 03/2007.
51. Williams RJ, Goodale LA, Shay-Fiddler MA, et al. Methlphenidate and dextroamphetamine abuse in substance-abusing adolescents. Am J Addict, 2004; 13:381–9.
52. Valverde-RC., Pastrana LS, Ruiz JA, et al. Neuroendocrine and electroencephalographic sleep changes due to acute amphetamine ingestion in human beings. Neuroendocrinology 1976; 22(1):57–71.
53. Shah R, Vankar GK, Upadhyaya HP. Phenomenology of gasoline intoxication and withdrawal symptoms among adolescents in India: a case series. Am J Addict 1999; 8(3):254–7.
54. Witek MW, Rojas V, Alonso C, et al. Review of benzodiazepine use in children and adolescents. Psychiatric Quarterly 2005; 76 (3):283–96.
55. Popoviciu L, Corfariu O. Efficacy and safety of midazolam in the treatment of night terrors in children. Brit J of Clin Pharmacology 1983; 16(Suppl):97S–102S.
56. Smith DE, Schwartz RH, Martin DM. Heavy cocaine use by adolescents. Pediatrics 1989; 83(4):539–42.
57. Estroff TW, Schwartz RH, Hoffman NG. Adolescent cocaine abuse. Clinical Pediatrics 1989; 28(12):550–5.
58. Johanson CE, Roehrs T, Schuh K, et al. The effects of cocaine on mood and sleep in cocaine-dependent males. Exp Clin Psychopharmacol 1999; 7(4):338–46.
59. Boyd CJ, McCabe SE, d'Arcy H. Ecstasy use among college undergraduates: gender, race and sexual identity. J Substance Abuse Treatment 2003; 24:209–15.
60. Wu LT, Schlenger WE, Galvin DM. Concurrent use of methamphetamine, MDMA, LSD, ketamine, GHB, and Flunitrazepam among American youth. Drug and Alcohol Dependence 2006; 84(1):102–11.
61. McGregor C, Srisurapanont M, Jittiwutikarn J, et al. The nature, course and severity of methamphetamine withdrawal. Addiction 2005; 100:1320–29.
62. Montoya AG, Sorrentino R, Lukas SE, et al. Long-term neuropsychiatric consequences of 'ecstasy' (NMDA): a review. Harv Rev Psychiatry 2002; 10(4):212–20.
63. Parrott AC, Sisk E., Turner JJ. Psychobiological problems in heavy "ecstasy" (MDMA) polydrug users. Drug and Alcohol Dependence 2000; 1, 60(1):105–10.
64. Baylen CA, Rosenberg H. A review of the acute subjective effects of MDMA/ecstasy. Addiction 2006; 101(7):933–47.
65. de. Win MM, Reneman L, Jager G, et al. A prospective cohort study on sustained effects of low-dose ecstasy use on the brain in new ecstasy users. Neuropsychopharmacology 2007; 32(2):458–70.
66. Buckley WE, Yesalis CE, Fried L, et al. Estimated prevalence of anabolic steroid use among male high school seniors. JAMA 1988; 260:3441–5.
67. Daly RC, SU TP, Schmidt PJ, et al. Cerebrospinal fluid and behavioral changes after methyltestosterone aministration: Preliminary findings. Arch Gen Psychiatry 2001; 58(2):172–7.

27 Overview of Pediatric Psychopharmacology

Sigita Plioplys[a], Jennifer Kurth[a], and Mary Lou Gutierrez[b]

[a]Department of Child and Adolescent Psychiatry, Children's Memorial Hospital and Department of Psychiatry and Behavioral Sciences at Feinberg School of Medicine, Northwestern University, Chicago, Illinois, U.S.A.
[b]Department of Psychiatry, Loyola Medical Center, Maywood, Illinois, U.S.A.

INTRODUCTION

Clinical practice of pediatric psychopharmacology is challenging for several reasons. Over the past 10 years, there has been significant increase in the use of psychotropic medications in the pediatric population. The largest increase was the use of atypical antipsychotics (138.4%), atypical antidepressants (42.8%), and selective serotonin reuptake inhibitors (18.8%) (1). Although treatment with psychotropic drugs is usually managed by a child and adolescent psychiatrist, a large proportion of children receive these medications from primary care doctors and pediatric specialists. Off-label medication use and constantly emerging new Food and Drug Administration (FDA) warnings and regulations issued by medical professional organizations require clinicians to have access and up-to-date training in clinical pharmacology.

The purpose of this chapter is to present an overview of the pharmacology and clinical principles of the most commonly used psychotropic medications in child and adolescent psychiatry. Each pharmacological category contains a significantly larger number of individual medications than are discussed in this chapter, but we selectively chose only those agents that either are approved by the FDA for use in pediatrics or have the most published evidence-based data or clinical experience. Thus, tricyclic antidepressants (TCAs) will not be discussed in this chapter due to their limited use in modern clinical psychiatric practice. Additionally, we discuss practical insights into the pediatric psychopharmacology practice from the child psychiatrist's perspective.

Most psychotropic medications that are effective and/or first line agents in the treatment of pediatric psychiatric disorders do not have FDA indications in the pediatric population. When available, specific information about the FDA indications and warnings is included. For more detailed and up-to-date information on FDA regulations, we refer the reader to the original source at http://www.fda.gov/medwatch/index.html (2). For detailed information on medication formulations, specific dosing strategies, drug–drug interactions and general side effects, please refer to the latest edition of the *Physician's Desk Reference* (3).

MEDICATIONS FOR ATTENTION DEFICIT HYPERACTIVITY DISORDER (ADHD)

Stimulants
Methylphenidate: Ritalin, Ritalin LA, Metadate CD, Concerta, Daytrana
Dexmethylphenidate: Focalin

Amphetamine Sulfate: Dextroamphetamines (Dexedrine), Mixed Amphetamine Salts (Adderall)

Selective Norepinephrine Reuptake Inhibitor
Atomoxetine Hydrochloride (Strattera)

Alpha-2-Adrenergic Agonists
Clonidine (Catapres, Catapres-Transdermal Therapeutic System), Guanfacine Hydrochloride (Tenex)

General Pharmacological Properties
Stimulants block the reuptake of norepinephrine and dopamine into the presynaptic neurons and increase their concentrations in the intrasynaptic space. Methylphenidate (MPH) is a racemic mixture of the *d*- and *l-threo* isomers. The *d*-isomer is more pharmacologically active than the *l*-isomer. Dexmethylphenidate (*d*-MPH) contains only the isolated active *d*-isomer. MPH and *d*-MPH are metabolized in the liver to *d*-ritalinic acid, which is inactive pharmacologically (4). Amphetamines are sympathomimetic amines and they are metabolized in the liver by oxidation to several active metabolites (4).

Atomoxetine increases norepinephrine in the synaptic cleft by inhibiting its presynaptic transporter (5). Atomoxetine is metabolized in the liver by cytochrome P450 enzymes, mostly by CYP2D6 to an active metabolite equipotent to atomoxetine. Children who are CYP2D6 "slow metabolizers" may experience atomoxetine's serum peak concentrations fivefold greater than fast metabolizers (6).

Alpha-2-adrenergic agonists modulate central noradrenergic activity by inhibiting the locus ceruleus and noradrenergic system (4). Guanfacine binds to the alpha 2A receptors more selectively than clonidine. About 50% of clonidine and guanfacine is excreted unchanged in the urine and the remaining 50% is metabolized in the liver. Alpha-2-adrenergic agonists should be used cautiously in patients with renal failure (3).

Indications and Usage
Stimulants have FDA indications for the treatment of ADHD and narcolepsy (2). MPH and *d*-MPH are approved for use in patients at least six years old, amphetamines in children over three years old. For detailed information on the use of stimulant medications in the treatment of ADHD in youths, please refer to the America Academy of Child and Adolescent Psychiatry (AACAP) Practice Parameters (7). Atomoxetine has FDA indication for the treatment of ADHD in individuals at least six years old (2). Atomoxetine's safety and efficacy have not been evaluated in pediatric patients younger than six years of age. Clonidine and guanfacine do not have FDA approval for treatment of any psychiatric disorders.

Major Warnings and Precautions
The FDA issued a Black Box Warning reporting sudden death in children prescribed stimulants (2), therefore stimulants should not be used in patients with

known structural cardiac abnormalities, cardiomyopathy, and serious heart rhythm abnormalities. Temporary slowing in growth has also been found in children medicated with stimulants (8). Administration of amphetamines for a prolonged period of time may lead to drug dependence, as amphetamines have potential for abuse. For atomoxetine, the FDA issued an alert about the increased risk of suicidal ideation in youth treated with this agent (2). Atomoxetine should be used with caution in patients with hepatic and renal impairment, hypertension or other cardiovascular disease, and patients with a history of urinary retention or bladder outlet obstruction. Clonidine and guanfacine are contraindicated in patients with significant cardiovascular diseases, depression, or a family history of a mood disorder (3).

Evidence Based and Clinical Experience

MPH has strong evidence supporting its use as the first line treatment for ADHD. The landmark Multimodal Treatment Study of Children with Attention-Deficit/Hyperactivity Disorder (MTA) was a 14-month multisite trial of four different treatment strategies for 579 children, aged 7–9.9 years (9). MTA compared the following treatments: (a) the fixed-dose of MPH titrated to the child's "best dose," (b) intensive behavioral treatment, (c) combined MPH and intensive behavioral treatment, and (d) standard community care. All four groups improved, but children in the MPH and combination groups improved significantly more than those in the intensive behavior treatment and standard community care groups. Core ADHD symptoms improved equally with the combined and with MPH treatment alone, however the combined therapy provided better outcomes for non-ADHD symptoms (e.g., oppositional and aggressive symptoms).

The Preschool ADHD Treatment Study (PATS) found that immediate-release MPH treatment was significantly more effective than placebo in decreasing ADHD symptoms in children ages 3–5.5 years (10). Statistically but not clinically significant elevations of blood pressure and pulse were associated with MPH treatment in this clinical sample. The most frequently reported adverse events were irritability, difficulty falling asleep, repetitive behaviors/thoughts, and decreased appetite. Moderate to severe adverse events were experienced by 25% to 30% of children receiving the highest total daily doses (15 and 22.5 mg/day) of MPH, compared with 15% to 20% of those on placebo (11).

Only a few studies have examined the long-term safety of stimulant use in pediatric populations (12). In a 15-month longitudinal study, amphetamine sulfate (dose 5 to 35 mg/day) was used in children aged six to 11 years, diagnosed with ADHD. Four boys developed hallucinations; three were receiving amphetamine sulfate and one was on placebo. Hallucinations rapidly ceased upon stopping medication or reducing the dose. Except for decreased appetite in the amphetamine group, there were no other significant differences in adverse effects in both groups.

Atomoxetine is a suggested second line treatment option for ADHD and is most commonly used as a complementary agent to the stimulants (4). A meta-analysis of long-term treatment (=2 years) with atomoxetine reported improvement in ADHD symptom severity in the first month of treatment, with continued improvement throughout the 24 months (13). Twenty-two percent of subjects reported abdominal pain and 21.3% reported decreased appetite. The optimal effective dose of atomoxetine is 1.2–1.3 mg/kg/day, administered once daily. The 1.8 mg/kg/day dose of atomoxetine did not provide any additional benefit.

Comparison studies of the efficacy and safety between stimulants and atomoxetine have been conducted. In a comparative study of dexmethylphenidate (d-MPH) and racemic MPH, d-MPH and MPH were found similarly effective in ADHD control, but d-MPH has a longer duration of action than MPH (14). Several studies compared the safety and efficacy of MPH and Adderall (15–17). Adderall was reported to exhibit longer lasting therapeutic effects than MPH (15,16), but more stomach aches and sad moods. Swanson et al. (16) reported that MPH had a faster onset of clinical effect than Adderall (1.8 hours and three hours respectively). Manos et al. (17) suggested that Adderall is clinically about twice as potent as MPH, as no significant differences in the ADHD symptom control was found in subjects taking optimal doses of MPH (19.5 mg/day) or Adderall (10.6 mg/day). Stimulants were found to be more efficacious in the treatment of ADHD than atomoxetine. OROS MPH (Concerta), and mixed amphetamine salts extended release (Adderall XR) were more effective than atomoxetine (Strattera) due to their extended duration of action and greater therapeutic efficacy (18,19).

Stimulants are available in short (four hour), intermediate (six to eight hour), and long-acting sustained-release (10–12 hour) formulations (3). A short-acting medication may be added to a sustained-release medication in the late afternoon to maintain ADHD symptom control in the evening. It is recommended that stimulants be given seven days per week (20), but patients with decreased appetite, irritability, or sleep problems may discontinue stimulants on weekends and holidays (21). Weight-based dosing guidelines are available, but effective maintenance dose of stimulants is guided by the clinical response and the side effects. For specific guidelines of ADHD management, please see ADHD Pocketcard (22).

For children who have difficulty swallowing pills, an MPH transdermal delivery system Daytrana has recently been approved by the FDA for children ages 6–12 years (23). MPH is delivered continuously while the patch is on and the therapeutic actions of the drug continue for up to two hours after removal. The patch may be removed before nine hours if a shorter duration of action is required or if late day adverse effects appear. Very few children removed the patch prematurely in clinical trials, and those who did had comorbid conduct disorder (23).

Effects on Sleep

Stimulants increase alertness and nocturnal wakefulness, and decrease REM, stage 3 and 4 sleep. Activation of dreaming has also been reported (24). Although parental reports suggest increased sleep difficulties in stimulant-treated children with ADHD compared with unmedicated children, actigraphy and polysomnography evidence do not consistently confirm these problems (25). Atomoxetine may cause insomnia in 16% of patients (4). The alpha agonists are often experienced as sedating medications. They reduce sleep latency, increase sleep maintenance, and decrease REM and stage 3 and 4 sleep (21).

ANTIDEPRESSANTS AND ANTIANXIETY MEDICATIONS

Selective Serotonin Reuptake Inhibitors (SSRIs)

Fluoxetine (Prozac), Sertraline (Zoloft), Citalopram (Celexa), Escitalopram (Lexapro), Fluvoxamine (Luvox), Paroxetine (Paxil)

Selective Serotonin-Norepinephrine Reuptake Inhibitors (SSNRIs)
Venlafaxine Hydrochloride (Effexor), Mirtazapine (Remeron), Duloxetine Hydrochloride (Cymbalta)

Other Antidepressants
Bupropion Hydrochloride (Wellbutrin)

Benzodiazepines (BZDs)
Chlordiazepoxide (Librium), Clonazepam (Klonopin), Diazepam (Valium), Lorazepam (Ativan)

General Pharmacological Properties
Whether classified as antidepressants or antianxiety medications, this group of medications predominantly increases serotonin, but also norepinephrine and dopamine in the neuronal synaptic cleft. Individual SSRIs are unrelated to each other chemically, except escitalopram, which is an isomer of racemic citalopram. Individual SSRI medications differ in their serotonergic selectivity and potency. Citalopram and escitalopram are the most selective serotonergic agents, as they have little or no effect on reuptake of norepinephrine and dopamine (26,27). Paroxetine and sertraline are the most potent serotonin reuptake inhibitors (28). SSNRIs increase intrasynaptic serotonin, norepinephrine and dopamine concentrations. Bupropion does not have any effect on serotonin, but increases norepinephrine and dopamine by blocking their reuptake (29). BZDs potentiate the inhibitory neurotransmitter γ-aminobuteric acid's (GABA) receptors in the brain and decrease neuronal excitability (30).

All antidepressants are metabolized in the liver by CYP450 enzymes, primarily CYP2D6 isoenzyme (31). Compared to adults, children are faster metabolizers and have shorter drug half-lives because of larger liver capacities relative to their body size. About 5% to 10% of children are "slow metabolizers" and may experience 10 to 15 times higher plasma concentrations after a single dose of medication (32). Medications that are metabolized to active metabolites (i.e fluoxetine) may exhibit their clinical effects and drug-drug interactions even after their discontinuation, because active metabolites have longer half-life duration than the parent compound (32).

BZDs are metabolized in the liver mostly by the cytochrome CYP450 3A isoenzyme via oxidation and dealkylation, and/or conjugation (33). CYP3A isoenzyme may be inhibited by certain medications (e.g., fluoxetine, fluvoxamine) or foods (grapefruit juice), which can result in increased BZDs' plasma concentrations causing augmented or prolonged BZDs effects (30). The clearance of diazepam can be reduced by 65% during concomitant administration with fluvoxamine. For this reason, administration of BZDs with fluvoxamine and grapefruit juice should be avoided (30).

Indications and Usage
In the pediatric population, the FDA has approved antidepressants for treatment of only two psychiatric conditions—major depressive disorder (MDD) and

obsessive-compulsive disorder (OCD) (2). Fluoxetine has FDA approval for use in children >8 years of age diagnosed with MDD and in children >7 years diagnosed with OCD, sertraline in children >6 years with OCD, and fluvoxamine in patients >8 years old with OCD (34–36). Remaining antidepressants are used off label and based on available evidence-based data and clinical experience in adults. The FDA has no indications for treatment of psychiatric disorders with BZDs in children (2).

In pediatric clinical practice, SSRIs, SSNRIs, and other antidepressants are widely used for treatment of anxiety disorders, selective mutism, premenstrual dysphoric disorder, posttraumatic stress and eating disorders (4). Bupropion was demonstrated to be effective for treatment of ADHD in several double blind placebo controlled studies (37). SSRIs are suggested as the first line agents for treatment of mood and eating disorders, with the SSNRIs and bupropion used as second line agents when SSRIs fail or are not effective (4). BZDs may be used as hypnotics and anxiolytics for short-term treatment of transient insomnia and anxiety (30), specifically during the initial treatment period with SSRIs, which may take 6–12 weeks for sufficient antidepressant/anxiolytic response.

Major Warnings and Precautions

In 2004, the FDA issued a Black Box warning regarding a twofold increased risk of suicidal thinking and behaviors in the pediatric population during the first months of treatment with antidepressants (4%) compared to placebo (2%) (38,39). Recently, a meta-analysis of 27 randomized, placebo-controlled trials of second-generation antidepressants in youth with mood and anxiety disorders was published (40). This study concluded that treatment with antidepressants provides much greater benefits than the risks from suicidal ideations and behaviors. The FDA has issued the antidepressant monitoring guidelines, which require weekly visits during the first month of treatment, and specific documentation of patient's mood, sleep, activation, suicidality, functional impairment, treatment response, and side-effects (39). Once the patient is stable, subsequent visits can be reduced to every two weeks for the following two months. An FDA-approved medication guide must be distributed to the families of children when dispensing a prescription of an antidepressant. Medication guides are available at http://www.fda.gov/cder/Offices/ODS/medicationguides.htm.

The major contraindication for use of second-generation antidepressants is concurrent administration with monamine oxidase inhibitors (MAOIs). SSRIs should be administered with caution in patients with impaired liver function (35). The contraindications for BZD use are pre-existing central nervous system (CNS) depression, narrow-angle glaucoma, and severe hypotension (3). As a precaution, BZDs should not be prescribed in large quantities for patients with suicidal tendencies, substance abuse disorders, with chronic pulmonary insufficiency, or sleep apnea (30).

Potentially fatal serotonin syndrome (agitation, confusion, hallucinations, hyper-reflexia, myoclonus, shivering, and tachycardia) may occur with concomitant use of serotonergic drugs (i.e., SSRIs/SNRIs, triptans, MAOIs, MAOI-like effects (i.e., linezolid), or with medications that impair SSRI metabolism (3). Specific warnings regarding increased seizure risk associated with the high doses of bupropion have been reported (41). Treatment with SSRIs may produce activation of mania or hypomania in susceptible patients, thus screening for risk of bipolar disorder is important prior to starting antidepressants (32).Treatment with BZDs is very limited in the pediatric population due to the possibility of paradoxical activation associated with hyperactivity, agitation, and aggression (30).

The BZD's withdrawal symptoms (i.e., anxiety, perceptual changes, seizures, insomnia, trembling, sweating, palpitations, dry mouth) may occur during the treatment and on the first day after discontinuation of the BZDs with short half-life (42). The onset of withdrawal from BZDs with a longer half-life can occur up to five days after its discontinuation. The severity of BZD withdrawal symptoms does not appear to correlate with the duration of drug taper (43). In general, a taper of SSRIs over a two to three week period is a safe recommendation to prevent dysphoria, anxiety, confusion, and dizziness that may follow withdrawal of treatment.

Evidence Based and Clinical Practice Experience

A large body of evidence supports the efficacy and safety of antidepressants in the treatment of pediatric mood and anxiety disorders. The multi-center Treatment Adolescent Depression Study (TADS) compared the efficacy of treatment with fluoxetine alone (10 to 40 mg/d), cognitive behavioral therapy (CBT) alone, CBT with fluoxetine (10 to 40 mg/d), and placebo (44). Combined treatment of fluoxetine and CBT was the most efficacious.

Recently, a meta-analysis was published of all available randomized clinical trials (27 studies, total of 4751 participants 19 years old) for second generation antidepressant treatment of MDD, OCD, and other anxiety disorders (40). The evidence for antidepressant treatment efficacy was found for all three clinical indications. The strongest effects were reported for the anxiety disorders, intermediate effects for OCD, and modest for MDD. Analysis of MDD studies found the pooled rates of response to treatment in 61% of patients receiving antidepressants and in 50% of those on placebo. For the OCD group, the pooled rates of response were found in 52% SSRI treated patients and in 32% receiving placebo. For other, non-OCD anxiety disorders, pooled rates of response were 69% in the antidepressant-treated group and 39% in the placebo group.

Effects on Sleep

The effects of SSRIs on sleep vary amongst agents (32). In children treated with fluoxetine, increased stage 1 sleep, the frequency of awakenings, REM latency, and suppression of REM sleep have been reported (45). Mirtazapine has a higher degree of sedation compared to all other antidepressants (32). Treatment with bupropion has caused insomnia in 11% to 20% of patients (32).

All BZDs have similar hypnotic potential, but vary in duration and potency. BZDs affect sleep architecture, increase the amount of stage 2 sleep, and duration of sleep, however it is not associated with feeling rested in the morning (30). During treatment with BZDs, the number of REM cycles increases, but the duration of cycles are shorter, thus the total REM time is decreased. BZDs suppress stage 4 sleep and may prevent night terrors. After discontinuation of BZDs, REM sleep may increase and a transitory period of vivid dreaming may occur (46). Patients taking BZDs with a relatively short half-life may experience rebound insomnia and develop tolerance to the hypnotic effect. BZDs with a longer half-life may produce residual daytime sleepiness, as the BZDs' concentrations and their metabolites gradually increase with chronicity of use (47).

ANTIPSYCHOTIC DRUGS

Typical (First Generation)
Haloperidol (Haldol), Chlorpromazine (Thorazine), Thioridazine (Mellaril)

Atypical (Second Generation)
Clozapine (Clozaril), Risperidone (Risperdal), Olanzapine (Zyprexa), Quetiapine (Seroquel), Ziprasidone (Geodon), Aripiprazole (Abilify)

General Pharmacological Properties
The antipsychotic effects of neuroleptic medications may be related to a decrease of dopamine levels in the neurons (48). Antipsychotics are classified based on their specific effects on dopamine receptors. The typical antipsychotics block postsynaptic dopamine (D_2) receptors and presynaptic dopamine autoreceptors. It is thought that extrapyramidal side effects and hyperprolactinemia are caused by D_2 blockade (49,50). In addition to dopamine receptors, the atypical antipsychotics (AAs) have affinity to a broader range of neuroreceptors, which determines their specific clinical characteristics (49,51). AAs with strong affinity to serotonin receptors (i.e., risperidone, ziprasidone, olanzapine) provide both antipsychotic and mood stabilizing effects. Clozapine is the most selective and potent AA due to its unique abilities to block dopamine (D_2) and (D_4) receptors as well as several serotonin receptors ($5\text{-}HT_{2A,\ 6,7}$) (49).

Antipsychotics are metabolized in the liver mostly by CYP450 system and also by hydroxylation, oxidation, demethylation, and conjugation (49). Haloperidol is well absorbed from the GI tract, but undergoes a significant first-pass metabolism (52). After oral intake, haloperidol's peak plasma concentration occurs within two to six hours. Following intramuscular administration, peak plasma concentration occurs after 10–20 minutes and peak pharmacologic action occurs within 30–45 minutes (53). This is an important factor to consider while selecting treatment intervention for acutely agitated patients.

Indications and Usage
AAs have a significantly safer side effect profile than typical antipsychotics, therefore, AAs are primarily used for treatment of psychiatric disorders. The use of typical antipsychotics is mostly reserved for acute or short-term treatment of aggression, delirium, or when treatment with AA fails. Until recently, there have been no FDA approved indications for use of AAs in patients 18 years old (2). Only risperidone has recently gained an FDA indication for treatment of irritability in Autistic Disorder in children ages 5–16 years (2). In clinical practice, AAs are suggested as first choice medications for childhood onset schizophrenia, other psychotic conditions, and Autistic disorder (4). Additionally, AAs are used for treatment of motor and vocal tics in Tourette's disorder, mood stabilization, short-term treatment of aggression, and delirium (54). Clozapine is indicated for the treatment of severe, treatment-resistant psychosis, although safety and efficacy of clozapine have not been established in children younger than 16 years of age (49). Risperidone, quetiapine, and olanzapine have indications for the management of

schizophrenia and the short-term treatment of acute manic or mixed episodes of Bipolar I disorder (54).

Major Warnings and Precautions

Potentially fatal agranulocytosis associated with the use of clozapine has been reported in 5% to 40% of adolescents (55); therefore this agent is indicated only for patients who have failed treatment with at least two other antipsychotics. Mandatory white blood cell counts should be monitored weekly for six months, then biweekly thereafter. Treatment should be discontinued if the WBC decreases 3000. Low-potency conventional antipsychotic agents and clozapine appear to be associated with the highest risk of seizures in children, therefore baseline electroencephalography (EEG) is recommended prior to starting treatment (54).

Antipsychotics are contraindicated for patients with severe cardiovascular abnormalities, such as ventricular tachycardia, QT prolongation, and arrhythmias, including torsade de pointes (PDR.net). Prior to treatment with all antipsychotics, baseline electrocardiogram (ECG) is recommended. If the QT_c interval exceeds 500 msec, typical antipsychotics should be discontinued. Thioridazine and ziprasidone are associated with the greatest risk of QT_c prolongation, although the correlation between the QT_c prolongation and ziprasidone's dose has not been clarified (56,57).

Neuroleptic malignant syndrome (NMS) is one of few known psychiatric emergencies and is associated with high mortality rate (5–20%) (58). NMS is characterized by acute onset of hyperthermia, muscle hypertonicity, altered mental status, autonomic instability, increased serum creatine kinase, rhabdomyolysis, and acute renal failure. NMS usually occurs early in the course of treatment with antipsychotics or with the dose increase. For more information, the reader is directed to the NMS Information Service (1-888-NMS-TEMP or www.nmsis.org).

Young age is a significant risk factor for the development of extrapyramidal side effects (EPS), which may be acute or chronic (49). Pool et al. (59) reported that about 70% of adolescents receiving treatment with typical antipsychotics developed EPS. Acute EPS are dystonic reactions, akathisia, and parkinsonian symptoms. Chronic EPS include tardive dyskinesia and dystonia. Acute dystonic reactions (spastic contractions of discrete muscle groups in the neck, face or extraocular muscles) develop acutely, but generally respond well to treatment with an anticholinergic agent (e.g., benztropine, trihexyphenidyl) or discontinuation of antipsychotic. Prophylaxis with an anticholinergic agent to prevent EPS may be considered for young patients, especially males (60). Akathisia is an inner sense of motor restlessness, inability to sit still, and sometimes insomnia. It usually subsides with treatment of low-dose propranolol or a benzodiazepine. Tardive dyskinesia (protrusion of the tongue, puffing of cheeks, chewing) usually occurs after prolonged treatment with antipsychotics, but in children this may occur following abrupt discontinuation of the antipsychotics (60). The risks of developing tardive dyskinesia and its irreversibility increase with the duration of treatment and cumulative dose of antipsychotic agent. Tardive dystonia is characterized by prolonged spastic muscle contractions and is associated with distress and physical discomfort.

Endocrinological side effects, such as increased serum prolactin in adult patients have been mostly associated with typical antipsychotics and to a lesser degree with AAs (61). Galactorrhea may develop in approximately 1–5% of adult patients and menstrual cycle changes (oligomenorrhea) in up to 20% of women treated with typical agents (61). Modest hyperprolactinemia was reported in children receiving olanzapine (61). Long-term effects of hyperprolactinemia in children are not known, but it may negatively affect further sexual development, fertility, maturation, and cause osteoporosis (62,63).

Weight gain occurs with all antipsychotic agents, although AAs seem to cause a greater increase than typical agents (64). The highest weight gain is associated with clozapine and olanzapine, closely followed by risperidone (49,64). Ziprasidone and aripiprazole are marketed as producing less weight gain, but studies in children are lacking to support this claim. Before starting treatment, baseline liver function test, fasting glucose, lipid profile, cholesterol, and triglyceride levels should be obtained and repeated every three months. During maintenance treatment with AAs, it is recommended not only to regularly monitor weight but also educate patients about the potential development of metabolic syndrome, type II diabetes, cardiovascular illness, and hypercholesterolemia.

Evidence Based and Clinical Practice Experience

There are only a few randomized controlled studies that provide evidence for use of antipsychotics in children. Only two controlled studies have been published on the use of typical antipsychotics in adolescents with schizophrenia (59,65). Both studies reported improvement of positive psychotic symptoms and higher rates of EPS and sedation, compared to placebo. In a comparison study, clozapine was significantly superior to haloperidol in treatment-resistant adolescents with childhood-onset schizophrenia (55). Comparison studies of risperidone, olanzapine, and haloperidol in adolescents with psychotic disorders reported that each of the three treatments produced significant clinical improvements, and risperidone was less sedating than olanzapine and haloperidol (66).

Risperidone was found to be effective and safe in the short-term treatment of children with autistic disorder, compared to placebo (67). Significant improvements in tantrums, aggression, self-injurious behavior, stereotypic behavior, and hyperactivity were noted in a risperidone-treated group of children with autism. Increased appetite, fatigue, dizziness, and drooling were significantly more frequent in the risperidone-treated group than in the placebo group, however the risk–benefit ratio was found favorable in this study.

Effects on Sleep

In general, sedation associated with treatment with antipsychotics is the second most common side effect. It may result from histamine receptor blockade. All antipsychotics decrease sleep onset latency, increase total sleep time and day time sedation (54). Clozapine may initiate immediate onset of REM after falling asleep and intensify dreams or nightmares may cause insomnia.

MOOD STABILIZERS

Lithium Carbonate
(Lithobid, Eskalith)

Antiepileptic drugs (AEDs)
Divalproex Sodium (Valproic Acid, Depakote, Depakene), Carbamazepine (Tegretol, Carbatrol, Equetro, Epitol), Oxcarbazepine (Trileptal), Lamotrigin (Lamictal), Topiramate (Topamax), Gabapentin (Neurontin)

General Pharmacological Properties
The mechanisms underlying lithium's mood stabilizing properties are complex and involve the second messenger system (68). Lithium blocks the activity of phospho-inositol (PI) (69) and inhibits cyclic adenosine monophosphate (cAMP) (70) intra-cellularly, which results in stabilization of neuronal excitation. Lithium and valproic acid may have neuroprotective effects due to regulation of glutamate excitotoxicity, activation of brain-derived neurotrophic factors, and mitogen-activated protein kinases (69,71). Lithium is not metabolized and 95% of its single dose is excreted by the kidneys (72). Compared to adults, children have higher lithium clearance and a shorter half life, thus serum steady-state (within five to eight days of treatment) and therapeutic levels can be reached quicker (68).

All AEDs exhibit modulating effects on the inhibitory (GABA) and/or excita-tory (glutamate) amino acids by blocking sodium, calcium and potassium channels, and stabilizing hyperexcited neural membranes (68). Most AEDs undergo a com-plete or near complete absorption when given orally, which may be significantly delayed by high fat meals. AEDs are metabolized in the liver by the CYPP450 system, mitochondrial ß-oxidation, hydroxylation and/or conjugation (73). Children have 50% higher clearance and shorter half-life of the AEDs than adults, thus doses have to be larger (mg/kg) than in adults (72). divalproex sodium (DVPX), carbamazepine (CBZ), and oxcarbazepine are metabolized to active metabolites then excreted by the kidneys. Gabapentin undergoes no metabolism and is excreted unchanged by the kidneys. CBZ is the only AED that produces induction of its own metabolism. Autoinduction stabilizes over three to five weeks at a fixed dose, therefore the dose titration should take over four weeks (72). For detailed discussion on the CYP450 mediated drug interactions with the AEDs, the reader is referred to Flockhart and Oesterheld's review of the subject (74).

Indications and Usage
Lithium and DVPX have FDA indications for treatment of acute manic episodes and maintenance therapy of bipolar disorder (BPD) in patients >12 years (lithium) and DVPX (patients>18 years) (72), and have been suggested as first line treatment for BPD in youth (75). In adults, CBZ, oxcarbazepine, and lamotrigine are indicated for acute and maintenance treatment of BPD type 1. CBZ is less potent compared to lithium and DVPX thus is often used as a third line medication for mood stabiliza-tion in rapid cycling mania and should be reserved for patients that failed treatment with lithium and DVPX (76,77). Lamotrigine is considered to be an alternative to first line maintenance therapies in the management of the rapid cycling BPD type 2, and may be more effective in preventing depressive than manic episodes (76).

Additionally, lithium, DVPX, CBZ, and oxcarbazepin are broadly used for treatment of irritability, impulsivity, and aggression, particularly reactive subtype (affect driven, explosive) in children and adolescents with disruptive behavioral disorders (77). Topiramate has a limited use for mood stabilization and control of aggression (72). Gabapentin is an anxiolytic and may be used as adjunctive in treatment of OCD, social phobia, and panic disorders (72).

Major Warnings and Precautions

Lithium
Contraindications for its use are significant renal and cardiovascular diseases, dehydration, hyponatremia, co-administration of diuretics and/or angiotensin converting enzyme (ACE) inhibitors. Symptoms of lithium toxicity (diarrhea, vomiting, tremor, ataxia, muscular weakness, arrhythmia, bradycardia, flattening or inversion of T-waves, drowsiness, coma) are closely related to high serum lithium levels (>3.5 mEq/L in12 hours after ingestion), but can occur at therapeutic levels as well (72). The most common side effects of lithium are gastrointestinal symptoms, polyuria, polydipsia, enuresis and fatigue (78). The most common CNS side effect is the fine hand tremor observed early in the treatment. Ataxia, choreoathetosis, EPS, slurred speech, blurred vision, psychomotor retardation, and seizures may develop upon toxic lithium serum levels. Osmotic diarrhea may occur due to decreased intestinal absorption of glucose and water, and may result in dehydration (72). Approximately 25% of patients experience a decrease in renal-concentrating ability during maintenance therapy and may develop nephrogenic diabetes insipidus (72). Sodium ion depletion results in lithium retention by the kidneys, potentially leading to toxicity. Lithium has a potent negative effect on the developing endocrine system and may cause euthyroid goiter and/or hypothyroidism (including myxedema) accompanied by lower T3 and T4 levels. Cardiac effects may result from lithium displacing potassium and causing reversible T-wave depression with therapeutic serum lithium levels (78). Lithium has teratogenic effects and causes Ebstein's anomaly. Baseline complete blood cell count (CBC) with differential, TSH, chemistry panel, pregnancy test, and ECG are mandatory, and monitoring of serum lithium levels, thyroid stimulating hormone, blood urea nitrogen (BUN) and creatinine at least every six months during maintenance treatment is recommended.

AEDs
DVPX can cause severe hepatotoxicity, including fatal hepatic failure, and young age (<2 years old) is a significant risk factor (68). The most common side effects are gastrointestinal symptoms, weight gain, drowsiness, and hair loss. Rare, but serious side effects include pancreatitis, thrombocytopenia, and polycystic ovaries (78). CNS side effects may range from mild irritability and somnolence to hyperamonemic encephalopathy (68). DVPX has teratogenic effects on embryo producing neural tube defects (72). Baseline CBC with differential, chemistry panel, including liver function tests (LFTS), and pregnancy test, are recommended prior to starting treatment. Monitoring serum DVPX levels, LFTs, and platelets at least every six months during maintenance treatment is recommended. The most common side effects associated with CBZ are transient leukopenia, rash, dizziness, diplopia, and headaches, although aplastic anemia and agranulocytosis have been reported (78). Thus baseline CBC with differential and pregnancy tests are suggested, with regular monitoring during maintenance treatment. Lamotrigine's side effects include dizziness, atacuia, somnolence, headache, blurred vision, GI symptoms, and rash, which can

progress to Stevens Johnson syndrome (78). The most common topiramate's side effects are weight loss, word-finding difficulties, poor concentration, and sedation, but case reports of renal calculi, depression, anxiety, and psychosis have been reported (78). Gabapentin produces somnolence, dizziness, ataxia, and nystagmus (78). DVPX, CBZ, and topiramate induce hepatic microsomal enzyme system and increase the metabolism of vitamin D, which impairs absorption of Ca, leading to decreased bone mineralization in healthy children, who received these med for >6 mos (77).

Evidence Based and Clinical Practice Experience

In a community based study of the medication use among youth with BPD, DVPX was found to be the most commonly used mood stabilizer (79%), followed by lithium (51%) and gabapentin (29%) (79).

Lithium has been consistently found to be effective in the acute treatment of mania with treatment response ranging from 42% to 68% (80,81). In youth, lithium is also effective in maintenance treatment of BPD. In an 18 month naturalistic prospective study of 37 adolescents stabilized on lithium, 92% of those who discontinued treatment with lithium experienced relapse compared to 38% of those continuing treatment (82). Lithium has also demonstrated effectiveness for treatment of both BPD and comorbid substance dependence disorders (83). Lithium may have protective effects against suicidality and relapse of BPD which may reduce future affective episodes (77). Lithium has been found to be more effective than placebo and similar to haldol (84) in the treatment of aggression in several placebo-controlled studies of the inpatient youth with conduct disorder (85). The recommended dose of lithium in youth is 30 mg/kg/day with therapeutic serum levels of 0.6–1.2 mEq/L (78).

DVPX has been effective in mood and behavioral stabilization of youths with a strong family history of BPD (86) and in those with mixed states of BPD (87). The recommended dose is 10–20 mg/kg/day with therapeutic serum levels >50 ug/mL (78). The response rate for treatment with DVPX in acute mania was reported from 46% to 83%, based on the various response criteria used (81,86). DVPX has demonstrated significant improvement compared to placebo in the number of temper outbursts, improvement in impulse control and mood swings in adolescents with oppositional defiant and conduct disorders (88).

In comparison studies, DVPX and lithium demonstrate similar efficacy in acute and maintenance treatment of BPD in youth (86), but DVPX is more effective than lithium in the treatment of mixed BPD states in youth (87). Other studies found comparable efficacy and response rates to treatment with DVPX (46%), lithium (42%), and CBZ (34%) (81). Data on the efficacy of OXBZ (89), gabapentine (90) and lamotrigine (91) in treatment of pediatric BPD are encouraging, but come from small case reports and open label studies, thus reports on topiramate's mood stabilizing effects are inconclusive (92).

Effects on Sleep

Lithium has chronopharmacological effects and lengthens the period of the circadian rhythms leading to a phase delay of circadian rhythms in adults with bipolar disorder and normal controls (93,94).

AEDs' effects on sleep result from their modulation of inhibitory and excitatory amino acids in the brain. AEDs with GABA-ergic properties (i.e., DVPX, CBZ, oxcarbazepine) have sedating effects; those that inhibit glutamate (i.e., lamotrigine) may produce activation, and AEDs with mixed mechanism of action (i.e., topiramate) may produce both sedating and activating effects on sleep. DVPX treatment has been associated the normalization of REM distribution during the night and stabilization of the sleep cycle. DVPX may produce mild sedation and increase in stages 3 and 4 sleep, but does not affect REM sleep (95). Many of the other AEDs delay REM onset or decrease the percent of time spent in REM sleep, improve sleep continuity, increased total sleep time and decrease fragmentation (95). CBZ decreases sleep latency and increases stages 3 and 4 sleep (95–97). It decreases REM density, but has no effect on REM latency or percentage. Gabapentin improves sleep and decreases awakenings by increasing the amount of time in stages 3 and 4 of sleep, decreasing the amount of stage 1 of NREM sleep, and increases the percentage and mean duration of REM sleep (98). Lamotrigine increases in the percentage of REM sleep from 8.5% to 13.6% with a decrease in the fragmentation of REM sleep (98). Lamotrigine and gabapentin may have stabilizing effects on sleep independently from their anticonvulsant effect.

REFERENCES

1. Martin A, Leslie D. Trends in psychotropic medication costs for children and adolescents, 1997–2000. Arch Pediatr Adolesc Med 2003; 157:997–1004.
2. http://www.fda.gov/medwatch/index.html (accessed May, 2007).
3. http://www.pdr.net (accessed April 2007).
4. Green WH, ed. Child and Adolescent Clinical Psychopharmacology, 4th edition. Philadelphia: Wolters Kluwer/Lippincott Willliams & Wilkins, 2007.
5. Spenser T, Biederman J, Wilens T, et al. Effectiveness and tolerability of atomoxetine in adults with attention deficit hyperactivity disorder. Am J Psychiatry 1998; 155:693–5.
6. Wernicke JF, Kratochvil CJ. Safety profile of atomoxetine in the treatment of children and adolescents with ADHD. J Clin Psychiatry 2002; 63(12):50–5.
7. Greenhill LL, Pliszka S, Dulcan MK, et al. American Academy of Child and Adolescent Psychiatry practice parameter for the use of stimulant medications in the treatment of children, adolescents, and adults. J Am Acad Child Adolesc Psychiatry 2002; 41(2 Suppl):26S–49S.
8. Swanson J, Greenhill L, Wigal T, et al. Stimulant-related reductions of growth rates in the PATS. J Am Acad Child Adolesc Psychiatry 2006; 45(11):1304–12.
9. MTA Cooperative Group, Moderators and mediators of treatment response for children with attention-deficit/hyperactivity disorder (ADHD), Arch Gen Psychiatry 1999; 56:1088–96.
10. Kollins SH, Greenhill LL, Swanson J, et al. Rationale, design, and methods of the Preschool ADHD Treatment Study (PATS). J Am Acad Child Adolesc Psychiatry 2006; 45(11):1275–83.
11. Wigal T, Greenhill LL, Chuang S, et al. Tolerability and safety of methylphenidate in preschool children with ADHD. J Am Acad Child Adolesc Psychiatry 2006; 45(11):1294–303.
12. Gillberg C, Melander H, von Knorring A, et al. Long-term stimulant treatment of children with attention-deficit hyperactivity disorder symptoms: A randomized, double-blind, placebo-controlled trial. Arch Gen Psychiatry 1997; 54(9): 857–64.
13. Kratochvil CJ, Wilens TE, Greenhill LL, et al. Effects of long-term atomoxetine treatment for young children with attention-deficit/hyperactivity disorder. J Am Acad Child Adolesc Psychiatry 2006; 45(8):919–27.

14. Wigal S, Swanson JM, Feifel D, et al. A double-blind, placebo-controlled trial of dexmethylphenidate hydrochloride and d,l-threo-methylphenidate hydrochloride in children with attention-deficit/hyperactivity disorder. J Am Acad Child Adolesc Psychiatry 2004; 43(11):1406–14.
15. Pliszka SR, Browne RG, Olvera RL, et al. A double-blind, placebo-controlled study of Adderall and methylphenidate in the treatment of attention-deficit/hyperactivity disorder. J Am Acad Child Adolesc Psychiatry 2000; 39(5):619–26.
16. Swanson JM, Wigal S, Greenhill LL, et al. Analog Classroom Assessment of Adderall® in Children with ADHD. J Am Acad Child Adolesc Psychiatry 1998; 37(5):519–26.
17. Manos MJ, Short EJ, Findling RL. Differential effectiveness of methylphenidate and Adderall in school-age youth with attention-deficit/hyperactivity disorder. J Am Acad Child Adolesc Psychiatry 1999; 38(7):813–19.
18. Kemner JE, Starr HL, Ciccone PE, et al. Outcomes of OROS® methylphenidate compared with atomoxetine in children with ADHD: A multicenter, randomized prospective study. Advances in Therapy 2005; 22:498–512.
19. Wigal SB, McGough JJ, McCracken JT, et al. A laboratory school comparison of mixed amphetamine salts extended release (Adderall XR) and atomoxetine (Strattera) in school-aged children with attention deficit/hyperactivity disorder. J Atten Disorder 2005; 9:275–89.
20. Dulcan M. Practice parameters for the assessment and treatment of children, adolescents, and adults with attention-deficit/hyperactivity disorder. J Am Acad Child Adolesc Psychiatry 1997; 36(9):85S–121S.
21. Martins S, Tramontina S, Polanczyk G, et al. Weekend holidays during methylphenidate use in ADHD children: A randomized clinical trial. J Child Adolesc Psychopharm 2004; 14(2):195–206.
22. http://www.myguidelines.com (accessed April 2007).
23. Pataki C, Suddath R. Transdermal methylphenidate: Patch designed for flexible, long-acting coverage. Current Psychiatry 2006; 5:95–101.
24. Mindell J, Owens J, Carskadon M. Developmental features of sleep. Child Adolesc Psychiatric Clin N Am 1999; 8(4):695–717.
25. Cohen-Zion M, Ancoli-Israel S. Sleep in children with attention-deficit hyperactivity disorder (ADHD): A review of naturalistic and stimulant intervention studies. Sleep Medicine Reviews 2004; 8(5):379–402.
26. Willetts J, Lippa A, Beer B. Clinical development of citalopram. J Clin Psychopharmacol 1999; 19(Suppl 1):36–46S.
27. Forest Pharmaceuticals, Inc. Lexapro® (escitalopram oxalate) tablets/oral solution prescribing information. St. Louis, MO; 2006 Sep.
28. Sanchez C, Hyttel J. Comparison of the effects of antidepressants and their metabolites on reuptake of biogenic amines and receptor binding. Cell Mol Neurobiol 1999; 19:467–89.
29. Cooper BR, Wang CM, Cox RF, et al. Evidence that the acute behavioral and electrophysiological effects of bupropion (Wellbutrin®) are mediated by a noradrenergic mechanism. Neuropsychopharmacology 1994; 11:133–41.
30. Barnett SR, Riddle MA. Anxiolytics: benzodiazepines, buspirone, and others. In: Martin A, Scahill L, Charney DS, Leckman JF, eds Pediatric Psychopharmacology: Principles and Practice. New York: Oxford University Press, 2003: pp. 341–50
31. Michalets EL. Update: clinically significant cytochrome P-450 drug interactions. Pharmacotherapy 1998; 18(1):84–112.
32. Chiu S, Leonard H. Antidepressants I: selective serotonin reuptake inhibitors. In: Martin A, Scahill L, Charney DS, Leckman JF, eds Pediatric Psychopharmacology. New York: Oxford University Press, 2003: pp. 274–83
33. Rall TW. Hypnotics and sedatives; ethanol: benzodiazepines and management of insomnia. In: Gilman AG, Rall TW, Nies AS eds Goodman and Gilman's The Pharmacological Basis of Therapeutics. 8th edn, New York: Pergamon Press, 1990: pp. 346–370.

34. Wagner KD, Ambrosini PJ. Childhood depression: Pharmacological therapy/treatment. J Clin Child Psychol. 2001; 30(1):88–97.
35. Committee on Safety of Medicines. Selective serotonin reuptake inhibitors (SSRIs): overview of the regulatory status and CSM advise relating to major depressive disorder (MDD) in children and adolescents including a summary of available safety and efficacy data [online]. Available from URL: http://medicines.mhra.gov.uk/ourwork/monitor-safetqualmed/safetymessages/ssrioverview_101203.pdf
36. Bridge JA, Iyengar S, Salary CB, et al. Clinical response and risk for reported suicidal ideation and suicidal attempts in pediatric antidepressant treatment. A meta-analysis of randomized controlled trials. JAMA 2007; 297:1683–96.
37. Barrickman LL, Perry PJ, Allen AJ, et al. Bupropion versus methylphenidate in the treatment of attention deficit hyperactivity disorder. J Am Acad Child Adolesc Psychiatry 1995; 34(5):649–57.
38. Hammad TA, Laughren T, Racoosun J. Suicidality in pediatric patients treated with antidepressant drugs. Arch Gen Psychiatry 2006; 63:332–9.
39. US Food and Drug Administration. Relationship between psychotropic drugs and pediatric suicidality: review and evaluation of clinical data. http://www.fda.gov/ohrms/dockets/ac/04/briefing/2004-4065b1-10-TAB08-Hammads-Review.pdf
40. Bridge JA, Iyengar S, Salary CB, et al. Clinical response and risk for reported suicidal ideation and suicidal attempts in pediatric antidepressant treatment. A meta-analysis of randomized controlled trials. JAMA 2007; 297:1683–96.
41. Van Wyck Fleet J, Manberg PJ, Miller LL, et al. Overview of clinically significant adverse reactions to bupropion. J Clin Psychiatry. 1983; 44(5, Sect 2):191–6.
42. Hobbs WR, Rall TW, Verdoorn TA. Hypnotics and sedatives; ethanol. In: Hardman JG, Limbird LE, Molinoff PB, Ruddon RW, Gilman AG, eds Goodman & Gillman's The Pharmacological Basis of Therapeutics, 9th edn New York: McGraw-Hill, 1996: pp. 361–396.
43. Rickels K, Case WG, Schweizer E, et al. Benzodiazepine dependence: Management of discontinuation. Psychopharmacol Bull 1990; 26:63–8.
44. March J, Silva S, Petrycki S, et al. Treatment for Adolescents with Depression Study (TADS) Team. Fluoxetine, cognitive-behavioral therapy, and their combination for adolescents with depression: Treatment for Adolescents with Depression Study (TADS) randomized controlled trial. JAMA 2004; 292(7):807–20.
45. Armitage R, Emslie G, Rintelmann J. The effect of fluoxetine on sleep EEG in childhood depression: A preliminary report. Neuropsychopharmacology 1997; 17:241–45.
46. Emslie GJ, Rush AJ, Weinberg WA, et al. A double blind, randomized, placebo-controlled trial of fluoxetine in children and adolescents with depression. Arch Gen Psychiatry 1997; 54:1031–7.
47. Shader RI, Greenblatt DJ. Use of benzodiazepines in anxiety disorders. N Engl J Med 1993; 328:1398–405.
48. Meltzer HY, Matsubara S, Lee LC. Classification of typical and atypical antipsychotic drugs on the basis of dopamine D1, D2 and serotonin2 pKi values. J Pharmacol Exp Ther 1989; 25:238–46.
49. Findling RL, McNamara NK, Gracious BL. Antipsychotic agents: traditional and atypical. In: Martin A, Scahill L, Charney DS, Leckman JF, eds. Pediatric Psychopharmacology: Principles and Practice. New York: Oxford University Press, 2003: pp. 328–40.
50. Nordstrom AL, Farde L. Plasma prolactin and central D2 receptor occupancy in antipsychotic drug-treated patients. J Clin Psychopharmacol 1998; 18:305–10.
51. Borison RL, Pathiraja AP, Diamond BI, et al. Risperidone: clinical safety and efficacy in schizophrenia. Psychopharmacol Bull 1992; 28:213–18.
52. Forsman A, Ohman R. Pharmacokinetic studies on haloperidol in man. Curr Ther Res 1976; 20:319–36.
53. Vasavan-Nair NP, Suranyi-Cadotte B, Schwartz G, et al. A clinical trial comparing intramuscular haloperidol decanoate and oral haloperidol in chronic schizophrenic patients: efficacy, safety, and dosage equivalence. J Clin Psychopharmacol 1986; 6(Suppl):30–7S.

54. Findling RL, Steiner H, Weller EB. Use of antipsychotics in children and adolescents. J Clin Psychiatry 2005; 66(Suppl 7):29–40.
55. Kumra S, Frazier JA, Jacobson LK, et al. Childhood-onset schizophrenia: a double-blind clozapine-haloperidol comparison. Arch Gen Psychiatry 1996; 53:1090–7.
56. Giles TD, Modlin RK. Death associated with ventricular arrhythmia and thioridazine hydrochloride. JAMA 1968; 205:108–10.
57. Blair J, Scahill L, State M, et al. Electrocardiographic changes n children and adolescents treated with ziprasidone: a prospective study. J Am Acad Child Adolesc Psychiatry 2005; 44(1):73–9.
58. Silva RR, Munoz DM, Alpert M, et al. Neuroleptic malignant syndrome in children and adolescents. J Am Acad Child Adolesc Psychiatry 1999; 38(2):187–94.
59. Pool D, Bloom W, Mielke DH, et al. A controlled evaluation of loxitane in seventy-five adolescent schizophrenic patients. Curr Ther Res Clin Exp 1976; 19:99–104.
60. McClellan J, Werry J. The Work Group on Quality Issues. Practice parameter for the assessment and treatment of children and adolescents with schizophrenia. J Am Acad Child Adolesc Psychiatry 2001; 40(Suppl 7):4–23S.
61. Wudarsky M, Nicolson R, Hamburger SD, et al. Elevated prolactin in pediatric patients on typical and atypical antipsychotics. J Child Adolesc Psychopharmacol 1999; 9:239–45.
62. Becker D, Liver O, Mester R, et al. Risperidone, but not olanzapine, decreases bone mineral density in female premenopausal schizophrenia patients. J Clin Psychiatry 2003; 64: 761–6.
63. Dunbar F, Kusumakar V, Daneman D, et al. Growth and sexual maturation during long-term treatment with risperidone. Am J Psychiatry 2004; 161:918–20.
64. Fedorowicz VJ, Fombonne E. Metabolic side effects of atypical antipsychotics in children: a literature review. J Psychopharmacology 2005; 19:533–77.
65. Realmuto GM, Erickson WD, Yellin AM, et al. Clinical comparison of thiothixene and thioridazine in schizophrenic adolescents. Am J Psychiatry 1984; 141:440–2.
66. Sikich L, Hamer RM, Bashford RA, et al. A pilot study of risperidone, olanzapine, and haloperidol in psychotic youth: a double-blind, randomized, 8-week trial. Neuropsychopharmacology 2004; 29:133–45.
67. McCracken JT, McGough J, Shah B, et al. Risperidone in children with autism and serious behavioral problems. New Engl J Med 2002; 347(5):314–21.
68. Danielyan A, Kowatch RA. Management options for bipolar disorder in children and adolescents. Pediatr Drugs 2005; 7(5):277–94.
69. Manji HK, Chen G PKC. MAP kinases and the bcl-2 family of proteins as long term targets for mood stabilizers. Mol Psychiatry 2002; 7(Suppl.1):S46–56.
70. Lenox RH, Hahn CG. Overview of the mechanism of action of lithium in the brain: Fifty year update. J Clin Psychiatry 2000; 61:5–15.
71. Nonaka S, Hough CJ, Chuang DM. Chronic lithium treatment robustly protects neurons in the central nervous system against excitotoxicity by inhibiting N-methyl-D-aspartate receptor-mediated calcium influx. Proc Nat Acad Sci USA 1998; 95:2642–7.
72. AHFS (American Hospital Formulary Service). Bethesda, MD: American Society of Health System Pharmacists, Inc., 2000.
73. Willmore, JL. A brief description of new AEDs. Neurology 2000, (55; Suppl 3), S18–24.
74. Flockhart DA, Oesterheld JR. Cytochrome P450-mediated drug interactions. Child Adolesc Psychiatr Clin North Am 2000; 9:43–76.
75. Kowatch RA, Fristad M, Birmaher B, et al. Treatment guidelines for children and adolescents with bipolar disorder. J Am Acad Child Adolesc Psychiatry 2005; 44:213–35.
76. American Psychiatric Association. Practice guideline for the treatment of patients with bipolar disorder (revision). Am J Psychiatry 2002; 159(Supp l): 1–50.
77. Lopez-Larson M, Frazier JA. Empirical evidence for the use of lithium and anticonvulsants in children with psychiatric disorders. Harv Rev Psychiatry 2006; 14(6): 285–304.

78. Davanzo P, McCracken J. Mood stabilizers: Lithium and anticonvulsants. In: Martin A, Scahill L, Charney DS, Leckman JF, eds. Pediatric Psychopharmacology: Principles and practice. New York: Oxford University Press, 2003: pp. 309–27.
79. Bhangoo RK, Lowe CH, Myers FS, et al. Medication use in children and adolescents treated in the community for bipolar disorder. J Child Adolesc Psychopharmacol 2003; 13:515–22.
80. Kafantaris V, Coletti DJ, Dicker R, et al. Lithium treatment of acute mania in adolescents: A large open trial. J Am Acad Child Adolesc Psychiatry 2003; 42:1038–45.
81. Kowatch RA, Suppes T, Carmody T, et al. Effect size of lithium, divalproex sodium, and carbamazepine in children and adolescents with bipolar disorder. J Am Acad Child Adolesc Psychiatry 2000; 39:713–20.
82. Strober M, Morrell W, Lampert C, et al. Relapse following discontinuation of lithium maintenance therapy in adolescents with bipolar illness: A naturalistic study. Am J Psychiatry 1990; 147:457–61.
83. Geller B, Cooper T, Sun K, et al. Double-blind placebo controlled study of lithium for adolescent bipolar disorders with secondary substance dependency. J Am Acad Child Adolesc Psychiatry 1998; 37:171–8.
84. Campbell M, Adams PB, Small AM, et al. Lithium in hospitalized aggressive children with conduct disorder. Arch Gen Psychiatry 1984; 41:650–6.
85. Malone RP, Delaney MA, Luebbert JF, et al. A double-blind placebo-controlled study of lithium in hospitalized aggressive children and adolescents with conduct disorder. Arch Gen Psychiatry 2000; 57:649–54.
86. Chang KD, Dienes K, Blasey C, et al. Divalproex monotherapy in the treatment of bipolar offspring with mood and behavioral disorders and at least mild affective symptoms. J Clin Psychiatry 2003; 64:936–42.
87. Pavuluri MN, Dove HB, Carbray JA, et al. Divalproex sodium for pediatric mixed mania: A 6-month open prospective trial. Bipolar Disord 2005; 7:266–73.
88. Steiner H, Petersen ML, Saxena K, et al. Divalproex sodium for the treatment of conduct disorder: A randomized controlled clinical trial. J Clin Psychiatry 2003; 64:1183–91.
89. Davanzo P, Nikore V, Yehya N, et al. Oxcarbazepine treatment of juvenile-onset bipolar disorder. J Child Adolesc Psychopharmacol 2004; 14:344–5.
90. Hamrin V, Bailey K. Gabapentin and methylphenidate treatment of a preadolescent with attention deficit disorder and bipolar disorder. J Child Adolesc Psychopharmacol 2001; 11:301–9.
91. Carandang CG, Maxwell DJ, Robbins DR. Lamotrigin in adolescent mod disorders. J Am Acad Child Adolesc Psychiatry 2003; 42:750–1.
92. DelBello MP, Findling RL, Kushner S, et al. A pilot controlled trial of topiramate for mania in children and adolescents with bipolar disorder. J Am Acad Child Adolesc Psychiatry 2005; 44:539–47.
93. Campbell M, Adams PB, Small AM, et al. Lithium in hospitalized aggressive children with conduct disorder: A double blind, and placebo controlled study. J Am Acad Child Adolesc Psyhiatry 1995; 34:445–53.
94. Klemfuss H. Rhythms and the pharmacology of lithium. Pharmacol Ther 1992; 1:53–78.
95. Declerck AC, Wauquier A. Influence of antiepileptic drugs on sleep patterns. In Degen R, Rodin EA, eds. Epilepsy, sleep and sleep deprivation, 2nd edn Amsterdam: Elsevier, 1991: pp. 235–9.
96. Obermayer WH, Benca RM. Effects of drugs on sleep. Neurol Clin 1996; 14:827–40.
97. Riemann D, Gann H, Bahro M, et al. The effects of carbamazepine on endocrine and sleep EEG variables in a patient with a 48 hour rapid cycling and healthy controls. Neuropsychobiology 1993; 27:163–70.
98. Placidi F, Diomedi M, Scalise A, et al. Effect of anticonvulsant on nocturnal sleep in epilepsy. Neurology 2000; 54(Suppl 1):S25–32.

28 Sleep and Obesity in Children

Riva Tauman

Sleep Disorders Center, Dana Children's Hospital, Tel Aviv Medical Center, Tel Aviv University, Tel Aviv, Israel

INTRODUCTION

The prevalence and severity of obesity in children and adolescents are dramatically increasing worldwide (1,2). The Center of Disease Control and Prevention (CDC) reports a rapid fourfold rise in child and adolescent obesity (ages 6–19) over the past 20 years (3). Thus, in parallel to the increase in obesity secular trends among the adult population, excessive ponderal indices currently affect 15–17% of all children and adolescents, with figures steadily rising (4). Concomitant with the increase in the prevalence of obesity, our society is facing a progressive reduction in sleep duration. Over the past 40 years, sleep duration of Americans has decreased significantly. Curtailment of sleep duration has become a widespread habit and a hallmark of modern society (5–7). Evidence suggests that short sleep duration and sleep disruption have a deleterious impact on glucose metabolism and appetite regulation and are associated with increased risk of obesity.

The increase in both the prevalence of obesity and its severity has also translated into a corresponding increase in the prevalence of obesity-associated morbidities, such as type 2 diabetes mellitus and insulin resistance, dyslipidemia, systemic hypertension, atherosclerosis and ischemic heart disease, non-alcoholic fatty liver/steatohepatitis, psychosocial complications and decreased quality of life, as well as obstructive sleep apnea syndrome (OSAS) and the obesity hypoventilation syndrome (8–11).

The short- and long-term morbid consequences of obesity stress the importance of increasing the public awareness to this problem, and prioritization of the overweight child and adolescent as a major public health concern and as an emergency. Indeed, we have increasingly become aware that many of the morbidities associated with obesity that have traditionally been viewed as problems of adults actually originate in childhood and adolescence.

OSAS may represent an important mechanism underlying the association between obesity and metabolic and cardiovascular morbidities through potentiation of inflammatory cascades. It is expected that the increased prevalence of obesity in children and adolescents in our society and worldwide will be accompanied by a steady increase in the incidence of OSAS. Indeed, the classic presentation of children with OSAS as underweight children with adenotonsillar hypertrophy is being substantially replaced by more and more patients being overweight (12).

OBSTRUCTIVE SLEEP APNEA SYNDROME

OSAS in children is characterized by recurrent events of partial or complete upper airway obstruction during sleep, resulting in disruption of normal gas exchange (intermittent hypoxia and hypercapnia) and sleep fragmentation (13). The clinical spectrum of obstructive sleep-disordered breathing includes OSAS, the upper airway resistance syndrome (UARS; traditionally associated with rather normal oxygenation patterns, but evidence for increased respiratory-related arousals, i.e., sleep fragmentation). At the low end of this spectrum, a condition that has been termed either primary or habitual snoring (i.e., habitual snoring in the absence of apneas, gas exchange abnormalities, and/or disruption of sleep architecture) and represents a relatively more benign manifestation of increased upper airway resistance during sleep. The usual nighttime symptoms and signs of OSAS in children include snoring, noisy breathing, snorting episodes, paradoxical chest and abdominal motion, retractions, witnessed apnea, difficulty breathing, cyanosis, sweating and restless sleep. Daytime symptoms can include mouth breathing, difficulty waking up, moodiness, nasal obstruction, daytime sleepiness, hyperactivity, and cognitive problems. More severe cases of OSAS may be associated with pulmonary hypertension and cor pulmonale, systemic hypertension, failure to thrive, developmental delay, and in extreme cases sudden unexpected death. The prevalence of OSAS in children is currently estimated at up to 3% among 2–8-year-old children (14,15). However, habitual snoring during sleep, the hallmark indicator of increased upper airway resistance is much more frequent in children and may affect up to 27% of children (16–18).

The pathophysiological mechanisms underlying the occurrence of obstructive sleep apnea are in many aspects quite different from those involved in adult OSAS. In the latter, OSAS is primarily, albeit not exclusively, associated with obesity, whereas the vast majority of cases of OSAS in children are due, at least to some extent, to enlarged tonsils and adenoids. The current understanding of childhood OSAS supports the existence of dynamic imbalance in upper airway function, whereby the combination of alterations in structural and anatomical characteristics, protective reflexes and neuromotor abnormalities of the upper airway are all implicated to a greater or lesser degree in any given particular child. Several reports suggest that pediatric OSAS may be more common in those children with family history of OSAS, children with allergy, children born prematurely, in African–American children, and in children with chronic upper and lower respiratory tract diseases (19–23).

OBESITY AS A RISK FACTOR FOR OSAS

The compelling evidence derived from the adult literature indicates that obesity is a risk factor for OSAS. In the pediatric population, overweight children are at increased risk for developing sleep-disordered breathing and the degree of OSAS is proportional to the degree of obesity (19, 24–29).

In the initial descriptions of OSAS in the modern era, Guilleminault and colleagues reported that 10% of 50 children who were diagnosed with OSAS were obese (24). Mallory and colleagues showed the presence of polysomnographic abnormalities in 24% of 41 obese children (27). Similarly, Silvestri and colleagues found evidence for partial airway obstruction in 66% and complete airway obstruction in 59% of the 32 obese children (28). In a case-control study design, Redline and colleagues examined risk factors for sleep disordered breathing in children aged 2–18 years, and found that the risk among obese children was increased four- to fivefold (19). In fact, for every increment in body mass index (BMI) by 1 kg/m^2 beyond the mean BMI for age and gender, the risk of OSAS increased by 12%. Similar trends demonstrating an increased risk of OSAS among obese and overweight children have been reported from all over the world (29–36). However, all of the above studies were performed on children who were referred for possible OSAS and therefore the prevalence of OSA may have been over estimated. When the prevalence of sleep disordered breathing was examined in the general obese population, 46% of obese children and adolescents showed evidence of abnormal polysomnographic findings and 27% had moderate to severe respiratory abnormalities during sleep (25). In addition, a positive correlation between obesity and apnea index and an inverse relation between obesity and oxygen saturation nadir were found (25). In another study from Singapore, 33% of obese children had OSAS (36), while in extremely overweight adolescents meeting eligibility criteria for bariatric surgery, polysomnographic findings compatible with the diagnosis of OSAS were found in 55% of patients (37).

Hence, childhood obesity is definitely associated with a higher risk for development of OSAS, with the wide difference in the prevalence rates among the various studies being related to a number of factors, namely, ethnic predisposition and different diagnostic criteria for OSAS and obesity. Moreover, most of the studies performed thus far had small sample sizes, thereby supporting the need for a prospective, well controlled large-scale assessment such as to shed light on the association between obesity and OSAS.

Adenotonsillar hyperplasia/hypertrophy is not always the main contributing factor to the development of OSA in obese children (25,38,39). Upper airway narrowing may also result from fatty infiltration of upper airway structures, while subcutaneous fat deposits in the anterior neck region and other cervical structures will also exert collapsing forces promoting increased pharyngeal collapsibility (40–42). Moreover, obesity can affect ventilation through mass loading of the respiratory system (43). Increased adipose tissue in the abdominal wall and cavity as well as surrounding the thorax increases the global respiratory load, and reduces intra-thoracic volume and diaphragm excursion, particularly when in the supine position (44), all of which may result in decreased lung volumes and oxygen reserve, while increasing the work of breathing during sleep (43).

In a series of recent studies involving both adult patients and rodent models, the potential role of leptin as an endocrine-mediated link between obesity, metabolic dysfunction, and sleep-disordered breathing has begun to emerge. Obesity is associated with peripheral and central leptin resistance, which in turn leads to relatively ineffective elevation of circulating leptin levels (45–48). The reduced bioavailability of leptin has been implicated in diminished hypercapnic responses (49), and in mechanisms underlying alveolar hypoventilation in obesity (50–53). Leptin is a potent respiratory stimulant, which in addition to its central chemoreceptor modulatory properties, appears to affect overall ventilatory drive (54–56), as well as influence overall peripheral chemoreceptor activity (57). Thus, in the context of obesity contributions to the emergence of sleep-disordered breathing in children, the role of adipokines in general, and more particularly that played by leptin, in the pathophysiology of upper airway dysfunction and altered ventilatory responses to increased upper resistance will require further investigation.

MORBIDITIES ASSOCIATED WITH OSAS: THE ROLE FOR OBESITY

While the clinical presentation of a child with OSA is usually vague and requires increased awareness of the primary care physician, the implications of OSA in children, especially obese, are broad and sometimes complex. If left untreated or alternatively if treated late, pediatric OSA may lead to substantial morbidity that affects multiple target organs and systems, and that may not be completely reversible with appropriate treatment, if the latter is instituted late. OSA in children can lead to behavioral disturbances and learning deficits, cardiovascular morbidity, compromised somatic growth, as well as decreased quality of life and depression.

NEUROBEHAVIORAL CONSEQUENCES

One of the now well established, long-term consequences of OSA in children is behavioral and neurocognitive morbidities. Schooling problems have been repeatedly reported in case series of children with OSA, and in fact may underlie more extensive behavioral disturbances such as restlessness, aggressive behavior, excessive daytime sleepiness and poor schooling (58–63) Furthermore, compelling evidence to support a causative association between OSA and hyperactivity and inattentive behaviors in children has emerged in the last two decades (64–71). In addition, daytime sleepiness, hyperactivity, and aggressive behaviors have all been documented in children who snore, even in the absence of OSA (72–74). As would be predicted from a mechanistic association, objectively measured sleep and respiratory disturbances were found to be relatively frequent among children with attention-deficit/hyperactivity disorder (ADHD)-like behaviors (75–77). However, the exact mechanisms by which OSA elicits hyperactivity and inattention remain unknown. It is possible that the sleep fragmentation and episodic hypoxia that characterize OSA lead to alterations within the neurochemical substrate of the prefrontal cortex with resultant executive dysfunction (78). Indeed, similar to adults, snoring children were found to perform poorly on measures of "executive functioning," i.e., the ability to develop and sustain an organized, future oriented and flexible approach to problem solving (79). Although overt excessive daytime sleepiness is not very common in children, it is more prominent among obese children (80). Furthermore, the manifestations of excessive daytime sleepiness differ in children compared to adults, such that both inattention and hyperactivity constitute behavioral correlates of sleepiness in younger patients. In a recent study examining the magnitude of sleep fragmentation induced by sleep disordered breathing in children, it was found that a numerical score, termed sleep pressure score, correlated with both cognitive and behavioral disturbances occurring in snoring children, independent from the degree of hypoxemia (81,82).

As a corollary to the above findings, improvements in learning and behavior have been reported following treatment for OSA in children (59,83–86), and suggest that the neurocognitive and behavioral deficits are at least partially reversible (87).

What about obesity and intellectual development? In a large study of 11,000 children attending kindergarten, overweight children had significantly lower math and reading scores compared to non-overweight children (88). In another large scale study on 7th–11th graders, obese children were more likely to be held back a grade and to consider themselves as poor students (89). Moreover, obesity at the age of 14 years was associated with lower school performance at age 16, and a lower level of education persisting until at least age 31 (90). Full scale IQ and performance IQ of obese children were found to be significantly lower compared to normal weight children in a study in China (91). Furthermore, an increased prevalence of behavioral and learning difficulties has been observed among children who are gaining weight rapidly (92). Although it is possible that obesity is a marker rather than a cause of low academic performance (88), and that mental health problems (low self esteem and depression) may predispose children both to increased weight gain and to lower school performance, we need to consider that both obesity and OSA are inflammatory diseases (93–95), and as such could potentiate each other in their downstream morbid effects. Indeed, Rhodes and colleagues showed that obese children with obstructive sleep apnea had substantial deficits in learning, memory, and vocabulary compared to obese non-apneic children, and that apneic/hypopneic events were inversely related to memory and learning performance in the entire sample (96). Unfortunately, this study was restricted to only 14 subjects, so that confirmation of either the additive or synergistic effects of obesity and OSA on end-organ related morbidities will have to await more extensive studies in the future.

QUALITY OF LIFE AND DEPRESSION

Obese children may be at risk for significant psychological distress. Obese children are more likely to display low self esteem and to suffer from higher rates of anxiety disorders, depression and other psychopathologies (97–99). These mental health conditions may be mediating factors for an overweight child to score poorly in school. Severely obese children and adolescents report many more missed school days than the general student population (100). Similarly, significant associations between obesity and depressive symptoms in childhood and later psychopathology in adulthood have been reported (101,102). Adults who had been diagnosed with clinically defined major depression during their youth had a greater BMI than adults who did not suffer from depression during their youth (103). Goodman and collegues examined 9374 adolescents in grades 7–12 and found that elevated BMI was related to depression at one year of follow up (104). Depressive overweight children may respond poorly to weight management programs, and are therefore in need of psychological treatment, in addition to strict weight-management programs (105,106).

Moreover, obese children will manifest a lesser quality of life when compared not only to non-obese children but also to children with chronic health conditions such as asthma or atopic dermatitis (107). In fact, children with morbid obesity report extreme reductions in their health-related quality of life (HRQOL), and their HRQOL scores are in fact similar to those of children with cancer (108).

The parallel between obesity and OSAS is further stressed by the findings that childhood OSA also leads to significant decreases in quality of life (109–113), and that quality of life scores will improve following adenotonsillectomy (111). In a recent study, Crabtree and colleagues have shown that snoring children are at higher risk for decreased HRQOL and for the presence of depressive symptoms, and that both of these appear to be unrelated to the presence of obesity (114). It is likely that the sleep disturbance associated with snoring increases fatigue, and that with increasing fatigue, snoring children will experience increased irritability, depressed mood, impaired concentration, and decreased interest in daily activities. These impairments in daily functioning may in turn interfere with other aspects of the child's life, including their relationships with family, school, and peers. Thus, a vicious cycle may develop and lead to more impaired global quality of life and to the presence of more depressive symptoms. Moreover, it is possible that some children with an underlying propensity for depression may develop overt clinical symptoms of this disorder if OSA is concurrently present. Thus, among the multiple morbidities associated with obesity, respiratory-related sleep disturbances may play an important role in further adversely affecting the already challenged and vulnerable well-being of an obese child.

CARDIOVASCULAR CONSEQUENCES

Childhood obesity is the leading cause of pediatric hypertension (115). Systolic blood pressure correlates positively with BMI, skinfold thickness, and waist-to-hip ratios in children and adolescents (116). In findings emanating from the Bogalusa Heart longitudinal cohort study, increased insulin and glucose levels in heavier children and adolescents were found as risk factors for increased left ventricular mass (117). Moreover, increasing evidence points to the occurrence of early endothelial dysfunction in obese children. Carotid intimal medial thickening, development of early aortic and coronary arterial fatty streaks and fibrous plaques and alteration of mechanical properties of the abdominal aorta have all been described in obese children (118,119). All of these early findings are known to increase the risk of myocardial infarction, stroke and other cardiovascular complications, and can be readily reversed following targeted interventions such as diet and exercise (120,121).

While genetic, metabolic, and hormonal factors such as insulin resistance or increased serum aldosterone levels have all been linked to the cardiovascular consequences of obesity, all of those studies did not consider the potential presence of OSAS and its contribution to such complications. Similar to obesity, pediatric OSAS has been associated with a higher risk for cardiovascular morbidity. Indeed, increased prevalence of systemic hypertension (122–124), alterations in blood pressure regulation (125), and changes in cardiac geometry (126,127), have been reported in children with OSAS, and have been ascribed, at least in part, to the presence of sustained sympathetic activation during both daytime and nighttime, as well as to increased sympathetic reactivity (128–130), and endothelial dysfunction (131,132). Parenthetically, when intermittent hypoxia exposures were conducted in postnatal rats during their sleep period, significant alterations in both the regulation of sympathetic responses and in baroreflex activity were found in adulthood, well after cessation of the intermittent hypoxic exposures, thereby suggesting that younger children with OSAS may be at increased risk for long-lasting vascular consequences if left untreated or if their treatment is delayed (133,134). The endothelial dysfunction associated with OSAS is most likely the result of initiation and propagation of inflammatory responses within the microvasculature (135). Indeed and similar to adults, plasma concentrations of C-reactive protein (CRP), an important circulating marker of inflammation and one of the best predictors for future cardiovascular morbidity, were found to be elevated in children and adolescents with OSAS, and to correlate with the severity of the OSAS independent of obesity (136,137). Of note, elevations of specific adhesion molecules that reflect endothelial dysfunction such as soluble P-selectin are frequently found in children with OSAS (132).

Since the prevalence of OSAS is higher in obese children, and since obesity constitutes one of the major risk factors for cardiovascular morbidity, it will be important to ensure that cardiovascular-related disease mechanisms thought to be secondary to obesity, are not in fact a consequence of OSAS in obese individuals. Furthermore, studies on the reversibility of cardiovascular complications following resolution of OSAS in obese children are needed, considering that significant decreases in CRP occur in non-obese children with OSAS after they are treated (138).

In addition to the systemic vascular effects of OSAS, the frequent oxygen desaturations during sleep that occur in children with more severe disease will result in sustained elevations of pulmonary artery pressures as a consequence of repetitive hypoxia-induced pulmonary vasoconstriction. Such elevations in pulmonary artery pressures may, potentially lead to *cor pulmonale*. While pulmonary hypertension is probably more frequent than predicted from the customary clinical assessment performed during the initial evaluation of the snoring child, the exact prevalence of this complication is unknown (139,140).

INSULIN RESISTANCE, TYPE 2 DIABETES AND METABOLIC SYNDROME

Over the past decade, an alarming increase in the prevalence of type 2 diabetes mellitus in children has been noted, and while in the past type 2 diabetes was a disease that occurred almost exclusively in adults, in recent years type 2 diabetes has surpassed type 1 diabetes to become the most frequent endocrine disorder affecting glucose homeostasis in children (141). Although universal screening is not yet recommended, the American Academy of Pediatrics and the American Diabetes Association recommended that all youngsters who are overweight and have at least two other risk factors should be tested for diabetes and insulin resistance beginning at age 10 years or at the onset of puberty and every two years thereafter (142). Insulin resistance is considered to be the greatest risk factor for the development of type 2 diabetes mellitus, and therefore provides an early intervention point for prevention of the disease and its consequences.

The term "metabolic syndrome," a known risk factor for cardiovascular disease in adults, refers to the clustering of insulin resistance, dyslipidemia, hypertension, and obesity. Although no clear cut definition of the metabolic syndrome has been agreed upon for the pediatric age group (143), the overall prevalence of the metabolic syndrome among 12–19-year-old children in the U.S. was found to be 4.2%, when using adult criteria (144). Using modified criteria, Weiss and colleagues found that the risk of the metabolic syndrome was nearly 50% in severely obese youngsters and risk increased with every 0.5 unit increment in BMI (converted to a Z score) (145). Elevation of fasting insulin levels and increased BMI during childhood emerged as the strongest predictors of the metabolic syndrome in adulthood (146,147). Moreover, insulin resistance in childhood is associated with an increased risk for later cardiovascular morbidity and mortality (148–150).

Similar to obesity, sleep-disordered breathing has been identified as an important risk factor for the metabolic syndrome in adult patients (151–154). Indeed, adults with OSAS share many features with the metabolic syndrome including systemic hypertension, central obesity, and insulin resistance. However, while several reports have found OSAS to be an independent predictor of insulin resistance, i.e., after controlling for BMI (155,156), this association was not confirmed by other reports (157,158), and the effect of treatment with continuous positive airway pressure (CPAP) on the metabolic disturbances associated with OSAS has yielded conflicting results (159–162).

In children, there are only three studies that have thus far examined the relations between OSAS, obesity and the metabolic syndrome. Two large cohort studies have shown that both insulin resistance and lipid dysregulation are primarily determined by the degree of adiposity, and that OSAS plays a minimal, if any, role in the occurrence of insulin resistance (34, 163). In another study conducted in obese children with OSAS, insulin resistance was found to correlate with the severity of the respiratory disease independently of the degree of obesity (164).

SOMATIC GROWTH IMPAIRMENT

Failure to thrive (FTT) used to be one of the common consequences of childhood OSAS (165–167). However, nowadays only a minority of children with OSAS will present with this problem, most probably because of earlier recognition and referral. Adenotonsillectomy and complete resolution of OSAS in children will induce significant improvements in growth in those children who present with FTT (168,169), but also in children with normal growth and OSAS (170). Interestingly, even obese children with OSAS will demonstrate weight gain after surgical removal of their enlarged tonsils and adenoids (171,172).

The suggested mechanisms for growth impairment in OSAS include decreased appetite possibly associated with reduced olfaction in children with adenoidal hypertrophy, dysphagia from tonsillar hypertrophy, decreased levels of insulin growth factor-1 (IGF-1), IGF binding proteins and possibly growth hormone release (171). Indeed, IGF-1 was found to increase following tonsillectomy and adenoidectomy parallel to the rebound growth that characterizes the response of children to surgery (171). Moreover, snoring children without OSAS were found to have stunted growth and disruption of circulating levels of IGF binding protein 3, suggesting that some of these children may suffer from disrupted sleep, which may affect growth hormone release (173). It is possible that disruption of non-rapid eye movement (NREM) sleep indeed plays a role in the stunting effects of OSAS, particularly when considering that GH release primarily occurs during delta NREM sleep (174,175).

Alternatively, changes in energy expenditure during sleep could account for the reduction in linear growth in children with OSAS. Indeed, Marcus and colleagues have shown increased metabolic requirements during sleep in children with OSAS that normalized following adenotonsillectomy with concomitant weight gain despite no change in caloric intake (176). These findings suggest that poor growth in some children with OSAS may be secondary to the increased energy expenditure that directly results from the increase in work of breathing during sleep. These findings however have been disputed by Bland and colleagues who found no evidence for increased daily energy requirements before and after adenotonsillectomy (177).

TREATMENT

As indicated above, tonsillar and adenoidal hypertrophy is the most common risk factor for OSAS in children. Many obese children with OSAS also have adenotonsillar hypertrophy further compromising upper airway patency (39,171). The relative contributions of obesity and adenotonsillar hypertrophy to pediatric OSAS among children where both problems co-exist is unclear, but one would expect that surgical removal of tonsils and adenoids in obese children would yield lesser improvements in sleep-disordered breathing compared to non-obese children. The efficacy of adenotonsillectomy in obese children with OSAS have thus far been evaluated in only a few studies, and most have surprisingly shown marked improvements in sleep-disordered breathing following surgery (178,179). A recent study by Mitchell and colleagues showed that adenotonsillectomy in obese children resulted in significant reductions of their respiratory disturbance indices with complete resolution of OSAS in 46% of patients (180). However, in a more recent study in a large pediatric cohort of 110 consecutively treated children (52% obese), the frequency of residual OSAS after adenotonsillectomy was higher among obese children compared to non-obese children, and that conversely, the frequency of complete cure was significantly lower among obese children compared to non-obese children (181). Thus, obesity appears to be a major determinant for adverse surgical outcome. Taken together, adenotonsillectomy is curative in some obese children with OSAS, leads to significant improvements in breathing during sleep in most patients, and therefore should remain the first line of treatment.

Notwithstanding such considerations, children with OSAS show an increased incidence of post-operative cardiac and respiratory complications, involving 23–27% of cases (182–184). Pre-existing medical conditions such as obesity should theoretically increase this risk even further. Indeed, morbid obesity is reported to a high risk for post-operative morbidity in general. However, it is not certain whether such increased risk is related to an underlying presence of undiagnosed OSAS or whether indeed obesity per se operates an independent risk factor for post-operative complications (185–187). Although the risks of surgery in pediatric obese patients with OSAS have yet to be conclusively defined, the American Academy of Pediatrics has already identified obesity as one of the risk factors for post-operative respiratory complications, and has recommended overnight hospitalization and monitoring after adenotonsillectomy (188).

In the presence of an obese child who snores, the diagnosis of OSAS and institution of adenotonsillectomy should not be based solely on clinical criteria, and pre-operative polysomnography should be conducted in this high risk group so as to anticipate underlying risks for respiratory and cardiac compromise in the immediate post-operative period. Moreover, since residual OSAS is more likely to occur after surgery in obese children, a follow-up polysomnographic evaluation would appear justified, to determine whether additional intervention might be needed.

Weight loss should also lead to improvement in the number and severity of apneic episodes. In adults, the beneficial effects of weight reduction programs on OSAS are so well recognized that this intervention constitutes one of the principal recommendations for management of OSAS in adults (189). While there is no doubt that in children, adenotonsillectomy should remain the primary approach for moderate and severe OSAS in obese children, every effort should be made to achieve significant weight reduction in these children (189). Indeed, Willi and colleagues reported resolution of sleep apnea after weight loss in five morbidly obese children (190), such that in special cases in whom surgery is not a viable option, intensive weight management may be particularly beneficial. Of note, weight loss improves not only the severity of sleep-disordered breathing, but that of other complications of childhood obesity and OSAS, such as vascular dysfunction (121,191). As mentioned above, an intensive weight reduction program is an important first line step towards a more definitive treatment for obese children with or without OSAS.

Another approach for the treatment of childhood obesity is multidisciplinary programs that combine dietary, behavioral, and physical activity intervention. These programs are reported to have short- and long-term beneficial effects (192). There are no studies examining the potentially beneficial role of an exercise/physical activity program in obese children with OSAS.

Another clearly more radical option for treatment of obesity and its potentially associated OSAS nowadays is bariatric surgery, particularly in morbidly obese adolescents who have serious obesity-related medical complications and who have failed other more conventional methods. In a preliminary study of 19 extremely obese adolescents meeting the criteria for bariatric surgery, Kalra and colleagues showed marked reductions in OSAS severity following weight loss (37).

OBESITY HYPOVENTILATION SYNDROME

This syndrome, also known as Pickwickian syndrome, is defined as a combination of obesity and awake arterial hypercapnia ($PaCO_2 > 45$ mmHg) in the absence of other known causes of hypoventilation. There are only a few reports of children with obesity hypoventilation syndrome (193–197). However with the recent increases in the prevalence of obesity in children and adolescents, this condition is likely to become increasingly frequent in children.

Patients with obesity hypoventilation syndrome will present, similar to OSAS, with hypersomnolence, fatigue, and/or morning headaches. However, the presence of daytime hypercapnia and hypoxemia may lead to polycythemia, pulmonary hypertension, and to right ventricular failure. Decreased ventilatory responses to hypercapnia and hypoxia are usually found during waking and during sleep, in contrast to pediatric patients with straightforward OSAS, who generally will have normal respiratory drive (198). In addition, decreased nocturnal alveolar ventilation, with or without obstructive sleep apnea/hypopnea events, will be present (199).

The pathogenesis of the disorder is not fully understood, and may represent a combination of mechanical loading of the respiratory system secondary to extreme obesity in the presence of susceptible individuals who may be predisposed due to genetically determined low sensitivity to chemoreceptor stimulation. The findings of elevated plasma leptin levels in obesity and in obstructive sleep apnea and the stimulatory role of leptin on respiratory control led to the hypothesis that obesity hypoventilation syndrome may be a result of central leptin resistance.

In children with obesity hypoventilation syndrome and OSAS, removal of the tonsils and adenoids was recommended as the initial therapeutic procedure (193). The reversibility of the blunted hypercapnic responsiveness following adenotonsillectomy in some of these children suggests that a component of the blunted response may be secondary to the mechanical effects of obesity on the respiratory system rather than a primary abnormality in neurological control of breathing. Since depressed ventilatory drive may occur in patients with significant hypoxia and hypercapnia in the immediate post-operative period following removal of tonsils and adenoids, mechanical ventilatory support may be required at least in the early post-operative period. For most of the patients however, tonsillectomy and adenoidectomy will not be sufficient to completely resolve the problem, and bilevel positive airway pressure (BiPAP) by nasal mask is necessary.

It should be emphasized that weight loss is the optimal and most efficient treatment for obesity-associated hypoventilation. Indeed, weight loss will reverse daytime hypercapnia and improve blood gases and lung volumes (200).

SHORT SLEEP DURATION AND OBESITY

Sleep plays an important role in energy balance. In rodents, food shortage or starvation results in decreased sleep (201), and conversely, total sleep deprivation leads to marked hyperphagia (202). Over the past 40 years, sleep duration in the U.S. population has decreased by 1.5 to two hours (5–7,203). The proportion of young adults reporting that they sleep fewer than 7 hours per night has increased from 15.6% in 1960 to 37.1% in 2001–2002 (5–7). Not surprisingly, reports of fatigue and tiredness are more frequent today than a few decades ago (204). Curtailment of bedtime has become a widespread habit and sleep loss has become a hallmark of modern society (204). Interestingly, the dramatic increase in the incidence of obesity seems to have developed over the same period of time as the progressive decrease in self reported sleep duration (205,206). The two secular trends mirror each other and it has been suggested that short sleep duration may be one of the modifiable contributing factors to the obesity pandemic.

There have been several epidemiologic studies in recent years reporting on an inverse relationship between sleep duration and body weight in both pediatric (207–211) and adult populations (212–216). Short sleep duration has been shown to be associated with increased risk of obesity in five-year-old children after controlling for television viewing and parental obesity (209,211). Significant negative correlation was found between total sleep time and risk of obesity in adolescents independent of other risk factors for obesity (210). In addition, a study of over 8000 children in the United Kingdom reported that sleep duration at the age of 30 months was associated with obesity at age seven years after adjusting for maternal education, energy intake at three years of age, and gender (207). The mechanism linking short sleep duration with weight gain is unknown, but there is growing evidence that the two key opposing hormones, leptin and ghrelin, are involved. In a series of elegant laboratory studies, Spiegel and colleagues have shown that recurrent partial sleep restriction in healthy young adults induced marked alterations in glucose metabolism concomitant with decrease of the levels of the anorexigenic hormone leptin and increase in the levels of the orexigenic factor ghrelin. Importantly, these neuroendocrine abnormalities were correlated with increased hunger and appetite, which ultimately may lead to overeating and increased weight gain (217).

SLEEP DISRUPTION AND GLUCOSE HOMEOSTASIS

Clinical and epidemiologic studies have suggested that sleep disruption which characterizes OSAS plays an important role in the development of the metabolic abnormalities associated with the disorder. Sleep disruption could contribute to the development of insulin resistance and type 2 diabetes mellitus either directly, through deleterious effects on components of glucose regulation, or indirectly, by its effects on appetite regulatory mechanisms leading to increased food ingestion, and consequent weight gain and obesity, the latter then providing a major risk factor for insulin resistance and diabetes.

Several epidemiologic studies in recent years have reported an association between short sleep duration and the development of diabetes, even after controlling for BMI (212,216,218,219).

Several mechanisms may underlie the association between sleep disruption and glucose homeostasis. Sleep restriction is associated with increased sympathetic activity, and since beta cell function is influenced by autonomic nervous system tone, it is possible that the altered insulin reactivity observed in sleep restriction conditions is related to the increase in tonic sympathetic activity associated with this condition. Another possible explanation involves disturbances in the secretory profiles of the counter-regulatory hormones, growth hormone, and cortisol. Indeed, short-term sleep restriction in normal subjects has been shown to worsen glucose tolerance, increase levels of evening cortisol, and heighten sympathetic activity (203,220).

Similarly to short sleepers, patients with OSAS display higher ghrelin levels, and these increased circulating ghrelin levels have been shown to decrease to nearly those of BMI-matched controls after only two days of CPAP treatment (212,221). However, in contrast to short sleepers, patients with OSAS have elevated leptin levels, which are corrected following treatment with CPAP (156,221–224).

One of the immediate acute and long-standing consequences of OSAS is sleep fragmentation. To date, there are only very few studies that have specifically examined the possible role of sleep fragmentation or altered sleep architecture on metabolic disturbances. It has been shown that sleep disruption is associated with increased metabolic rate throughout the night compared with nondisrupted sleep (225). In another experimental study, using acoustic stimuli in healthy subjects, sleep fragmentation and suppression of slow wave sleep resulted in elevation of plasma catecholamine levels that correlated with the degree of sleep fragmentation (226). Moreover, sleep fragmentation was also associated with increased morning cortisol levels and hyperlipidemia, with a positive correlation between arousal frequency and morning levels of serum and salivary cortisol (227). Thus, activation of the HPA axis and the presence of abnormally high sympathetic output due to sleep fragmentation (228) have been proposed as the most likely mechanism underlying the metabolic abnormalities observed in OSAS. Further studies are needed to validate the hypothesis that sleep fragmentation without reduction in total sleep time may adversely affect metabolic and endocrine function, and play a pathogenetic role in the metabolic abnormalities observed in patients with OSAS.

REFERENCES

1. Magarey AM, Daniels LA, Boulton TJ. Prevalence of overweight and obesity in Australian children and adolescents: Reassessment of 1985 and 1995 data against new standard international definitions. Med J Aust 2001; 174:561–4.
2. Lobstein T, Baur L, Uauy R; IASO International Obesity TaskForce. Obesity in children and young people: a crisis in public health. Obes Rev 2004; suppl 1:1-4.
3. Centers for Disease Control and Prevention, National Center for Health Statistics. Percentage of children ages 6 to 18 who are overweight by gender, race and Hispanic origin, 1976-1980,1988-1994 and 1999-2002. National Health and Nutrition Examination Survey; 2003.
4. Dietz WH, Robinson TN. Clinical practice. Overweight children and adolescents. N Eng J Med 2005; 352:2100–09.
5. National Sleep Foundation. "Sleep in America" Poll. Washington, DC: National Sleep Foundation, 2000.

6. National Sleep Foundation. "Sleep in America" Poll. Washington, DC: National Sleep Foundation, 2001, Executive summary.
7. National Sleep Foundation. "Sleep in America" Poll. Washington, DC: National Sleep Foundation, 2002.
8. Pinhas-Hamiel O, Dolan LM, Daniels SR, Standiford D, Khoury PR, Zeitler P. Increased incidence of non-insulin-dependent diabetes mellitus among adolescents. J Pediatr 1996; 128:608–15.
9. Luepker RV, Jacobs DR, Prineas RJ, Sinaiko AR. Secular trends of blood pressure and body size in a multi-ethnic adolescent population: 1986 to 1996. J Pedaitr 1999; 134:668–74.
10. Daniels SR, Arnett DK, Eckel RH, Gidding SS, Hayman LL, Kumanyika S, Robinson TN, Scott BJ, St Jeor S, Williams CL. Overweight in children and adolescents: Pathophysiology, consequences, prevention, and treatment. Circulation 2005; 111:1999–2012.
11. Barlow SE, Dietz WH. Obesity evaluation and treatment: Expert Committee recommendations. The Maternal and Child Health Bureau, Health Resources and Services Administration and the Department of Health and Human Services. Pediatrics 1998; 102:e29.
12. Kelly A, Marcus CL. Childhood obesity, inflammation and apnea: What is the future of our children? Am J Respir Crit Care Med 2005; 171(3):202–03.
13. American Thoracic Society. Standards and indications for cardiopulmonary sleep studies in children. Am J Crit Care Med 1995; 153:866–78.
14. Ali NJ, Pitson DJ, Stradling JR. Snoring, sleep disturbance, and behaviour in 4-5 year olds. Arch Dis Child 1993; 68:360–3.
15. Gislason T, Benediktsdottir B. Snoring, apneic episodes, and nocturnal hypoxemia among children 6 months to 6 years old. An epidemiologic study of lower limit of prevalence. Chest 1995; 107:963–6.
16. Corbo GM, Fuciarelli F, Foresi A, De Benedetto F. Snoring in children: Association with respiratory symptoms and passive smoking. BMJ 1989; 299:1491–4.
17. Owen GO, Canter RJ, Robinson A. Snoring, apnoea and ENT symptoms in the paediatric community. Clin Otolaryngol Allied Sci 1996; 21:130–4.
18. Ferreira AM, Clemente V, Gozal D, Gomes A, Pissarra C, Cesar H, Coelho I, Silva CF, Azevedo MH. Snoring in Portuguese primary school children. Pediatrics 2000; 106:e64.
19. Redline S, Tishler PV, Schluchter M, Aylor J, Clark K, Graham G, Risk factors for sleep-disordered breathing in children. Associations with obesity, race, and respiratory problems. Am J Respir Crit Care Med 1999; 159:1527–32.
20. Redline S, Tishler PV, Hans MG, Tosteson TD, Strohl KP, Spry K, Racial differences in sleep-disordered breathing in African–Americans and Caucasians. Am J Respir Crit Care Med 1997; 155:186–92.
21. Urschitz MS, Guenther A, Eitner S, Urschitz Duprat PM, Schlaud M, Ipsiroglu OS, Poets CF. Risk factors and natural history of habitual snoring. Chest 2004; 126:790–800.
22. Mitchell EA, Thompson JM. Snoring in the first year of life. Acta Pediatr 2003; 92:425–9.
23. Rosen CL, Larkin EK, Kirchner HL, Emancipator JL, Bivins SF, Surovec SA, Martin RJ, Redline S. Prevalence and risk factors for sleep-disordered breathing in 8- to 11-year-old children: Association with race and prematurity. J Pediatr 2003; 142:383–9.
24. Guilleminault C, Korobkin R, Winkle R. Review of 50 children with obstructive sleep apnea syndrome. Lung 1981; 159:275–87.
25. Marcus CL, Curtis S, Koerner CB, Joffe A, Serwint JR, Loughlin GM.. Evaluation of pulmonary function and polysomnography in obese children and adolescents. Pediatr Pulmonol 1996; 21:176–83.
26. Young T, Peppard PE, Gottlieb DJ. Epidemiology of obstructive sleep apnea – A population health perspective. Am J Respir Crit Care Med 2002; 165:1217–39.

27. Mallory GB Jr, Fiser DH, Jackson R. Sleep-associated breathing disorders in morbidly obese children and adolescents. J Pediatr 1989; 115:892–7.
28. Silvestri JM, Weese-Mayer DE, Bass MT, Kenny AS, Hauptman SA, Pearsall SM. Polysomnography in obese children with a history of sleep-associated breathing disorders. Pediatr Pulmonol 1993; 16:124–9.
29. Sogut A, Altin R, Uzun L, Ugur MB, Tomac N, Acun C, Kart L, Can G. Prevalence of obstructive sleep apnea syndrome and associated symptoms in 3–11-year-old Turkish children. Pediatr Pulmonol 2005; 39:251–6.
30. Sulit LG, Storfer-Isser A, Rosen CL, Kirchner HL, Redline S. Associations of obesity, sleep-disordered breathing, and wheezing in children. Am J Respir Crit Care Med 2005; 171:659–64.
31. Chay OM, Goh A, Abisheganaden J, Tang J, Lim WH, Chan YH, Wee MK, Johan A, John AB, Cheng HK, Lin M, Chee T, Rajan U, Wang S, Machin D. Obstructive sleep apnea syndrome in obese Singapore children. Pediatr Pulmonol 2000; 29:284–90.
32. Rosen CL. Clinical features of obstructive sleep apnea hypoventilation syndrome in otherwise healthy children. Pediatr Pulmonol 1999; 27:403–9.
33. Reade EP, Whaley C, Lin JJ, McKenney DW, Lee D, Perkin R. Hypopnea in pediatric patients with obesity hypertension. Pediatr Nephrol 2004; 19:1014–20.
34. Tauman R, O'Brien LM, Ivanenko A, Gozal D. Obesity rather than severity of sleep-disordered breathing as the major determinant of insulin resistance and altered lipidemia in snoring children. Pediatrics 2005; 116:e66–73.
35. Tauman R, O'Brien LM, Gozal D. Plasma CRP in an extended cohort of snoring children: The role of hypoxemia and obesity. Sleep suppl A: 266
36. Wing YK, Hui SH, Pak WM, Ho CK, Cheung A, Li AM, Fok TF. A controlled study of sleep related disordered breathing in obese children. Arch Dis Child 2003; 88:1043–7.
37. Kalra M, Inge T, Garcia V, Daniels S, Lawson L, Curti R, Cohen A, Amin R. Obstructive sleep apnea in extremely overweight adolescents undergoing bariatric surgery. Obes Res 2005; 13:1175–9.
38. Kahn A, Mozin MJ, Rebuffat E, Sottiaux M, Burniat W, Shepherd S, Muller MF. Sleep pattern alterations and brief airway obstructions in overweight infants. Sleep 1989; 12:430–8.
39. Shine NP, Coates HL, Lannigan FJ. Obstructive sleep apnea, morbid obesity, and adenotonsillar surgery: A review of the literature. Int J Ped Otolaryngol 2005;69:1475–82.
40. Horner RL, Mohiaddin RH, Lowell DG, Shea SA, Burman ED, Longmore DB, Guz A. Sites and sizes of fat deposits around the pharynx in obese patients with obstructive sleep apnoea and weight matched controls. Eur Respire J 1989; 2:613–22.
41. Suratt PM, Wilhoit SC, Atkinson RL. Elevated pulse flow resistance in awake obese subjects with obstructive sleep apnea. Am Rev Respir Dis 1983; 127:162–5.
42. White DP, Lombard RM, Cadieux RJ, Zwillich CW. Pharyngeal resistance in normal humans: Influence of gender, age, and obesity. J Appl Physiol 1985; 58:365–71.
43. Mallory GB Jr, Beckerman RC. Relationships between obesity and respiratory control abnormalities. In: Beckerman RC, Brouillette RT, Hunt CE, eds Respiratory Control Disorders in Infants and Children. Baltimore: Williams & Wilkins, 1992:342–51.
44. Naimark A, Cherniack RM. Compliance of the respiratory system and its components in health and obesity. J Appl Physiol 1960; 15:377–82.
45. Aygun AD, Gungor S, Ustundag B, Gurgoze MK, Sen Y. Proinflammatory cytokines and leptin are increased in serum of prepubertal obese children. Mediators Inflamm 2005; 2005(3):180–3.
46. Reinehr T, Kratzsch J, Kiess W, Andler W. Circulating soluble leptin receptor, leptin, and insulin resistance before and after weight loss in obese children. Int J Obes (Lond) 2005; 29:1230–5.
47. Celi F, Bini V, Papi F, Contessa G, Santilli E, Falorni A. Leptin serum levels are involved in the relapse after weight excess reduction in obese children and adolescents. Diabetes Nutr Metab 2003; 16:306–11.

48. Huang KC, Lin RC, Kormas N, Lee LT, Chen CY, Gill TP, Caterson ID. Plasma leptin is associated with insulin resistance independent of age, body mass index, fat mass, lipids, and pubertal development in nondiabetic adolescents. Int J Obes Relat Metab Disord 2004; 28:470–5.

49. Polotsky VY, Smaldone MC, Scharf MT, Li J, Tankersley CG, Smith PL, Schwartz AR, O'Donnell CP. Impact of interrupted leptin pathways on ventilatory control. J Appl Physiol 2004; 96:991–8.

50. Phipps PR, Starritt E, Caterson I, Grunstein RR. Association of serum leptin with hypoventilation in human obesity. Thorax 2002; 57:75–6.

51. Yee BJ, Cheung J, Phipps P, Banerjee D, Piper AJ, Grunstein RR. Treatment of obesity hypoventilation syndrome and serum leptin. Respiration 2006; 73:209–12.

52. Saaresranta T, Polo O. Does leptin link sleep loss and breathing disturbances with major public diseases? Ann Med 2004; 36:172–83.

53. Shimura R, Tatsumi K, Nakamura A, Kasahara Y, Tanabe N, Takiguchi Y, Kuriyama T. Fat accumulation, leptin, and hypercapnia in obstructive sleep apnea-hypopnea syndrome. Chest 2005; 127:543–9.

54. Wolk R, Johnson BD, Somers VK. Leptin and the ventilatory response to exercise in heart failure. J Am Coll Cardiol 2003; 42:1644–9.

55. O'Donnell CP, Schaub CD, Haines AS, Berkowitz DE, Tankersley CG, Schwartz AR, Smith PL. Leptin prevents respiratory depression in obesity. Am J Respir Crit Care Med 1999; 159:1477–84.

56. Tankersley CG, O'Donnell C, Daood MJ, Watchko JF, Mitzner W, Schwartz A, Smith P. Leptin attenuates respiratory complications associated with the obese phenotype. J Appl Physiol 1998; 85:2261–9.

57. Groeben H, Meier S, Brown RH, O'Donnell CP, Mitzner W, Tankersley CG. The effect of leptin on the ventilatory response to hyperoxia. Exp Lung Res 2004; 30:559–70.

58. Weissbluth M, Davis AT, Poncher J, Reiff J. Signs of airway obstruction during sleep and behavioral, developmental, and academic problems. J Dev Behav Pediatr 1983; 4:119–21.

59. Gozal D. Sleep-disordered breathing and school performance in children. Pediatrics 1998; 102:616–20.

60. Ali NJ, Pitson D, Stradling JR. Sleep disordered breathing: Effects of adenotonsillectomy on behaviour and psychological functioning. Eur J Pediatr 1996; 155:56–62.

61. Urschitz MS, Eitner S, Guenther A, Eggebrecht E, Wolff J, Urschitz-Duprat PM, Schlaud M, Poets CF. Habitual snoring, intermittent hypoxia, and impaired behavior in primary school children. Pediatrics 2004; 114:1041–8.

62. Owens J, Opipari L, Nobile C, Spirito A. Sleep and daytime behavior in children with obstructive sleep apnea and behavioral sleep disorders. Pediatrics 1998; 102:1178–82.

63. Guilleminault C, Winkle R, Korobkin R, Simmons B. Children and nocturnal snoring: Evaluation of the effects of sleep related respiratory resistive load and daytime functioning. Eur J Pediatr 1982; 139:165–71.

64. Kaplan BJ, McNicol J, Conte RA, Moghadam HK. Sleep disturbance in preschool-aged hyperactive and nonhyperactive children. Pediatrics 1987; 80:839–44.

65. Stein MA, Mendelsohn J, Obermeyer WH, Amromin J, Benca R. Sleep and behavior problems in school-aged children. Pediatrics 2001; 107:e60.

66. Chervin RD, Dillon JE, Bassetti C, Ganoczy DA, Pituch KJ. Symptoms of sleep disorders, inattention, and hyperactivity in children. Sleep 1997; 20:1185–92.

67. Chervin RD, Archbold KH. Hyperactivity and polysomnographic findings in children evaluated for sleep-disordered breathing. Sleep 2001; 24:313–20.

68. Chervin RD, Archbold KH, Dillon JE, Panahi P, Pituch KJ, Dahl RE, Guilleminault C. Inattention, hyperactivity, and symptoms of sleep-disordered breathing. Pediatrics 2002; 109:449–56.

69. O'Brien LM, Mervis CB, Holbrook CR, Bruner JL, Klaus CJ, Rutherford J, Raffield TJ, Gozal D. Neurobehavioral implications of habitual snoring in children. Pediatrics 2004; 114:44–9.

70. O'Brien LM, Mervis CB, Holbrook CR, Bruner JL, Smith NH, McNally N, McClimment MC, Gozal D. Neurobehavioral correlates of sleep-disordered breathing in children. J Sleep Res 2004; 13:165–72.

71. O'Brien LM, Gozal D. Sleep in children with attention deficit/hyperactivity disorder. Minerva Pediatr 2004; 56:585–601.

72. Gottlieb DJ, Vezina RM, Chase C, Lesko SM, Heeren TC, Weese–Mayer DE, Auerbach SH, Corwin MJ. Symptoms of sleep-disordered breathing in 5-year-old children are associated with sleepiness and problem behaviors. Pediatrics 2003; 112:870–7.

73. Montgomery-Downs HE, Jones VF, Molfese VJ, Gozal D. Snoring in preschoolers: Associations with sleepiness, ethnicity, and learning. Clin Pediatr 2003; 42:719–26.

74. Melendres MC, Lutz JM, Rubin ED, Marcus CL. Daytime sleepiness and hyperactivity in children with suspected sleep-disordered breathing. Pediatrics 2004; 114:768–75.

75. Corkum P, Tannock R, Moldofsky H, Hogg-Johnson S, Humphries T. Actigraphy and parental ratings of sleep in children with attention-deficit/hyperactivity disorder (ADHD). Sleep 2001; 24:303–12.

76. Corkum P, Tannock R, Moldofsky H. Sleep disturbances in children with attention-deficit/hyperactivity disorder. J Am Acad Child Adolesc Psychiatry 1998; 37:637–46.

77. O'Brien LM, Holbrook CR, Mervis CB, Klaus CJ, Bruner JL, Raffield TJ, Rutherford J, Mehl RC, Wang M, Tuell A, Hume BC, Gozal D. Sleep and neurobehavioral characteristics of 5- to 7-year-old children with parentally reported symptoms of attention-deficit/hyperactivity disorder. Pediatrics 2003; 111:554–63.

78. Beebe DW, Gozal D. Obstructive sleep apnea and the prefrontal cortex: Towards a comprehensive model linking nocturnal upper airway obstruction to daytime cognitive and behavioral deficits. J Sleep Res 2002; 11:1–16.

79. Gozal D, Holbrook CR, Mehl RC, Nichols KL, Raffield TJ, Burnside MM, Mervis CB. Correlation analysis between NEPSY battery scores and respiratory disturbance index in snoring 6-year old children: a preliminary report. Sleep 2001 suppl: A206- G.

80. Gozal D, Wang M, Pope DW Jr. Objective sleepiness measures in pediatric obstructive sleep apnea. Pediatrics 2001; 108:693–7.

81. Tauman R, O'Brien LM, Holbrook CR, Gozal D. Sleep pressure score: A new index of sleep disruption in snoring children. Sleep 2004; 27:274–8.

82. O'Brien LM, Tauman R, Gozal D. Sleep pressure correlates of cognitive and behavioral morbidity in snoring children. Sleep 2004; 27:279–82.

83. Stradling JR, Thomas G, Warley AR, Williams P, Freeland A. Effect of adenotonsillectomy on nocturnal hypoxaemia, sleep disturbance, and symptoms in snoring children. Lancet 1990; 335:249–53.

84. Ali NJ, Pitson D, Stradling JR. Sleep disordered breathing: effects of adenotonsillectomy on behaviour and psychological functioning. Eur J Pediatr 1996; 155:56–62.

85. Friedman BC, Hendeles-Amitai A, Kozminsky E, Leiberman A, Friger M, Tarasiuk A, Tal A. Adenotonsillectomy improves neurocognitive function in children with obstructive sleep apnea syndrome. Sleep 2003; 26:999–1005.

86. Montgomery-Downs HE, Crabtree VM, Gozal D. Cognition, sleep and respiration in at-risk children treated for obstructive sleep apnoea. Eur Respir J 2005; 25:336–42.

87. Gozal D, Pope DW Jr. Snoring during early childhood and academic performance at ages thirteen to fourteen years. Pediatrics 2001; 107:1394–9.

88. Datar A, Sturm R, Magnabosco JL. Childhood overweight and academic performance: National study of kindergartners and first-graders. Obes Res 2004; 12:58–68.

89. Falkner NH, Neumark-Sztainer D, Story M, Jeffery RW, Beuhring T, Resnick MD. Social, educational, and psychological correlates of weight status in adolescents. Obes Res 2001; 9:32–42.

90. Laitinen J, Power C, Ek E, Sovio U, Jarvelin MR. Unemployment and obesity among young adults in a northern Finland 1966 birth cohort. Int J Obes Relat Metab Disord 2002; 26:1329–38.

91. Li X. A study of intelligence and personality in children with simple obesity. Int J Obes Relat Metab Disord 1995; 19:355–7.

92. Mellbin T, Vuille JC. Rapidly developing overweight in school children as an indicator of psychosocial stress. Cta Pediatr Scand 1989; 78:568–75.

93. Zaldivar F, McMurray RG, Nemet D, Galassetti P, Mills PJ, Cooper DM. Body fat and circulating leukocytes in children. Int J Obes (Lond) 2006; 30(6):906–11.

94. Cindik N, Baskin E, Agras PI, Kinik ST, Turan M, Saatci U. Effect of obesity on inflammatory markers and renal functions. Acta Paediatr 2005; 94:1732–7.

95. Gozal D, Kheirandish L. Oxidant stress and inflammation in the snoring child: Confluent pathways to upper airway pathogenesis and end-organ morbidity. Sleep Med Rev 2006; 10:83–96.

96. Rhodes SK, Shimoda KC, Waid LR, O'Neil PM, Oexmann MJ, Collop NA, Willi SM. Neurocognitive deficits in morbidly obese children with obstructive sleep apnea. J Pediatr 1995; 127:741–4.

97. Zametkin AJ, Zoon CK, Klein HW, Munson S. Psychiatric aspects of child and adolescent obesity: A review of the past 10 years. J Am Acad Child Adolesc Psychiatry 2004; 43:134–50.

98. Vila G, Zipper E, Dabbas M, Bertrand C, Robert JJ, Ricour C, Mouren-Simeoni MC. Mental disorders in obese children and adolescents. Psychosom Med 2004; 66:387–94.

99. Mustillo S, Worthman C, Erkanli A, Keeler G, Angold A, Costello EJ,.Obesity and psychiatric disorder: developmental trajectories. Pediatrics 2003; 111:851–9.

100. Schwimmer JB, Burwinkle TM, Varni JW. Health-related quality of life of severely obese children and adolescents. JAMA 2003; 289(14):1813–19.

101. Sheslow D, Hassink S, Wallace W, DeLancey E. The relationship between self-esteem and depression in obese children. Ann N Y Acad Sci 1993; 699:289–91.

102. Mills JK, Andrianopoulos GD. The relationship between childhood onset obesity and psychopathology in adulthood. J Psychol 1993; 127:547–51.

103. Pine DS, Goldstein RB, Wolk S, Weissman MM. The association between childhood depression and adulthood body mass index. Pediatrics 2001; 107(5):1049–56.

104. Goodman E, Whitaker RC. A prospective study of the role of depression in the development and persistence of adolescent obesity. Pediatrics 2002; 110(3):497–504.

105. Barlow SE, Dietz WH. Obesity evaluation and treatment: Expert Committee recommendations. The Maternal and Child Health Bureau, Health Resources and Services Administration and the Department of Health and Human Services. Pediatrics 1998; 102:e29.

106. Jonides L, Buschbacher V, Barlow SE. Management of child and adolescent obesity: Psychological, emotional, and behavioral assessment. Pediatrics 2002; 110:215–21.

107. Ravens-Sieberer U, Redegeld M, Bullinger M. Quality of life after in-patient rehabilitation in children with obesity. Int J Obes Relat Metab Disord 2001; suppl 1: s63–5.

108. Schwimmer JB, Burwinkle TM, Varni JW. Health-related quality of life of severely obese children and adolescents. JAMA 2003; 289:1813–9.

109. Franco RA Jr, Rosenfeld RM, Rao M. First place – resident clinical science award 1999. Quality of life for children with obstructive sleep apnea. Otolaryngol Head Neck Surg 2000; 123:9–16.

110. Mitchell RB, Kelly J, Call E, Yao N. Quality of life after adenotonsillectomy for obstructive sleep apnea in children. Arch Otolaryngol Head Neck Surg 2004; 130:190–4.

111. Goldstein NA, Fatima M, Campbell TF, Rosenfeld RM. Child behavior and quality of life before and after tonsillectomy and adenoidectomy. Arch Otolaryngol Head Neck Surg 2002; 128:770–5.

112. Friedlander SL, Larkin EK, Rosen CL, Palermo TM, Redline S. Decreased quality of life associated with obesity in school-aged children. Arch Pediatr Adolesc Med 2003; 157:1206–11.

113. Rosen CL, Palermo TM, Larkin EK, Redline S. Health-related quality of life and sleep-disordered breathing in children. Sleep 2002; 25:657–66.

114. Crabtree VM, Varni JW, Gozal D. Health-related quality of life and depressive symptoms in children with suspected sleep-disordered breathing. Sleep 2004; 27:1131–8.
115. Speiser PW, Rudolf MC, Anhalt H, Camacho-Hubner C, Chiarelli F, Eliakim A, Freemark M, Gruters A, Hershkovitz E, Iughetti L, Krude H, Latzer Y, Lustig RH, Pescovitz OH, Pinhas-Hamiel O, Rogol AD, Shalitin S, Sultan C, Stein D, Vardi P, Werther GA, Zadik Z, Zuckerman-Levin N, Hochberg Z; Obesity Consensus Working Group. Childhood obesity. J Clin Endocrinol Metab 2005; 90:1871–8.
116. Lurbe E, Alvarez V, Redon J. Obesity, body fat distribution, and ambulatory blood pressure in children and adolescents. J Clin Hypertension 2001; 3:362–7.
117. Urbina EM, Gidding SS, Bao W, Elkasabany A, Berenson GS. Association of fasting blood sugar level, insulin level, and obesity with left ventricular mass in healthy children and adolescents: The Bogalusa Heart Study. Am Heart J 1999; 138:122–7.
118. Freedman DS, Dietz WH, Tang R, Mensah GA, Bond MG, Urbina EM, Srinivasan S, Berenson GS. The relation of obesity throughout life to carotid intima-media thickness in adulthood: The Bogalusa Heart Study. Int J Obes Relat Metab Disord 2004; 28:159–66.
119. Tounian P, Aggoun Y, Dubern B, Varille V, Guy–Grand B, Sidi D, Girardet JP, Bonnet D. Presence of increased stiffness of the common carotid artery and endothelial dysfunction in severely obese children: A prospective study. Lancet 2001; 358:1400–1.
120. Watts K, Beye P, Siafarikas A, O'Driscoll G, Jones TW, Davis EA, Green DJ. Effects of exercise training on vascular function in obese children. J Pediatr 2004; 144:620–5.
121. Woo KS, Chook P, Yu CW, Sung RY, Qiao M, Leung SS, Lam CW, Metreweli C, Celermajer DS. Effects of diet and exercise on obesity-related vascular dysfunction in children. Circulation 2004; 109:1981–6.
122. Marcus CL, Greene MG, Carroll JL. Blood pressure in children with obstructive sleep apnea. Am J Respir Crit Care Med 1998; 157:1098–103.
123. Kohyama J, Ohinata JS, Hasegawa T. Blood pressure in sleep disordered breathing. Arch Dis Child 2003; 88:139–42.
124. Enright PL, Goodwin JL, Sherrill DL, Quan JR, Quan SF; Tucson Children's Assessment of Sleep Apnea study. Blood pressure elevation associated with sleep-related breathing disorder in a community sample of white and Hispanic children: The Tucson Children's Assessment of Sleep Apnea study. Arch Pediatr Adolesc Med 2003; 157:901–4.
125. Amin RS, Carroll JL, Jeffries JL, Grone C, Bean JA, Chini B, Bokulic R, Daniels SR. Twenty-four-hour ambulatory blood pressure in children with sleep-disordered breathing. Am J Respir Crit Care Med 2004; 169:950–6.
126. Amin RS, Kimball TR, Bean JA, Jeffries JL, Willging JP, Cotton RT, Witt SA, Glascock BJ, Daniels SR. Left ventricular hypertrophy and abnormal ventricular geometry in children and adolescents with obstructive sleep apnea. Am J Respir Crit Care Med 2002; 165:1395–9.
127. Amin RS, Kimball TR, Kalra M, Jeffries JL, Carroll JL, Bean JA, Witt SA, Glascock BJ, Daniels SR. Left ventricular function in children with sleep-disordered breathing. Am J Cardiol 2005; 95:801–4.
128. Aljadeff G, Gozal D, Schechtman VL, Burrell B, Harper RM, Ward SL. Heart rate variability in children with obstructive sleep apnea. Sleep 1997; 20:151–7.
129. Baharav A, Kotagal S, Rubin BK, Pratt J, Akselrod S. Autonomic cardiovascular control in children with obstructive sleep apnea. Clin Auton Res 1999; 9:345–51.
130. O'Brien LM, Gozal D. Autonomic dysfunction in children with sleep-disordered breathing. Sleep 2005; 28:747–752.
131. Chin K, Nakamura T, Shimizu K, Mishima M, Nakamura T, Miyasaka M, Ohi M. Effects of nasal continuous positive airway pressure on soluble cell adhesion molecules in patients with obstructive sleep apnea syndrome. Am J Med 2000; 109:562–7.
132. O'Brien Lm, Serpero LD, Tauman R, Gozal D. Plasma adhesion molecules in children with sleep-disordered breathing. Chest 2006; 129(4):947–53.

133. Soukhova-O'Hare GK, Cheng ZJ, Roberts AM, Gozal D. Postnatal intermittent hypoxia alters baroreflex function in adult rats. Am J Physiol Heart Circ Physiol. 2006; 290:H1157–H1164.

134. Soukhova-O'hare GK, Roberts AM, Gozal D. Impaired control of renal sympathetic nerve activity following neonatal intermittent hypoxia in rats. Neurosci Lett. 2006; 399(3):181–5.

135. Hansson GK. Inflammation, atherosclerosis and coronary artery disease. N Eng J Med 2005; 352:1685–95.

136. Tauman R, Ivanenko A, O'Brien LM, Gozal D. Plasma C-reactive protein levels among children with sleep-disordered breathing. Pediatrics 2004; 113:e564–9.

137. Larkin EK, Rosen CL, Kirchner HL, Storfer-Isser A, Emancipator JL, Johnson NL, Zambito AM, Tracy RP, Jenny NS, Redline S. Variation of C-reactive protein levels in adolescents: Association with sleep-disordered breathing and sleep duration. Circulation 2005; 111:1978–84.

138. Kheirandish-Gozal L, Capdevila OS, Tauman R, Gozal D. Plasma C-reactive protein in non obese children with obstructive sleep apnea before and after adenotonsillectomy. J Clin Sleep Med 2006; 2(3):301–4.

139. Shiomi T, Guilleminault C, Stoohs R, Schnittger I. Obstructed breathing in children during sleep monitored by echocardiography. Acta Pediatr 1993; 82:863–71.

140. Tal A, Leiberman A, Margulis G, Sofer S. Ventricular dysfunction in children with obstructive sleep apnea: radionuclide assessment. Pediatr Pulmonol 1988; 4:139–43.

141. Vivian EM. Type 2 diabetes in children and adolescents – the next epidemic? Curr Med Res Opin 2006; 22:297–306.

142. Gahagan S, Silverstein J; American Academy of Pediatrics Committee on Native American Child Health; American Academy of Pediatrics Section on Endocrinology. Prevention and treatment of type 2 diabetes mellitus in children, with special emphasis on American Indian and Alaska Native children. American Academy of Pediatrics Committee on Native American Child Health. Pediatrics 2003; 112:e328.

143. Tresaco B, Bueno G, Pineda I, Moreno LA, Garagorri JM, Bueno M. Homeostatic model assessment (HOMA) index cut-off values to identify the metabolic syndrome in children. J Physiol Biochem 2005; 61:381–8.

144. Cook S, Weitzman M, Auinger P, Nguyen M, Dietz WH. Prevalence of a metabolic syndrome phenotype in adolescents: Findings from the third National Health and Nutrition Examination Survey, 1988-1994. Arch Pediatr Adolesc Med 2003; 157:821–7.

145. Weiss R, Dziura J, Burgert TS, Tamborlane WV, Taksali SE, Yeckel CW, Allen K, Lopes M, Savoye M, Morrison J, Sherwin RS, Caprio S. Obesity and the metabolic syndrome in children and adolescents. N Eng J Med 2004; 350:2362–74.

146. Srinivasan SR, Myers L, Berenson GS. Predictability of childhood adiposity and insulin for developing insulin resistance syndrome (syndrome X) in young adulthood: The Bogalusa Heart Study. Diabetes 2002; 51:204–9.

147. Steinberger J, Moorehead C, Katch V, Rocchini AP. Relationship between insulin resistance and abnormal lipid profile in obese adolescents. J Pediatr 1995; 126:690–5.

148. Bao W, Srinivasan SR, Berenson GS. Persistent elevation of plasma insulin levels is associated with increased cardiovascular risk in children and young adults. The Bogalusa Heart Study. Circulation 1996; 93:54–9.

149. Berenson GS, Srinivasan SR, Bao W, Newman WP 3rd, Tracy RE, Wattigney WA. Association between multiple cardiovascular risk factors and atherosclerosis in children and young adults. The Bogalusa Heart Study. N Eng J Med 1998; 338:1650–5.

150. Cruz ML, Huang TT, Johnson MS, Gower BA, Goran MI. Insulin sensitivity and blood pressure in black and white children. Hypertension 2002; 40:18–22.

151. Strohl KP, Novak RD, Singer W, Cahan C, Boehm KD, Denko CW, Hoffstem VS. Insulin levels, blood pressure and sleep apnea. Sleep 1994; 17:614–8.

152. Strohl KP. Diabetes and sleep apnea. Sleep 1996; 19:S225–S228.
153. Grunstein RR, Stenlof K, Hedner J, Sjostrom L. Impact of obstructive sleep apnea and sleepiness on metabolic and cardiovascular risk factors in the Swedish Obese Subjects (SOS) Study. Int J Obes Relat Metab Disord 1995; 19:410–18.
154. Grunstein RR. Metabolic aspects of sleep apnea. Sleep 1996; 19:S218–S220.
155. Punjabi NM, Sorkin JD, Katzel LI, Goldberg AP, Schwartz AR, Smith PL. Sleep-disordered breathing and insulin resistance in middle-aged and overweight men. Am J Respir Crit Care Med 2002; 165:677–82.
156. Ip MS, Lam B, Ng MM, Lam WK, Tsang KW, Lam KS. Obstructive sleep apnea is independently associated with insulin resistance. Am J Respir Crit Care Med 2002; 165:670–6.
157. Stoohs RA, Facchini F, Guilleminault C. Insulin resistance and sleep-disordered breathing in healthy humans. Am J Respir Crit Care Med 1996; 154:170–4.
158. Davies RJ, Turner R, Crosby J, Stradling JR. Plasma insulin and lipid levels in untreated obstructive sleep apnoea and snoring; their comparison with matched controls and response to treatment. J Sleep Res 1994; 3:180–5.
159. Harsch IA, Schahin SP, Radespiel-Troger M, Weintz O, Jahreiss H, Fuchs FS, Wiest GH, Hahn EG, Lohmann T, Konturek PC, Ficker JH, Continuous positive airway pressure treatment rapidly improves insulin sensitivity in patients with obstructive sleep apnea syndrome. Am J Respir Crit Care Med 2004; 169:156–62.
160. Brooks B, Cistulli PA, Borkman M, Ross G, McGhee S, Grunstein RR, Sullivan CE, Yue DK. Obstructive sleep apnea in obese noninsulin-dependent diabetic patients: Effect of continuous positive airway pressure treatment on insulin responsiveness. J Clin Endocrinol Metab 1994; 79:1681–5.
161. Saarelainen S, Lahtela J, Kallonen E. Effect of nasal CPAP treatment on insulin sensitivity and plasma leptin. J Sleep Res 1997; 6:1460147.
162. Smurra M, Philip P, Taillard J, Guilleminault C, Bioulac B, Gin H, CPAP treatment does not affect glucose-insulin metabolism in sleep apneic patients. Sleep Med 2001; 2:207–13.
163. Kaditis AG, Alexopoulos EI, Damani E, Karadonta I, Kostadima E, Tsolakidou A, Gourgoulianis K, Syrogiannopoulos GA. Obstructive sleep-disordered breathing and fasting insulin levels in nonobese children. Pediatr Pulmonol 2005; 40:515–23.
164. de la Eva RC, Baur LA, Donaghue KC, Waters KA. Metabolic correlates with obstructive sleep apnea in obese subjects. J Pediatr 2002; 140(6):641–3.
165. Everett AD, Koch WC, Saulsbury FT. Failure to thrive due to obstructive sleep apnea. Clin Pediatr 1987; 26:90–92.
166. Ahlqvist-Rastad J, Hultcrantz E, Melander H, Svanholm H. Body growth in relation to tonsillar enlargement and tonsillectomy. Int J Pediatr Otolaryngol 1992; 24:55–61.
167. Freezer NJ, Bucens IK, Robertson CF. Obstructive sleep apnoea presenting as failure to thrive in infancy. J Pediatr Child Health 1995; 31:172–5.
168. Brouillette RT, Fernbach SK, Hunt CE. Obstructive sleep apnea in infants and children. J Pediatr 1982; 100:31–40.
169. Bar A, Tarasiuk A, Segev Y, Phillip M, Tal A. The effect of adenotonsillectomy on serum insulin-like growth factor-I and growth in children with obstructive sleep apnea syndrome. J Pediatr 1999; 135:76–80.
170. Lind MG, Lundell BP. Tonsillar hyperplasia in children. A cause of obstructive sleep apneas, CO2 retention, and retarded growth. Arch Otolaryngol 1982; 108:650–4.
171. Soultan Z, Wadowski S, Rao M, Kravath RE. Effect of treating obstructive sleep apnea by tonsillectomy and/or adenoidectomy on obesity in children. Arch Pediatr Adolesc Med 1999; 153:33–7.
172. Roemmich JN, Barkley JE, D'Andrea L, Nikova M, Rogol AD, Carskadon MA, Suratt PM. Increases in overweight after adenotonsillectomy in overweight children with obstructive sleep-disordered breathing are associated with decreases in motor activity and hyperactivity. Pediatrics 2006; 117:e200–e208.

173. Nieminen P, Lopponen T, Tolonen U, Lanning P, Knip M, Lopponen H. Growth and biochemical markers of growth in children with snoring and obstructive sleep apnea. Pediatrics 2002; 109:e55.

174. Van Cauter E, Leproult R, Plat L. Age-related changes in slow wave sleep and REM sleep and relationship with growth hormone and cortisol levels in healthy men. JAMA 2000; 284:861–8.

175. Obal F Jr, Krueger JM. The somatotropic axis and sleep. Rev Neurol 2001; 157:S12–S15.

176. Marcus CL, Carroll JL, Koerner CB, Hamer A, Lutz J, Loughlin GM. Determinants of growth in children with the obstructive sleep apnea syndrome. J Pediatr 1994; 125:556–62.

177. Bland RM, Bulgarelli S, Ventham JC, Jackson D, Reilly JJ, Paton JY, Total energy expenditure in children with obstructive sleep apnoea syndrome. Eur Respir J 2001; 18:164–9.

178. Kudoh F, Sanai A. Effect of tonsillectomy and adenoidectomy on obese children with sleep-associated breathing disorders. Acta Otolaryngol Suppl 1996; 523:216–18.

179. Wiet GJ, Bower C, Seibert R, Griebel M. Surgical correction of obstructive sleep apnea in the complicated pediatric patient documented by polysomnography. Int J Pediatr Otolaryngol 1997; 41:133–43.

180. Mitchell RB, Kelly J. Adenotonsillectomy for obstructive sleep apnea in obese children. Otolaryngol Head Neck Surg 2004; 131:104–8.

181. Tauman R, Gulliver TE, Krishna J, Montgomery-Downs HE, O'Brien LM, Ivanenko A, Gozal D. Persistence of obstructive sleep apnea syndrome in children after adenotonsillectomy. J Pediatr 2006; 149(6):803–8.

182. Strauss SG, Lynn AM, Bratton SL, Nespeca MK. Ventilatory response to CO2 in children with obstructive sleep apnea from adenotonsillar hypertrophy. Anesth Analg 1999; 89:328–32.

183. McColley SA, April MM, Carroll JL, Naclerio RM, Loughlin GM, Respiratory compromise after adenotonsillectomy in children with obstructive sleep apnea. Arch Otolaryngol Head Neck Surg 1992; 118:940–3.

184. Rosen GM, Muckle RP, Mahowald MW, Goding GS, Ullevig C, Postoperative respiratory compromise in children with obstructive sleep apnea syndrome: Can it be anticipated? Pediatrics 1994; 93:784–8.

185. Spector A, Scheid S, Hassink S, Deutsch ES, Reilly JS, Cook SP. Adenotonsillectomy in the morbidly obese child. Int J Pediatr Otolaryngol 2003; 67:359–64.

186. Walker P, Whitehead B, Rowley M. Criteria for elective admission to the paediatric intensive care unit following adenotonsillectomy for severe obstructive sleep apnoea. Anesth Intensive Care 2004; 32:43–6.

187. Price SD, Hawkins DB, Kahlstrom EJ. Tonsil and adenoid surgery for airway obstruction: Perioperative respiratory morbidity. Ear Nose Throat J 1993; 72:526–31.

188. American Academy of Pediatrics. Clinical practice guideline: Diagnosis and management of childhood obstructive sleep apnea syndrome. Pediatrics 2002; 109:704–12.

189. Man GC. Obstructive sleep apnea. Diagnosis and treatment. Med Clin North Am 1996; 80: 803–20.

190. Willi SM, Oexmann MJ, Wright NM, Collop NA, Key LL Jr, The effects of a high-protein, low-fat, ketogenic diet on adolescents with morbid obesity: body composition, blood chemistries, and sleep abnormalities. Pediatrics 1998; 101:61–7.

191. Ng DK, Lam YY, Chan CH. Dietary intervention combined with exercise improves vascular dysfunction but also obstructive sleep apnea in obese children. Circulation 2004; 110:e314.

192. Nemet D, Barkan S, Epstein Y, Friedland O, Kowen G, Eliakim A. Short- and long- term beneficial effects of a combined dietary-behavioral-physical activity intervention for the treatment of childhood obesity. Pediatrics 2005; 115:e445–e449.

193. Ward SL, Marcus CL. Obstructive sleep apnea in infants and young children. J Clin Neurophysiol 1996; 13:198–207.

194. Spier N, karelitz S, The Pickwickian syndrome: Case in a child. Am J Dis Child 1960; 99:822–7.
195. Cayler GG, Mays J, Riley HD Jr. Cardiorespiratory syndrome of obesity (Pickwickian syndrome) in children. Pediatrics 1961; 27:237–45.
196. Riley DJ, Santiago TV, Edelman NH. Complications of obesity-hypoventilation syndrome in childhood. Am J Dis Child 1976; 130:671–4.
197. Bourne RA, Maltby CC, Donaldson JD. Obese hypoventilation syndrome of early childhood requiring ventilatory support. Int J Pediatr Otolaryngol 1988; 16:61–8.
198. Marcus CL, Gozal D, Arens R, Basinski DJ, Omlin KJ, Keens TG, Ward SL. Ventilatory responses during wakefulness in children with obstructive sleep apnea. Am J Respir Crit Care Med 1994; 149:715–21.
199. Olson AL, Zwillich C. The obesity hypoventilation syndrome. Am J Med 2005; 118:948–56.
200. Rapoport DM, Garay SM, Epstein H, Goldring RM. Hypercapnia in the obstructive sleep apnea syndrome. A reevaluation of the "Pickwickian syndrome." Chest 1986; 89:627–35.
201. Danguir J, Nicolaidis S. Dependence of sleep on nutrients' availability. Physiol Behav 1979; 22(4):735–40.
202. Everson CA, Bergmann BM, Rechtschaffen A. Sleep deprivation in the rat: III. Total sleep deprivation. Sleep 1989; 12(1):13–21.
203. Spiegel K, Knutson K, Leproult R, Tasali E, Van Cauter E. Sleep loss: A novel risk factor for insulin resistance and Type 2 diabetes. J Appl Physiol 2005; 99:2008–19.
204. Biliwise DL. Historical change in the report of daytime fatigue. Sleep 1996; 19:462–4.
205. Flegal KM, Carroll MD, Kuczmarski RJ, Johnson CL. Overweight and obesity in the United States: Prevalence and trends, 1960-1994. Int J Obes Relat Metab Disord 1998; 22:39–47.
206. Flegal KM, Carroll MD, Ogden CL, Johnson CL. Prevalence and trends in obesity among US adults, 1999-2000. JAMA 2002; 288(14):1723–7.
207. Reilly JJ, Armstrong J, Dorosty AR, Emmett PM, Ness A, Rogers I, Steer C, Sherriff A; Avon Longitudinal Study of Parents and Children Study Team. Early life risk factors for obesity in childhood: cohort study. Br Med J 2005; 330 (7504):1357.
208. Sekine M, Yamagami T, Handa K, Saito T, Nanri S, Kawaminami K, Tokui N, Yoshida K, Kagamimori S. A dose-response relationship between short sleeping hours and child-hood obesity: Results of the Toyama Birth Cohort Study. Child Care Health Dev 2002; 28:163–70.
209. Locard E, Mamelle N, Billette A, Miginiac M, Munoz F, Rey S. Risk factors of obesity in a five year old population. Parental versus environmental factors. Int J Obes Relat Metab Disord 1992; 16:721–9.
210. Gupta NK, Mueller WH, Chan W, Meininger JC. Is obesity associated with poor sleep quality in adolescents? Am J Hum Biol 2002; 14:762–8.
211. von Kries R, Toschke AM, Wurmser H, Sauerwald T, Koletzko B. Reduced risk for over-weight and obesity in 5- and 6-y-old children by duration of sleep – a cross-sectional study. Int J Obes Relat Metab Disord 2002; 26(5):710–6.
212. Taheri S, Lin L, Austin D, Young T, Mignot E. Short sleep duration is associated with reduced leptin, elevated ghrelin, and increased body mass index. PLos Med 2004; 1:e62.
213. Hasler G, Buysse DJ, Klaghofer R, Gamma A, Ajdacic V, Eich D, Rossler W, Angst J. The association between short sleep duration and obesity in young adults: A 13-year prospective study. Sleep 2004; 27:661–6.
214. Vioque J, Torres A, Quiles J. Time spent watching television, sleep duration and obesity in adults living in Valencia, Spain. Int J Obes Relat Metab Disord 2000; 24:1683–8.
215. Vorona RD, Winn MP, Babineau TW, Eng BP, Feldman HR, Ware JC. Overweight and obese patients in a primary care population report less sleep than patients with a normal body mass index. Arch Intern Med 2005; 165:25–30.

216. Ayas NT, White DP, Al-Delaimy WK, Manson JE, Stampfer MJ, Speizer FE, Patel S, Hu FB. A prospective study of self-reported sleep duration and incident diabetes in women. Diabetes Care 2003; 26:380–4.
217. Spiegel K, Tasali E, Penev P, Van Cauter E. Brief communication: Sleep curtailment in healthy young men is associated with decreased leptin levels, elevated ghrelin levels, and increased hunger and appetite. Ann Intern Med 2004; 141:846–50.
218. Nilsson PM, Roost M, Engstrom G, Hedblad B, Berglund G. Incidence of diabetes in middle-aged men is related to sleep disturbances. Diabetes Care 2004; 27:2464–9.
219. Meisinger C, Heier M, Loewel H; MONICA/KORA Augsburg Cohort Study. Sleep disturbance as a predictor of type 2 diabetes mellitus in men and women from the general population. Diabetologia 2005; 48:235–8.
220. Spiegel K, Leproult R, Van Cauter E. Impact of sleep debt on metabolic and endocrine function. Lancet 1999; 354:1435–9.
221. Harsch IA, Konturek PC, Koebnick C, Kuehnlein PP, Fuchs FS, Pour Schahin S, Wiest GH, Hahn EG, Lohmann T, Ficker JH. Leptin and ghrelin levels in patients with obstructive sleep apnoea: Effect of CPAP treatment. Eur Respir J 2003; 22:251–7.
222. Chin K, Shimizu K, Nakamura T, Narai N, Masuzaki H, Ogawa Y, Mishima M, Nakamura T, Nakao K, Ohi M. Changes in intra-abdominal visceral fat and serum leptin levels in patients with obstructive sleep apnea syndrome following nasal continuous positive airway pressure therapy. Circulation 1999; 100:706–12.
223. Sanner BM, Kollhosser P, Buechner N, Zidek W, Tepel M. Influence of treatment on leptin levels in patients with obstructive sleep apnoea. Eur Respir J 2004; 23:601–4.
224. Shimizu K, Chin K, Nakamura T, Masuzaki H, Ogawa Y, Hosokawa R, Niimi A, Hattori N, Nohara R, Sasayama S, Nakao K, Mishima M, Nakamura T, Ohi M. Plasma leptin levels and cardiac sympathetic function in patients with obstructive sleep apnoea-hypopnoea syndrome. Thorax 2002; 57:429–34.
225. Bonnet MH, Berry RB, Arand DL. Metabolism during normal, fragmented, and recovery sleep. J Appl Physiol 1991; 71:1112–8.
226. Tiemeier H, Pelzer E, Jonck L, Moller HJ, Rao ML. Plasma catecholamines and selective slow wave sleep deprivation. Neuropsychobiology 2002; 45:81–6.
227. Ekstedt M, Akerstedt T, Soderstrom M. Microarousals during sleep are associated with increased levels of lipids, cortisol, and blood pressure. Psychosom Med 2004; 66:925–31.
228. Somers VK, Dyken ME, Clary MP, Abboud FM Sympathetic neural mechanisms in obstructive sleep apnea. J Clin Invest 1995; 96:1897–904.

Index